Human Sexuality

1817

HARPER & ROW, PUBLISHERS, New York
Cambridge, Philadelphia, San Francisco,
London, Mexico City, São Paulo, Sydney

HUMAN SEXUALITY

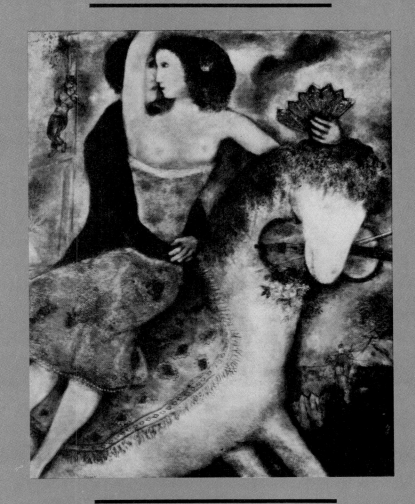

Morton G. Harmatz
Melinda A. Novak

University of Massachusetts, Amherst

This book is dedicated to Mark Harmatz, Harry and Louise Harmatz, Jerry Meyer, and the many students who have been our sources of inspiration.

Sponsoring Editor: Kathy Robinson
Development Editor: Claudia Kohner
Project Editor: Nora Helfgott
Designer: Gayle Jaeger
Production Manager: Willie Lane
Photo Researcher: June Lundborg
Compositor: Black Dot, Inc.
Printer and Binder: R. R. Donnelley & Sons Company
Art Studio: J&R Art Services, Inc.
Positions Drawings: Stuart Weiss/FreelanCenter

Library of Congress Cataloging in Publication Data

Harmatz, Morton G.
  Human sexuality.

  Bibliography: p. 571
  Includes index.
  1. Sex. 2. Sex customs—History. 3. Sex
(Biology) 4. Sex (Psychology) 5. Birth control.
I. Novak, Melinda A. II. Title
HQ21.H328 1983   612.6   82-15871
ISBN 0-06-042632-2

Credits

(The numbers in **boldface** preceding each credit are page numbers in this text.)

Cover and title page art Marc Chagall. *Equestrian*, 1931. Collection, Stedelijk Museum, Amsterdam.

TEXT

5 Mead quotation Margaret Mead: *Sex Temperament in Three Primitive Societies.* Copyright © 1935 by William Morrow & Co. Inc. Reprinted by permission of William Morrow & Co. Inc. **6 Ostow quotation** Mortimer Ostow: *Sexual Deviation/ Psychoanalytic Insights.* Copyright © 1974 by Quadrangle/The New York Times Book Co. Reprinted by permission of Times Books, a division of Quadrangle/The New York Times Book Co., Inc. **6–7 Bengis quotation** Ingrid Bengis: *Combat in the Erogenous Zone.* Copyright © 1972 by Ingrid Bengis. Reprinted by permission of The Julian Bach Literary Agency, Inc. **10 Beach quotation** F. Beach: *Human Sexuality in Four Perspectives.* Reprinted by permission of The Johns Hopkins University Press.
12 Letter Excerpted from the book *The Redbook Report on Female Sexuality* by Carol Tavris and Susan Sadd. Copyright © 1975, 1977 by the Redbook Publishing Company. Used by permission of Delacorte Press. **31–32 Schlessinger quotation** A. Schlessinger: "An informal history of love, USA." Reprinted from *The Saturday Evening Post.* Copyright © 1966 by The Curtis Publishing Company. Reprinted by permission of *The Saturday Evening Post.* **229–230 Bem quotations** Sandra Bem: "Androgyny vs. fluffy women and chesty men." Reprinted from *Psychology Today* Magazine, September 1975. Pp. 59–62. Copyright © 1975 by Ziff-Davis Publishing Company. Reprinted by permisssion of Ziff-Davis Publishing Company. **248 Hunt quotation** Morton Hunt: *Sexual Behavior in the Seventies.* Originally appeared in *Playboy* Magazine. Copyright © 1973 by Morton Hunt. Reprinted by permission of PEI Books, Inc., and of The Lescher Agency. **261 Levinger list** George Levinger: "Toward the analysis of close relationships," *Journal of Experimental Social Psychology*, 1980, vol. 16, pp. 510–544. Reprinted by permission of Academic Press. **264–265 Box 10.1, "The chemistry of love"** Based on Jane O'Reilly: "Isolating the chocolate factor," pp. 44–46, in *Ms.* Magazine, August 1980. Used with permission from the *Ms.* Foundation for Education and Communications. Copyrighted August 1980. **277 Hite quotations** Reprinted with permission of Macmillan Publishing Co., Inc., from *The Hite Report* by Shere Hite. Copyright © 1976 by Shere Hite. **302 Belson quotations** A. A. Belson: "Erotic fantasies: The new therapy," *Harper's Bazaar*, August 1980, pp. 153ff. Copyright © 1980 The Hearst Corporation. Courtesy of *Harper's Bazaar.* **358–359 Peplau quotations** Letitia Anne Peplau: "What homosexuals want." Reprinted from *Psychology Today* Magazine, March 1981, pp. 28–38. Copyright © 1981 by Ziff-Davis Publishing Company. Reprinted by permission of Ziff-Davis Publishing Company. **370 "Dear Abby" letters** Used by permission of Abigail Van Buren. **398–399 Frank, Anderson, and Rubinstein quotations** Ellen Frank, Carol Anderson, and Debra Rubinstein: "Frequency of sexual dysfunction in 'normal' couples," *The New England Journal of Medicine*, vol. 299, pp. 111–115, 1978. Reprinted by permission of *The New England Journal of Medicine.* **413 and 415 Kaplan lists** Adapted from Helen S. Kaplan: *The New Sex Therapy.* New York: Brunner/Mazel, 1974. Used by permission of Brunner/Mazel Publishers. **422 Krafft-Ebing quotation** Copyright © 1965 by Franklin S. Klaf. From the book *Psychopathia Sexualis* by Richard von Krafft-Ebing. Reprinted by permission of Stein and Day Publishers. **425 and 432 Stoller quotations** R. Stoller: *Sex and Gender: The*

Saunders Co. and of Dr. S. S. C. Yen. **124 *Figure 6.4 (left and right)*** Courtesy Robert H. Glass, M.D. **125 *Figure 6.5*** Redrawn from *Principles of Anatomy and Physiology, Third Edition,* by Gerard J. Tortora and Nicholas P. Anagnostakos. Copyright © 1981 by Gerard J. Tortora and Nicholas P. Anagnostakos. Used by permission of Harper & Row, Publishers, Inc. **130 *Figure 6.6*** Redrawn from C. Faiman and J. S. D. Winter: "Diurnal cycles in plasma FSH, testosterone, and cortisol in men," in the *Journal of Clinical Endocrinology and Metabolism,* 1971, vol. 33, pp. 186–192. Copyright © 1971 by The Endocrine Society. Used by permission of The Williams & Wilkins Company and of Dr. C. Faiman. **133 *Figure 6.7*** Redrawn from J. Richard Udry and Naomi M. Morris: "Distribution of coitus in the menstrual cycle," in *Nature,* 1968, vol. 220, pp. 593–596. Copyright © 1968 Macmillan Journals Limited. Used by permission of *Nature* and of Drs. J. Richard Udry and Naomi M. Morris. **144 *Figure 7.2*** Landrum B. Shettles. **145 *Table 7.1*** Redrawn from J. MacLeod and R. Z. Gold: "The male factor in fertility and infertility: VI. Semen quality and certain other factors in relation to ease of conception," in *Fertility and Sterility,* vol. 4., 1953, pp. 10–33. Reproduced with the permission of the publisher, The American Fertility Society. **151 *Figure 7.3*** Redrawn from D. R. Mishell, Jr., L. Wide, and C. A. Gemzell: "Immunologic determination of human chorionic gonadotropin in serum," in the *Journal of Clinical Endocrinology and Metabolism,* 1963, vol. 23. Copyright © 1963 by The Endocrine Society. Used by permission of The Williams & Wilkins Company and of Drs. D. R. Mishell, Jr., L. Wide, and C. A. Gemzell. **153 *Figure 7.4*** Wide World Photos. **154 *Figure 7.5*** From *From Conception to Birth: The Drama of Life's Beginnings* by Robert Rugh and Landrum B. Shettles. Copyright © 1971 by Robert Rugh and Landrum B. Shettles. Reprinted by permission of Harper & Row, Publishers, Inc. **155 *Figure 7.6*** From *Human Reproduction* by Eric Golanty. Copyright © 1975 by Holt, Rinehart and Winston, Inc. Used by permission of Holt, Rinehart and Winston, CBS College Publishing. **156 *Figure 7.7*** Landrum B. Shettles. **189 *Figure 8.1*** © Ken Heyman. **195 *Figure 8.2*** Courtesy Alan Guttmacher Institute. **195 *Figure 8.3*** Redrawn from *Womancare: A Gynecological Guide to Your Body* by Lynda Madaras and Jane Patterson, M.D., F.A.C.O.G. Copyright © 1981 by Lynda Madaras. Illustrations copyright © 1981 by Avon Books. Used by permission of Avon Books, New York. **196 *Figure 8.4 (top)*** Courtesy Alan Guttmacher Institute. ***Figure 8.4 (bottom)*** Redrawn from *Womancare: A Gynecological Guide to Your Body* by Lynda Madaras and Jane Patterson, M.D., F.A.C.O.G. Copyright © 1981 by Lynda Madaras. Illustrations copyright © 1981 by Avon Books. Used by permission of Avon Books, New York. **198 *Figure 8.5 (left)*** Courtesy Alan Guttmacher Institute. **200 *Figure 8.6*** Courtesy Alan Guttmacher Institute. **206 *Figure 8.7*** Redrawn from Howard I. Shapiro, M.D.: *The Birth Control Book.* Copyright © 1977 by Howard I. Shapiro. Used by permission of St. Martin's Press, Inc., New York. **208 *Figure 8.8*** Redrawn from R. A. Hatcher et al.: *Contraceptive Technology, 1980–1981.* Breakdown from *National Disease and Therapeutic Index* and from information from *The Association for Voluntary Sterilization, September, 1977.* Reprinted by permission of Irvington Publishers, Inc. **209 *Figure 8.9*** Redrawn from Howard I. Shapiro, M.D.: *The Birth Control Book.* Copyright © 1977 by Howard I. Shapiro. Used by permission of St. Martin's Press, Inc., New York. **210 *Figure 8.10 (left)*** Redrawn from V. Osathanondh: "Minilaparatomy for internal female sterilization," in J. C. Sciarra et al., Eds., *Advances in Female Sterilization Techniques.* Copyright © 1976 by Northwestern University. Used by permission of Harper & Row, Publishers, Inc. ***Figure 8.10 (right)*** Redrawn from Howard I. Shapiro, M.D.: *The Birth Control Book.* Copyright © 1977 by Howard I. Shapiro. Used by permission of St. Martin's Press, Inc., New York. **262 *Figure 10.1*** Based on data from George Levinger and J. Diedrick Snoek: *Attraction in Relationships: A New Look at Interpersonal Attraction* (1972). It was adapted in *Social Psychology,* copyright © 1980 by Random House, Inc. Used by permission of CRM Books, a Division of Random House, Inc. **263 *Figure 10.2*** Redrawn from George Levinger and J. Diedrick Snoek: *Attraction in Relationships: A New Look at Interpersonal Attraction.*

Morristown, NJ: General Learning Press, 1972. Copyright © 1978 by George Levinger and J. Diedrick Snoek. Used by permission of George Levinger and J. Diedrick Snoek. **272 Table 10.1** Reprinted with permission of authors and publisher from: Cimbalo, R. S., Faling, V., and Mousaw, P. "The course of love: A cross-sectional design." *Psychological Reports*, 1976, vol. 38, pp. 1292–1294. **286 Figure 11.5** Redrawn from Masters, W. H., and Johnson, V. E.: *Human Sexual Response*. Boston: Little, Brown, 1966. Copyright © 1966 by William H. Masters and Virginia E. Johnson. Used by permission of the Masters and Johnson Institute and of Little, Brown and Company. **310, 311, 313, 323, 324, and 325 Tables 12.1, 12.2, 12.3, 12.5, 12.7, 12.9, and 12.10** Based on data in Morton Hunt: *Sexual Behavior in the Seventies*. Originally appeared in *Playboy* Magazine. Copyright © 1973 by Morton Hunt. **312, 314, 323, 325, and 329 Tables 12.4, 12.6, 12.8, 12.11, and 12.12** Excerpted from the book *The Redbook Report on Female Sexuality* by Carol Tavris and Susan Sadd. Copyright © 1975, 1977 by The Redbook Publishing Company. Used by permission of Delacorte Press. **322 Figure 12.1** Adapted from *Human Sexualities* by John H. Gagnon. Copyright © 1977 by Scott, Foresman and Company. Reprinted by permission. **341 Table 13.1** Adapted from E. E. Levitt and A. Klassen: "Public attitudes toward homosexuality," in the *Journal of Homosexuality*, 1974, vol. 1 (1), pp. 29–45. Used by permission of the *Journal of Homosexuality*. **374 Figure 14.1** Redrawn from S. S. C. Yen: "The biology of menopause," in the *Journal of Reproductive Medicine*, 1977, vol. 18, pp. 287–296. Used by permission of the *Journal of Reproductive Medicine*. **385 Figure 14.2** Redrawn from Clyde E. Martin: "Sexual activity in the aging male," in J. Money and H. Musaph, Eds: *Handbook of Sexology*. Copyright © 1977 by Elsevier Biomedical Press B.V. Used by permission of Elsevier Biomedical Press B.V. and of Dr. Clyde E. Martin. **417 Table 15.1** Based on data from Masters, W. H., and Johnson, V. E.: *Human Sexual Inadequacy*. Boston: Little, Brown, 1970. Copyright © 1970 by Little, Brown and Company. Used by permission of the Masters and Johnson Institute and of Little, Brown and Company. **447 Table 17.1** Reprinted from Altrocchi: *Abnormal Behavior*, published by Harcourt Brace Jovanovich. Adapted from B. D. Townes, W. D. Ferguson, and S. Gillam: "Differences in psychological sex adjustment and familial influences among homosexual and nonhomosexual populations," in the *Journal of Homosexuality*, 1976, vol. 1, pp. 261–272. Used by permission of the *Journal of Homosexuality*. **459 Figure 17.1** © Erika Stone 1982. **467 Figures 18.1 and 18.2** Redrawn from the contribution by P. J. Wiesner, O. G. Jones, and J. H. Blount to the chapter on "World trends in sexually transmitted diseases," which was published by the Royal Society of Medicine in its book entitled *Sexually Transmitted Diseases* (1976), pp. 5–13 inclusive. Used by permission of the Royal Society of Medicine and of the Department of Health & Human Services. **470, 473, and 475 Figures 18.3, 18.4, and 18.5** Courtesy Nicholas J. Fiumara, M.D., M.P.H., Director, Division of Communicable and Venereal Diseases, Massachusetts Department of Public Health. **484 Figure 18.6** Redrawn from a brochure on breast self-examination published in spring 1980 by the University of Massachusetts Health Center/Amherst. Used by permission of the University of Massachusetts Health Center/Amherst. **501 Figure 19.1** Redrawn from G. G. Abel et al.: "The components of rapists' sexual arousal," in the *Archives of General Psychiatry*, 1977, vol. 34, pp. 895–903. Copyright © 1977, American Medical Association. Used by permission of the American Medical Association and of Gene G. Abel, M.D.

ILLUSTRATIVE ART   **3** Pablo Picasso. *Meditation (Contemplation)*. Paris, late 1904. Watercolor and pen, $13\frac{5}{8}$ × $10\frac{1}{8}$ in. Collection, Mrs. Bertram Smith, New York. **14 (top)** The Bettmann Archive. **(bottom)** Courtesy of the American Museum of Natural History, Drummond Collection. Photograph, J. Kirschner. **17** Masaccio. *Expulsion of Adam and Eve*. Brancacci Chapel, Florence. Photograph, Alinari/EPA. **19** Museum of Natural History, Vienna. **22** The Bettmann Archive. **26** The Bettmann Archive. **28** The New York

Brief contents

Detailed contents

Preface

Few subjects generate as much interest as sexuality. In the past 20 years the myths and misinformation that characterized much of the knowledge of sexuality have been replaced by a science of human sexuality devoted to a systematic investigation of the subject. This research, pioneered by a few dedicated and courageous individual investigators, has uncovered important and exciting findings. We wrote *Human Sexuality* to present this information to today's undergraduate students—both for its academic and personal value.

Although modern research has supplied the answers to many questions, by no means have all the questions, let alone all the answers, been found. We are in the early years of the era of scientific research into human sexuality. In this text we present not only what has been learned but how it has been studied. This text provides a framework to help students *think about* the personal and social issues that relate to sexuality. How do the results of research affect their own behavior and feelings? What effect does this information have on their attitudes toward those people who differ? How much control should society have over individuals' personal lives? What options—and conflicts—do today's students have that their parents didn't? Which of today's "facts" may be tomorrow's myths?

Human Sexuality is designed to provide balanced and comprehensive coverage of the subject of sexuality. The biological, psychological, and sociological aspects of sexuality are each given full treatment. As an author team of a biopsychologist (Novak) and a clinical psychologist (Harmatz), we combine complementary academic points of view. In addition, as representatives of both genders, we combine and balance the male and female views.

Human Sexuality is written for the undergraduate college or university student with no prior college courses in psychology or biology. All major technical terms are defined, and concepts are explained. However, we felt that just because a book is scientifically sound, it need not be dry and uninteresting. We have tried to make this text as dynamic as the subject itself. Classroom response to this material at the University of Massachusetts, Amherst, indicates that we have succeeded.

ORGANIZATION OF THE TEXT

The organization of *Human Sexuality* provides a framework for the balanced and comprehensive coverage of the biological, psychological, and sociological aspects of human sexuality. Though we believe this structure provides optimal presentation of the material, the text is written so that chapters can be used in any sequence or combination that suits the individual instructor.

This text is divided into five parts: "Introduction," "Human Sexual Biology," "Human Sexuality Across the Life Span," "Human Sexual Problems," and "Issues and Trends in Human Sexuality."

Part One begins with a chapter that raises basic questions about sexual behavior through the use of a group of vignettes. This chapter is followed by one on the history of sexual attitudes and practices. The chapter on the scientific approach to sexual behavior, Chapter 3, is a logical continuation of the history chapter. We also felt that it was important to place the coverage of the scientific methodology early in the text so that students would be aware of the methods scientists use—and the limitations of these methods—as they read about the results of research in later chapters.

The next part of the text, "Human Sexual Biology," presents unusually complete coverage of the anatomy and physiology of sexual behavior and reproduction. In addition to explaining how each anatomical structure contributes to sexuality, Chapter 4, "The Anatomy of Human Sexuality," lays to rest many of the myths that are associated with the sex organs. Chapter 5 is unique in providing a full chapter on the process by which individuals develop male and female characteristics during prenatal development. Also included in this chapter is coverage of errors in sexual differentiation. Throughout this part physiological and anatomical factors are related to behavior. An extensive program of pedagogically useful drawings and photographs supplements this part.

Part Three is titled "Human Sexuality Across the Life Span." It treats sexuality as a lifelong experience affecting us as individuals and as members of society. Unlike many textbooks that include a chapter on the physiology of sexual arousal among the biology chapters, we include this chapter between the chapter on love and attraction and the chapter on marital status and sexual behavior—a rather natural place in terms of the mores in today's society. The part begins with a chapter titled "Sexuality in the Early Years" that covers the development of sexuality from infancy through adolescence from the following perspectives: (1) the development of sexual behavior, (2) the development of gender roles, and (3) the development of sexual awareness and attitudes. The chapter on homosexuality is included in this part, and this topic is treated as a normal sexual variation. The final chapter in this part, which covers sexuality and aging, is unique in its discussion of how societal beliefs and expectations have influenced the expression of sexuality in the elderly. Throughout this part, the emotional, biological, and behavioral aspects of sexuality are explored.

Part Four, "Human Sexual Problems," includes coverage of sexual dysfunction, sexual variance, clinical treatment, and sex-related diseases and disorders. The first chapter in the part covers sexual dysfunctions; the focus is on dysfunctions that affect many people at certain points in their lives. The next chapter is on sexual variance; in this chapter, the focus is on sexual behaviors that differ markedly from society's usual patterns. These chapters cover the causes of these disorders, as well as descriptions and evaluations of the various treatment approaches. Next, Chapter 17 focuses on two types of individuals seeking change: dissatisfied homosexuals and transsexuals. Dissatisfied homosexuals are that small segment of the homosexual population who are unhappy with their sexual orientation. This chapter provides in-depth coverage of these two clinical phenomena. The final chapter in this part covers sexually transmitted diseases and other medical problems that relate to sexual activity or the sexual organs. The modes of transmission and treatment of various sexually transmitted diseases are presented. Also discussed are nonvenereal sexual disorders, self-help information, and sex and the handicapped.

Part Five covers issues and trends in human sexuality. The first chapter, "Rape," forms a bridge between Parts Four and Five. Although rape is a form of variant behavior, legal issues play an important role in how both the victim and the rapist are viewed and treated by the public. Thus, this chapter concerns not only the act of rape as it is perpetrated against a woman or a man but also the legal-social issues and the legal processes. The next chapter deals with various aspects of sexuality, such as pornography and prostitution, that interact with the legal system. Some speculation about future trends in sexuality is presented in the last chapter.

SPECIAL
FEATURES

This text includes several features that will greatly enhance its value to students. Throughout the text there are "boxes" that present especially relevant and recent findings. The coverage in the boxes will spark student interest and broaden their exposure to the subject of human sexuality. The text coverage is amplified by an extensive art program including pedagogical and illustrative art. Each chapter concludes with a summary that recapitulates the major points in the chapter; these summaries will help students organize the material for study. Annotated bibliographies follow the summaries. In addition, key terms are highlighted in boldface within the text, and they are defined in an extensive glossary at the back of the book. Pronunciations accompany difficult terms in the glossary. Accompanying this text is an *Instructor's Manual*, which is divided into three parts. The first part provides a general guide to developing a course in human sexuality. Included among the features of this part is a list of suggested audiovisual aids. The second part is organized by chapter. For each chapter there is an outline summary, definitions of key terms, and discussion questions. The third part is a test bank.

ACKNOWLEDGMENTS

A textbook of this scope is helped along by many people. It is impossible to thank them enough, so we feel that at least we should thank them publicly. At the University of Massachusetts, Amherst, thanks go to Bruce Kerr and Gilda Morelli, who, in the midst of their very busy graduate studies, also served as research assistants to this project. The voluminous amount of material to be covered was made more manageable by their efforts. Sally Ives typed almost all of the manuscript, sometimes at speeds approaching the incredible and with an eye for improving our prose.

We thank the following reviewers, who made helpful suggestions throughout the development of this project:

Paul Abramson, University of California, Los Angeles
Mary Kay Biaggio, University of Idaho
Professor James F. Calhoun, University of Georgia
Spurgeon Cole, Clemson University
Eva E. Conrad, San Bernardino Valley College
Joseph W. Critelli, North Texas State University
Patricia Cronin, Bradford College
Gertrude V. DiFrancesco, Bucks County Community College
David A. Edwards, Emory University
Robert J. Feiguine, University of Denver
Anita Fisher, College of San Mateo
Irene Hanson Frieze, University of Pittsburgh
Alan G. Glaros, Wayne State University
Charles W. Hager, Texas Wesleyan College
Harry M. Hoberman, University of Oregon
Ethel Kamien, University of Lowell
Richard Maslow, San Joaquin Delta College
Henry J. Oles, Southwest Texas State University
Ollie Pocs, Illinois State University
Bernard Saper, Florida International University
Dayton M. Spaulding, Plymouth State College of The University of New
    Hampshire
Judith E. Steinhart, Brooklyn College of The City University of New York
Beverly E. Thorn-Gray, The Ohio State University
Michael G. Walraven, Jackson Community College
Erik Wright, University of Kansas

Several people at Harper & Row played important roles in seeing this project through to completion. Neale Sweet and Claudia Wilson were responsible for our working with Harper & Row in the first place. Their initial belief and continuing faith in the project were of great help. We thank Kathy Robinson, the psychology editor, who joined the project midway, for adopting and nurturing us as her own. Claudia Kohner was the central person in seeing every phase of the project through to completion, and to her we express our deepest thanks and affection—even for keeping us to those deadlines, which seemed so impossible at the time. Special thanks go to Jackie Estrada for her work on the summaries, the boxes, and the text itself. The readability of the final product benefited from her efforts. Nora Helfgott has been responsible for seeing the manuscript through the various stages of production, and she has handled a most difficult job with apparent ease. Finally, we wish to thank the designer, Gayle Jaeger, who has done an outstanding job. The art program runs the gamut from highly technical and detailed figures to photographs to reproduction of fine art. Even the briefest perusal of the text indicates what a fine art package has been realized. There are many other people at Harper & Row who contributed to this text whom we do not know directly, and we wish to thank them all for a textbook of which we are very proud.

Morton G. Harmatz
Melinda A. Novak

Introduction

one

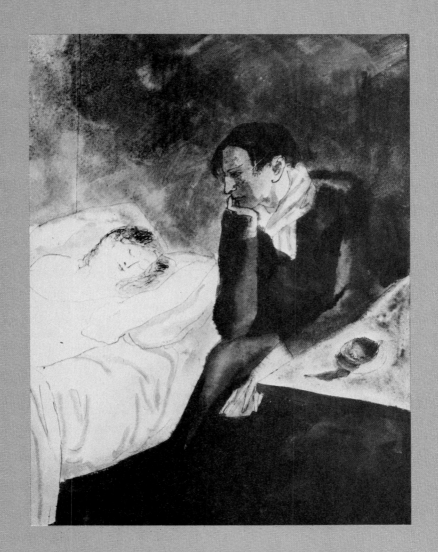

Inquiry into human sexuality

1

chapter

1

Sexual issues are involved at every stage of our lives and in almost every interaction. Our work, our family lives, our play, our entertainment, our friendships—all are influenced to some extent by the fact that we are sexual beings. The great variety of ways in which sexuality can have an impact on people's lives is illustrated through the following five examples. Each of these vignettes, while totally different from the others, demonstrates the importance of sexual issues in everyday life.

Example 1   *Sally and Dave: A Problem of Sexual Satisfaction*

Sally and Dave have been seeing each other since they met at a party in Sally's dorm at the beginning of the semester. They came from the same suburb of a nearby city, knew each other vaguely in high school, but never dated or showed particular interest in each other in those days. Now, in their sophomore year in college, they have found each other attractive and have spent a great deal of time together. They like each other in many ways and have even begun to talk in terms of serious commitment to each other.

Along with their increasing involvement in the relationship, they have experienced a parallel increase in their physical feelings. Recently their petting activities became so intense that sexual intercourse seemed to be the logical next step—a step on both of their minds almost constantly. Both Sally and Dave have mild ethical feelings against promiscuous sexual intercourse, but they also believe that sex is acceptable between people who feel deeply about each other and are likely to have a continuing relationship. The fact is, however, that up to this point neither had engaged in a sexual relationship before, and, while excited about the possibility, both were also fearful, unsure, and anxious about what would happen and how they would function in a sexual role.

Dave and Sally's anxiety was well founded. Neither had any real knowledge about sexuality. The "sex-ed" course they took in high school had not been helpful; their parents had avoided the issue entirely; and their peers had bragged about sexual exploits but basically demonstrated their own ignorance. Neither Dave nor Sally knew about the other's inexperience. Sally assumed that Dave was experienced from the way he talked about sex. Dave hoped that Sally was a virgin but also hoped she had enough experience to know what to do.

One night after a party, and with the facilitating effects of some mild drinking, Dave and Sally's lovemaking finally took that ultimate step—intercourse. In a mixture of excitement and fear, Dave and Sally went through some fumbling, clumsy activities that approximated what each thought sexual intercourse was supposed to be like. It was over very quickly. After saying how wonderful it was, each lay in bed thinking about the experience. These were not warm afterglow thoughts of how beautiful the experience had been.

Sally felt mostly discomfort and confusion. She wondered what she had done wrong. Where were the fireworks? Why hadn't the earth moved? Had she somehow turned Dave off and ruined it for both of them? Didn't he love her after all?

Dave thought it had been over all too fast, and he felt none of the pleasure he had anticipated. Masturbation had been much better than this! He was disappointed and a little embarrassed about the whole experience and also blamed Sally for not helping him out. He even wondered about his "manhood" and his future sexual functioning with other women.

Sally and Dave were both left wondering whether sex was oversold or whether there was something wrong with them, either as individuals or in their feelings toward each other. Overall, it was far from the peak experience they had been led to expect.

Example 2   *Sexuality in the Arapesh Culture*

Anthropologist Margaret Mead (1935) studied the sexual behavior of a group of people called the Arapesh and described what she came to understand about their sexual lives. One of the things she learned was that the Arapesh accept sexual intercourse only within the bonds of marriage. As Mead noted, "The casual encounter, the liaison, a sudden stirring of desire that must be satisfied quickly—these mean nothing to them. Their ideal is essentially a domestic one, not a romantic one. Sex is a serious matter, a matter that must be surrounded with precautions; a matter above all in which the two partners must be of one mind" (p. 77).

The Arapesh exclude erotic feelings and passion from their sexual activity. Satisfactory sexual intercourse is predictable, routinized, and without intense pleasure or emotion. Sex should meet expected patterns, and there should not be experimentation or variation. Women indicate that the ideal mate is one who approaches sex with "ease and lack of difficulty of sex-relationships." Women are not expected to have orgasms, and no such response is reported. Men thus do not try to satisfy their wives. Even the climax in men is unimportant and is only reported as the loss of erection.

Example 3   *Bill and Kathy W.'s Attempts to Conceive a Child*

Bill and Kathy W. tried to have a baby for more than 2 years before they sought professional advice. They were confused and upset by what was happening to them and were afraid that something was really wrong. They never thought they would have problems conceiving, and in fact had taken great pains to avoid a pregnancy before they were ready.

Bill and Kathy had a good marriage and were generally happy with their lives. However, their inability to conceive was beginning to strain their relationship. Each silently accused the other of being the "defective" partner in the marriage. And each felt increasingly insecure about his or her worth as a person. Bill in particular feared he was sterile; the thought alone was a damaging blow to his masculinity. Kathy felt that she would never be a mother—a role that was an important part of her identity. Having come from traditional backgrounds, the couple also felt family and peer pressure to start a family. Bill and Kathy brought their questions to the family physician.

In order to get to the bottom of the problem, the doctor ordered a series of tests for both Kathy and Bill. The tests showed that they could have children, although conditions were far from ideal. Bill's sperm count was below normal, and Kathy had a highly irregular menstrual cycle.

In discussions with Bill and Kathy the doctor also discovered another problem: Neither knew much about the mechanics of conception. They had no idea when ovulation occurs in the woman's cycle or how important it is to have intercourse around the time of ovulation. They only knew what their parents, friends, and clergy had told them when they were growing up—that pregnancy happened all too easily. Using this "advice" as a guide, they had frequent sexual contact in the hope that Kathy would become pregnant. The urgency they began to feel took much of the romance, spontaneity, and joy out of their sexual lives.

Example 4   *Variant Sexual Responses: The Case of Frank B.*

Frank B. was a **masochist**—a person who derives sexual pleasure from experiencing physical and psychological pain. Ostow (1974) reported that Frank engaged in his version of masochism by seeking prostitutes who would hurt him during sex. He approached them by asking, "What is the worst thing you have ever done with a man?" If the answer appealed to him, he would insist that the prostitute perform that act with him. He most preferred to have the woman humiliate him in some way, such as walking on him, scolding him, and ordering him around like a servant. He also liked to have another prostitute present to "observe his degradation." According to Ostow:

> The women had to show contempt, amusement, and enjoyment of his plight before he became excited. After the humiliation had been completed to his satisfaction and he was sufficiently aroused, [Frank] would perform a conventional act of intercourse. If, at the same time, the prostitute described humiliations she planned for the next time, his excitement would be heightened. After an experience of this kind, the orgasm would give him a sense of total relief. (Ostow, 1974, p. 67)

Frank B. was being treated for this problem behavior because he found he could not control his desire for pain and humiliation and was concerned about his mental health.

Example 5   *Experiences with Love and Trial Marriage*

Ingrid Bengis (1972), the author of the well-known feminist essay *Combat in the Erogenous Zone*, was left wondering about her reactions after the break-up of an important relationship. This led to the self-inquiry that she described as follows:

> Having concluded that trial marriages were the only way to find out whether you could work things out with a man, it never occurred to me that a trial marriage might not succeed, that affairs might end, that love might die, not on the railroad tracks, but in arguments that were supposed to be settled by making love, or in the resolutions about "freedom"

and "nonpossessiveness," which tore the very heart out of intimacy. For
years I had an upward and onward view of life, believing that growth
inevitably led to more growth. Living with someone, I thought, was
supposed to make you love each other even more.

 . . . I didn't count on . . . the power of sex. I didn't realize that sex
made a difference, or at least not that kind of a difference. I thought sex
was an expression of love, a part of love. What I didn't think was that it
transformed everything, that for me and for most women, making love
with a man several times created unpredictable bonds—which weren't
broken by saying: "This was a trial marriage for which the contract has
expired." I didn't realize that intimacy, physical intimacy, had unknown
properties, that it created deepening needs, created highly unprogressive
bursts of possessiveness and jealousy, created some balance between tension and satisfaction that became the mirror of every other aspect of a
relationship. I didn't realize that sex deepened love and love deepened
sex, even when love was on its way out. I didn't realize that love could
reverse itself, could be withdrawn, or that the consequences of such a
withdrawal could be so powerful as to crush vast expanses of one's own
potential for feeling. I didn't realize there actually was such a thing as
falling apart over the loss of love, nor that the difference between waking
up next to a man you loved and not waking up next to him could be all
the difference in the world.

 What I discovered in the midst of my drive toward emancipation was
that sex, love, hurt, and hate were the real stuff I was made of; that
fairness, rationality, and the willingness to discard or give away what one
had never been sure of possessing in the first place were all secondary
characteristics, carefully cultivated to be sure, but capable of collapsing
the moment stronger passions reared their heads. (pp. 151–152)

SCIENCE—ONE APPROACH TO INQUIRY ABOUT HUMAN SEXUALITY

As we read these examples of human sexual functioning, hundreds of
questions come to mind: How can we ever impose any order on something
that involves so many important issues with such a variety of ways of affecting
people's lives? Where do those who seek to understand human sexuality begin
their quest?

One place to begin is with scientific inquiry—the search for knowledge
based on posing questions and then attempting to answer those questions. But
how could even the process of scientific inquiry make sense of such a complex
topic? Some relief comes from the fact that such inquiry is not approached
randomly. Science is, however, a relative newcomer to inquiry about human
sexuality. As we will see in Chap. 2, religion, law, philosophy, and other such
disciplines have provided frameworks for the posing and answering of questions about sexuality throughout human history. But since the nineteenth
century, science has been making the major contribution to our knowledge of
this complex subject.

Up to this point we have spoken of science as if it were a single approach
to inquiry. The fact is that the scientific approach to human sexual behavior is
multidisciplinary—it is the province of several subfields of science. The exis-

tence of separate scientific disciplines is science's way of simplifying the inquiry process by sorting the great number and variety of questions into the disciplines most likely to contribute answers. One way of dividing the questions is to look at them in terms of levels, moving from within the person (biology-physiology) to person-world interaction (psychology) to interaction of large groups of people (sociology). Let us look at each of these disciplines to see what kinds of questions might fall within their jurisdiction and to see how they might deal with or explain the cases presented in our five examples.

Biology is the study of living organisms. Physiology is the study of the systems within biological organisms. Together they provide knowledge of the living system as it functions sexually. Sexual intercourse is the surface manifestation of two tremendously complex biological systems functioning in very special ways—individually and in interaction. What is it about human anatomy that makes sexual behavior possible? How do the feelings of arousal relate to physiological events? What do we know about the nature of orgasm? These are some of the questions appropriate to biological-physiological analysis.

For Bill and Kathy, understanding the biological-physiological aspects of conception was crucial to improving their chances of having a baby. What actually occurs during conception? When is conception most likely during Kathy's menstrual cycle? Are there physiological indicators that would help them time their sexual activity? Are some positions more conducive to impregnation than others? Considering Bill's low sperm count and Kathy's irregular cycles, it was not surprising that they had trouble conceiving a child. However, it is a bit surprising that they were still unsuccessful after 2 years of trying. It became clear that Bill and Kathy's lack of knowledge was what reduced their small chances even further. They had no way of knowing how they could maximize their chances with careful timing or how other preplanning measures might have helped. In fact, some of their activities were counterproductive. Common sense told them that the more sex they had, the better their chances of conceiving a baby. They did not realize that their high frequency of intercourse actually kept Bill's sperm count low. Kathy's emotional state also worked against them, in that her nervousness probably accentuated the irregularity of her cycle. In her case, less concern would have been more conducive to conception.

It is clear from this assessment that Bill and Kathy needed counseling on the biological and physiological aspects of reproduction. They also needed practical advice for using this information. Bill and Kathy contributed to their lowered probability of conception, and only through altering their behavior could they increase their chances of having a child.

Sally and Dave also suffered from a lack of information. They had little knowledge of their own or their partner's sexual anatomy and even less understanding of the physiology of sexual arousal and intercourse. They were forced to function through trial and error, trying to answer their questions about their own and their partner's sexual response in the midst of the sexual act. It is no wonder that their sexual experience was negative. We left them posing questions in their minds that should have been answered long before they ever became sexually involved.

Ingrid Bengis's writings, in which she struggled with love and attachment, seem rather removed from the biological-physiological sphere. But are her concerns so remote? Is there not a biological-physiological level to the intense feelings she describes? Certainly feelings affect the functioning of the physical organism. All those love songs in which the heart skips a bit, breathing falters, sleep is lost, and hunger disappears represent physiological effects. Is it possible that there are important biological-physiological events involved in creating or supporting emotional attachments?

From the questions we have raised, it is obvious that knowledge of the biological-physiological basis of sexuality is necessary for a thorough understanding of sexual behavior. Not only can we learn more about how we function but also about how sexual systems became part of the human organism in the first place. Such subdisciplines as evolutionary biology, animal physiology, and sociobiology are devoted to explaining this type of question and can greatly expand our knowledge about human sexual behavior.

*Psychological
issues*

When people think of psychotherapy, they often picture a patient lying on a couch talking in tortured terms about his or her sex life—or lack of one— while the therapist sits nearby, patiently nodding. Although this stereotype is certainly not representative of the way therapy is performed today, we cannot deny that issues of sexuality are high on the list of problems for which people seek therapeutic solutions. What are the psychological aspects of sexual functioning that create such problems? The answers to that question will take up much of the rest of this book. However, it would be valuable to mention a few of the questions here.

Consider Sally and Dave's situation. Many psychological questions arise as we examine their case. What effect does anxiety have on the sexual response? What psychological learning is going on in the situation that may prove maladaptive to future sexual behavior? How have their expectations and psychological sex roles affected their behavior? What will this initial negative experience mean to their relationship and to their self-esteem? Sally and Dave's psychological history, the psychological pressures of the moment, and their psychological futures have all come together around this one experience.

The Arapesh sexual behavior, as we noted, calls for inhibiting much of the passion that Western society associates with sexual behavior. What kind of psychosexual development must have been part of the Arapesh child-rearing process to permit such a lack of feeling? Can repressing what we think of as strong, "natural" emotional responses be accomplished at no psychological cost? Even our supposedly permissive society has been accused of creating psychological maladjustment by excessive repression of natural sexual feelings. It would thus be valuable to try to assess the effects that differing child-rearing practices have on adult sexual behavior.

Frank B.'s masochistic behavior is already considered to be a psychological problem. In fact, his story comes from the record of his treatment for sexually variant behavior; it is a clinical case study. Some psychological theories would attribute Frank's problem to distortions that developed during his childhood such that he felt the need to be punished for his sexual urges. Other psychological theories would ascribe his behavior to incorrect learning such that inappropriate associations were made between punishment and sexual gratification early in Frank's life. These approaches are discussed in detail later in this book.

Sociological issues

According to Beach (1976), the control of sexual behavior is a fundamental law in all societies:

> *The general law states simply that every society shapes, structures, and constrains the development and expression of sexuality in all of its members. This is universally achieved by social training from infancy and by constant social reward and punishment throughout life. There is not, and can never have been, a true society without sexual rules. (p. 116)*

The questions raised by society are concerned with the relationship of sexuality to the social structure. What is socially acceptable sexual behavior? Who should define what is acceptable? What is attractive and desirable? What are the appropriate sex roles? What are the models for marriage? For child rearing? What are the consequences of deviating from the group norm?

Depending on the society, each and every aspect of an individual's life, from birth to death, may be specified and directed. Among the Shakers, for example, all sexual expression was totally prohibited. A society's definition of sexuality thus can be every bit as important as the biological-physiological factors that control sexual behavior.

The relationship between society and sexuality is an interdependent one, however. The sexual nature of human beings provides important determinants in the formation of societies. The structure and rules of society have to take into account the strong nature of sexuality. As a result, many of the elements within the social structure are really reactions to people's sexual needs. Marriage and family patterns, social stratification and dominance, rites of passage to adulthood, sex roles, and so on are all aspects of society shaped by the existence of sexual drives. The interplay of sexuality and society becomes a contributor to the development of both.

You can see the mutual relationship between society and sexuality in each of the five examples that began our discussion. Social expectations influenced Bill and Kathy's desire for a baby. When they did not succeed in fulfilling this desire, the expectations turned into social pressures, which made conception even more difficult. In addition, the couple's lack of knowledge about sexual matters can be seen as a failure of society, since it failed to transmit the necessary sexual information to them. Understanding why and how this happened is important to investigators of human sexuality.

In the case of Sally and Dave, our society heightened the probability of sexual problems in several ways. They were raised to believe that sex is desirable but forbidden, were given no information about how to function sexually, but were told that their identity as "male" and "female" would depend on how well they functioned sexually. With all these pressures and their lack of knowledge, they were then thrown together to "have sex." Given this common experience, we must question society's view of sex education, social sex-role identity issues, and numerous other societal impositions on sexual functioning.

The case of Frank B. raises several social issues regarding sexual variance—a very important aspect of the interaction between sexual behavior and society. In our society Frank's behavior is not considered "normal" regardless of how he feels about it himself. Yet we cannot be certain how our society will react to this or to any other form of sexual behavior in the future. We may become more tolerant, or we may react more harshly. Neither can we assume that other societies share our definition of sexual abnormality. What is unacceptable in our society may be considered perfectly normal in another, and vice versa.

We saw such a difference in cultural definitions of normality in the example of the Arapesh. As we noted, "normal" Arapesh couples do not experience the arousal and excitement we assume to be an element of sexual intercourse. Their sexual training has been such that they do not experience feelings we consider to be almost a reflexive part of our own sexual contact. How would Ingrid Bengis fit in to Arapesh society? Her concerns about love and passion would have no meaning. She would, in fact, be considered "abnormal" by the Arapesh. These examples help us see that we can never understand much about sexual behavior without understanding the social context in which it occurs.

The example of Ingrid Bengis also shows that changes *within* a society can influence sexual interactions. Ingrid entered a relationship with many traditional expectancies that were perhaps appropriate to the lives of her parents but inappropriate to the changing morality of Ingrid's generation. What happens when a society is changing rapidly? What are the effects on individuals whose roles are in flux and whose formerly clear social relationships become clouded? These are particularly important questions to all of us, living as we do in such a rapidly changing society.

THE PERSONAL LEVEL OF INQUIRY

The inquiry process, as we have described it, is the process of forming appropriate questions and then trying to find answers for them. Science's approach to that process can seem highly intellectualized and removed from personal experience. This deliberate objectivity is sought by scientists to avoid the dangers of imposing their own opinions, interests, desires, and so on, upon their observations. Acquiring knowledge for its own sake is often expressed as an ideal of scientific inquiry. But it is an ideal, not an accomplished reality, and as a student, you (like most scientists) should not avoid the personal relevance and importance of the questions posed and the answers suggested by scientific research. Humans have been called the "inquiring animal" not because of idle curiosity but because of the control that knowledge gives us over ourselves and our environment. There are few topics as personally relevant to each of us as the topic of human sexuality. Your personal desire for knowledge —*your* inquiry—not only is appropriate but also is a valuable component in the journey you are about to take into the subject. Your personal involvement will make the subject all the more important and interesting and, it is hoped, will engage you in the excitement of discovery that is very much a part of the advances science is making in the study of human sexuality.

The personal relevance of the topic also creates some problems. We noted that objectivity and distance are often desirable. The scientific investigator in such a self-relevant area must be careful to reduce the subjective elements as much as possible. Each of us must also watch for that loss of objectivity that may undermine our own approach to this topic. Imagine how Frank B. might react to the section of the textbook on masochism. Would he fail to recognize himself? Would he angrily denounce any book that would devalue such an obviously "normal" behavior? Or would he be distraught to find that he is driven to engage in behaviors that are formally labeled "variant" and that are considered to be psychiatric problems?

By looking through Frank's eyes, we can see how difficult it would be to accept other people's views, no matter how objective, in areas of such personal sensitivity. Here, for example, is a letter written in response to a popular magazine's national survey of women's sexual attitudes and behavior (Tavris and Sadd, 1977):

> *Before I got married, I was like all other women, panting to experience the ecstasy of sex. I had read and heard (from men) the wonders of it. Well, I married a wonderful man and we have been married almost 30 years. From the first night it was just unpleasant. I endured it, but I have always resented my husband's flight to the heights while I experience "blah." Thank goodness the last three years he has slowed down so I don't have to act the part of enjoying something so repulsive. I really love my husband but he is a man and to him sex is food.*
>
> *Now what I want to tell you is I am not alone in this. In all of my life I have* never *talked to a woman who did not feel as I do. Not once have I heard a woman say she enjoys sex. I hear them call it repulsive, tell things they do to get out of it (sitting up late to avoid it, stealing into bed without waking their husbands). They shudder at the thought of this going on into their sixties, seventies.*
>
> *Okay, who is kidding whom?*
>
> *P.S. I think this women's liberation is silly, mostly, but I'm all for the part that says we can stop faking orgasms. (pp. 29–30)*

This letter is extreme, but it does indicate how personal feelings can dominate one's whole view of this subject. We all experience reactions of this sort at one point or another in the study of sexuality. When you find yourself asking, like the letter writer, "Who's kidding whom?" that may be a good point to stop yourself, look at the topic again, and ask whether you are being as objective as you should be on that particular issue.

THE NEED FOR
REAL KNOWLEDGE

The numerous questions we have posed, and the many more you may have posed for yourself, indicate how great the need is for knowledge about sexual behavior. But what kind of knowledge? Until recently, it was not acceptable to study sexual behavior directly. Without such direct study, we were left with an information gap—a gap filled by distortions, folklore, misinformation, and advice from self-appointed experts. All too often these myths were accepted as true, producing serious social problems and great individual pain. Table 1.1 lists some of the most flagrant myths concerning sexual behavior. Each has the potential to interfere with an individual's optimal sexual adjustment. Without factual information to replace these distortions, too many people are forced to build their sex lives on the shakiest of foundations.

TABLE 1.1

*Ten myths
exploded*

1 The only acceptable sexual position is the male superior (man-on-top) position.
2 Sex during menstruation is unclean and harmful.
3 Sex should be avoided during pregnancy.
4 A small penis is less satisfying to a woman than a large one.
5 Prostitutes are either frigid or homosexual (or both).
6 Anal intercourse is perverted and dangerous.
7 It's good to sublimate the sex drive for long periods of time.
8 An excessively amorous woman is a nymphomaniac.
9 Advancing age means the end of sex.
10 Any man who can't make it with a woman is suffering from severe psychiatric problems.

Source: Masters and Johnson (December 1970), pp. 124ff.

The need is for *real* knowledge, that is, reliable and valid knowledge that can only be obtained through direct study of the problem. Science, the institution devoted to such objective appraisal of the world, is one way of acquiring real knowledge. Investigators are beginning the kind of deliberate, intensive, and cautious studies that will lead to the accumulation of factual information. What they learn will help increase our understanding of human sexual responses, and it will help make our personal sexual lives more fulfilling. For the first time, our society is open to the idea of using knowledge to enhance sexual growth. It becomes even more important, then, that the information disseminated is reliable and valid.

LOVE,
ATTACHMENT,
AND HUMAN
SEXUALITY

Different cultures in different parts of the world possess remarkably similar folktales about the origin of men and women. Early Greek stories referred to mythological beings with four arms, four legs, two faces, and the sex organs of both men and women. These "he-she" beings were split in half by Zeus to lessen their considerable strength and ability. The two halves then wandered in search of each other, seeking to reestablish the perfect union they had once known.

This medieval woodcut shows Eve emerging from the body of Adam. This illustrates the Judeo-Christian view of the original unity of the sexes.

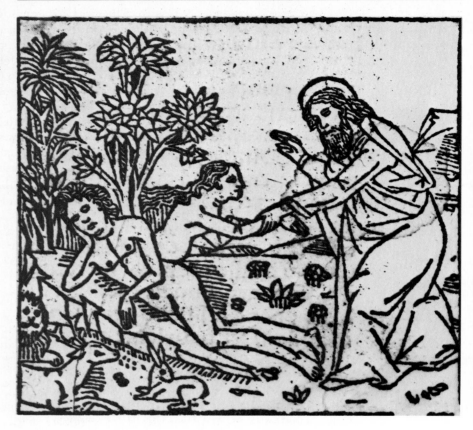

The center of this jade amulet contains the yin (female)-yang (male) symbol. Together they form a perfect whole.

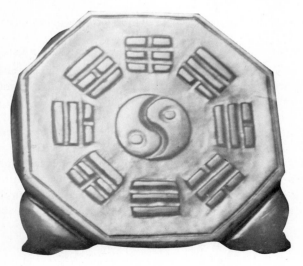

The Old Testament of the Judeo-Christian world tells the story of Eve being made from Adam's rib. Thus, they too were once a single whole being. The Chinese describe their world in terms of Yin and Yang. When these qualities are combined, they create the perfect harmony of nature. Heaven and earth and the sun and moon are Yin-Yang combinations. So are man and woman, who together produce perfect harmony.

These folktales provide a useful theme as we embark upon our study of human sexuality, for as we shall see, this highly complex subject is basically about the perfect harmony people seek by joining together. Much of our discussion will be an exploration of the coming together involved in sexual behavior, but now would be a good time to remind ourselves that such coming together has always meant more than the physical union of sexual intercourse. Human sexuality goes far beyond the act of mating. It includes the various aspects of emotional bonding—attachment and love—as well. These related aspects of human sexuality have as much, and sometimes more, meaning and power than the physical act of sex. In our study of human sexuality, we must not forget the emotional dimensions. Learning about sexual behavior without examining attachment and love would leave us as incomplete as one of the half-beings of mythology. Like them, we aspire to wholeness.

SUMMARY

1 Knowledge of sexual behavior is gleaned from scientific inquiry—the posing and answering of relevant questions. The scientific approach to sexuality is multidisciplinary; questions in this area are directed to many different subfields, including biology-physiology, psychology, and sociology.

2 Biology deals with questions about the relationship of physiological events to sexual behavior. Psychology deals with the role that emotional, motivational, and cognitive factors play within the individual in sexual behavior and sexuality and with the problems people may experience in these areas. At the level of sociology and anthropology, questions are raised about the relationship between sexuality and the social structure.

3 Those who study sexuality must maintain a balance between scientific objectivity and personal involvement.

4 Because myths abound in the sexual realm, there is a need for reliable and valid knowledge upon which people can base their actions and decisions.

5 Any study of sexual behavior must take into account the emotional as well as the physical aspects involved.

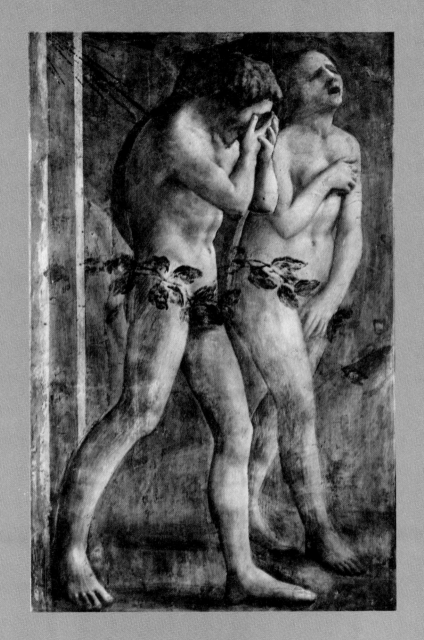

Human sexuality:
A historical perspective

2

chapter
2

Nothing is so much to be shunned as sex relations.

—ST. AUGUSTINE

Sexual pleasure, wisely used and not abused, may prove the stimulus and liberator of our finest and most exalted activities.

—HAVELOCK ELLIS

Which of these two attitudes—sexual repression or sexual liberation—has dominated the history of Western civilization? It would be easy to point to the Puritans and the Victorians to make a case for a history of sexual repression. But it would be equally valid to cite the open sexuality of Greece and Rome and liberalized attitudes toward sexuality in Renaissance Europe to justify an argument in favor of permissiveness. The truth is that both of these attitudes have predominated at different times in Western culture, and in many cases they have coexisted. Today we find that elements of both these attitudes color our views of human sexuality. In fact, our current views are very much the product of the sexual rules and mores of all of the historical periods and cultures that have preceded our own.

In this chapter we will take a brief look at how sexuality was viewed during some of the major periods of Western history. For each period we will examine the prevailing rules of sexual behavior, how they came about, and the institutions that dominated sexual knowledge and its dissemination through the society. We will see that there have been many cycles in sexual thought and behavior, with periods of repression typically followed by periods of greater freedom, and vice versa. As you read about these historical periods, try to note which patterns have had an influence on today's sexual attitudes and behavior.

PREHISTORIC
SEXUAL LIFE

Unfortunately, we have little information on the sexual behavior of prehistoric humans. While relics, paintings, and other artifacts are suggestive, we must be cautious about imposing our own views of sexual behavior in interpreting the meaning of these objects.

There is some evidence that primitive humans lived in nuclear family groups, much as we do today. Richard Leakey, the anthropologist, discovered the remains of such a family group in Africa. The group, which included a father, mother, and three children, is believed to be about 5 million years old. Is this family structure somehow natural to the species? Is it dictated by the necessity of caring for the highly dependent human infant? Current primitive cultures also show similar family structures, which seems to indicate that there may indeed be forces that lead human beings to such groupings.

Among the oldest artifacts left to us from prehistorical cultures are the so-called Venus figures. The Venus of Willendorf, found in Austria, and the Venus of Lespugue, found in France, are estimated to be 20,000 years old. The interesting feature of these carved figures, and of similar ones found more recently, is the overemphasis on the sexual and childbearing characteristics of women. The figures all have exaggeratedly large breasts, buttocks, hips, and

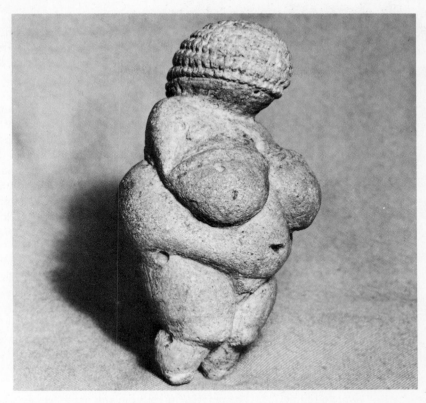

The Venus of Willendorf. The early depiction of the female. We can only guess at its meaning or purpose.

thighs and carefully detailed genitals. Many anthropologists feel that these figures are fertility symbols. This possibility is supported by other indications of primitive cultures' great concern with reproduction. *Fertility*—the renewal of life—was a major issue of survival, whether it involved crops, animals, or the next generation of humans.

But perhaps these figures did not have quite so serious a meaning. One cannot help but wonder whether they could have been examples of an early erotic art form—could the Venus figures have been the *Playboy* centerfolds of their day?

EARLY CULTURES

The roots of Western culture can be traced back to the cultures of the Middle East. The peoples of this region settled down from nomadic life to become stock breeders and farmers in the rich valleys of the Nile, Euphrates, and Tigris rivers. They eventually differentiated into the Egyptian, Mesopotamian, Assyrian, Babylonian, and Hebrew cultures. In each of these cultures, the dominant view of life was mystical, and the dominant social institutions were religious. These societies were theocratic—ruled by religious dogma based on worship of one or more gods. The rulers on earth were often considered to be gods themselves or claimed to have some divine connection. The Egyptian pharaohs, for example, claimed direct descent from the gods. Rule was established by religious law and was maintained through the divine rulers and their priests.

The earliest written laws said little about sexual behavior, although they did deal with family relationships. The Babylonian Code of Hammurabi, written in the twentieth century B.C., contained the first known written laws governing sexual behavior. It stated that incest (sex with a blood relative) and bestiality (sex with animals) were forbidden and punishable by death. The code indicated that males dominated all social interactions, and it outlined rules governing the number of wives a man could have, as well as financial arrangements for acquiring wives and inheriting property. Other documents of the time suggested that sex was generally approved of in the context of procreation. Strong rules were also set forth concerning the maintenance of family structures.

The ancient Egyptians appear to have had a positive attitude toward sexuality. Sexual activity with the goal of procreation was permitted and encouraged. The Egyptians approached sexual behavior as a natural process but with much ritual attached to it. According to written records, they favored the female superior sexual position, with the woman straddling the reclining man. This position was symbolic of their religious belief that a male god represented the earth and a female god represented the sky above. Egyptian males were sexually privileged and could commit adultery, divorce their wives, and use slaves for childbearing if their wives proved barren. Both males and females were circumcised. (The practice of circumcising male babies was probably adopted by the Jews during their enslavement in Egypt.)

The pharaohs had a sexual life different from that of the people they ruled. We know from documented evidence that the pharaohs engaged in nonprocreative sexual relations. Indeed, they were known for their sexual intrigues, ideas of heightened sexual pleasure, and perfumes and makeup. They had incestuous relationships in the form of marriage between brother and sister, thus breaking the prevailing law against incest. As we will see in our exploration of other historical eras, this kind of double standard was not unusual. The rules of sexual behavior often varied from social class to social class.

The generally permissive, sex-positive sexual attitudes of the Tigris-Euphrates and Nile valleys were changed by the invasion of the Persians in the sixth century B.C. (Bullough, 1976). The Persians followed the Zoroastrian religion, which defined everything in terms of good and evil. This religion was probably the source of the concept of the "wicked flesh in conflict with the divine spirit" that soon dominated this part of the world.

One of the major demons of Zoroastrianism was Jeh, the primeval whore. She brought out the evil sexual impulses in men. She made women menstruate; thus, the Persians believed menstruating women were dangerous and to be feared. This belief may well be the basis for the Judaic view of menstruating women as "unclean."

According to Zoroastrianism, any sexual activity not leading to procreation was a sin of the flesh. Ejaculation, for example, was considered a grave sin unless it occurred during intercourse with a woman. Therefore, coitus interruptus, homosexual activity, bestiality, masturbation, and even nocturnal emissions ("wet dreams") were considered sinful. The Zoroastrian view eventually found its way into the Judeo-Christian religions.

EARLY JUDAISM   The Hebrews were distinguished from other peoples of the Middle East by their belief in a single god as opposed to the many gods of other religions. The Hebrew code of behavior, the Deuteronomic legislation of 640 B.C., provided a generally positive view of sexual activities. Within the marital relationship, few restrictions were placed on sexual behavior. Women were viewed as more sexual by nature, and men were duty-bound to satisfy their wives by bringing them to orgasm. Parents were entrusted with the responsibility of passing on sexual information to their children.

The influence of Zoroastrianism appeared in the new laws that governed the Jewish people upon their return from Egypt. The Holiness Code (Exodus and Leviticus) and the Ten Commandments reflected a more restrictive attitude toward sex. Because of God's commandment to "go forth and multiply," procreation dominated the new laws, and the Hebrews sought to increase the birth rate. Although a high value was placed on virginity before marriage, there were only mild restrictions against premarital sex, particularly for men. Adultery, however, was forbidden in the Ten Commandments. Because menstruation was regarded as unclean, a menstruating woman was isolated and was forbidden to engage in sex.

There were rules against nakedness, and coitus interruptus, masturbation, and homosexuality were strongly forbidden because of the rule against "spilling of the seed." Although homosexuality was not mentioned at all in the earlier Hebrew codes, homosexual acts were made punishable by death in later documents.

In general, the Judaic period represented a transition from the generally positive view of sexual behavior in ancient times to the more restrictive views that characterized the rise of Christianity. Many of the laws of ancient Judaism are still reflected in modern attitudes as part of the Judeo-Christian tradition.

ANCIENT GREECE   Early Greece was dominated by a base of religious beliefs that governed all aspects of life, including sexuality. However, the gods of Greek mythology were a sexually rambunctious group, at least by usual religious standards, and their lusty and positive approach to sexual behavior remained embedded in Greek culture as it moved in a more secular direction.

During the classical period, the so-called Golden Age (beginning at about the fifth century B.C.), Greece was governed by political rather than religious

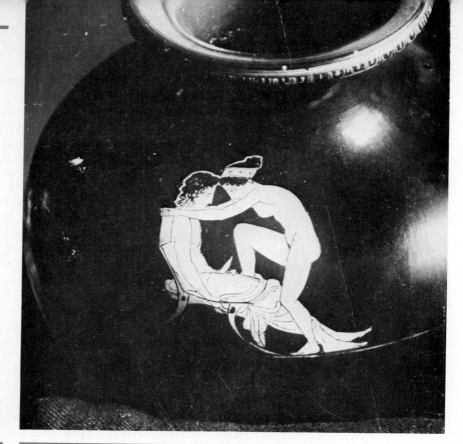

Greek vases were often decorated with erotic scenes.

leaders, and, off and on, democratic rule prevailed. **Naturalism**, the idea that events could be explained in terms of the laws of nature, became the dominant cultural view. This philosophy provided a sharp contrast to the religious views that controlled other cultures of the time—most religions supported the belief that events in the world were the result of forces beyond human comprehension and control.

Several important institutions controlled sexual behavior. Laws were used to control marital, contractual, and monetary aspects of sexual life. The more personal aspects of sexual behavior were the province of art and aesthetics. The human form was studied as a work of art to be admired. In general, sexual relationships were governed by the rules of reason, and excesses were avoided. This emphasis on beauty and moderation pervaded much of the Greek view of the ideal life.

At the height of the Golden Age, the ideal of beauty was exemplified by the young man. Both physically and intellectually, the young man was seen to be at the ideal point of all nature. Art, sculpture, drama, and poetry were devoted to **homoerotic expression**—the sensual desire of men for men. The view that man was bisexual by nature began to dominate Greek society and was given free expression. Homoerotic attachments between older and younger men were considered important. The younger man was brought into adulthood by his mentor, who himself was restored to greater vigor by the relationship.

Homosexual acts were less clearly a part of the relationship. Historians suggest that homosexual contact was indeed a major part of sexual life, but such activities were not written about directly in documents of the time. Greek writers tended to idealize the male-male relationships, and they considered the sexual aspect to be less than ideal. Male prostitution existed, but it was not an admired activity for seller or buyer. Although homosexual activity was probably a prevalent sexual behavior, it may not have been as universally accepted a part of Greek life as we have come to believe.

The sexual attitudes of Greece continued to become freer over time. Nudity became a regular part of sports and dramatic presentations. Plato wrote that free love would be a legal right in his idealized society, the Republic.

So far we have described male sexuality in ancient Greece. Unfortunately, we know much less about the behavior code for Greek women. The Greeks, male-dominated as they were, did not write much about women's lives. Among the upper classes, wives were managers, whereas concubines and prostitutes provided companionship, entertainment, and sexual satisfaction for the husbands. Greek literature does tell of female homosexuality, or lesbianism. In fact, the term *lesbianism* comes from the island of Lesbos, where the poetess Sappho conducted a school for women. Sappho is said to have killed herself over unrequited love for one of her students. Despite such stories, historians tell us that lesbianism was not widely practiced in Greece.

ROMAN CIVILIZATION

Roman civilization spanned several centuries. Because sexual rules and customs changed greatly during that period, no single Roman approach to sexual behavior can be identified. In the earliest recorded periods, Roman sexual codes were highly restrictive, but as the society evolved it became freer and more permissive.

The Roman citizen's life was ruled by secular laws and legal codes rather than by religion. The best-known laws were the Twelve Tables (457–449 B.C.) and the Patrician Code. These documents outlined the various laws of Roman society, including those governing sexual practices. However, these codes did not seem to be greatly concerned with sexual behavior, and even sexual excesses and deviations were not given any special consideration.

In the Roman family, sexual activity began early—at about age 12 for girls and age 14 for boys. The parents were responsible for instructing their children in sexual matters. Mothers taught daughters; fathers taught sons. As with the Hebrews, sexual teaching was an important duty of the parents.

Toward the end of the Roman Empire, interest in the romantic aspects of sexuality increased. The great poets of love flourished and were widely read. Ovid's *Ars Amatoria (The Art of Love*, 10 B.C.) was the Roman version of a best-seller. In it, Ovid discussed the true delights of love through the conquest of women—primarily married women. This advocacy of adultery brought Ovid widespread criticism, which indicates that the Romans may have been far less decadent than they are usually depicted.

Prostitution was an accepted practice in Rome. Houses of prostitution existed throughout Rome, and their numbers greatly increased in the waning years of the Empire. These latter years also saw an increase in the practice of more unusual sexual behaviors, which are probably the basis for our current stereotyped view of Roman sexual decadence. Sexual activities joined violence in the Roman Circus of gladiator fame. Animals were trained to have sexual intercourse with humans and were turned loose on captured people in the coliseum for the amusement of the audience. Bulls, leopards, horses, large dogs, bears, and other animals would brutally attack women and men to the cheers of the crowd.

Although homosexuality was never considered a deviation under the law, it was generally viewed negatively and was referred to derogatorily as "the Greek way." Homosexual activity did increase somewhat in the final period of the Empire, primarily among the upper classes.

Some historians cite the loosening of morality in general and of sexual morality in particular as the basis for the fall of Rome. Others have claimed that the fact that Christianity took such a strong hold reflected the higher standards of the populace relative to those of the leaders. While we can never really know which, if either, of these views is correct, we do know that Roman society changed greatly, particularly with regard to sexual behavior, when it adopted Christianity.

THE RISE OF CHRISTIANITY

At the time of Christ's birth, Judaism was already undergoing changes toward greater restrictions of sexual behavior. Jesus, a Palestinian Jew, was raised at a time when sexual behavior was being greatly debated. While he had few negative things to say about sex in his own teachings, Jesus was concerned about sexual excess. He himself was presumed to be celibate, a behavior that was counter to the prevailing Jewish view. He was concerned about the laxity of Jewish divorce laws and preached against adultery for both men *and* women.

The writings of Christ's disciples indicate clearly negative views of sexual behavior. This negativity was particularly emphasized in the early writings of Paul. He wrote that chastity and celibacy were superior to marriage, and he encouraged men not to engage in sex at all: "It is good for a man not to touch a woman." (1 Corinthians 7:1) If, however, a man's drive was too strong (that is, if the man was too weak!), he could resort to sexual intercourse—but only in marriage ("It is better to marry than to burn."—Paul). This **asceticism** toward sexuality was the most extreme version of a negative approach to sexuality represented by the early Christians. These ideas were generally disregarded by the Jews, but they hit responsive chords elsewhere and developed a following.

Although in Rome social order and sexual behavior had been the province of the legal-political system rather than the religious system, this situation began to change. When Rome was experiencing its greatest social disruption, Christian preachers came from the East calling for moral reform. They told people to think less of this life and more of their souls in eternity. Because the Christian teachings were viewed as critical of the prevailing rule, the Christians were violently suppressed. However, as Roman society faltered, Christian doctrine answered people's need for some sense of order. Eventually, Christianity came to dominate Rome through the Catholic church.

With the Middle Ages, the church came to control all aspects of life. Between the fifth and fifteenth centuries, the restrictive views of the early Christians were strengthened. St. Augustine, whom we quoted at the beginning of this chapter, wrote at the end of the fourth century: "Behold I was conceived in inequity and in sin hath my mother conceived me." This statement of sexual guilt, which is still part of the evening prayer of the Catholic church, was to characterize the Catholic view of sexual behavior for several centuries.

Chastity was considered a virtue. When chastity was not possible, sexual behavior was to be engaged in without pleasure. Church documents of the eighth century specified that only one sexual position was to be used (the male superior position) since other positions might be enjoyable. Different penalties were given for engaging in different sexual positions. The most forbidden was rear-entry, which carried a penalty of seven years' penance. The documents also called for abstinence on Sundays and on certain important church occasions. When added together, these occasions amounted to about 5 months out of the year during which sexual intercourse was not permitted.

Chastity for priests was imposed in the year 1050; all heterosexual, homosexual, and autosexual behaviors were forbidden. Furthermore, any nonprocreative activity hinting of sexuality was forbidden for lay people. Dancing, singing, touching each other, viewing parts of the body—all were designated as sins. Even thoughts had to be totally nonsexual, thus closing off the outlet of fantasy during this period.

As time passed, church control grew. Secular legislation came to be administered through ecclesiastical courts. In the twelfth century, the church took control of marriage laws and imposed rules forbidding divorce. Any deviations from the church-established rules were severely punished.

In the midst of this repression, the phenomenon of courtly love managed to develop among the nobility. From the fifteenth century on, knights and their ladies carried on amorous relationships, although it is not clear whether these affairs actually involved sexual activity. (Once again we are reminded that the standards of behavior for the upper classes were different from those for the lower classes.) The admiration and respect for women contained in the code of the knights raised the status of women from that of possessions to idolized individuals. Women were placed on pedestals. This period of courtly love eventually changed the idea of man-woman relationships for all of Western culture. The activities of the knights and their fair maidens laid the historical groundwork for the idea of romantic love as it is practiced today.

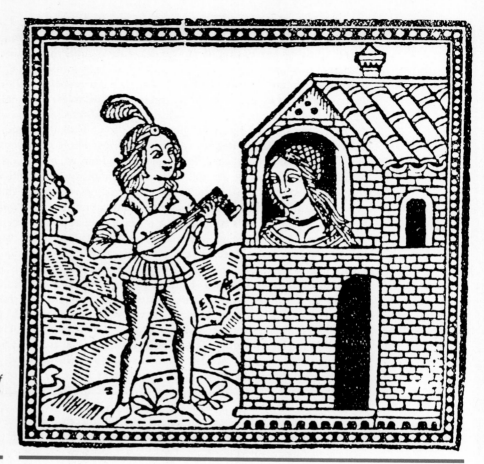

This medieval scene illustrates the idealization of the female new to the history of Western male-female relationships.

THE RENAISSANCE

One of the central themes of the Renaissance was a renewed interest in the artistic display of the human body. Nude statuary from the Roman era showing the human body as high art inspired Renaissance painters and sculptors. At first these artistic creations were placed in a religious context and were actually commissioned by the church. The church reasoned that art was meant for spiritual enhancement, not earthly pleasure.

During the fourteenth century, erotic art and literature slowly began to appear, particularly in Venice. Leonardo da Vinci, Michelangelo, and others produced works that went far beyond church-held standards. The literature of the time set a new moral tone, speaking of unfulfilled sexual desire seeking expression in a restrictive environment. Stories of lovers overcoming hurdles to have a sexual affair gained great popularity.

Within the church itself other reformers were raising theological and philosophical questions centered around standards of sexual behavior. Debates over the celibacy of priests, for example, shook the church to its very core. Martin Luther was one of the strongest voices of dissent. He argued that most of the upper administration of the church was not celibate—that in fact these powerful men were quite promiscuous. Luther disliked this deception and wrote (in the sixteenth century) that if celibacy could not work (and he knew from personal experience that it could not), the church should give it up. Luther also argued for the acceptance of sexual activity as a natural and pleasurable act. He felt that the church should accept sexual behavior as appropriate for married individuals, and he insisted that marriage should be a civil not a religious ceremony. In several ways, then, Luther pressed the church to separate itself from such broad control over people's sexual lives.

The church was also buffeted by the actions of the king of England, Henry VIII, who was outraged by the church's views on divorce. Henry had petitioned Rome for a divorce in 1528, but his request had been refused. Shocked by the church's decision not to absolve him—a member of the ruling class—from the sexual rules governing the masses, Henry decided to set up his own church with himself as its leader. With one bold stroke, Henry broke with Rome and established the Church of England.

PURITANISM

Other new religious orientations emerged from the Protestant movements of the Renaissance. Some of those seeking reform were disturbed by the liberal climate of Europe and sought greater rather than lesser control over human sexual behavior. John Calvin, for example, designed a highly restrictive life for his followers in Geneva in the middle of the sixteenth century. Calvin and others were "fundamentalists" in their interpretation of the teachings of the Bible. This meant living by the Bible *as written*. The Puritans of England also held such beliefs and were persecuted for them. They emigated to America, where they felt they could practice their religion freely.

During the seventeenth and eighteenth centuries, America was dominated by the Puritan ethic. Puritan views of sexual behavior were not totally negative. Puritans believed that sexual activity was normal and should not require or demand abstinence. They also felt that husbands had the responsibility of physically satisfying their wives. They placed few restrictions on marital sexual relations; most rules concerned maintaining the family structure.

The Puritans were not antisex. However, it is not without justification that we associate the word *Puritan* with a grudging attitude toward sexual pleasure. The Puritans stood for hard work, self-discipline, and no pleasure except that achieved through religious experience. The earth was a test for these "chosen people," and a hard, unpleasant life only enhanced their chances of earning a desirable afterlife.

Because the church elders were the administrators of the community, there was no distinction between church and state. The law served the religious goals set forth in the Bible. The interpretations of the church elders made sin a crime as well as a source of religious guilt, and many of the sins-crimes were related to sexual behavior. Just about every kind of sexual expression

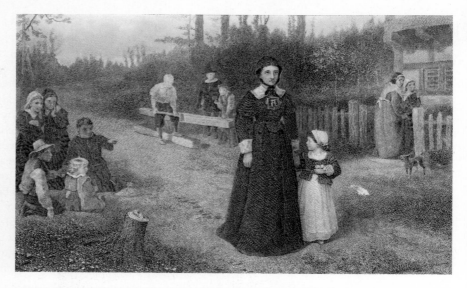

The famous scarlet letter of adultery during the Puritan era. The Puritans had an extremely narrow view of what was acceptable human sexual behavior.

except behaviors confined to marriage was forbidden. Abuses were met with severe penalties. The Jamestown Laws of 1607, for example, indicated the death penalty for sodomy, bestiality, and adultery.

The Puritan view of sexual behavior continues to have a lasting influence on American society. The all-pervasive sex laws still on the books in many states are one legacy of our Puritan forefathers. We still find, for example, that in some communities it is illegal to kiss on Sunday. Such laws may seem humorous by today's standards, and they are rarely enforced. Unfortunately, not all of these leftover laws are treated as a joke; as recently as 1978 a husband was prosecuted for engaging in "sodomy" with his wife. It is amazing that laws designed by fundamentalists in small communities in the sixteenth and seventeenth centuries are still influencing the sexual behaviors of individuals in a major industrial nation in the 1980s (see Chap. 20).

THE EMERGENCE OF SCIENCE

In the late seventeenth century, science began to emerge as a method of inquiry into the natural world. The study of anatomy provided the first extensions of scientific inquiry into sexual behavior. As scientists described the human reproductive system for the first time, it became clear that human birth was not something set apart from the birth of other creatures in the animal world. This fall from a divine view of birth in humans was comparable to the discovery that the earth was not the center of the universe.

The growing field of medicine was called upon more and more to deal with sexual disorders and deviations. When the clergy's prayers, incantations, and punishments failed to control deviant sexual behavior, other methods were employed. As science looked for and found answers in natural events rather than in religious dogma, sexual behavior began to be viewed as part of the natural world. Slowly, during the eighteenth century, the knowledge and control base of human sexual behavior shifted from religion to science.

The shift to science did not necessarily mean that the new interpretations were always correct or that the rules of sexual conduct that followed from them were more humane. In fact, during the nineteenth century, scientific explanations were used by society as a new basis for sexual repression. The idea that sexual stimulation of any kind, but especially orgasm, sapped a human's "vital forces" led to the bizarre Victorian view of sexuality, as we will see shortly. Nevertheless, the gradual movement of sexual behavior from the religious to the scientific sphere of influence is one of the major turning points in the development of our contemporary approach to human sexuality.

THE
VICTORIAN
ERA

Queen Victoria's name and her own restrictive attitudes about sexual behavior were given to the period that spanned her lifetime (1837–1901). To the Victorians, sexual feelings represented the animal side of human nature and had to be controlled rather than expressed. The "good and evil" dichotomy of the Puritans still prevailed, but now motivation came out of a perverse concern for health and decorum rather than out of religious or moral convictions.

Women, especially mothers, had a special place in the Victorian age. Yet sexual activity—the route to becoming a mother—was considered a highly unpleasant necessity. Sexual intercourse was performed with both parties clothed in several layers so that nudity and the tactile pleasure of human flesh would not provide excessive stimulation. Any woman who enjoyed sexual feelings and activities was considered perverted; only prostitutes made lusty sexual partners. Thus, two types of Victorian woman emerged: the sensitive, delicate wife and mother and the lusty prostitute.

Men were seen as being just the opposite of women. Victorians viewed men as animals with insatiable appetites, which they imposed on women. Men had to be controlled—they were never to be enticed or sexually stimulated. In fact, Victorian society went to great lengths to avoid any such sexual stimulation. Women's clothing styles were designed to disguise the body. Women's legs were covered at all times by numerous hoops and petticoats. In fact, legs could never be referred to in speech. (Even piano legs were fitted with special covers.) When a Victorian woman went to a physician, she pointed to body areas on a mannequin to indicate where she experienced problems. The physician did not touch her. If an examination was absolutely necessary, the woman's mother or husband had to be present. Nonhuman sexual displays were treated similarly: Statues in museums were covered, and animals wore appropriate "clothing" over their sex organs.

Victorian medicine supported these views. Bullough (1976) notes that there was a "renewal of the traditional Western hostility toward sex with a scientific foundation" (p. 546). In the work of Benjamin Rush, the founder of American psychiatry, all diseases were reducible to either an increase or a decrease in

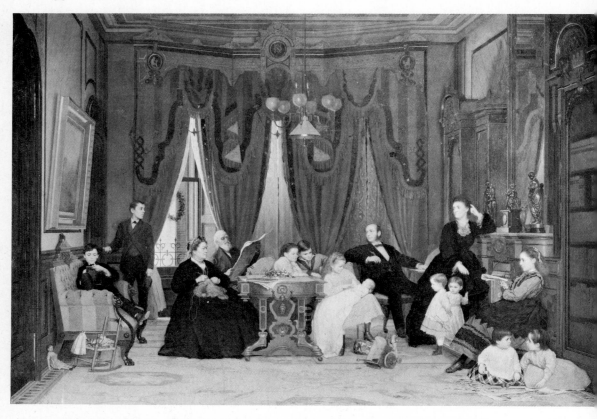

nervous energy. According to Rush, sexual involvement increased energy and reduced the body's ability to withstand illness. He therefore believed that sexual contact should not be too exciting for men and not exciting at all for women—women's natures were already too delicately balanced. You can imagine what these influential ideas did to restrict sexual arousal, foreplay, and variations in sexual positions.

One of the most interesting and influential medical theories of the time was that semen was part of the vital (life) force or animal essence of a man. Using it diminished that life force. And excessive use could be unhealthy and even life threatening. According to this theory, a man's available supply of semen should be used solely for procreation. Any other use of male ejaculation was strongly discouraged. We now see the Biblical rule against "spilling the seed" dressed in distorted medical-scientific reasoning. Sylvester Graham, inventer of graham flour, went so far as to argue that for adequate health maintenance people should not have sexual relations more than 12 times a year.

The preservation of the vital force became a major issue of the time. Since masturbation was the most likely way for men to excessively drain their vital energy, it was cited as the cause of many illnesses and disorders. The most serious problem ascribed to the effects of excessive masturbation was mental illness. Medical books of the time claimed that those who masturbated could be "diagnosed" on the street by their short stature, red, runny eyes, and slackness of posture.

The discovery that syphilis was a sexually transmitted disease gave credence to the connection between sexual behavior and ill health, particularly "madness." The dangers of sex, especially pleasurable sex, now included a serious disease. This fact became a strong weapon in the arsenal against sexuality.

The restrictive sexual attitudes of the Victorian period showed strong socioeconomic class differences. As in other periods, the rich and ruling classes ignored the rules and went about their lives with relative freedom. Although Queen Victoria led a conservative personal life, her royal court was noted for sexual excesses and intrigue. The very poor were also absolved from the rules. The Victorian intellectuals considered the lower classes to be nonrational and animalistic in their desires. It was the large and growing middle classes who were expected to conform to the strict moral code, and on the surface at least, it appeared that they did.

A Victorian home scene. The ideals of family, motherhood, and the avoidance of all "animal" tendencies, especially sexuality, typified this time.

As in other highly repressive societies, Victorian society provided safety valves for sexual expression. In Victorian Europe there developed an underground of erotic literature and art that provided a large body of pornographic material. Prostitution flourished, with great vitality and variety in the types of services offered. There were also sexual casualties of the repressive society—those who experienced sexual disorders and deviations in the attempt to maintain the delicate balance between sexual expression and repression. The Victorian period is known for the numerous sexual "deviates" described in the medical literature of the era. Richard von Krafft-Ebing wrote his famous *Psychopathia Sexualis* (1886), in which he detailed many of these cases (with the descriptive sections in Latin to protect public sensibilities). In the late 1800s, Leopold von Sacher-Masoch described his sexual practices, which centered around physical pain as a prelude to sexual satisfaction. Krafft-Ebing dubbed this type of sexual activity *masochism*. Sexual deviations became a central focus for the developing psychiatry of the day, and this focus was seminal in the development of Sigmund Freud's theories.

The end of the Victorian era may have been speeded by the excessive sexual repression. In effect, the period exerted too much control over natural aspects of sexuality, and eventually the pendulum had to swing in the opposite direction. The separation of feelings from sexuality was a particularly difficult distinction to maintain. Schlessinger (1966) summarized the Victorian effect in America as follows:

Yet the pursuit of happiness through a passionless marriage was generating a lurking, nagging frustration. By barring the joy of sex from wedlock, the

Victorian code at once degraded the sexual impulse and weakened the marital tie. By transferring romantic love to the fantasy world of the sentimental novel and emptying serious literature of adult sexual content, it misled the national imagination and impoverished the national sensibility. The Victorians' unsatisfactory pursuit of happiness thus ended half on Main Street and half on Back Street, with marriage denied passion and passion denied legitimacy.

This untenable dichotomy of passion and marriage could not be maintained. The Victorian grip on sexual behavior began to loosen, but we are still left with residues of the period today, as many of our current attitudes, laws, and even medical and scientific views reflect Victorian ideas.

THE TWENTIETH CENTURY

It would have been perfect had the Victorian period ended with the turn of the century, as Queen Victoria herself so conveniently did by dying in 1901. Periods are rarely so accommodating, and the Victorian era died slowly. What was left of it ended in 1914, at the start of World War I. After the war, the Roaring Twenties emerged with a much freer view of sexual behavior. This was the jazz age—the period of the flapper and ultrashort skirts. The emotional aspects of love were pursued with an intensity never known to the Victorians. It was the beginning of the age of love.

Scientists interested in studying the life sciences had worked quietly through the last part of the nineteenth century. They had focused their inquiry on the areas of reproduction and sexual functioning and had been accumulating a large body of knowledge in cell biology, cellular reproduction, animal and human sexual anatomy, and microscopic biology of related areas. Slowly the general picture of reproductive biology of the various species was being filled in. The work was not necessarily aimed at understanding human sexual functioning, but at the turn of the century science began to look more directly at human sexual behavior. The distortions of the "semen theories" at the end of the nineteenth century did not give way easily, but little could be found to support such ideas in the twentieth century.

Medical research on various diseases provided some of the most exciting breakthroughs of the time. Syphilis and other venereal diseases were more accurately diagnosed, and cures were found for some of them. This work proved that they were infectious diseases, not disorders of excessive sexual behavior.

Interest in the various medical illnesses extended to other problems as well. People with sexual disorders could now seek help from physicians. Men like Jean Charcot and Krafft-Ebing, who were highly respected physicians, made it possible to work with the so-called sexual deviates, and they contributed greatly to the emerging understanding of variant sexual behaviors. The British psychologist Havelock Ellis, whom we quoted at the beginning of the chapter, did much to bring sexual behavior into the psychological sphere of influence by writing the six-volume *Studies of the Psychology of Sex*, published between 1897 and 1910. His nonjudgmental writings about sexual disturbances set a new tone for scientific treatises on sexual behavior.

What had been a quiet revolution, moving inquiry about sexual behavior into the scientific arena, became a much noisier one with the dissemination of the theories of Sigmund Freud. Freud's work will be discussed in greater detail in Chaps. 9 and 16, but we should note here that he shocked both his scientific colleagues and the public with his theories about the sexual nature of human development.

Most of the work done on the psychology of human sexuality at the beginning of the twentieth century was based on pathological populations—people with sexual problems. Unfortunately, these studies provided little insight into normal sexual functioning, and it was years before inroads in this area were made. It was not until the pioneering work of Alfred Kinsey, halfway into the century, that any substantial knowledge about "normal" men and women became available. Revolutions in science can sometimes be very slow indeed.

Attempts to perfect contraceptive techniques were also expanded at the turn of the century. These attempts helped spur basic research on human sexuality, since in order to prevent conception, scientists first had to understand sexual functioning. These efforts produced great clashes between the political, religious, and scientific forces of society.

The early attempts at scientific inquiry into sexuality laid the groundwork for the scientific contributions that have taken place in recent years—contributions that will be discussed throughout this text. Unfortunately, attitudes change much more slowly than science would like. Kinsey was severely criticized for daring to research people's sexual behavior. William Masters and Virginia Johnson, who discovered much of what we know about the physiology of sexual intercourse, have found it hard to continue their work, even today. It is difficult for scientists to approach sexual research without having eyebrows raised as to their "real" motivations, and they must often proceed without the blessings of their institutions, colleagues, or funding agencies. It is to the credit of a dedicated group of scientists that advances have been made at all.

Our brief examination of the historical patterns of sexual repression and permissiveness has taken us through an interesting and varied landscape. We have found that humankind has used a number of methods to seek a balance between sexual expression and social control of that expression. That all these methods have proved wanting to a greater or lesser degree should not surprise us. Whether there can ever be a perfect solution to the problem of how sexual behavior should exist in a structured social order must itself remain an open question. As George Bernard Shaw so succinctly stated the issue, "Unless we gratify our sex desire, the race is lost; unless we restrain it, we destroy ourselves."

We like to think that the recent turn toward science will help us achieve a more fulfilling sexual adjustment, striking this important balance between gratification and restraint. However, it is important to remember that people in other historical periods were convinced that the institutions controlling sexual behavior in their time were the appropriate ones. It will be for future historians to give us an unbiased perspective on the contributions of the late twentieth century to establishing the proper role for sexuality in society.

SUMMARY

1 Our knowledge of sexuality in prehistoric humans comes solely from relics and artifacts, such as the Venus figures. It appears that prehistoric peoples lived in family groups and were highly concerned with reproduction.

2 Middle Eastern cultures, such as the Egyptians, were governed by religious dogma. Many of the societies approved of sex for procreational purposes and generally gave special privileges to males. Permissive attitudes changed with the coming of the Persians, whose Zoroastrian religion saw any sexual activity not leading to procreation as a sin of the flesh.

3 The early Hebrews had a generally positive view of sexual activities as long as they occurred within marriage, but with the appearance of the Holiness Code, more restrictive rules were introduced. Menstruating women were seen as unclean, and adultery was forbidden. There were rules against nudity, masturbation, and homosexuality.

4 Greece during its Golden Age was dominated by *naturalism* as opposed to religious dogma. Although laws controlled marital, contractual, and monetary aspects of sexual life, most people were left to their own devices in the personal realm. The emphasis was on beauty and moderation, and the arts often centered around male *homoerotic expression*.

5 Roman civilization began with highly restrictive sexual codes, but over the centuries this society became freer and more permissive. In fact, toward the end of this period, prostitution, bizarre sexual practices, and bestial sexual acts in the Roman Circus increased greatly.

6 The early disciples of Christ, such as Paul, had clearly negative views about sexuality. Paul wrote that chastity and celibacy were superior to marriage and encouraged sexual *asceticism*. In the Middle Ages the Catholic church dominated all aspects of life, and sexual behavior was strictly controlled. In no way were people to derive pleasure from this act. In the midst of this repression the idea of courtly love arose among the nobility, laying the groundwork for today's notion of romantic love.

7 During the Renaissance, erotic art and literature slowly began to appear, and within the church people like Martin Luther were beginning to question many of the restrictions on people's sexual lives. The church's control was further eroded by individuals such as Henry VIII, who founded the Church of England in reaction to Rome's denial of his request for a divorce.

8 The Puritans of England brought their Puritan ethic to America in the seventeenth century. The Puritans were not antisex, but they believed that they would receive greater rewards in the afterlife if they denied themselves pleasure in the present. They did, however, restrict sexual activity to marriage, and transgressors were severely punished. The Puritans also managed to link Church and State, so that many of their religious beliefs were enacted into laws, some of which remain today.

9 During the eighteenth century, the knowledge and control base of

human sexual behavior shifted from religion to science. However, many of the "scientific" ideas of the time were highly erroneous.

10   Sexual repression dominated the Victorian era, during which sexual feelings were seen as representing the animal side of human nature and as requiring control rather than expression. Although motherhood was extolled, the route to becoming a mother was considered a highly unpleasant necessity. Women who enjoyed sex were considered perverted, whereas men were seen as animals with insatiable appetites who must not be encouraged. These codes applied primarily to the middle classes of the time.

11   In the twentieth century, scientific advances in the areas of reproduction and sexual functioning have contributed to the sexual revolution in which we have been embroiled for the past few decades. Increased knowledge in such fields as psychology, contraceptive technology, and sociology has added fuel to the fire of this revolution.

**ADDITIONAL
READING[1]**

Bullough, Vern L. Sexual Variance in Society and History. New York: Wiley, 1976.
   An exceptionally well-written history of human sexual practices and attitudes with an emphasis on how we got to where we are today. Comprehensive and enjoyable to read.

Hunt, Morton, M. The Natural History of Love. New York: Minerva Press, 1965.
   An interesting history of the role of love and sexual conduct across the ages.

Tannahill, Reay. Sex in History. New York: Stein & Day, 1980.
   An unusually wide-ranging discussion of how human sexuality both shaped and was in turn shaped by the history of humankind. Discusses prehistoric and Eastern practices as well as the development of those in the West.

Taylor, G. Rattray. Sex in History. New York: Harper & Row, 1973.
   A shorter work which traces the development of contemporary Western sexual attitudes from the medieval period on. Emphasizes the distinction between the sexual ideals of various groups and their actual practices.

[1] An asterisk indicates that the book is available in a paperback edition.

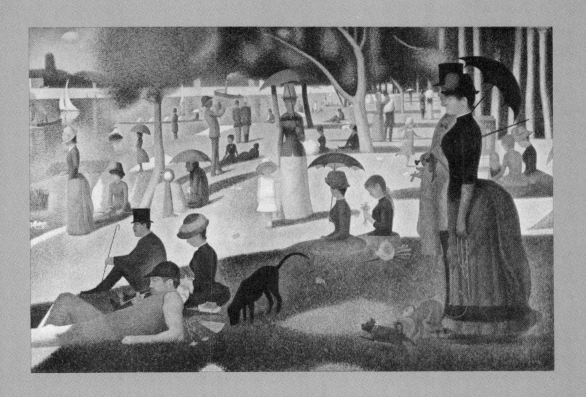

Human sexuality:
A scientific perspective

3

chapter

3

"There is no man or woman who does not face in his or her lifetime the concerns of sexual tensions. Can that one facet of our lives, affecting more people in more ways than any other physiologic response other than those necessary to our very existence, be allowed to continue without benefit of objective, scientific analysis?" So wrote William Masters and Virginia Johnson in the preface to their pioneering work, *Human Sexual Response* (1966). They were concerned with the continuing resistance in our society to full scientific study of sexual behavior and the resultant timidity of researchers to commit themselves to such scientific study.

Masters and Johnson attributed part of the scientific timidity to fear—fear of public opinion, of social consequences, of religious intolerance, of political pressure, and of bigotry and prejudice. Scientists are people, too, and they carry with them the same heritage of Judeo-Christian and Victorian attitudes that characterize the rest of society. For many, the topic of human sexuality continues to create feelings of discomfort. Fortunately, as a result mainly of the efforts of researchers such as Masters and Johnson, these attitudes have slowly given way to a much more objective approach to the study of sexual behavior.

But there are those in society who tend to be concerned by the fact that science studies sexuality at all. Some think that science, with its tedious presentation of facts and figures, will diminish or destroy the romantic mystique of human sexuality. Yet this fear is unfounded. When we replace misinformation with *real* knowledge, we gain a greater understanding of our own sexuality, and this understanding tends to enhance, rather than detract from, the sexual mystique. Using scientific information, we can free ourselves of the problems created by misinformation, and we can reach a higher and more satisfying level of sexual expression.

Other people resist the scientific inquiry into sexuality because they believe that science is dull. They think that science will reduce the wonders of sexuality to a boring school subject—something to be memorized, tested on, and forgotten. Nothing could be further from the truth. The study of sexual behavior is an active field of inquiry, not a finished subject ready to be presented as a series of accepted facts. Furthermore, the investigation of human sexuality has reached the most dynamic, exciting phase in its history. Never before has there been such an openness to the exploration of human sexuality. And never before have we had the technical sophistication to enable us to make rapid, often dramatic strides. As you will see throughout this book, many recent scientific discoveries have already significantly altered our thinking about sexual behavior. Such knowledge only enhances our ability to predict and change behavior. Nevertheless, the scientific study of sexual behavior is still in its infancy, and many important questions about human sexuality remain to be answered.

In this chapter we will be examining the broad range of questions about human sexuality that scientists from a number of disciplines raise, and we will be looking at the techniques scientists use in their efforts to answer these questions.

QUESTIONS
ABOUT
HUMAN
SEXUALITY

If we reflect for a moment on the phrase *human sexuality*, we will discover that it encompasses a multitude of elements. Sexuality can be interpreted to include our attractiveness to partners, our pattern of sexual behavior, our masculinity or femininity, our ability to reproduce and have offspring, and our capacity for sexual arousal and response. It is not surprising, then, that the study of human sexuality covers an amazing array of human behaviors, not just sexual behavior per se.

All these elements of human sexuality can be studied from four different perspectives: biological, psychological, sociological, and anthropological. At the *biological* level, scientists are interested in determining how internal bodily factors influence our sexuality. At the *psychological* level, scientists are concerned with the extent to which our experiences, attitudes, and beliefs shape our sexuality. At the *sociological* level, scientists examine the importance of societal rules on sexuality. Finally, at the *anthropological* level, scientists compare and contrast the sexual attitudes and behaviors of various cultures.

The biological perspective

Biologists are particularly interested in the extent to which factors present *within* the individual contribute to sexual expression. The focus of their work has been on three aspects of physiology: genes and chromosomes (hereditary material), hormones (chemicals produced by the sex glands), and the nervous system (particularly the brain).

The chromosomes and the genes they contain play a role in the development of sexuality. For one thing, the sex chromosomes determine whether a person is genetically male or genetically female. Under ordinary circumstances, humans possess two sex chromosomes—an XX arrangement for females and an XY arrangement for males. In some rare cases, however, a person is born with just one sex chromosome, an X, in an arrangement represented as XO. (The YO arrangement appears to be fatal.) An XO female shows normal external genitals but has no internal reproductive organs and will not go through puberty unless she receives hormone treatments. (See Chap. 5 for a discussion of Turner's syndrome, the official name for XO cases.)

Hormones also have a role in human sexuality. As we shall see in Chap. 6, the presence or absence of the male sex hormone, testosterone, determines whether a penis and scrotum or a clitoris and vagina will form during early fetal development. Increases in certain hormones in individuals with lower-than-average levels have been associated with enhanced sexual performance. Nevertheless, humans can often function quite effectively in the sexual realm in the absence of sex hormones.

In a general sense, the brain and other parts of the nervous system underlie all aspects of sexuality. Our brain allows us to perceive and respond to sexual stimuli. Parts of the brain also control the release of the sex hormones and the maintenance of the menstrual cycle in females (see Chap. 6).

While we have only scratched the surface in looking at the biological basis of human sexuality, we can perhaps achieve a broader view by mentioning a few representative questions about sexuality that biologists pose. For example: To what extent is male sexual behavior dependent on male hormones or female sexual behavior dependent on female hormones? What is the sequence of biological events that leads to the production of sperm (male sex cells) and the release of eggs (female sex cells)? Knowledge in this realm might be used to solve the problem of infertility, such as that experienced by Bill and Kathy described in Chap. 1. Still other questions could include: Is there a biological explanation for transsexuals (people who feel they are trapped in the body of the wrong sex)? What kinds of distortions in sexuality are produced by genetic defects? What are the physiological processes that underlie sexual arousal and orgasm? Does a woman's desire for sexual activity change across her menstrual cycle? Biologists have discovered at least partial answers for most of these questions, but the opportunities for increased knowledge abound.

The psychological perspective   Psychology is concerned with all those experiences and environmental factors that contribute to an individual's sexual behavior. These factors can vary from the influence of parents and peers to the arousal that might be produced by erotic literature or pictures. Psychology is also concerned with the alteration of sexual behavior through therapy. Given this broad orientation, it is not surprising that the psychology of sexuality is pursued from many different avenues. As examples of the psychological perspective, let us review just three of these approaches: developmental, social, and clinical.

Developmental psychology   Developmental psychologists are particularly interested in how an individual's sexuality develops from infancy on. They ask questions such as: To what extent does our sexuality change as we get older? What events contribute to such changes? How do sex roles develop?

Some researchers have argued for a "stage" view of sexuality; that is, they see individuals as passing through a series of stages in childhood and adolescence in order to develop "normal" sexuality. Such stages are often differentiated on the basis of subtle types of interactions with parents and peers. Failure to pass through a stage is often thought to result in abnormal adult sexual behavior. Perhaps the most famous of these stage theories was proposed by Sigmund Freud; it is discussed in detail in Chap. 9.

Developmental psychologists also want to know the extent to which sex roles in our culture stem from actual biological differences between the sexes and to what extent they result from cultural stereotypes of masculinity and femininity. Feminist writers, for example, argue that sex-role differences can be attributed to the expectations of parents and teachers and to the prejudicial content of books, films, and television. The controversy over the basis of sex-role differences is examined in greater detail in Chap. 9.

Social psychology   Social psychologists are more concerned with the various social stimuli or personal experiences that lead to attraction, love, and sexual arousal. When two people meet, what determines whether they will be attracted to each other? Are people more likely to be attracted to others with similar attitudes and beliefs, or is it more common that opposites attract? Do physical characteristics—"good looks"—play an important part in attraction? And what about the more complex phenomenon called love? What produces this elusive state that can make a person suicidal at one moment, euphoric the next? Why is it that each love relationship seems unique and bound to last forever when in reality people commonly fall in and out of love several times in their lives? What is the relationship between love and sex?

Social psychologists are also interested in the environmental cues that trigger sexual arousal. It has often been said that men can be aroused by explicit (pornographic) sexual scenes, whereas women require more romantic themes to be aroused. Recent evidence suggests, however, that both men and women can be aroused by a wide variety of sexually provocative material (see Chap. 11).

Clinical psychology   Clinical psychologists, who are particularly concerned with the difficulties of sexual functioning, ask what causes sexual problems and try to determine the forms of therapy that might prove helpful with such problems. Because sexual behavior is so rich and varied in the human species, clinical psychologists are often faced with the difficulty of separating so-called normal from abnormal sexual behavior. In many instances the determination of abnormal sexual behavior is made not by the psychologists but by the individuals seeking professional help. In such cases the psychologist might try to help the client change his or her sexual patterns or might concentrate on altering the client's perception of what is normal and abnormal. Some people need to learn to accept situations they cannot change, while others may need to be assured that their behavior is, in fact, within the normal range.

For the clinical psychologist, problematic sexual behavior such as masochism, fetishism, and voyeurism may be seen as tied to early experiences such as childhood sexual encounters or to problems in learning sexual behavior. Helping individuals with these problems might involve undoing the effects of early experiences or at least understanding them, or it might mean altering deviant learning patterns (see Chap. 16).

In addition, the clinical sex researcher seeks to understand how the typical patterns of sexual activity are altered. Various crises can precipitate such sexual dysfunctions as erectile failure in men and inhibited sexual desire in women. The clinical researcher is interested in developing and using techniques that will restore and enhance sexual activity.

The psychology of sexuality is an exceedingly broad topic. It encompasses the development of sexuality in infants, adults, and elderly persons; the relationship between sex and love; the nature and description of sexual arousal; assessment of the behavioral similarities and differences between men and women; examination of the causes of sexual problems; and development of various therapies that can be used to aid those with maladaptive or dysfunctional sexual behaviors.

The sociological perspective

In contrast to psychology, which concentrates on the behavior of individuals, sociology emphasizes group behavior and processes. Sociologists examine those societal factors that influence sexuality and contribute to sex-related differences in behavior. Because *society* is such an all-encompassing term, it is not surprising that the sociological basis of human sexuality is approached from several different vantage points.

Some sociologists are concerned with the way that sexual behavior is shaped by societal institutions such as religious, legal, and educational institutions. Sociologists might ask about the extent to which such institutions control or alter sexual behavior. For example: How much do birth rates vary among religious groups that either do or do not prohibit the use of artificial birth control techniques? How do various religious systems disseminate information about sexual behavior? Do legal punishments alter the sexual behavior of sex offenders? Does sex education decrease the occurrence of teenage pregnancy? Some of these issues are discussed in Chaps. 19 and 20.

Other sociologists might be interested in the influence of social structure on sexual behavior. Social structure may be examined in terms of socioeconomic status (upper, middle, and lower class), life-style (married with children, living together, homosexual couple, single, and so on), or racial and ethnic background. This interest in social structure might give rise to such questions as: Are the sexual activities of middle-class people different from those of lower-class people? Is the life of the single "bachelor" male as romantic as it is often portrayed? What percentage of couples who live together eventually marry? Are the relationships of cohabiting couples more durable than more traditional marriage relationships? What is the nature of attraction and sexuality for people who frequent singles' bars? These types of issues are discussed to some extent in Chap. 12.

Still other sociologists are interested in the roles that individuals play in society at large. Such roles are often defined by the kinds of jobs people hold, such as police officer, prostitute, professor, or politician. In this regard, sociologists might ask what kinds of sexual problems are faced by politicians or police officers. Does sexual behavior change when it is bought and paid for? How open about their sexual activity are people in these roles? Other roles may actually be defined by sexual preference. Sociologists might be interested in contrasting homosexual and heterosexual life-styles and relationships. The differences, as indicated in Chap. 13, are not all that great.

The anthropological perspective

The science of anthropology is concerned with the study of the cultures of diverse peoples currently living on the earth as well as those of our ancestors. Anthropology differs from other sciences in that it emphasizes cross-cultural comparisons. Such comparisons are often made between our own Western industrial culture and some nonindustrialized primitive cultures, such as the Arapesh studied by Margaret Mead (see Chap. 1).

Three of anthropology's four subfields delve into studies related to sexuality: cultural anthropology, archaeology, and physical anthropology. (The fourth subfield is linguistics.)

Cultural anthropologists are particularly interested in the contrasts between sexual practices and sex roles in different cultures. Mead found, for example, quite a few major differences between Arapesh sexual behavior and

American sexual behavior. Cultural anthropologists look for similarities between cultures as well as for differences. One universal aspect of sexual behavior, for example, is the incest taboo. Other aspects of sexual behavior, such as homosexuality, may vary widely from culture to culture.

Archaeologists are interested in the material culture of the peoples of the past. Surprisingly enough, such materials as tools, weapons, dwellings, ornaments, and burial places can tell us something about the role of sexuality in these cultures. For example, the size of a dwelling can give some indication of the number of people in an average household. Pottery may contain drawings of sexual acts or marriage rites. As we saw in Chap. 2, many early cultures left behind artifacts that have revealed something of the sexual mores of the time. Whereas the cultural anthropologist is interested in comparing contemporary cultures, the archaeologist compares present-day cultures with past ones.

Physical anthropologists study the biological characteristics of past and present humans and of their nearest primate relatives, the monkeys and apes. In the realm of sexual behavior, the physical anthropologist is interested in comparing the sexual behavior of humans, apes, and monkeys. Such comparisons often reveal interesting differences. For example, face-to-face intercourse is rare in monkeys and apes but common in humans. Such comparisons may tell us something about how human sexual behavior evolved.

The interaction between perspectives

We have treated each of the four perspectives as separate from one another. Yet in actuality there is a great deal of overlap between these fields. There are psychologists, for example, who are particularly interested in the impact of physiology and hormones on sexual behavior. Such scientists are referred to as *biopsychologists* or *psychobiologists*. Social psychologists share many interests with sociologists, just as sociologists do with anthropologists. Anthropologists, in turn, have ties with biologists and psychologists. In fact, there is less distinction between these perspectives than one might at first think. This is consistent with the viewpoint that an understanding of human sexuality requires an integration of all four of these perspectives. Expressed another way, an explanation of any facet of human sexuality is incomplete if it ignores any of these perspectives.

METHODS OF SCIENTIFIC INQUIRY

The aim of science lies not only in the formulation of questions about a phenomenon but also in the search for the answers to these questions. This process consists of obtaining useful information in the form of **verifiable data**— verifiable in the sense that other investigators can obtain the same results under similar circumstances. As we shall see, there are a number of different data-gathering methods that sex researchers can use to collect desired information. These methods require orderliness and precision and cannot be used haphazardly. Furthermore, interpretation of the results requires great care. The researcher must refrain from asserting a causal connection between two events if the data have been derived from any method other than experimentation. Only under some experimental conditions can investigators feel relatively safe in drawing conclusions of cause and effect.

There are a number of ways in which sex researchers can collect information about human sexuality. They may ask individuals about their sexual attitudes and behaviors through the use of ***interviews*** and ***questionnaires***. They may rely on ***observation*** of sexual activity and of sex differences in behavior and the like in either naturalistic or laboratory settings. Or they can study specific individuals in great depth, using the ***case-study*** approach.

Interviews   The interview technique was made famous in sexual research by Alfred Kinsey. From the late 1930s to the 1940s, Kinsey interviewed thousands of subjects to obtain information about their sexual attitudes, beliefs, and behavior (see Box 3.1). The outcome of these interviews was two landmark works: *Sexual Behavior in the Human Male* (1948) and *Sexual Behavior in the Human Female* (1953). These two books formed the foundation for the modern study of sexuality.

In interviews, subjects are asked to respond to a series of questions posed by an interviewer. The responses are either written down or taped for later scrutiny. Interviewers often have flexibility in the questioning process—they can develop or expand upon points raised by the subject or return to comments made earlier in the interview. As such, the interview can be a rich and varied source of information.

There are, however, a few problems associated with interviews: interviewer bias, subject bias, and interviewer-subject interaction. To see how these problems can affect research, let us use a hypothetical example of interview research. Suppose that Professor X wants to characterize the sexual activities of college students. Her curiosity is motivated by her perception that parents often think of the college environment as one that fosters sexual activity. Thus, Professor X decides to interview college students about their sexual behavior and attitudes to determine whether such parental views are accurate.

Researchers often have expectations about the outcome of their research, and Professor X is likely to have already formed some opinions about the sexual practices of students before beginning her study. Such expectations and opinions can form ***interviewer biases***, and researchers must be careful not to let such biases interfere with the interview process. Thus, Professor X must avoid asking leading questions or hinting at appropriate answers. She must also refrain from smiling when she hears answers that are consistent with her viewpoint and frowning or being passive when she hears answers that don't fit with her views. In fact, we might suggest that Professor X use interviewers other than herself.

Just as interviewer bias can affect research results, so, too, can ***subject bias*** alter outcomes; that is, subjects might respond with what they think are typical or standard answers rather than honestly state what they actually do or do not feel. In response to the question "How frequently do you engage in sexual intercourse in a week?" students may exaggerate or minimize their rate of sexual intercourse. It is the responsibility of the interviewer to encourage an honest report. To do so, he or she must establish an atmosphere of trust and

BOX 3.1

How Kinsey did his research

Alfred Kinsey became instantly famous in 1948 with the publication of his pioneering work Sexual Behavior in the Human Male. *The book contains data on the sex lives of 5300 white males, detailing such behaviors as masturbation; childhood sexuality; premarital, marital, and extramarital intercourse; homosexuality; and animal contacts. In 1953 Kinsey and his colleagues published a companion volume,* Sexual Behavior in the Human Female, *based on interviews with 5940 white females and covering the same topics as the male research.*

How did a shy, quiet entymologist, a professor at Indiana University well-known for his elaborate studies of the gall wasp, end up as a controversial sex researcher immersed in study of the intimate sex lives of 18,000 Americans?

It all began in 1937 when Indiana University asked Kinsey, then a distinguished professor of zoology, to chair a faculty committee responsible for establishing a noncredit marriage course for seniors. As part of the course, Kinsey, a married man with three children, conducted individual conferences with students. These students often had questions about sex that he could not answer, simply because of the lack of scientific information on sexuality. In order to gather data to try to answer some of these questions, Kinsey asked students about their sexual histories and compiled summaries of their answers for use in marriage course lectures. Eventually he began to supplement these student case histories by conducting off-campus interviews, and in the fall of 1940 he put his full effort into this research, leaving his gall wasps behind.

During the next few years Kinsey perfected the interviewing technique that he was to use for the thousands of case studies he and his co-workers were to gather. In 1943 he hired Wardell Pomeroy, who with Kinsey conducted about 85 percent of the ultimate 18,000 case histories. Also on the team was Clyde Martin, a statistical analyst, and Paul Gebhard, an anthropologist. A few other interviewers were also involved in the course of the next 10 years.

Kinsey had his interviewers memorize all the questions to be administered to subjects. The number of questions ranged from a minimum of 350 to a maximum of 521, depending on the number of follow-up questions needed with specific subjects. The interviewers also had to master a complex system of codes to be used in taking the histories and in filing them. These codes allowed the interviewers to record the equivalent of 25 typewritten pages of material on just 1 page, and they also protected the privacy of the subjects. These codes were never written down; only the researchers knew them.

Some of the interviews were done in soundproof offices at Indiana University, but a great majority were conducted on field trips all over the country. Subjects varied from suburban matrons to imprisoned prostitutes, from highly placed executives to underworld characters. In all cases the interviews were conducted with the utmost privacy, sometimes even in Kinsey's car. All interviewees were volunteers; no one was ever forced to take part in the study.

Kinsey often entered small communities (such as Nicodemus, Kansas) or visited organizations in hopes of per-

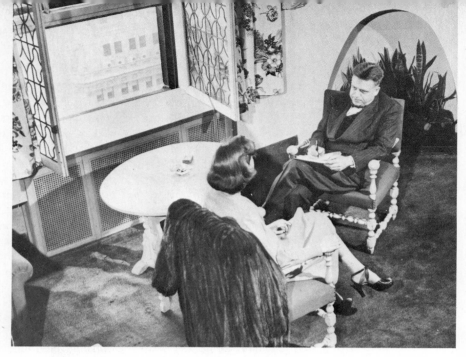

Pioneer sex researcher Alfred Kinsey used interviews to generate information about human sexual behavior.

suading 100 percent of the population or members to participate in his research. Apparently his powers of persuasion were great—he once convinced a whole group of psychiatrists who were hostile to his research to take part in it. On another occasion he decided to learn about the world of homosexual prostitution in the Times Square area of New York City. Without contacts and looking like the studious midwestern professor that he was, he hung around gay bars on Eighth Avenue looking for men to interview. He finally went up to one man and said, "I am Dr. Kinsey from Indiana University, and I'm making a study of sex behavior. Can I buy you a drink?" (quoted in Pomeroy, 1972). Obviously the man was quite skeptical. But after being subjected to Kinsey's persuasive powers, the man not only provided his case history but convinced other male prostitutes to volunteer interviews as well.

Kinsey's interviewing technique was based on sound psychological principles. The interviewers were trained to be direct in their questioning, never hesitating or apologizing. They did not use euphemisms such as "touching yourself" for masturbation or "relations with other persons" for sexual intercourse. Furthermore, they never asked whether a subject had engaged in a particular activity but rather when he or she had first done it. In this way the interviewers conveyed the idea that they would not be surprised if the subject had engaged in the activity. They were also trained to not ask leading questions and to avoid suggesting possible answers.

Because there were so many questions, the interviewers asked them as rapidly as possible. This pace also made it difficult for subjects to make up answers, and they were likely to be more spontaneous in their responses. As Pomeroy put it, "We looked our subjects squarely in the eye and fired the questions at them as fast as we could. These were two of our best guarantees against falsifying." The question sequence was also carefully designed so that a series of cross-checks was built in to detect falsehoods and cover-ups. In addition, Kinsey did some follow-up interviews 2 or more years after the initial ones to see how consistent people were in their answers.

A typical interview took about 2 or 3 hours. It began with general conversation between the subject and the interviewer. For the first 15–20 minutes of the interview, the questions were routine ones about age, birthplace, religion, health, hobbies, education, marriages, and family background. This nonthreatening phase prepared people to answer more intimate questions. Next came questions about early sex education and then early sex experiences. After that came the heart of the interview: questions about masturbation, homosexuality, sexual intercourse, and so on. The sequence of questions was varied, depending on the sex and socioeconomic level of the subject.

The recording techniques used by the interviewers were highly complex, because they took down not only the subject's responses but also his or her voice inflections. To be sure that all interviewers recorded these inflections in the same way, some sessions were conducted with two researchers recording the responses. Kinsey and Pomeroy found, for example, that they were able to record an individual's history simultaneously with about 98 percent accuracy.

The most important aspects of conducting the interviews seemed to be (1) guaranteeing absolute confidentiality, (2) staying in control of the interview (not letting the subject lie or evade questions), and (3) dealing with

people on their own level. In this last regard, Kinsey often used a person's own vernacular, from slang to the language of prostitutes and pimps, in order to gain his or her confidence.

According to one of Kinsey's physician colleagues, Kinsey himself was a consummate master of the interview technique: "The subject is aware from the first that he is being dispassionately studied by a sincere but shrewd and extremely well-informed scientific man —well-informed in the ways of the world and of the underworld as well." It is said that Kinsey even took up moderate smoking and drinking in order to improve his rapport with interview subjects (Wallechinsky and Wallace, 1975). As Pomeroy put it, Kinsey was "never the rigid, academic college professor, but a scientist whose pragmatism and willingness, even urge, to experiment at any time gave him the flexibility to handle any kind of problem that arose."

Kinsey's goal was to reach 100,000 interviews. He never got that far. He died in 1956 of heart problems brought on by overwork. But Kinsey's name will be linked forever with the scientific study of human sexuality. Upon his death the New York Times ran an editorial praising the conscientiousness and comprehensiveness of his work. "In the long run," the editorial said, "it is probable that the value of his contribution to contemporary thought will lie much less in what he found out than in the method he used and his way of applying it." Kinsey had shown that sexual behavior could be studied scientifically and dispassionately, producing results of value both to science and to the general public.

acceptance, devoid of embarrassment or awkwardness. Such an atmosphere will produce more accurate answers and more valid research results.

Finally, some subtle interactions between the interviewer and subject may affect the outcome of the interview. The answers of the subject may vary as a function of the age and sex of the interviewer. For example, female subjects may reveal more to female interviewers than to male ones, and college students may reveal more to graduate student interviewers than to professors.

If interviewer bias, subject bias, and interactional factors between interviewer and subject are carefully controlled, the interview technique can be a powerful one. Its strength depends on the skills of the interviewer: The greater his or her skills, the more useful the information obtained.

Questionnaires and surveys   Within recent years the questionnaire or survey has become much more popular than the interview as a method for assessing sexual attitudes and behavior. Some questionnaires cover only specific aspects of behavior, such as homosexuality, or involve only a limited number of subjects. More broadly based questionnaires administered to many different subjects located in different geographical regions are called **surveys**. Among the most famous of these surveys are the Hunt (1974) report, the *Redbook* survey (Levin and Levin, 1975), and the Hite reports on female and male sexuality (1976, 1981). Because the Hunt and *Redbook* reports in particular are frequently cited, let's look a little more closely at how the research was conducted.

The Hunt report, which was published in book form as *Sexual Behavior in the 1970s*, was originally commissioned by the Playboy Foundation, conducted by an independent research organization called the Research Guild, and written up by Morton Hunt, a professional writer. The purpose of this survey was to provide up-to-date data on sexual behavior that could be compared to Kinsey's data to see how behaviors may have changed in the intervening 30 years. To conduct the study, the Research Guild began by calling people at random from the phone book in 24 American cities. These people were asked to participate in a small-group discussion on human sexuality. Of those who were called, only 20 percent agreed to participate, yielding a subject sample of 1044 women and 982 men. After the subjects met for their small-group discussion, they were given a questionnaire to fill out. The questionnaires contained over 1000 questions and differed depending on whether the person was male or female, married or unmarried. About 10 percent of the subjects were also chosen for in-depth interviews. All the questionnaires were administered in 1972, and the results were serialized in *Playboy* before being published in book form in 1974.

The *Redbook* survey consisted of a questionnaire that was included in the October 1974 issue of this women's magazine. The survey was originally conceived of by a *Redbook* magazine editor, Robert Levin, and the questions were designed by Robert Bell, a sociologist. A surprising 100,000 responses were received for this 60-item survey of female sexuality. The results were summarized and analyzed by Robert Levin and his wife Amy in the September and October 1975 issues of *Redbook* (Levin and Levin, 1975). Robert Levin died in 1976, and the data were further analyzed and discussed in detail by Carol Tavris and Susan Sadd, two social psychologists. They published the book version of the survey titled the *Redbook Report on Female Sexuality* (1977), which provides the basis for our discussion of this important report. Because the sample consisted entirely of female *Redbook* magazine readers, the respondents tended to be married, young, educated, white, and middle- to high-income. Thus, the results are representative of only a limited segment of the American population. An additional *Redbook* survey was conducted in 1980 and is discussed in Chap. 21.

The questionnaire technique involves providing subjects with a list of questions and asking them to answer the questions to the best of their knowledge. Whereas interview questions are often open-ended ("What was your first sexual experience?), the questionnaire items are usually set up so that the subject has a limited choice of answers. Here are some sample questionnaire items:

Q   *Do you ever engage in oral sex?*
A   *1   Yes*
    2   No
Q   *On the average, how frequently do you engage in sexual intercourse per week?*
A   *1   0 times*
    2   1–3 times
    3   4–6 times
    4   7–9 times
    5   10 or more times
Q   *How acceptable to you is intercourse before marriage?*
A   *Totally   Somewhat   Very*
    acceptable   acceptable   acceptable
        1   2   3   4   5

Although the interview and questionnaire techniques are similar, they differ in the kinds of information they obtain. With questionnaires, the subjects answer only the questions provided. Thus, answers can be quickly and easily tabulated (even machine scored) and the results readily analyzed. In interviews, on the other hand, more areas can be explored and more information generated, even though the replies cannot be easily tabulated or compared.

Many researchers studying sexual behavior favor questionnaries over interviews because fewer problems occur. Experimenter expectations have less of an effect because the researcher is not usually present when the subject fills out the questionnaire. Potential interactions between the researcher and the subject are also minimized, although in the Hunt study the use of small-group discussions prior to filling out the questionnaire may have affected the way subjects responded. Subject bias is still a problem with questionnaires, however, because subjects may either exaggerate or minimize their sexual activities and not provide an accurate self-report. However, the fact that the questionnaire procedure provides a great degree of anonymity may help reduce subject bias.

The advantage of the questionnaire (its standardized questions) can be its very downfall if the questions are not formulated appropriately. In this regard, the *Redbook* survey in particular has been criticized for containing poorly designed questions. Kahn (1981) notes that there was not a wide enough range of responses to allow the participants to make intelligent choices. In addition, the choices provided ("often," "occasionally," "never") might have led to a variety of interpretations by the respondents. For example, the woman who finds oral-genital contact somewhat unpleasant might indicate that a twice-per-month request from her partner is "often," whereas a woman who enjoys oral sex might rate a twice-per-month occurrence as "occasional."

An additional problem with surveys, as we noted with the *Redbook* survey, is that the sample may not be representative of the population as a whole. This problem is discussed in greater detail later in this chapter.

Observation　Researchers sometimes use direct observation as a method for studying any and all facets of sexuality. Observation can be used in two different settings. Naturalistic observation, as the term implies, takes place in a natural or real-life setting where the free flow of behavior is recorded. Observation can also occur in a more controlled laboratory setting, where the researcher can make use of sophisticated equipment and can control extraneous factors.

The extent to which researchers use naturalistic observation in the study of actual sexual intercourse is minimal. Sexual intercourse usually occurs in the privacy of a bedroom, thus reducing the possibility of direct observation. Sexual intercourse is only one aspect of sexuality, however. Naturalistic observation can be and is frequently used in studying other aspects of sexual behavior, such as sex differences in the behavior of children, courtship patterns in teenagers, and the behavior of swingers at a party. The goal of the observer is to capture the free flow of behavioral activity in as unobtrusive a manner as possible. Anthropologists also use naturalistic observation to study the sexual customs of primitive cultures. They may observe child sex play, pubertal rites of passage, courtship, marriage, family life, and sexual intercourse itself.

Although naturalistic observation is an important tool for researchers, it has some potential problems. How should the observer interact with the people that he or she is watching? Should the observer watch the group without interacting? Or should he or she become a member of the group and watch from within? This latter technique is called **participant observation.** Both strategies have their strengths and weaknesses. If the observer remains a stranger, he or she may not get an opportunity to observe certain private behaviors or customs. In addition, some groups may view the observer with hostility and may act differently in his or her presence. On the other hand, use of participant observation may change the group or culture. As a researcher watches a group of people, they will in turn be watching him or her. These people might then proceed to inadvertently act in a way designed to produce some reaction in the researcher or might copy or imitate the behaviors of the observer. In this way bias can be introduced into the observational method.

Until recently, observation in the laboratory seemed out of the question as a method for studying sexual intercourse and other sexual behaviors. However, with the pioneering work of Masters and Johnson, the study of sexual behavior in the laboratory has become a reality (see Box 3.2). Although their early work was somewhat biased because some of the subjects were prostitutes, the earlier findings have been confirmed by more refined studies using "nonprofessionals," including married and unmarried couples. (Their results are provided in detail in Chap. 11.)

Many other aspects of sexuality can be studied through observations conducted in a laboratory setting. For example, sex researchers have examined sexual arousal patterns in men and women as a function of viewing erotic materials or listening to erotic tapes. We will examine the extent to which the sexual arousal of rapists differs from that of other people in Chap. 19. Still other researchers have observed the interaction patterns (verbal communication, body language, and physical closeness) of lovers under specific conditions in the laboratory. Finally, investigators may use a laboratory setting to examine differences in the attitudes and behavior of men and women.

One of the major disadvantages of studying sexual behavior in the laboratory is the artificiality of this setting. People do not typically make love in a laboratory. Nor do they watch erotic material for the benefit of scientists. To do so may seem strange or bizarre to some people, which may affect their behavior as subjects. On the other hand, there is one powerful advantage to observing sexual behavior in the laboratory. Under these conditions scientists can often use sophisticated instruments to provide additional information on behavior and physiology. The importance of Masters and Johnson's work was not so much that they were able to observe and describe the behavior of couples engaging in sexual intercourse but rather that they were able to correlate specific physiological changes with this sexual behavior. Their ability to catalog these physiological events depended on the use of several measuring instruments. In addition to the simple measurement of anatomical changes during different phases of sexual arousal, they developed intrauterine electrodes to measure uterine contractions and plastic penises with cinematographic attachments to film the physiological changes occurring within the vagina. Information was also gathered on such basic physiological measures as heart rate, blood pressure, and respiration.

Researchers who study sexual arousal responses to erotic material use several devices to measure sexual excitement in men and women. The ***vaginal photoplethysmograph*** (Sintchak and Geer, 1975) measures pulse amplitude and blood volume. It is a clear acrylic tube 4.5 centimeters (1.76 inches) long and 1.2 centimeters (0.47 inch) in diameter. The device contains a small lamp, photocell, and connecting wires. When it is inserted into the vagina, the indirect light reflected back to the photocell from the vaginal wall is affected by changes in the vagina associated with sexual arousal (namely, vasocongestion; see Chap. 11). The ***circumferential penile transducer*** is an unobtrusive

BOX 3.2

Masters and Johnson

With the publication of their first book, Human Sexual Response, *in 1966, William Masters and Virginia Johnson broke through the barrier preventing observation of sexual behavior and became famous overnight. The interest of the public was fully justified, for* Human Sexual Response *described in great detail (albeit in dry scientific language) how the human body responds to erotic stimulation during masturbation and sexual intercourse. This information was gleaned from direct laboratory observation of 10,000 orgasms—it was not based on speculation or on randomly collected data.*

Their second book, Human Sexual Inadequacy, *represented a monumental contribution in the area of sexual therapy. In it they reported on the causes of sexual inadequacy in the male and female and presented a series of therapeutic techniques for overcoming sexual dysfunction. A third book,* The Pleasure Bond *(1975), described how couples could strengthen and intensify their sexual relationship over time.*

How did William Masters and Virginia Johnson get involved in such controversial research? Masters probably first became interested in sex research in his first year of medical school at the University of Rochester School of Medicine and Dentistry. At that time he was working in the laboratory of George Washington Corner, a famous anatomist who was studying the biology of sex. Dr. Corner assigned Masters the problem of learning about the reproductive cycle of the female rabbit. From this initial experience, Masters developed a keen interest in the study of human sexual behavior, a topic about which little was known back in the early 1940s when he was a medical student. Dr. Corner approved of Masters' decision to study sexual behavior, but he warned him to (1) wait until age 40 before undertaking the study of human sexuality, (2) first earn a scientific reputation in other areas, and (3) wait until his research could be sponsored by a major university. Dr. Corner knew that general prejudice against sex research was strong, both within the scientific community as well as among the general public. He was concerned that Masters would be attacked and that his career might be endangered if he began his sexuality research too soon.

Masters received his M.D. in 1943 and then moved to Washington University School of Medicine in St. Louis, where he went through the stages of internship and residency and ultimately became a professor. From 1948 to 1952 Masters developed a scientific reputation in a "respectable" area: the use of hormone replacement therapy for aging women. In the course of this work, Masters acquired his clinical but compassionate attitude toward the study of human sexuality.

In 1954, Masters was ready to embark on the study of human sexuality. He had followed Dr. Corner's suggestions by establishing a respectable name for himself, becoming associated with a major university, and nearing age 40. In addition, Kinsey's studies in the late 1940s and early 1950s helped pave the way for the kind of research Masters had in mind: a comprehensive

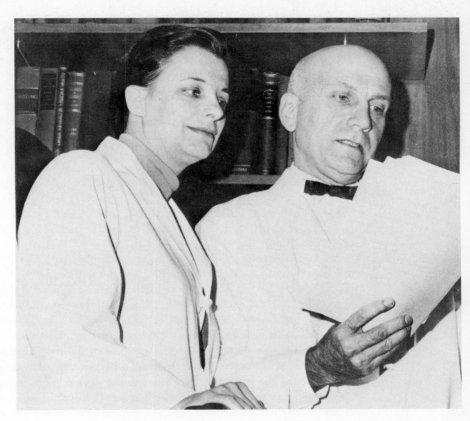

The famous sex research team of William H. Masters and Virginia Johnson.

study of physiological sexual responses, from initial stimulation to orgasm to quiescence. Masters often acknowledged his debt to Kinsey for "opening the previously closed doors of our culture to the definitive investigation of human sexual response."

When Masters began his task of studying the physiological responses underlying human sexual activity, he realized that he needed a woman to assist him in the interviewing. Virginia Johnson answered his ad for an interviewer, and she has been with him ever since. Mrs. Johnson had already developed a keen interest in psychology and sociology while at the University of Missouri. She turned out to be one of those unusual individuals who can maintain objectivity under even the most trying of circumstances. She brought to Masters' research an invaluable perspective and level of compassion. Masters and Johnson set out to understand human sexual response, to destroy many of the myths about human sexual behavior, and to discover techniques that might restore dysfunctional sexuality to normal levels. To say that they have done remarkably well in achieving these goals would be an understatement.

ring that encircles the penis just behind the coronal ridge. As erection occurs, the increased circumference is displayed on an oscilloscope. Still other kinds of instruments, when used in a laboratory setting, can contribute to our understanding of human sexuality. For example, measuring hormone levels and observing the effects of these levels on the quality and quantity of sexual activity can help us to better understand the role of hormones in sexual behavior.

Observation, whether in a natural or laboratory setting, has several advantages over the various self-report techniques. First, subject bias may be reduced substantially. It is probably not eliminated completely, however, as subjects may react differently when they know they are being watched. Second, this technique allows the observer to record behaviors or obtain information that might appear to be irrelevant at first but might later turn out to be important; that is, the observer has few preconceived notions about what he or she will find. Such preconceptions are inherent in both the interview and questionnaire techniques.

Perhaps the greatest disadvantage of direct observation is that few people may be willing to have their sexual activities monitored. Those who *are* willing to be observed may have sexual attitudes and practices different from those of the population as a whole. Thus, direct observation research may involve a marked bias in choice of subjects.

Case studies   The case-study method usually involves an intensive examination of a specific person, including a review of the individual's past sexual behavior as well as current life situation. Often used by clinical psychologists, this technique can provide useful clues to the development of maladaptive behavior, including problem sexual behavior. The psychologist might start by asking about the current problem as perceived by the patient and might administer psychological tests such as the Rorschach inkblot test. The psychologist might also consult the client's medical and school records and might seek information from parents, siblings, and friends.

The case study is valuable because it provides a total view of the many possible factors that influence a person's behavior. In some cases it might be the only method that can be used to assess these factors. Consider the example of Frank B. described in Chap. 1. The description of Frank B.'s masochistic behavior is only a small part of a larger case study that also included information on Frank's early childhood, adolescence, and current life situation. Most of this information was gleaned from his reminiscences, reports of dreams, and reactions to psychological tests.

The mere collection of information, whatever the technique used, does not allow us to establish cause and effect. To understand the casual mechanisms underlying human sexuality, one must conduct experiments.

Experiments   The experiment is the method of choice for many researchers because of its power to detect causal relationships. The primary advantage of experiments is that they permit the researcher to control conditions and thus eliminate as much as possible all influences on the subjects' behavior except those factors that are being studied. In this manner, the researcher can infer causal relationships from the results. The main disadvantage of experiments is the element of control. By controlling all extraneous influences, one may create an unnatural situation, and behavior as measured in such unnatural situations may have little relevance to the real world.

The basic procedures used in the **experimental method** can best be demonstrated through example. One sexual problem that can occur in men is the loss of the ability to achieve or sustain an erection—a problem termed *erectile dysfunction* (the older term *impotence* may be more familiar). Let's suppose that we are looking for a cure for this problem and that we have access to a group of men who experience erectile dysfunction. Let us also assume that these men share other characteristics: They are all married, and they all have stressful occupations (for example, air traffic controller, business executive). A working hypothesis (hunch) might be that injections of the male hormone testosterone will restore erections. In order to test this hypothesis, we would design an experiment to see whether men given testosterone do actually show improvement in their erectile functioning.

Our experiment could be set up as follows. The men with the erectile problem would be divided into two groups. The first group would come to the laboratory to receive injections of testosterone; they would constitute the **experimental group**. An experimental group consists of those subjects who receive the experimental treatment. The second group of men would come to the laboratory and would get injections, but these injections would not contain testosterone. This group, the **control group**, would provide a means of comparison for assessing the effects of the testosterone treatment.

The next step would be to ensure that placement of subjects in the experimental and control groups be done completely at random. This procedure eliminates the possibility that any observed differences in the behavior of the two groups might be due to systematic differences between the subjects assigned to each group. It would not be suitable, for example, to put all air traffic controllers in the experimental group and all business executives in the control group. Nor would it be proper to put all men between ages 40 and 50 in one group and men between 30 and 40 in the other group.

The final step would be to measure the actual effects that the testosterone has on erections and sexual intercourse. We might ask the men to fill out weekly questionnaires about their sexual responses or to attend weekly interviews. In this way we could determine whether the experimental condition has had any effect. Scientists generally refer to the experimental condition as the **independent variable** in the experiment. In essence, it is the factor that the experimenter manipulates to create a difference between the experimental group and the control group. In our experiment, the independent variable is the injection of testosterone. That which the investigator measures to assess the effect of the independent variable is called the **dependent variable**. In our example, the dependent variable is the frequency of erections experienced by the subjects. It is important to recognize that the words *independent* and *dependent* refer to the relationship between the variables. Changes in the independent variable are controlled by the experimenter and are unaffected by the dependent variable. Changes in the dependent variable, however, reflect changes in the independent variable.

Experiments like the one in our example can be hampered by two potential flaws: possible **experimenter bias** and **placebo effects**. Because experimenters usually have some idea of how the experiment will turn out, their expectations may influence the actual outcome of the study. In fact, in some cases the experimenter may unwittingly create the expected results. This effect has been termed self-fulfilling prophecy. If the researcher shows approval when the subject describes results that are consistent with the hypothesis and frowns when the subject's descriptions do not coincide with the hypothesis, these expressions will undoubtedly influence the subject's responses. One way to eliminate this potential source of error is to have the experimenter "blind" to the treatment group of the subjects. During the interview, the researcher would not know whether a particular subject had received the testosterone or not. The assignment of subjects to groups could be made by someone other than the person who does the actually interviewing.

Just as the experimenter brings certain expectations to the experiment, so do the subjects. In our experiment, the subjects who receive testosterone injections might expect to see an improvement in their sexual behavior, and this expectation might be a self-fulfilling prophecy. To control for this possibility, the control group is given a **placebo**—an injection that the subjects think is testosterone but is really an inert, physiologically inactive substance, such as the oil in which testosterone is usually dissolved. If the control group reports an increased frequency in erections despite the lack of testosterone in their injections, placebo effects are said to be at work. If experimenter bias and placebo effects are controlled for and we find that the testosterone-treated subjects do indeed show an increased frequency of erections when compared to the control group subjects, we can conclude that the testosterone therapy *caused* a change in sexual functioning.

Correlation studies   Under some circumstances, scientists cannot use an experiment to study the question at hand. Even though subject characteristics such as sex, race, socioeconomic status, and age are known to have profound effects on behavior, they cannot be manipulated by the researcher. In other cases, experiments cannot be performed for ethical reasons. Consider, for example, our subjects in the experiment on erectile dysfunction. It would be interesting to determine whether the stressful jobs they hold (air traffic controller and so on) cause their erectile dysfunctions. To do so, however, we would have to start out with two equivalent groups of men similar in age, education, socioeconomic status, and medical history. The men in the control group would receive no manipulation, while the men in the experimental group would be subjected to on-the-job stress for several years (the independent variable). Only then could the men be tested, and any differences in the incidence of erectile failure (the dependent variable) be directly attributed to job stress. Clearly, no one would want to participate in this study because of the unpleasant circumstances, and scientists' own ethical beliefs would restrain them from conducting such an experiment. Scientists faced with such a dilemma sometimes resort to animals as subjects. And, in fact, many animal studies have indicated that stress does indeed have a profound effect on a wide range of behaviors, including sex. We must recognize, however, that animals are not exactly identical to human beings and that any comparisons may therefore be limited.

An approach that can be used when actual experiments are not possible is **correlational research**. In this kind of research, the investigator determines the extent to which two variables are related (vary with respect to each other). In the foregoing example, we might examine the extent to which sexual problems are related to (not necessarily caused by) job stress. In yet another example, Professor Y might be interested in the relationship between the amount of knowledge pregnant women have about the birthing process and the extent to which they fear it. To find out, Professor Y would select a number of pregnant women at random and interview them about their knowledge of labor and delivery. Have they taken Lamaze classes? Have they been seeing an obstetrician regularly? He might even administer a factual exam. He would then test their fearfulness about the anticipated birth with a standard anxiety test. Finally, Professor Y would calculate a correlational statistic, called a **correlation coefficient**, that would establish the strength of the relationship between knowledge about birth and fear of it.

Basically, two types of relationships can emerge from correlational research: positive correlations and negative correlations. When the relationship between two variables is such that high scores in one tend to be associated with high scores in the other (or low scores with low scores), a positive correlation is said to exist. Researchers have discovered, for example, that extensive knowledge about sexual behavior is associated with high levels of sexual satisfaction. A negative correlation occurs when high scores in one variable tend to be associated with low scores in another and vice versa. For example, there is a negative relationship between knowledge about birth and fear of it. The *more* knowledgeable women are about birth, the *less* they fear it. There is also a negative correlation between the frequency of intercourse in men and their age past retirement; that is, frequency of intercourse declines as the age of the retired person increases. In many instances of scientific investigation, however, the investigator may find no relationship at all between the variables being studied.

The major problem with correlational research is a tendency on the part of both scientists and the public to make causal inferences. It is important to realize that although correlational research can tell us *whether* two variables are related, it cannot tell us *how* they are related; that is, a strong positive correlation between variable A and variable B does not tell us that A causes B or that B causes A. It may be that both A and B are related to some third factor that causes both. Consider, for example, the fact that every year in the Northern Hemisphere the trees lose their leaves in the fall. Other changes, such as a decrease in temperature, also occur at this time. However, the loss of leaves is not caused by the reduced temperature. Rather, a third factor, the movement of the earth away from the sun, with the associated decrease in day length, causes both the change in the temperature and the loss of leaves.

Another problem in inferring causal relationships from correlational studies is that it may be difficult to determine which of the two variables is the causative agent. Suppose, for example, that Professor Z is interested in determining the cause of promiscuity among teenagers. Because Professor Z suspects that some childhood experience or exposure may condition children to become sexually promiscuous, she decides to examine the backgrounds of both promiscuous and nonpromiscuous teenagers. Through interviews with adolescents and their parents, Professor Z discovers that parents of promiscuous teenagers tend to have fewer negative attitudes toward premarital sex than do parents of less sexually active teenagers. On the basis of these data, Professor Z might be tempted to conclude that teenage promiscuity is fostered, at least in part, by the sexual attitudes of parents. However, such a conclusion is not justified at this stage of the investigation. It is possible, for instance, that parents of sexually promiscuous adolescents might have changed their attitudes about premarital sex because they did not want to think of their children as having committed unacceptable acts. Therefore, even if a causal relationship does exist between teenage promiscuity and parental attitudes, it would not be clear which factor was the cause and which the effect. Do permissive parental attitudes cause promiscuity, or does promiscuity cause a change in parental attitudes? This example demonstrates that scientists must use caution in interpreting their initial observations and must be careful not to use correlation to determine causation.

Many areas of sexual behavior are just beginning to come under scientific scrutiny. In areas where investigators have not yet progressed beyond the correlational research phase, they must be careful not to jump to hasty conclusions from the data they have gathered or to make unwarranted causal inferences. Even in those few areas where experiments have actually been performed, it is not uncommon for accepted ideas to fall by the wayside with the addition of new information. Even the results of an experiment are not final. Thus, although many of the recent discoveries presented in this book will still be applicable years from now, others will have been modified or replaced by new knowledge.

ISSUES IN THE SCIENTIFIC STUDY OF SEXUALITY

The study of human sexuality—whether conducted by means of an experiment or by means of correlational studies using observations, questionnaires, or interviews—poses some important concerns for the scientist. One of these concerns is sampling bias. Another is the ethical aspects involved in using human subjects in sex research.

Subject sampling

One of the goals of sex research is to be able to make some general predictions about the sexual behavior of a large population of individuals. Because of the diversity of individuals in the world, scientists rarely try to make predictions that would be applicable to the entire human population.

Instead, they usually identify a smaller population to study and apply their generalizations. For example, a psychologist might be interested in the sex roles of white, middle-class elementary school students or might be concerned with the sexual behavior of rapists.

In the best of all possible worlds, the scientist would study the behavior of each member of the population and then make some general predictions about that population. However, cost, time, and the sheer number of individuals contained within any population make this impossible. As a result, researchers select a small number of individuals from the population for study—a process called **subject sampling**. To be valid, the sample must be truly representative of the population being studied. If the sample is biased in any way, the predictions cannot be generalized from the sample to the larger population. In the *Redbook* survey, for example, the 100,000 respondents might have been representative of the readers of that particular magazine, but they were not representative of women in America as a whole.

There are two basic problems with sampling that can give rise to biases. First, appropriate procedures must be used to identify representative subjects. Second, the scientists must get a majority of the sample subjects to agree to participate in the study. To demonstrate these problems, let's use a hypothetical example. Suppose that Professor L is interested in describing the sexual practices of college students. He decides to interview students at the large university where he teaches. One thing he has to keep in mind is that the sexual activities of these college students are probably not representative of the activities of young teenagers, middle-aged adults, married couples, or even students in small colleges. How does Professor L select a sample of 100 students to interview out of the more than 15,000 students on his campus? Perhaps he could use students enrolled in courses on human sexuality. They might prove to be eager and attentive subjects. However, students taking a course in sexuality may have sexual propensities different from those of students not taking such a course. Or perhaps the professor could use all sophomores or all students from the same dorm. But these, too, would be potentially biased samples.

The solution to Professor L's dilemma is to select a truly random sample of college students. In a **random sample**, subjects are not selected in a systematic way. Random samples can literally be achieved by drawing names out of a hat. More typically, the professor might place all the names of the students into a computer, which would then shuffle the names and produce a random list. By using random samples, psychologists reduce the risk of having a group of subjects that is not representative of the population as a whole.

But merely selecting a random sample is not sufficient. Professor L must now get the randomly identified subjects to participate in his study. Herein lies one of the major problems of conducting sexual research: Many potential subjects refuse to be included. As we noted earlier, only 20 percent of those asked to participate in the Hunt study agreed to do so. While subjects often have perfectly good reasons for refusing, such as not having enough time or wanting to maintain their privacy, their failure to participate essentially destroys the random sample that has been generated. The study of human sexuality is thus limited by sampling biases. Data on human sexual activities have often been obtained from subjects who want to participate in such research, and their sexual behaviors and beliefs may differ from those of the larger population to which they belong.

These problems plague most areas of sexual research. The subjects studied by Masters and Johnson are probably not representative of the majority of Americans. After all, these subjects were willing to be observed during very private events—sexual intercourse and masturbation. And in the Hunt study, not only did a small percentage agree to participate, but the use of telephone listings to produce the sample may have created a bias by excluding those with unlisted numbers or without telephones. At present, then, sampling biases occur in most studies of human sexuality.

Ethical concerns

Most sex researchers are acutely aware of the ethical problems and implications of their research. People may be asked to reveal highly personal experiences to complete strangers. In some rare cases, these revelations may be rather painful or may bring back unpleasant memories.

In order to minimize the harm to subjects, researchers always use three important standards for conducting studies of human subjects. The first precaution is ***informed consent***. Subjects must be informed about the nature of the experiment prior to their participation in it. Even if subjects agree to participate, they can still withdraw at any time if they so desire. The second standard is protection of the subject's ***anonymity***. In many studies the subject is given a number and is known only by that number. In studies where the subject's name is known or used, the information obtained is confidential and cannot be released without the subject's permission. The third standard is ***peer review*** of potential research on human subjects. Proposals of experiments must be reviewed and evaluated by a "human subjects committee" before the research can be conducted. The committee usually consists of scientists, lay people in the community, and lawyers. It is the burden of the researchers to convince this committee that their experiments will be ethical and humane.

SUMMARY

1   Human sexuality can be studied from four different perspectives: biological, psychological, sociological, and anthropological.

2   The biological perspective focuses on three main areas: the role of chromosomes, the role of homones, and the role of the brain and nervous system in human sexuality.

3   The psychological perspective offers many approaches. Developmental psychologists are interested in how an individual's sexuality develops from infancy on, including sexual behavior and sex roles. Social psychologists are concerned with interactional factors between people that lead to attraction, love, and arousal. Clinical psychologists focus on problems with sexuality, such as variant behavior and sexual dysfunctions.

4   The sociological perspective concentrates on societal factors that influence sexuality and that contribute to sex-related differences in behavior. Sociologists may examine the effects of social institutions, social structure, and social roles.

5   The anthropological perspective focuses on cross-cultural comparisons of sexual behavior. Cultural anthropologists are interested in the contrasts between sexual practices in currently existing cultures. Archaeologists examine the material culture of peoples of the past to determine the role of sexuality in their lives. Physical anthropologists are concerned with comparing past and present humans with other primate species.

6   Among the major methods scientists use to gather *verifiable data* are interviews, questionnaires, observation, and case studies. In *interviews*, subjects are asked to respond to a series of questions posed by an interviewer. This process can be a rich source of information, but it is subject to *interviewer biases*, *subject bias*, and the effects of interviewer-subject interaction.

7   *Questionnaires* are made up of questions with limited-choice answers that respondents may fill out without a researcher present. *Surveys* are questionnaires administered to many different subjects in many different geographical regions. Although experimenter expectations and experimenter-subject interactions are reduced with this method and the results are easily quantified, subject bias can still occur, and problems can be created if the questions are not well formulated.

8   *Observation* may occur in real-life settings *(naturalistic observation)* or in the laboratory. Naturalistic observation may be done within the group being studied *(participant observation)* or from outside the group. Laboratory observation allows the researcher to carefully control conditions and to make precise measurements, but its artificiality may influence results. Furthermore, subjects may react differently when being watched or may be unwilling to be watched.

9   *Case studies* are intense examinations of specific individuals—their history, their current life situations, their sexual background, and any sexual problems.

10   An *experiment* is designed to detect causal relationships. In an experiment, the researcher randomly assigns subjects to the *experimental group* and to the *control group*. Then the experimental group is subjected to the experimental condition (the *independent variable*), and the control group is not. Finally, both groups are assessed for any changes that have occurred as a result of manipulating the independent variable. The factor that is measured is called the *dependent variable*. Experiments are subject to *experimenter bias* and to *placebo effects*. Both may be explained in terms of self-fulfilling prophecy.

11   In *correlational studies*, the researcher determines the extent to which two variables are related. High values in one variable associated with high values in the other (or low values in each) suggest a positive correlation; high values in one and low values in the other suggest a negative correlation. Investigators doing correlational studies and others interpreting the results must be careful not to draw causal inferences from them.

12   For research results to be valid, *subject sampling* must not be biased; that is, the subjects chosen must be truly representative of the population being studied. Sampling bias can occur because incorrect procedures are used to choose subjects and because a majority of those chosen refuse to participate in the study. So far, sampling bias seems to have been an unavoidable part of most studies of human sexuality.

13   Sex researchers must use three important standards for conducting studies of human subjects: *informed consent*, protection of the subjects' *anonymity*, and *peer review* of suggested research projects using human subjects.

ADDITIONAL READING

* **Brecher, Edward.** *The Sex Researchers.* New York: Signet, 1969.

  An interesting blend of science and history. Gives an in-depth look at the work of some of the major sex researchers, their methodologies, and their results.

  Pomeroy, Wardell. *Dr. Kinsey and the Institute for Sex Research.* New York: Harper & Row, 1972.

  Written by one of the original members of Kinsey's research team, this book provides a portrait of one of the pioneers of sex research and his efforts to bring the study of human sexuality into the realm of scientific inquiry.

* **Sagan, Carl.** *Broca's Brain: Reflections on the Romance of Science.* New York: Random House, 1979.

  A well-written series of essays that both discusses and demonstrates the utility of scientific thinking in a number of areas. Interesting and easy to read.

* **Weinberg, Martin (Ed.).** *Sex Research: Studies from the Kinsey Institute.* New York: Oxford University Press, 1976.

  Presents not only an overview of the original work of Kinsey but also that of later researchers at the institute, such as Gebhard, Bell, and Weinberg and Williams. Also traces the development of, and changes in, the application of the scientific method to the study of sexuality at the institute.

two

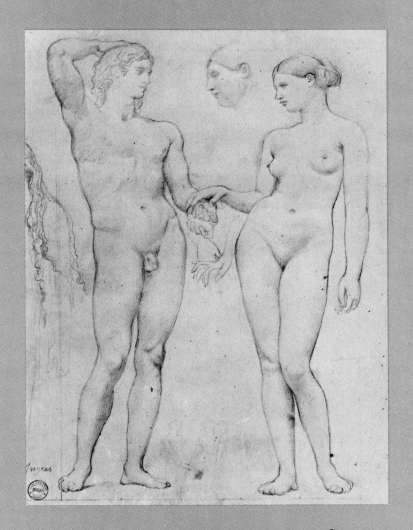

The anatomy of
human sexuality

4

chapter

4

From childhood onward people in our society are fascinated with sexual anatomy. This fascination is evidenced by the popularity of magazines, films, and TV programs that provide glimpses of normally hidden body parts and by the attention immediately paid to people wearing revealing outfits. Yet despite this keen interest in sexual anatomy, few people know all about sexual structures and how they work. The privacy of sexual activities, paired with the reticence and even embarrassment of many people when they try to discuss sex, may account for this lack of knowledge. As a result, the information people acquire about sexual anatomy and behavior is sometimes false, misleading, and inaccurate. Consider the following myths, which are thought to be "facts" by many people:

A woman's sexual satisfaction is directly related to the size of her partner's penis. The larger the penis, the greater the satisfaction.
The size of the penis in the unaroused state is correlated with the size of the fully erect penis. Thus, a small flaccid penis becomes a small erect penis.
A man's penis can sometimes become trapped in a woman's vagina, and a doctor may be required to separate the couple.
The absence of a hymen means that the woman is not a virgin.

Consider further what happens if people actually believe these myths. The man with a small penis may feel inadequate. A woman whose hymen was stretched through vigorous exercise may feel guilty. We can see, then, that it is important for people to have a thorough knowledge of sexual structures and functions. The purpose of this chapter is to examine sexual anatomy, to explain how each anatomical structure contributes to human sexuality, and to lay to rest various myths that are associated with the sex organs.

As we describe the functions of the various sexual structures, it is important to keep in mind that these organs function on two levels. On one level, they are organs of sexual arousal, which respond to sexual stimulation. On another level, they are organs of reproduction, which are concerned with producing and bringing together the sex cells that can lead to the development of a new human being. In this chapter we will be concerned with both the sexual and reproductive aspects of the sexual anatomy. However, a more thorough discussion of the role of sexual anatomy in arousal and sexual intercourse is provided in Chap. 11.

THE FEMALE SEX ORGANS

Unlike the male sex organs, which are readily available for self-inspection, the female organs are difficult to see. Because much of our self-knowledge of sexual anatomy comes from examining our own genitals, women tend to be less informed about such anatomy than men. Within the last decade, many writers who have placed emphasis on women learning more about their bodies have suggested that women use mirrors to inspect their genitals. By looking in the mirror, a woman can see those structures that form her external sexual anatomy, as shown in Fig. 4.1

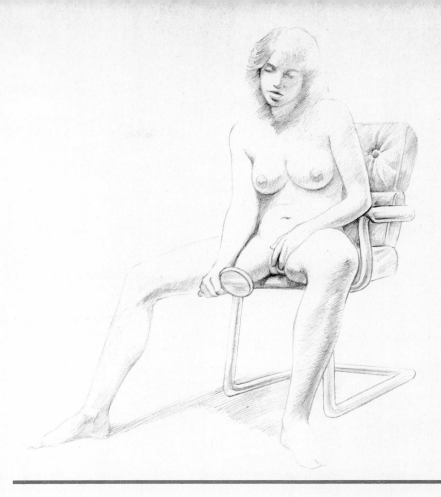

*FIGURE 4.1
Self-inspection of
the genitals is one
way in which
women can learn
about their sexual
anatomy.*

*Female external
anatomy*

The entire genital region of the female is known as the **vulva**. Contained
within the vulva are a number of structures that can be readily identified,
including the mons pubis, the major and minor lips, the clitoris, and the
vaginal opening (see Fig. 4.2).

Mons pubis　The **mons pubis** or **mons veneris** (from the Greek, meaning
"mound of Venus") is a fatty pad of tissue located in the most forward or
frontal part of the vulva. This tissue rests on top of the pubic bones where they
fuse together (the **pubic symphysis**). At puberty the mons pubis becomes
covered with hair and is generally the most noticeable part of the female
genitals.

Labia majora (major lips)　Extending down and back from the mons pubis
are the **labia majora** (major lips), the female counterpart of the scrotum. These
are fatty folds of skin that are quite distinct near the pubis but that flatten out
and meld into the surrounding tissue near the anus. There may be considerable
variation in the thickness of these folds from woman to woman. As with the

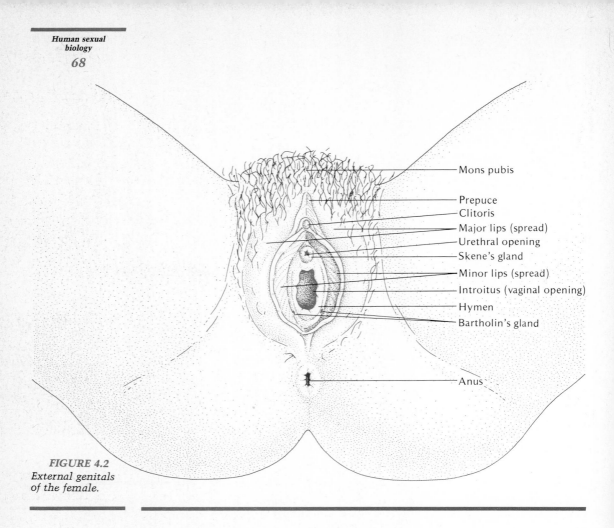

Mons pubis

Prepuce
Clitoris
Major lips (spread)
Urethral opening
Skene's gland
Minor lips (spread)
Introitus (vaginal opening)
Hymen
Bartholin's gland

Anus

*FIGURE 4.2
External genitals
of the female.*

mons pubis, the outer side of the major lips becomes covered with hair at puberty. However, the inner side of the major lips remains hairless. In the absence of sexual stimulation, the major lips normally meet at the midline and provide protection for the clitoris and for the urinary and vaginal openings. During sexual arousal, these lips undergo a change in shape and position. In childless (***nulliparous***) women, the lips become thin and flatten out, thereby exposing the vaginal opening. In ***parous*** women (who have borne children), however, the lips become engorged and distended with blood and only partially reveal the vaginal opening.

Labia minora (minor lips) Contained within the major lips and separated from them by the ***pudendal cleft*** are the ***labia minora*** (minor lips). These are thin sheets of soft reddish pink skin that run from the clitoris to the bottom of the vaginal opening. The minor lips make contact with the clitoris in two ways. First, the topmost part of the folds merges and forms a single layer of skin surrounding the top of the clitoris. This skin is referred to as the ***prepuce*** of the clitoris. Second, both folds meet beneath the clitoris to form another structure, the **frenulum** of the clitoris.

The minor lips undergo marked changes with sexual stimulation. During intercourse, the lips increase two to three times in thickness and become vividly colored. As is the case with the major lips, the changes vary as a function of the birth history of the woman. In nulliparous women, the color changes from a pink to a bright red. In parous women, the typical bright red color of the minor lips increases to deep wine as the result of sexual stimulation.

Clitoris   The **clitoris** is one of the most important structures for the female sexual response, because direct or indirect stimulation of the clitoris produces orgasm—that pulsating wave of sensation that climaxes sexual activity. Coming from a word meaning "that which is closed in," the clitoris is a small shaftlike structure that juts out from the vulva just below the mons pubis. The clitoris is somewhat similar to the penis of the male in that it contains erectile tissue. During sexual excitement, the clitoris becomes engorged with blood; however, its attachment to the body prevents it from becoming erect. The clitoris is divided into two parts: the **shaft**, which is surrounded by the prepuce formed by the minor lips, and the **glans**, or head. Both the shaft and the glans are sensitive to oral, manual, and other stimulation. The glans is so sensitive, however, that direct contact may be unpleasant. As a result, stimulation of the shaft with occasional stroking of the glans, along with stimulation of the mons pubis, is often most effective in producing orgasm. The sensation of orgasm comes from the rich nerve network contained within the clitoris.

Urinary opening   Immediately below the clitoris and between the minor lips is the **urethral** (urinary) **opening**, through which urine passes. Because of the lack of knowledge about the female anatomy and because the female genitals are difficult to observe, many people mistakenly think that the source of urine flow is the clitoris or the vagina.

Vaginal opening and hymen   Located below the urinary opening is the **introitus**, or entrance, to the vagina. The introitus is surrounded by an exterior muscle, the **bulbocavernosus**, which acts as a sphincter for the vagina. The introitus is highly reactive to both pain and pleasure. If a woman is anxious about intercourse or experiences some physical pain, the bulbocavernosus may involuntarily contract, thereby tightening the vaginal opening and producing additional pain. In some cases such vaginal spasms can be so intense that the vagina cannot be penetrated by the penis, a condition called **vaginismus** (see Chap. 15). At a slightly deeper muscular level, the introitus and outer one-third of the vaginal barrel are surrounded by a muscular ring called the **pubococcygeus**.

The entrance to the vagina may be partially obstructed by a thin, delicate membrane called the **hymen**. There are different types of hymen, as shown in Fig. 4.3. Although the hymen appears to have no biological function, it has tremendous cultural significance. In a majority of cultures, an intact hymen or "maidenhead" has been an important indicator of virginity. Presumably, during

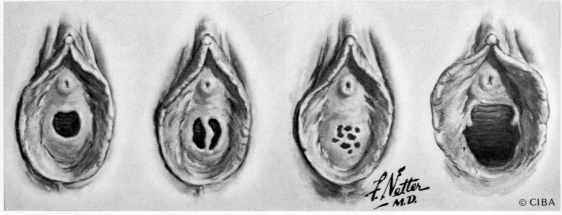

Annular hymen   Septate hymen   Cribriform hymen   Introitus (after intercourse)

FIGURE 4.3
The appearance of the hymen varies considerably from individual to individual. In some cases, it encircles the entire rim of the vagina (annular), and in others it may have several smaller openings (septate and cribriform). In the sexually experienced woman, the introitus appears larger, although remnants of hymen tissue are still present.

the first act of intercourse this thin membrane is stretched or torn because the vaginal opening is generally not large enough to accept an erect penis when the hymen is present. Using this line of reasoning, only women with intact hymens might be assumed to be virgins. However, there are actually a number of ways in which a hymen can be stretched or torn other than through sexual intercourse. Females may "lose" their hymens through vigorous activity or participation in certain kinds of sports, and some females may actually be born without a hymen. Nevertheless, many women have been unnecessarily discriminated against, humiliated, or even tortured because of a "missing" hymen. We might also note that the presence of a hymen does not necessarily signify virginity. Indeed, in some women the hymen may not be torn at all until the woman gives birth to a child.

Considerable cultural ritual may also be associated with the removal of the hymen, the act of "defloration." During medieval times, lords often deflowered the brides of men living as serfs on their land. This "plucking of the maidenhead," as it was called, took place on the wedding night. In other cultures, such as certain Australian tribes, defloration has been performed by older women who stretch or tear the hymen of young women 1 week prior to marriage. In yet other cultures, a variety of instruments, such as animal horns or stone penises, have been used in ritual defloration. Today, the hymen has less cultural significance, particularly in the United States, than it had in the past. The possession of an intact hymen is not of great importance. Women who have exceptionally large hymens or who are particularly anxious about possible pain with their first intercourse, however, sometimes seek surgery. This surgery, which is rarely performed, involves cutting the hymen tissue, thereby making penile penetration easier. Instead of surgery, some doctors recommend that the woman mechanically stretch her hymen by inserting two fingers into the vagina and spreading them; this process is to be repeated several times a day for several weeks (Lanson, 1975). Graduated inserters—rods of progressively larger diameter—which are used in cases of vaginismus, may also be recommended. However, such procedures are usually unnecessary, as the first experience in intercourse is usually not painful for most women.

Bartholin's glands   The **Bartholin's glands** are a pair of glands located just inside the inner lips on either side of the vaginal entrance. Prior to Masters and Johnson's research it was assumed that these glands produced the lubrication for the vaginal opening and barrel. They found, however, that these glands produce neither enough secretion nor any amount early enough in arousal to be primarily responsible for vaginal lubrication. A small amount of fluid is produced by these glands, but only after a woman is thoroughly aroused and the act of intercourse has been particularly prolonged.

Skene's glands   Located within the inner lips on either side of the urinary opening are the **skene's glands**. These glands secrete a small amount of fluid that helps to keep the urinary opening moist. They are similar in origin to the male prostate.

*Female internal
anatomy*

The internal sex organs are, of course, not available for visual self-inspection. Instead, we must rely on pictures and drawings to enhance our understanding of sexual anatomy. As Fig. 4.4 shows, the internal sex organs of the female consist of the ovaries, fallopian tubes, uterus, and vagina.

Ovaries   The ovaries are small oval bodies (4 centimeters × 3 centimeters, or 1.56 inches x 1.17 inches) located in the lower abdomen next to the fallopian tubes on either side of the uterus. The ovaries are not directly connected to the fallopian tubes but are held in place by suspensory elements such as the **ovarian ligaments**, which are attached to the uterus, and other ligaments attached to the abdominal wall.

The ovaries have two important functions. First, they are responsible for the manufacture and release of female **gametes**—the **eggs**, or **ova** A second function of the ovaries is the production of female sex hormones (estrogen and progesterone), which play a role in sexual behavior and are important in the preparation of the uterus for the implantation of fertilized eggs.

Each ovary consists of two layers: the inner **medulla** and the outer **cortex** The medulla is rich in blood vessels, whereas the cortex contains numerous **follicles**, each of which serves as a container for a single immature ovum. The maximum number of follicles (about 1 million) is established by the fifth prenatal month of life. Thus, long before the female is born, all of the eggs that she will carry in her ovaries have been formed. These eggs are not fully mature but must go through a maturation process.

For the most part, very few eggs reach full maturity. If we could look at the follicles within the ovary, we would see eggs at different stages of development and regression. Some groups of eggs would be maturing while others would be deteriorating (Fig. 4.5). This inexorable process of partial maturation

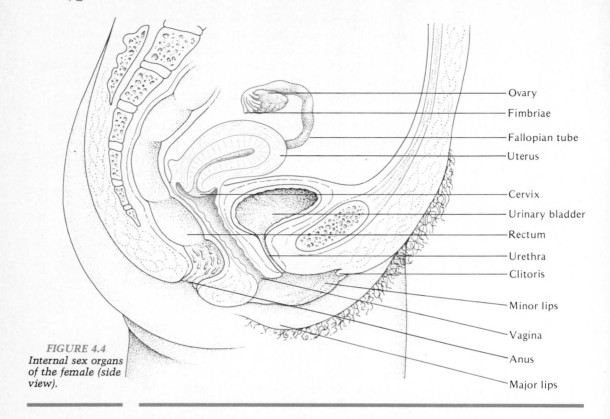

Ovary

Fimbriae

Fallopian tube

Uterus

Cervix

Urinary bladder

Rectum

Urethra

Clitoris

Minor lips

Vagina

Anus

Major lips

*FIGURE 4.4
Internal sex organs
of the female (side
view).*

and **atresia** (deterioration) begins before the female is born (Shepard, 1979). By the time the female reaches puberty, many of her eggs have already deteriorated. In fact, of the original 1 million eggs, only about 400,000 remain (Baker, 1963). At puberty, the maturation process changes in that a few of the eggs (usually 1 per month) become fully mature and are actually released by the ovary to make their way down the fallopian tube to the uterus. The process by which the ovary releases eggs is called **ovulation**.

Despite the presence of thousands of follicles in the ovary, only 400–500 eggs are actually released for the purposes of reproduction. This figure is based on the assumption that the average woman ovulates 13 times a year and is reproductively active for about 35 years. By the time of menopause, few eggs remain (Block, 1952). Although there are 2 ovaries, only 1 egg is released each month. Essentially, the egg that develops most rapidly in a given cycle is the one ultimately released, regardless of whether it is from the left or right ovary. Thus, the removal of 1 ovary does not necessarily reduce ovulation.

At puberty the ovary has a white and glistening appearance. But as each egg ruptures the ovarian wall, the ovary becomes progressively scarred and

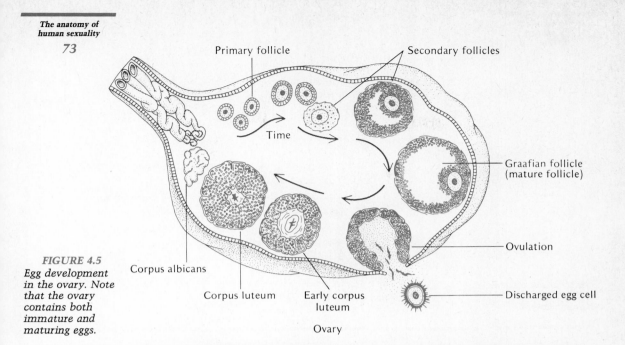

Primary follicle

Secondary follicles

Graafian follicle (mature follicle)

Time

Ovulation

Discharged egg cell

Corpus albicans

Corpus luteum

Early corpus luteum

Ovary

FIGURE 4.5
Egg development in the ovary. Note that the ovary contains both immature and maturing eggs.

pitted. Even the empty follicles undergo change. Immediately after the release of the egg, the empty follicle becomes a yellowish structure, called a ***corpus luteum***, which secretes hormones (see Chap. 6). About 12 days later, if pregnancy has not occurred, the structure starts to regress and becomes a ***corpus albicans***.

Fallopian tubes   The ***fallopian tubes*** are thin structures about 10 centimeters (3.90 inches) long that extend from the ovaries to the uterus, through which eggs are carried. The end located nearest the ovaries is cone-shaped and is called the ***infundibulum*** (Fig. 4.6). The edges of the infundibulum contain irregular cilialike projections called ***fimbriae***, which may touch but are not directly attached to the ovary. Because there is no direct path between ovary and fallopian tube, some researchers have postulated that there is a chemical affinity between fallopian tube and egg that serves to draw the egg to the fimbriae, which catch it and direct it into the tube. They point to the fact that pregnancy has been known to occur in women who have an intact ovary but no fallopian tube on one side and no ovary but an intact fallopian tube on the other side. Thus, the egg had to travel from the ovary *across* the body to the fallopian tube on the other side.

The next portion of the fallopian tube after the infundibulum is the ***ampulla***, which in turn becomes the ***isthmus***, a slender cord running to the uterus. The last section consists of the ***intramural portion***, which is contained in the walls of the uterus. The fallopian tubes themselves consist of three layers. The internal ***mucosa*** contains cells that are believed to participate in the nutrition of the egg. The second layer, the ***muscularis***, produces wavelike

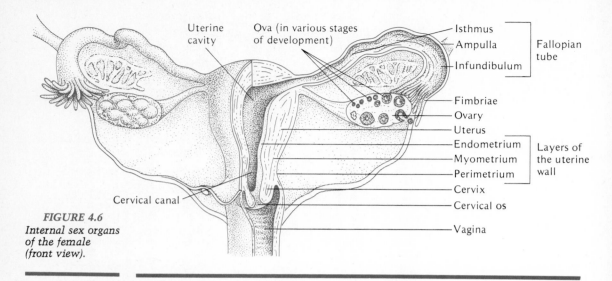

Isthmus
Ampulla
Infundibulum
}
Fallopian tube

Uterine cavity
Ova (in various stages of development)

Fimbriae
Ovary
Uterus
Endometrium
Myometrium
Perimetrium
}
Layers of the uterine wall

Cervix
Cervical os
Vagina

Cervical canal

FIGURE 4.6
*Internal sex organs
of the female
(front view).*

contractions of the tube that progressively move the egg toward the uterus. The third layer is simply a membrane surrounding the tube. Conception—the meeting of sperm and egg—usually takes place in the infundibular portion of the tube. From there, the fertilized egg is moved along slowly through the ampulla, isthmus, and intramural portion, and on into the uterus. The process is essentially the same for both fertilized and unfertilized ova.

Uterus The **uterus** is an upside down, pear-shaped hollow organ situated between the urinary bladder and rectum which is used to nourish a developing organism. Before the first pregnancy, the uterus is 7.5 centimeters (2.93 inches) long, 5 centimeters (1.95 inches) wide, and 1.75 centimeters (0.68 inch) thick. Like the other internal sex organs, it can be divided into distinct parts. The four main parts are the **fundus** (the rounded wider portion of the pear that lies above the level of the fallopian tubes), the **body**, the narrower **isthmus**, and the **cervix** (the neck of the uterus that projects into the vagina).

The wall of the uterus is uniquely designed to be able to provide nutrients for developing offspring, to stretch to accommodate a fetus, and to forcefully expel a baby after it is fully developed. The uterine wall is made up of three layers. The inner layer, or **endometrium**, contains many glands and blood vessels that carry nutrients from the mother to the fetus (see Fig. 4.6). The thickness of the endometrium varies with the menstrual cycle. Prior to ovulation, the endometrium is developing and becomes thickly engorged with blood vessels. This process reaches its peak several days after ovulation. If an egg is not fertilized, the endometrium begins to deteriorate, and eventually the vascular tissue is shed through the vagina to the outside. This sloughing of uterine vascular tissue, or **menstruation**, is discussed further in Chap. 6.

The second layer of the uterine wall, the **myometrium**, consists of interconnected sheets of smooth muscle. These muscles have great strength and elasticity—characteristics they need to be able to carry and then expel a fetus. Given the size of a full-term infant compared to the typical size of the uterus, the uterine wall has to be capable of expansion to 10 times its original size. And yet, the muscles must be sufficiently strong to push the baby out at birth. This expulsion is accomplished through powerful contractions of the myometrium.

The third layer, the **perimetrium**, forms the external cover of the uterus. It does not have the importance or significance of the inner two layers.

Cervix   The **cervix** is actually that part of the uterus which extends into the vagina. The **cervical os** is the small opening at the center of the cervix. The cervix contains glands that secrete different types of mucous at different points in the menstrual cycle. During ovulation, for example, the cervix produces a mucous that can be readily penetrated by sperm. At other times, however, the mucous secretions are thick enough to form a plug.

Vagina   The **vagina** is the female organ that accepts the erect penis during the act of intercourse. The vagina also serves as the passageway for sperm, for menstrual tissue from the uterus, and for the baby during birth.

The vagina is a highly flexible and expandable muscular tube. Under most conditions, the vaginal space is quite small, and the vaginal walls touch each other. The vagina varies in length from 7 to 8 centimeters (2.73 to 3.12 inches) in the unstimulated female. During sexual arousal, however, it increases in both length and width to accommodate the penis. Maximal width of the vagina is obtained during birth, when the vaginal wall must expand and stretch to allow for the passage of the newborn's rather large head.

The vaginal walls, like those of the uterus, consist of three layers. The innermost layer, or **mucosa**, resembles the soft pink skin found inside the mouth. But unlike smooth cheek tissue, the mucosa has a corrugated appearance. This corrugation is particularly distinctive in nulliparous women. It becomes less noticeable after repeated childbirth, and it disappears entirely after menopause. The middle vaginal layer is muscular, but it is much less developed than the muscular layer of the uterine wall. The outer layer consists of thin elastic fibrous tissue. Both of these layers aid in vaginal contractions.

The vaginal walls are poorly supplied with nerve endings. As a result, the vagina is rather insensitive except for the introitus and the outer inch of the vaginal barrel, which are richly innervated and highly sensitive to tactile stimulation. This insensitivity is especially significant during childbirth, when the baby's head greatly stretches the vaginal walls. Childbirth would be even more painful if the vagina were sensitive to tactile stimulation.

During arousal and intercourse, the walls of the vagina become heavily lubricated. With arousal, individual mucoid drops begin to appear in the corrugations of the vaginal wall. This "sweating" phenomenon, as Masters and Johnson (1966) have called it, provides complete lubrication for the vaginal barrel during arousal and intercourse.

Because the vagina is the primary female organ used during sexual intercourse, there is some concern about the relative fit of the vagina and penis.
Being the elastic organ that it is, the vagina can accommodate a penis of nearly
any size. However, some men have described vaginas as being "tight" or
"loose," depending on how snugly the vaginal barrel and opening fit around the
penis. Men tend to prefer tight vaginas, as there is increased friction on the
head of the penis during thrusting. However, the vagina is not an actual space
or volume but rather a *potential* space that enlarges to accommodate the penis.
Thus, the issue is not the largeness of the vagina but the tone of the vaginal
muscles. In women who have had children, for instance, the pubococcygeal
muscles may be somewhat relaxed. Such women can regain vaginal elasticity
and strength through what is called the **Kegel exercise**. This involves a muscular contraction similar to that used to hold back urine after urination has
begun. Women are instructed to contract the pubococcygeal muscles and relax
them about 20 times in a row. This process is repeated 10 times a day for at
least a month, by which time the woman should note a change in the muscular control potential of the vagina (Kegel, 1952).

A number of myths are associated with the vagina. One of the most
common modern folktales is that of the couple who were making love only to
discover that the man's penis had become trapped in his partner's vagina. As
the story goes, the couple had to go to the hospital to be separated. Despite
this interesting tale, there is absolutely no evidence to suggest that the penis
can become trapped in the vagina. For one thing, if the vaginal opening were
extremely tight to begin with, as with vaginismus, the penis would not be able
to penetrate the vagina in the first place. And if the vagina became tight after
penetration (which is highly unlikely), the man would lose his erection and his
penis would quickly slide out of the vaginal barrel. It is difficult to imagine
that a man could maintain an erection if he thought his penis were trapped or
if he were on his way to the hospital to be separated from his partner.

Although the trapping of the penis is essentially impossible for humans,
something like this does happen in dogs. During sexual intercourse, the penis
of the dog becomes locked in the vagina. Initial penetration of the vagina
occurs when the dog's penis is only partially erect and is aided by a bone along
the length of the penis. After penetration, the penis expands and becomes
locked in the vagina. Dog breeders call this a "tie." During this time, which
can last a half hour or more, the male and female dog cannot be separated.
After semen is released, the penis becomes flaccid and slides out of the vagina.
Thus, dogs can get stuck together, but humans can't.

Other myths concern the belief that dangerous elements lurk within the
vaginal barrel. Many primitive cultures describe the vagina as containing teeth,
thorns, blades, or other objects that can injure the penis. Perhaps this notion is
used to prevent teenage experimentation in such cultures. The Pomo Indians of
California believe that young virgin women have thorns surrounding the vagina that must be broken off by their intended husbands before marriage. Need-

The breasts

less to say, no physical examination of the female vagina has ever revealed the
presence of such objects.

The **breasts** have a unique position in our study of sexual anatomy. Techni-
cally, they are not directly involved in the sexual act, nor do they have a role
in reproduction prior to birth. And in some cultures breasts have little if any
sexual significance. However, in certain societies, such as our own, breasts are
considered to play an important role in sexual arousal. One need only look at
clothing styles or posters of female sex symbols to realize that many men are
aroused by the sight of the partially or fully exposed breast. And many women
become sexually excited when their breasts are fondled or caressed. Thus,
breasts are important sexually to both men and women in our culture.

The breasts (see Fig. 4.7), which are located over the chest muscles between the second and sixth ribs, contain **mammary** (milk) **glands** that can be
used to nourish infants. Each breast consists of 15–20 clusters of mammary
glands leading into ducts that open onto the nipple. The soft consistency of the
breast is the result of fatty tissue, which is loosely packed between each
cluster. The nipple contains smooth muscle fibers that when touched cause
the nipple to become erect. The area of skin around the nipple is called the
areola; it becomes permanently darkened with pregnancy.

Like the clitoris and major and minor lips, the breasts respond to sexual
arousal. Nipple erection is the first indication of the breast's reaction to sexual

*FIGURE 4.7
The breast (front
and side views).*

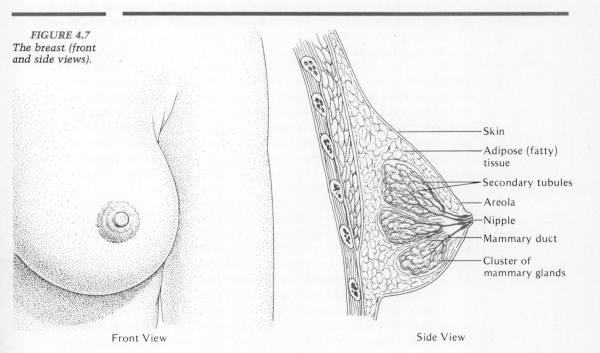

Skin

Adipose (fatty)
tissue

Secondary tubules

Areola

Nipple

Mammary duct

Cluster of
mammary glands

Front View   Side View

stimulation. As sexual tension increases, the breasts show obvious enlargement, which is caused by the engorgement of the veins within the breast. This
breast enlargement is greater for women who have never suckled babies.

Many women are concerned about the size of their breasts. Some think
that their breasts are too small, while others feel that theirs are too large.
Some people link the size of the breasts with the degree of sexual reactivity,
the argument being the larger the breasts the more sexually reactive they are.
This is clearly a myth. What differentiates small from large breasts is not the
number of nerve endings but rather the amount of fatty tissue. Because the
number of nerve endings in all breasts is approximately the same, small breasts
have more nerves per square inch than do large breasts.

Our culture places a premium on large, nicely shaped breasts. Women with
very small or even very large breasts may feel dissatisfied. As a result, they
may seek to have their breast size increased or decreased through surgery. A
reduction in breast size can be accomplished by removing some of the fatty
tissue, and an increase is usually achieved through implants. At one time
breast enlargement involved injections of liquid silicone. Because of unsatisfactory results (the silicone became lumpy) and other complications, this technique is no longer in use. Today, soft silicone implants, in which the silcone is
encased in an inert sac, are used. This approach appears to entail little risk and
does not interfere with lactation.

THE MALE SEX ORGANS

In contrast to the female sex organs, much of the male sexual anatomy is
readily visible (see Fig. 4.8). As we shall discover, however, there is a great deal
of similarity between the male and female sexual structures.

Male external anatomy

The external sexual anatomy of the male consists of the penis and scrotum.

Penis   The *penis* (see Figs. 4.9 and 4.10) is a pendulous, rodlike organ used
for copulation and the elimination of urinary wastes. The tip of the penis is
called the **glans**, the rod is referred to as the **body**, and the point of attachment
to the trunk is called the **root**. The opening in the glans through which urine
and semen pass is called the **meatus**. The glans is separated from the body of
the penis by the **coronal ridge**. Although the penis as a whole is quite sensitive
to sexual stimulation, the coronal ridge and glans are considered to be the
most sexually excitable parts of the penis. The penis, like the clitoris, is the
primary site of orgasmic response.

In females, orgasmic stimulation and sexual intercourse are not related to
the release of eggs, but in males they usually coincide with the release of
sperm. We use the word *usually* because orgasm can occur without **ejaculation**
(release of sperm) and vice versa. For example, sexually immature men may
experience orgasm without sperm release. A few mature males may exhibit a
phenomenon called **retrograde ejaculation**, in which the sperm are carried
backward in the ejaculatory ducts instead of out through the urinary meatus.

One of the most interesting feats of the penis is its ability to change from
a soft, flaccid state to a firm, erect one. Erection is accomplished by anatomical
structures within the penis. Internally, the penis consists of three parallel

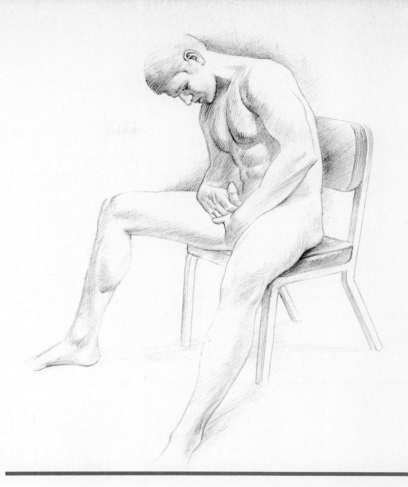

*FIGURE 4.8
Self-inspection of
the genitals can
also help men
understand their
sexual anatomy.*

cylinders of spongy tissue that traverse its length (see Fig. 4.10). Two of the
cylinders are called the ***corpora cavernosa*** (cavernous bodies), and the third is
called the ***corpus spongiosum*** (spongy body). Each cylinder is surrounded by a
fibrous coat, and an additional fibrous coat encloses all three cavernous bodies,
making them appear to be a single structure. As the words *cavernous* and
spongy imply, these cylinders consist of many irregular spongelike spaces
mixed with blood sinuses. Erection is accomplished by a vasocongestive reaction. During sexual arousal, the arteries of the penis dilate, and large amounts
of blood enter the sinuses of the cavernous and spongy bodies. The expansion
of these sinuses presses against the veins, and most of the entering blood is
retained. This increase in blood flow creates pressure within the spongy tissue,
and the penis becomes firm. The mechanism of ***detumescence***, or loss of
erection, is less well understood. Apparently, the arteries begin to constrict,
pressure is removed from the veins, and the blood is drained from the sinuses.

An additional anatomical characteristic, the ***prepuce***, or ***foreskin***, is surgically removed in an operation called ***circumcision*** (see Fig. 4.11). In the uncircumcised male, the foreskin encloses the glans at all times except during

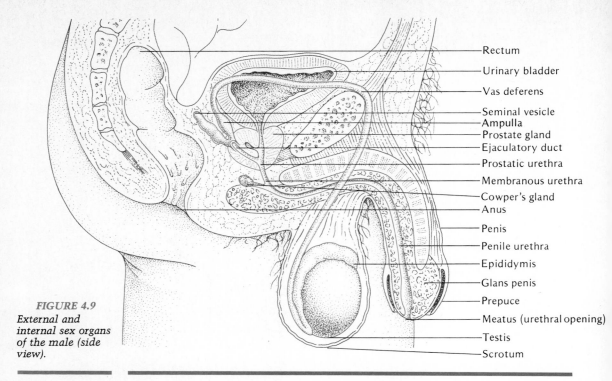

Rectum
Urinary bladder
Vas deferens
Seminal vesicle
Ampulla
Prostate gland
Ejaculatory duct
Prostatic urethra
Membranous urethra
Cowper's gland
Anus
Penis
Penile urethra
Epididymis
Glans penis
Prepuce
Meatus (urethral opening)
Testis
Scrotum

FIGURE 4.9

External and internal sex organs of the male (side view).

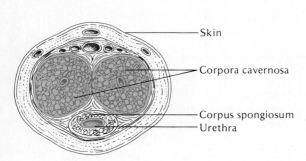

Skin
Corpora cavernosa
Corpus spongiosum
Urethra

Cross Section

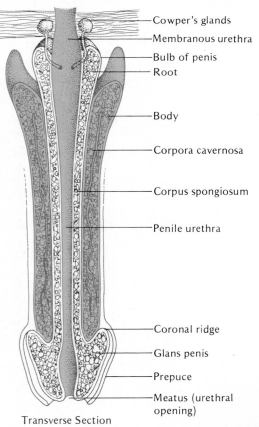

Cowper's glands
Membranous urethra
Bulb of penis
Root
Body
Corpora cavernosa
Corpus spongiosum
Penile urethra
Coronal ridge
Glans penis
Prepuce
Meatus (urethral opening)

Transverse Section

FIGURE 4.10

The internal structure of the penis as viewed from a cross section and transverse section.

sexual arousal, when the enlargement of the penis pushes the foreskin back, exposing this highly sensitive structure. Some argue that circumcision increases sensitivity because the glans is more fully exposed. Others suggest that circumcision decreases sensitivity because constant exposure to minor kinds of stimulation, such as the pressure from underwear, causes adaptation of the glans to mild stimulation. Whatever the case, both circumcised and uncircumcised males seem able to achieve high levels of sexual satisfaction (Masters and Johnson, 1966). Indeed, only the sexually experienced men who have undergone circumcision as adults have a basis for comparison, and they are not the ones making the arguments.

Circumcision is often performed for religious or hygienic reasons and is widely practiced throughout the world. In the United States it is routine to circumcise newborn male infants. Concerns about hygiene focus on the cheese-like material called **smegma** that is produced by several glands located beneath the foreskin in uncircumcised males. If allowed to accumulate, smegma can become quite odorous. Thus, uncircumcised men must be careful to retract the foreskin and cleanse this area as they clean the rest of their bodies.

Evidence suggests that circumcision might be related to lower incidence of penile cancer among circumcised men and to a lower incidence of cervical cancer in women married to circumcised men (Hand, 1970; Licklider, 1961). Because this evidence is based only on correlational studies, it would be unwise to draw any major conclusions from these findings, however.

Culturally and psychologically, the penis has received considerable attention throughout history. In primitive cultures, the male genitals assumed such

FIGURE 4.11
The circumsized (left) and uncircumsized (right) penis. Note the foreskin in the picture on the right.

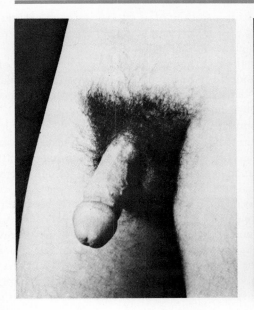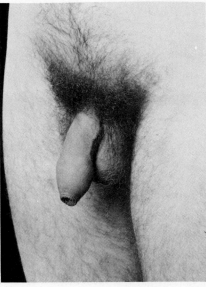

importance that they sometimes became the object of religious fervor. The Greeks and Romans saw the male genitals as symbols of fertility and revered them for their reproductive capabilities. In present-day American culture, much attention has been focused on penis size. It has commonly been assumed that the man with a large penis is a better lover and can provide a woman with more satisfaction than can a man with a smaller penis. This belief is not true, according to Masters and Johnson (1966), who found that women respond more to such factors as ardor and touch than to penile size. Indeed, because the vaginal barrel has so few nerve endings and is relatively insensitive, extremely deep penetration does not necessarily increase stimulation or enhance sexual responsiveness, except in those women who find pressure on the cervix pleasurable.

Penis size does vary from man to man, but such variation is apparently greater in the flaccid state than in the erect state. When flaccid, the average penis is 6.5–10.5 centimeters (2.53–4.10 inches) long. Because small penises tend to enlarge more in the erect state than large penises do, there is little correlation between the size of the penis when flaccid and when erect. The average erect penis is 15 centimeters (5.85 inches) long, although penis lengths of over 30 centimeters (11.70 inches) have been recorded. Because the average depth of the vagina is limited to a little over 15 centimeters (5.85 inches), there seems to be little advantage to an exceptionally long penis, although there may be some advantage to increased thickness (Bennett, 1972).

Scrotum The other part of the external male genitals is the **scrotum** (see Fig. 4.9). The scrotum is a soft, pouchlike structure from the abdominal wall that contains the testes. Unlike the penis, the scrotum may be lightly covered with hair.

*Male internal
anatomy*

The internal sex organs of the male consist of the testes and accessory structures, including the vas deferens, seminal vesicles, epididymis, prostate gland, and Cowper's glands (see Fig. 4.9).

Testes Despite the fact that the **testes** are carried outside of the body cavity, they are considered to be internal sex organs. The singular word *testis*, meaning "witness," dates back to a time when men declared their oath to truth by placing their hands on their genitals.

The testes are similar in function to the ovaries, in that they produce hormones and manufacture gametes. Although both testes are similar in size, about 4.6 centimeters (1.79 inches) long and 2.6 centimeters (1.01 inches) wide, the left one generally hangs lower than the right one, thereby giving the appearance of unequal size.

The testes are located outside the body, apparently because the production of viable sperm is dependent on the maintenance of a constant temperature slightly lower than normal body temperature (about 93°F). However, the outside temperature is hardly constant, and the testes can be subject to such temperature-changing situations as immersion in cold water and high body fevers. Nevertheless, the testes remain at a fairly constant temperature as a result of a muscular system in the scrotum that pulls the testes closer to the

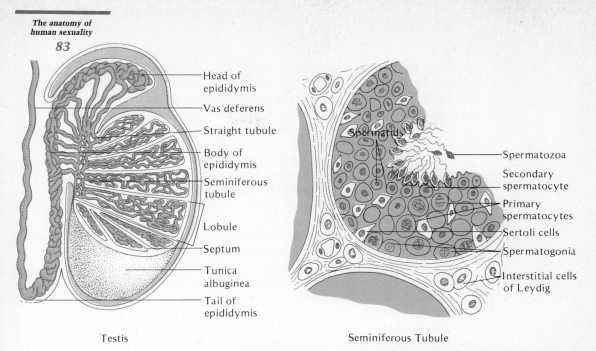

Testis

Seminiferous Tubule

FIGURE 4.12

The internal structure of the testis and cross section of seminiferous tubule.

body to warm them or pushes them away from the body to cool them. The shriveling of the scrotum after entering cold water is caused by reflexive movement of the **dartos muscle**, which pulls the testes closer to the body. Other movements of the dartos may cause the testes to hang low in the scrotum and away from body heat. The dartos muscle also responds to involuntary sexual excitement, fear, and danger. When the inner surface of the thigh is stroked, the dartos contracts slightly. Another muscle from the spermatic cord, the **cremaster muscle**, elevates the testes when they are exposed to the cold and lowers them upon exposure to warmth. This is referred to as the **cremasteric reflex**.

Each testis is encapsulated by a thin, white sheath called the **tunica albuginea** (see Fig. 4.12). The sheath not only surrounds the testis but courses through it, dividing the testis into numerous lobes. Each of these lobes contains **seminiferous tubules**, the structures that produce sperm. Certain types of sterility appear to be related to the tunica albuginea and its inability to expand during swelling. When sexually mature men contract mumps, for example, the seminiferous tubules swell and may become crushed by the tight, inflexible sheath, thereby causing sterility. Prior to sexual maturity, the tubules are not well developed and damage is unlikely. Mumps cannot lead to sterility in sexually mature women, since the comparable organ, the ovary, is not surrounded by a tight inflexible sheath.

The seminiferous tubules are responsible for the manufacture and storage of the male gametes, the **sperm**. Unlike the ovaries, which contain a full complement of eggs prior to birth, the testes continuously manufacture sperm after puberty. Nevertheless, the sperm are formed from primordial cells that are present before birth. The process of sperm production, **spermatogenesis**, will be discussed a little later in this chapter. The seminiferous tubules, which look like long, thin strands, are curled and packed densely together. There are over 1000 tubes; if spread end to end, they would be about 31 meters long.

The **interstitial cells**, or **Leydig's cells**, are involved in the other primary function of the testes, the production of the male sex hormone, testosterone. Located in the connective tissue between the seminiferous tubules near the blood vessels, the interstitial cells produce testosterone and then secrete it into the bloodstream.

The duct system   An extensive system of ducts carries the sperm that are manufactured in the testes to the penis and then to the outside of the body during ejaculation. These ducts include the *epididymis*, the *vas deferens*, the *ejaculatory duct*, and the *urethra*. These ducts are shown in Fig. 4.9.

Epididymis   The **epididymes** are located outside each testis. Each epididymis consists of a long tube about 6 meters long that is coiled into a region at the top and side of the testis. The epididymis receives sperm from the testis, stores them for ripening (a period that may last 6 weeks or more), and then transports them into the vas deferens during ejaculation by contractions of the muscular wall.

Vas deferens   The **vas deferens** begins at the epididymis and moves upward into the abdomen. From there it broadens into an enlarged area, the **ampulla**, and connects with the seminal vesicles. These tubes, which are 45 centimeters long (17.55 inches), serve not only to transport sperm but to store them for periods of time in the ampulla. The vas deferens also plays an important role in male sterilization. **Vasectomy** refers to a procedure in which the two vasa deferentia are severed. Following this rather simple surgery, sperm cannot be transported to the penis. The testes and penis, however, continue to function in the same way as they did prior to surgery. (See Chap. 8 for further discussion.)

Ejaculatory duct   Behind the urinary bladder, each vas deferens empties its contents into the **ejaculatory duct**. The ejaculatory ducts are about 2 centimeters long and in turn empty their contents into the *urethra*.

Urethra   The **urethra**, which serves as a passageway for both sperm and urine, is the final duct in the system. It can be subdivided into three parts. The **prostatic urethra** is 2–3 centimeters (0.78–1.17 inches) long and passes through the prostate. The **membranous urethra** is about 1 centimeter (0.39 inch) in length. The final 15 centimeters (5.85 inches) of the urethra is known as the **penile urethra**. This portion enters the root of the penis and ends at the urethral opening, the meatus. Despite the fact that the urethra can carry both sperm and urine, urine is not expelled during ejaculation, nor is semen deposited in the urinary bladder. This is because the muscle sphincter at the base of the bladder is closed at the time of ejaculation.

Accessory glands   Various secretions are added to the sperm as they traverse the duct system. This mixture of sperm and secretions is called **semen**. These additional secretions are produced by several glands that are located near and empty their contents into the ducts. These glands include the *seminal vesicles*, the *prostate*, and the *Cowper's glands*.

Seminal vesicles The paired **seminal vesicles** are saclike organs located behind the bladder and in front of the rectum. They secrete a substance containing a high percentage of the sugar fructose, which is believed to aid in sperm motility. The seminal vesicles make a significant contribution to the volume of the semen.

Prostate Just below the bladder lies a walnut-shaped structure, the **prostate**. Its function is to provide a milky alkaline fluid that makes up the major proportion of the semen. This fluid is rich in proteins and cholesterol, thereby providing a nutrient medium for the sperm. The prostate secretions also contain prostaglandins and another biochemical substance, **fibrinogenase**, which produces a temporary coagulation of the semen within the vagina so that the sperm do not leak out. Within a few minutes, the semen liquefies. The prostate produces secretions continuously during adulthood; this production, however, is accelerated during sexual arousal. In the normal course of development, the prostate enlarges with the onset of puberty and shrinks with old age. It may, however, enlarge very rapidly from age 40 to 75. Under some conditions, the prostate may become so enlarged during this period that it interferes with or disrupts urination. In such cases, all or part of the gland may require surgical removal.

Cowper's glands **Cowper's glands** are tiny, pea-shaped glands located on either side of the base of the penis. During sexual excitement, they release a small amount of alkaline fluid that lubricates and reduces the acidity of the urethra in preparation for the passage of sperm. Sperm are easily destroyed by acid conditions. The fluid from Cowper's glands is often found on the tip of the penis during sexual arousal. Because this secretion may contain sperm, it is possible for a woman to become pregnant as a result of penile penetration even if the man does not ejaculate within the vagina.

Semen Once the sperm have received their contributions from the seminal vesicles, prostate, and Cowper's glands, they are ready for expulsion from the penis. The average amount of semen released during ejaculation is about 4 milliliters, and the average number of sperm contained within the semen varies from 50 to 100 million per milliliter. When the number of sperm falls below 20 million per milliliter, the man may be sterile (i.e., unable to fertilize the female's egg). Scientists have recently discovered that semen contains an antibiotic, called *seminalplasmin*, which has an action similar to that of penicillin and streptomycin. Because the vagina contains bacteria, it has been hypothesized that seminalplasmin keeps these bacteria under control so as to aid in fertilization.

Semen varies in consistency from man to man and from the same man as a function of sexual frequency. Sometimes the semen appears to be thick and viscous, and at other times it is thin and watery. The more often a man ejaculates, the more watery his semen becomes. Nonetheless, there is no truth to the myth that men can become weakened or debilitated through the loss of "precious body fluids" as a result of ejaculation.

Spermatogenesis   Sperm are manufactured in the seminiferous tubules and then proceed through stages of maturation. The tubules contain two types of cells that are important in sperm production: the **spermatogenic cells**, which actually produce the sperm, and the **Sertoli cells**, which nurture the sperm at various stages of development. As a male reaches maturity, the seminiferous tubules come to contain an increasing number of cells known as **primitive spermatogonia**. Each spermatogonium then divides and produces daughter cells, each with a full complement of chromosomes (46). One of these daughter cells remains a spermatogonium, ready to produce future spermatogonia. The other daughter cell becomes a **primary spermatocyte**, which constitutes the next stage in the development of sperm. This cell then undergoes reduction division to form two smaller **secondary spermatocytes**, each containing only half the chromosome complement (23). The X and Y chromosomes found in the primary spermatocyte are divided so that one cell receives the X chromosome and the other, the Y chromosome. In this way equal numbers of X-carrying and Y-carrying sperm are produced. These secondary spermatocytes then divide to produce two daughter cells, called **spermatids**, which then develop gradually into the highly motile **spermatozoa** that are used to fertilize eggs produced in the ovary. The entire spermatogenesis cycle takes about 74 plus or minus 6 days to complete. About 500 million spermatozoa are manufactured each day in an adult male.

A mature sperm is extremely small and can only be seen with the aid of a microscope. Interestingly, a sperm is the smallest human cell, whereas the egg is the largest. A sperm cell is divided into four sections: head, neck midsection, and tail (see Fig. 4.13).

When sperm and egg unite, the full set of 46 chromosomes is restored, with 23 provided by each gamete. Each fertilized egg contains 2 sex chromosomes. If the 2 are XX, the child will be a girl; if they are XY, the child will be a boy. Because each gamete contains only half of the chromsomes, each contributes only 1 sex chromosome to the child. The egg always provides an X chromosome, but the sperm, as we have seen, may carry either an X or a Y chromosome. Thus, it is the genetic contribution of the father that determines the sex of the child.

Recent evidence suggests that there are major differences between X-carrying and Y-carrying sperm and that these differences may be used to assist couples in predetermining the sex of their child (Shettles, 1972). Y sperm have smaller heads and longer tails, which makes them lighter and more mobile than X sperm. Y sperm are also more susceptible to destruction and thus tend to have a life span shorter than that of X sperm. Accordingly, couples desiring to have female offspring must engage in activities that favor the differential survival of X-carrying sperm. These actions include:

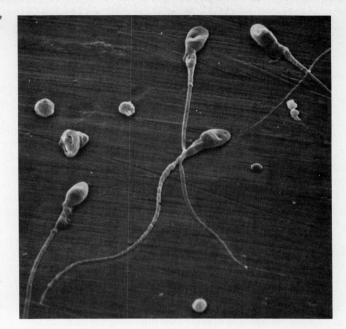

*FIGURE 4.13
Scanning electron
micrograph of sev-
eral spermatozoa
at a magnification
of 2000X.*

1   Using an acid douch prior to intercourse. Acidic conditions can kill sperm,
    so that the weaker Y sperm should die off more readily.
2   Employing specific positions that prevent deep penile penetration of the
    vagina. In this way, the Y sperm will have to travel further, thereby
    increasing their susceptibility to destruction. The woman should avoid
    orgasm, as that would help propel the weak Y sperm further.
3   Having intercourse regularly, ceasing 2 days before ovulation. Because X
    sperm tend to live longer and the average life span for sperm is about 48
    hours, the weaker Y sperm will die off before the egg arrives in the
    ampulla of the fallopian tube.

For those couples who want male babies, the procedures should be reversed.
These include:

1   Using an alkaline douche prior to intercourse to help sustain the life of the
    Y sperm.
2   Using positions that provide deep penetration, such as the man-above
    position, and bringing the woman to orgasm, so that the distance the
    sperm must travel is shorter. Also, the vaginal contractions associated
    with orgasm may help propel the sperm through the cervix and into the
    uterus.
3   Refraining from intercourse for several days prior to ovulation and engag-
    ing in intercourse on the day of ovulation, as abstinence tends to be
    associated with an increase in the percentage of Y sperm in the semen.

Despite these precautions, it is only fair to note that one cannot guarantee the
sex of the child. One can merely increase the probabilities.

SUMMARY

1   The external female genital region is known as the *vulva*. Structures of the vulva include the *mons pubis*, the *labia majora*, the *labia minora*, the *clitoris*, the *urethral opening*, the vaginal *introitus*, and the *Bartholin's glands*. The entrance to the vagina is partially blocked by the *hymen*.

2   The internal female sex organs consist of the ovaries, fallopian tubes, uterus, and vagina. The *ovaries* are responsible for the production of *ova* and of sex hormones. Ova mature in individual follicles and are released once a month in the process of *ovulation*. After the egg is released, the follicle becomes a *corpus luteum*.

3   The *fallopian tube* extends from the ovaries to the uterus. Eggs released from the ovary are captured by the *fimbriae* on the *infundibulum* of the tube and move through the *ampulla, isthmus*, and *intramural portion* of the tube.

4   The *uterus* consists of the *fundus, body, isthmus*, and *cervix*. The uterine wall is made up of three layers: the inner *endometrium*, the middle *myometrium*, and the outer *perimetrium*.

5   The *vagina* is a highly flexible muscular tube able to accommodate the male penis or a full-term fetus. The vaginal walls have few nerve endings and can become heavily lubricated during arousal and intercourse.

6   Although not sex organs, the *breasts* play an important role in sexual behavior in our culture. Each breast consists of clusters of *mammary glands* and fatty tissues. The area around the nipple is called the *areola*.

7   The external genitals of the male consist of the penis and the scrotum. The *penis* can be divided into three parts: the *glans*, the *body*, and the *root*. The glans is separated from the body by the *coronal ridge*. The tissue in the penis that accomplishes erection consists of the *corpora cavernosa* and the *corpus spongiosum*. In our culture, the *foreskin* of the penis is commonly removed at birth by *circumcision*. The *scrotum* contains the testes.

8   The internal male sex organs consist of the testes and other organs. The *testes* produce of sperm and male sex hormones. Within the testes are the *seminiferous tubules*, where sperm are produced. The *epididymes*, long tubes just outside the testes, receive sperm and store them before transporting them to the *vas deferens*. From there, the sperm enter the *ejaculatory duct* and then the *urethra*. Other structures include the *seminal vesicles, prostate gland*, and *Cowper's glands*, which all contribute to the production of *semen*.

9   In the process of *spermatogenesis, spermatogenic cells* within the seminiferous tubules produce sperm, and *Sertoli cells* nurture them. The process begins when a *primitive spermatogonium* produces a *primary spermatocyte*, which in turn produces a *secondary spermatocyte*. This divides into two *spermatids*, which develop into *spermatozoa*. Each sperm contains either an X chromosome or a Y chromosome and determines whether the new organism it creates will be male or female.

ADDITIONAL
READING

Boston Women's Health Book Collective. Our Bodies, Ourselves (2nd ed.). New York: Simon & Schuster, 1976.

An easy-to-read presentation of female sexual anatomy. Also includes a wealth of information on female sexuality in general, pregnancy, birth, birth control, and STD.

Netter, Frank. Reproductive System. The Ciba Collection of Medical Illustrations (vol. 3). Summit, N.J.: Ciba, 1965.

A superb set of illustrations of male and female sexual and reproductive anatomy. Includes brief explanations of illustrations.

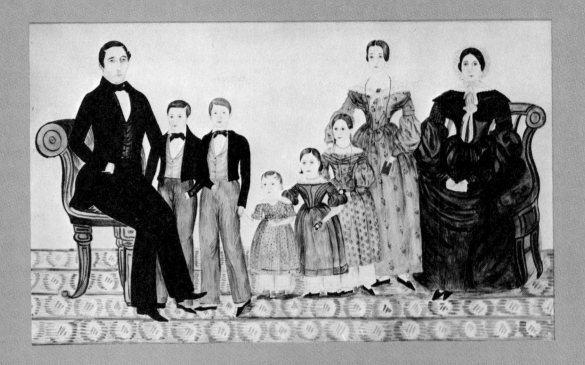

*Sexual differentiation
and determination*

5

chapter

5

From the very moment of birth, human infants are identified as either male or female. This assignment of sex is based on an inspection of the newborn infant's external sex organs. If the child has a penis and scrotum, it's a boy. If it has a clitoris, labia, and vagina, it's a girl. No other pronouncement will have such far-reaching effects and consequences in the life of this new human being as this simple indication of sex.

In the years following birth, the child is fitted with the trappings of his or her sex. Little girls are dressed in pink and are given dolls to play with. Little boys are dressed in blue and are given trucks to play with. As they grow older, girls become the ones who wear dresses and act "ladylike," while boys are the ones who wear pants and like to "roughhouse." Although much lip service has been paid recently to changing these childhood stereotypes, they still persist.

In adults, sex assignment has even more important biological and cultural consequences. Men are expected to be "masculine" and to be sexually attracted to women. Women are expected to be "feminine" and to be sexually attracted to men. What this has meant for our culture is that men must be strong, assertive, and unemotional, whereas women must be weak, passive, and emotional. The basic assumption underlying these social roles is that men and women are different and that these differences are what has led to the well-established rules.

In the last few decades, however, people have begun to challenge this assumption and the roles it supports, and the behaviors of many men and women have begun to change accordingly. The cracks in the foundation of these taken-for-granted social roles have come from two main sources. First, there has been a marked switch in emphasis from the differences between the sexes to the similarities. This switch has been a result of the efforts of many researchers coupled with the highly visible work of the feminist movement, and it has had profound social, political, and legal repercussions. Given the similarities between men and women, it is argued that women ought to be able to train for and seek traditionally masculine jobs, to receive equal pay for equal work, to play traditional male sports if they so desire, and to cast off the role of housewife if it does not fit. That this viewpoint has found a receptive audience is evidenced by the significant numbers of women who are exploring these options. Similarly, but on a smaller scale, many men are exploring traditional feminine activities, particularly child rearing.

The second source of questioning about the foundation of sex differences comes from the exposure of the public to people who do not fulfill society's expectations of their sex. In the last decade, for example, many homosexuals, bisexuals, transsexuals, and transvestites have emerged from their closet existence to face public scrutiny and demand their rights, including the right to live as they are without penalty, persecution, or legal prosecution.

Both of these sources of challenge to the traditional sex roles raise some baffling questions. The shift of focus from the differences between the sexes to the similarities raises the question of what the real differences are between males and females and what these differences mean. The existence of homosexuality and other such variant orientations raises the question of how masculine and feminine characteristics arise. What is the basis for sexual orientations? Why do transsexuals experience a profound conflict between their sexual identity (their psychological sex) and their sexual anatomy (their biological sex)? Before we can begin to answer these questions, we must understand more about how sex is biologically determined.

THE BIOLOGICAL ORGINS OF THE SEXES

If we are to examine the origins of sex and masculine and feminine characteristics, we must start very early in the life of the individual. In fact, we must start with the **prenatal period**, which begins with conception and ends with birth. Sex is not simply a matter of having a certain combination of sex chromosomes as a result of a sperm fertilizing an egg. Rather, there must occur an elaborate sequence of events that ultimately leads to the formation of penis and scrotum or clitoris and vagina. Early in prenatal development, the embryo possesses no anatomical characteristics that signify its sex. But just as the various organs of the body unfold and develop, so, too, does the sex of the organism emerge. The process by which an organism develops the anatomical and physiological characteristics of its sex is termed **sexual differentiation**.

Physiological elements involved in sexual differentiation

The process of sexual differentiation primarily involves the sex chromosomes, the gonads, the genitals, the connecting ducts, and the brain.

Sex chromosomes The **chromosomes** are thin, strandlike structures made up of **genes**, the basic hereditary units. Humans have 23 pairs of chromosomes, and these same 23 pairs are found in every cell of the body. It is the twenty-third pair, the **sex chromosomes**, that play an important role in the process of sexual differentiation. As we saw in Chap. 4, in women the sex chromosomes are identical and are designated as XX. In men the sex chromosomes are different and are denoted as XY. These designations are actually based on the appearance of these chromosomes under the microscope. The Y chromosome is much smaller than the X chromosome and is incomplete or fragmentary, so that many genes found on the X chromosome are missing from the Y chromosome (Ohno, 1967). The significance of these chromosomes will be further discussed later in this chapter.

The gonads The word **gonad** is a general term for the internal sex glands (ovaries and testes) and can be applied equally to males and females. The gonads have two important functions. The first is to secrete hormones that are carried in the bloodstream and that affect both physiology and behavior. **Testosterone**, the main hormone secreted by the testes, has many different effects. It is responsible for the developmental changes that occur in males at puberty, including deepening of the voice, appearance of facial hair, and so on. It also plays an important role in sexual arousal (see Chap. 6). **Estrogen** and **progesterone**, the major ovarian hormones, also stimulate changes in sexual characteristics at puberty, including growth of the breasts, uterus, and vagina. These hormones are responsible for the menstrual cycle and play a fundamental role in reproduction (see Chap. 6).

The prenatal effects of hormone secretion are crucial to sexual differentiation. Both the fetal testis and the fetal ovary manufacture hormones. But, as we shall see, whereas testosterone production is absolutely essential to the development of masculine sex organs, estrogen is not necessary to the development of feminine sex organs (Wilson, George, and Griffin, 1981).

The second function of the gonads is to produce *gametes,* the sex cells that are used to create offspring. As we saw in Chap. 4, the testes produce many extremely small but highly mobile gametes called *sperm.* The ovaries produce a limited number of large immobile gametes called *eggs* or *ova.*

The genitals The term **genitals** refers to the external sex organs, the most acknowledged indicators of sex. In females, the genitals consist of the labia or lips, the clitoris, and the vagina. In males, the genitals consist of the penis and scrotum. These structures were described in detail in Chap. 4.

The connecting ducts The connecting ducts consist of an internal set of connections between the gonads and the external genitals. In males, the epididymis, vas deferens, ejaculatory duct, and urethra serve to carry sperm from the testes to the penis. The fetal precursors to these connections are called the **Wolffian ducts.** In females, eggs are transported from the ovary through the fallopian tube to the uterus. The fetal precursors to the fallopian tubes and uterus are the **Mullerian ducts.** During early prenatal development the growing organism possesses *both* sets of ducts. But as we shall see, depending on certain complex events, one set of ducts begins to develop more fully while the other regresses.

The brain The brain is a powerful structure that controls and modulates our behavior and perhaps regulates sex differences in behavior. Despite the fact that the intense pleasures of intercourse are experienced in the genitals, this process is mediated centrally in the brain. The brain also controls our level of sexual arousal as well as physiological events, such as hormone secretion by the ovaries and testes.

One particularly intriguing question is the extent to which hormonal events in the fetus affect development of the brain. Does testosterone, for instance, masculinize the brain and in turn produce differences in the behavior of men and women? Although brain differences do exist to some extent in males and females, the significance of these differences in humans is unknown. Studies have been done with rats and monkeys that show distinct effects of hormones on sex differences in the brain. Such studies are described a little later in the chapter.

The process of sexual differentiation

Sexual differentiation involves a complex sequence of events that ultimately leads to the formation of gonads, ducts, and genitals. In addition, it may include subtle brain alterations that perhaps form the basis for certain behavioral sex differences. The growing organism is initially termed an **embryo** during the first 8 weeks of life and then is referred to as a **fetus** until birth. In this section we will examine this sequence of events in prenatal development to see how sexual differentiation actually occurs.

Embryonic development Except for the difference in sex chromosome composition, there is no way to recognize the sex of the embryo during the

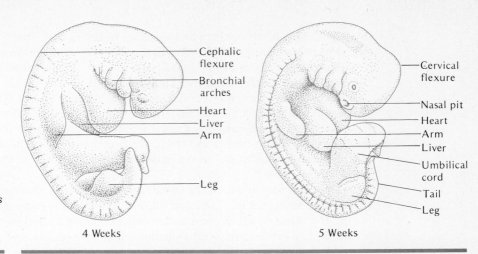

FIGURE 5.1
*Human embryos
of 4 weeks and 5
weeks look little
like human beings
and cannot be
differentiated by
sex.*

first weeks of life. This is not surprising, as the embryo bears little resemblance to a human being. At the moment of conception, the sperm and egg unite to form a single cell. Shortly thereafter, this single cell undergoes successive division and doubling so that a multicelled organism is formed. At the end of 28 days, the developing embryo has a discernible head, trunk, and tail but is not humanlike in appearance (see Fig. 5.1). Despite this activity during the first month, the embryo remains undifferentiated with respect to anatomical sexual characteristics.

Sexual differentiation does not really get underway until about the fifth to sixth week of embryonic development. At this point a generalized genital system makes its appearance. It is generalized in the sense that it is the same in potential males and females. The genital system consists of three primordial, or primitive, components, which will eventually become the mature gonads, ducts, and genitals. The first component is the **gonadal tissue**, which consists of two parts: the **medulla** and the **cortex**, which eventually differentiate into either the testes or ovaries. The second component, the **rudimentary external genitals**, bear little resemblance to mature genitals. Consisting of three parts, a **genital tubercle**, **genital folds**, and a **genital swelling** these embryonic structures must undergo considerable further alteration in order to be fashioned into a clitoris and vagina or penis and scrotum. The third component is the two distinct pairs of ducts. The Wolffian ducts will develop into structures connecting the testes with the penis, and the Mullerian ducts will develop into structures connecting the ovaries with the vagina. Although both ducts are present during early prenatal development, only one pair is found at the time of birth. After the sex of the organism is well established, the primitive ducts of the opposite sex regress and largely disappear.

The developmental phase in which a generalized genital system makes its appearance has been termed the **indifferent period** because the sex of the embryo cannot be determined by inspection of the genitals. Even internally, the gonads are identical, with both male and female ducts present.

The differentiation of the genital system begins in the seventh to eleventh week of embryonic development. The first important event is initiated by the sex chromosomes, which direct the primordial gonads to begin the process of differentiation. In an XY individual, the medulla of the gonad develops into testes while the cortex atrophies and disappears. In an XX individual, it is the cortex that becomes ovaries and the medulla that regresses. The differentiation of the gonads occurs earlier in the male (seventh week) than in the female (eleventh week).

The exact way in which the chromosomes direct this process is unknown. It has been suggested that genes on the Y chromosome produce a substance called **H-Y antigen**, which controls testicular differentiation (Jost, 1970). Recent evidence, however, would seem to indicate that an interaction of genes on the X and Y chromosomes leads to the development of H-Y antigen, which then controls the development of the testes (Silvers and Wachtel, 1977; Hazeltine and Ohno, 1981). In the absence of this H-Y antigen, the primitive gonad becomes an ovary.

The second pivotal event in sexual differentiation is not controlled by the chromosomes. Rather, the development of the ducts and external genitals is controlled by hormones. Of particular significance is the testosterone produced by the newly formed testes.

Overwhelming evidence indicates that the presence or absence of testosterone determines the direction of development of the genitals. If testosterone is present, a penis and scrotum will form. If testosterone is absent, a clitoris and vagina will form. Thus, the appearance of female genitals is not dependent on estrogen or even on the presence of an ovary, for that matter (Jost, 1972). Researchers have concluded, then, that the basic pattern of sexual differentiation is female and that stimulation in the form of testosterone is necessary to

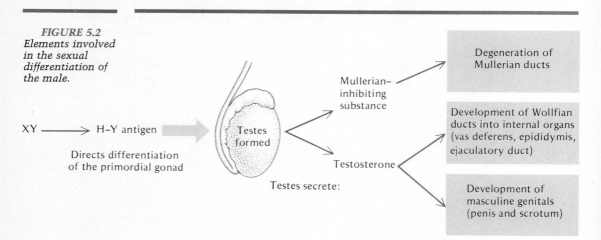

FIGURE 5.2
Elements involved in the sexual differentiation of the male.

XY ⟶ H–Y antigen

Directs differentiation
of the primordial gonad

Testes formed

Testes secrete:

Mullerian-inhibiting substance

Testosterone

Degeneration of Mullerian ducts

Development of Wollfian ducts into internal organs (vas deferens, epididymis, ejaculatory duct)

Development of masculine genitals (penis and scrotum)

divert the process of sexual differentiation from the female path (Wilson, George, and Griffin, 1981).

We can trace the development of the ducts and genitals from the primitive genital system with some precision. In the male, a ***Mullerian-inhibiting substance*** from the testes causes the regression of the Mullerian ducts. As the Mullerian ducts degenerate, the Wolffian ducts, under the influence of testosterone, elaborate to form the epididymis, the vas deferens, and the ejaculatory duct (see Fig. 5.2). A short time after the ducts undergo modification, the primitive external genitals are altered by testosterone stimulation. The genital tubercle becomes the head of the penis, the genital fold is molded into the shaft of the penis, and the genital swellings become the scrotum.

In the absence of testosterone secretion, differentiation proceeds in another direction, and female anatomical structures begin to form. The Wolffian ducts regress, and now it is the Mullerian ducts that are modified into the fallopian tubes, the uterus, and the upper part of the vagina (see Fig. 5.3). The primitive external genitals are also being altered at this time. The genital tubercle is molded into the clitoris. The genital folds are shaped into inner lips and the lower part of the vagina, and the genital swelling forms the outer lips. By the end of 4 months, the genitals have become completely differentiated, and the sex of the newly developing organism can be established by genital inspection (see Fig. 5.4).

Movement of the ovaries and testes   During prenatal development, the newly formed ovaries and testes are changing not only in shape but in position. Initially, both types of gonads are located at the top of the abdominal cavity. By the end of the tenth week, however, they have migrated to a position in the lower abdomen. The ovaries remain in this position until after birth. The testes, on the other hand, have to travel from the abdomen to the scrotum by

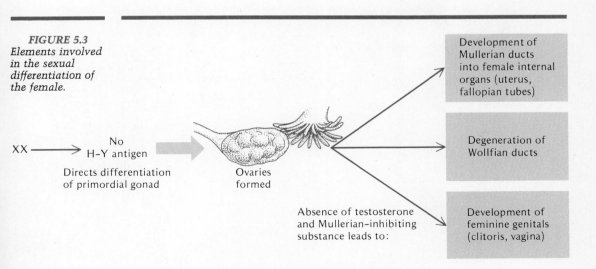

*FIGURE 5.3
Elements involved
in the sexual
differentiation of
the female.*

XX ——→ No
H–Y antigen

Directs differentiation
of primordial gonad

Ovaries
formed

Development of
Mullerian ducts
into female internal
organs (uterus,
fallopian tubes)

Degeneration of
Wolffian ducts

Absence of testosterone
and Mullerian-inhibiting
substance leads to:

Development of
feminine genitals
(clitoris, vagina)

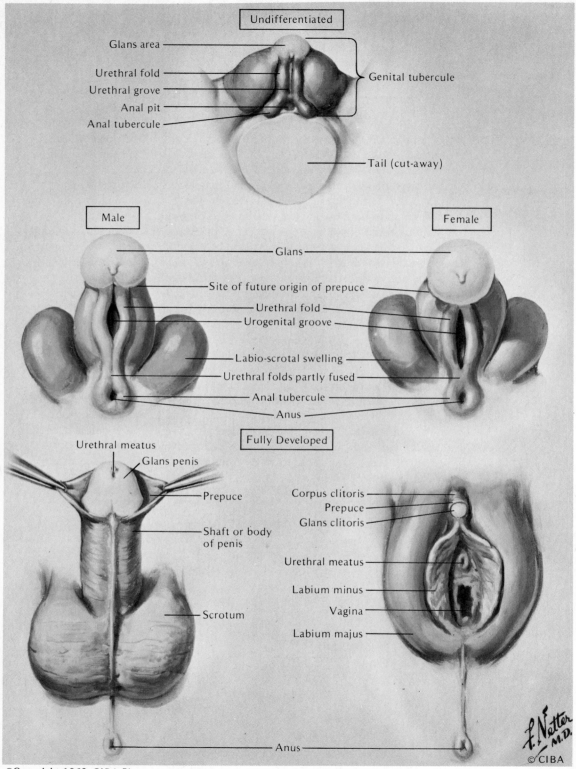

Undifferentiated

Glans area
Urethral fold
Urethral grove
Anal pit
Anal tubercule
Genital tubercule

Tail (cut-away)

Male

Female

Glans
Site of future origin of prepuce
Urethral fold
Urogenital groove
Labio-scrotal swelling
Urethral folds partly fused
Anal tubercule
Anus

Fully Developed

Urethral meatus
Glans penis
Prepuce
Shaft or body of penis
Scrotum

Corpus clitoris
Prepuce
Glans clitoris
Urethral meatus
Labium minus
Vagina
Labium majus

Anus

F. Netter
M.D.
© CIBA

way of the ***inguinal canal.*** The descent of the testes into the scrotum is usually completed by the fourth prenatal month, at which time the inguinal canal is reduced in size. In 2 percent of all male births, the testes fail to travel down the inguinal canal to the scrotum, a condition called ***undescended testes***, or ***cryptorchidism.*** In some instances the testes will descend by puberty. In other instances hormone treatment or surgery may be required to correct the problem.

Sexual differentiation and the brain   The last stage of sexual differentiation involves the brain and occurs after the circulatory system is well formed (at about 4 months). At this point, hormones secreted by the newly formed gonads circulate through the bloodstream and find their way to the brain. This hormonal stimulation results in a subtle alteration of brain functioning. As in the case with differentiation of the genitals, testosterone appears to play a pivotal role. In the absence of any hormone stimulation, the brain is differentiated in the female pattern. But if testosterone is present, the brain is subtly altered into the male pattern.

Because it is often assumed that the male and female brains are identical, we should ask what is meant by sexual differentiation of the brain. Scientists typically focus on two general differences between the sexes that may be traced to brain functioning. The first is hormonal cyclicity. Simply stated, female hormone levels increase and decrease in a cyclic fashion after sexual maturity, whereas male hormone levels remain relatively constant. The regulation of these hormone levels is controlled by a small structure in the forebrain, the ***hypothalamus.*** Evidence suggests that the hypothalamus may be altered by early developmental events. In rats, the adult pattern of hormone production is laid down early in development as a result of the presence or absence of testosterone. This testosterone is presumably carried through the bloodstream to the brain, where it alters neural tissue, thereby producing the constant pattern of hormone production. The cyclic pattern of hormone production is produced in the absence of any stimulation from testosterone. Anatomical studies of the hypothalamus indicate that hypothalamic cells do indeed differ in male and female rats. Thus, early hormonal events may actually alter the brain and its functioning (see Box 5.1). The extent to which this applies to humans, however, may be seriously questioned. Research on a closely related species, the rhesus monkey, suggests that early hormonal events do not underlie the development of cyclic as opposed to constant hormonal secretion patterns (Knobil et al., 1980).

A second and more controversial question is the extent to which the brain may be sexually differentiated with respect to behavior and personality. Are there masculine and feminine traits that are governed by brain differentiation? Researchers studying monkeys think there are. Male and female rhesus monkeys differ behaviorally, especially with respect to play, aggression, and sexual mounting patterns. Male juvenile monkeys, for example, show higher levels of play initiation, more vigorous forms of rough-and-tumble play, and higher levels of aggression and mounting patterns than do females. Alterations of hormones during prenatal development, however, can affect this difference. If

*FIGURE 5.4
External genital
differentiation in
the human fetus.*

BOX 5.1

Male and female brains

Are male and female brains basically different? The answer is yes, at least for rats. A number of biological studies have shown that the brains of male and female rats differ significantly both in the distribution of nerve connections and in the size of certain structures in the preoptic area. Furthermore, it is thought that these morphological differences give rise to behavioral differences. And hormones appear to be at the bottom of it all.

To put it as nontechnically as possible, researchers have discovered that the synaptic connections—the connections between nerve cells—in the preoptic area (near the hypothalamus) in rats' brains differ in males and females. These researchers found that if newborn male rats are castrated, they develop a female pattern of synaptic connections and that if newborn females are given testosterone (the male hormone), they develop a male pattern of synaptic connections (Kolata, 1979).

Other researchers have identified a structure in the rat brain's preoptic area that they call the sexually dimorphic nucleus. This structure, which is visible to the naked eye, is five times larger in male rats than in female rats. Yet in newborn males that are castrated, the nucleus is smaller, and in newborn females given testosterone, this nucleus is larger. Thus, hormones play an important role in these sexual brain differences.

How do hormones cause these differences? The question has not yet been answered. It is known, however, that the preoptic area is a principal binding site for estrogen (the female hormone). Interestingly enough, because of complex biochemical processes, estrogen causes the development of male—not female—brain differentiation in rats. This has been shown by the fact that newborn female rats given high doses of estrogen actually develop masculine characteristics.

Research on the role of estrogen in sexual differentiation of the rat brain is focusing on two areas: the nature of estrogen receptor sites in the preoptic area and the nature of the "critical period" during which such differentiation takes place. In rats, the critical period seems to start a few days before birth and ends 4 or 5 days after birth. If, for example, rats are castrated or given high doses of hormones after this period, they do not show the sexual reversal that occurs when these alterations are made during the critical period.

What does all this mean for human beings? If these kinds of differences are discovered in the brains of human males and females, it could mean that men and women think differently. In rats, for example, a high concentration of estrogen receptors is found in the cerebral cortex during the critical brain differentiation period. And since this area of the brain controls speech, hearing, and cognitive functions, basic neurological differences here could influence basic patterns of learning and thought.

genetic (XX) female fetuses receive doses to testosterone via injections to the pregnant mother, then such females differ from normal females during postnatal development. Tostosterone-treated females show higher levels of play initiation, more rough-and-tumble play, and higher levels of aggression and mounting. In essence, these treated females exhibit masculine types of behavior. Thus, prenatal hormonal events may play a role in the development of sex-specific patterns of behavior (Goy, Wolf, and Eisele, 1977).

Because human sexual behavior is more variable than that of monkeys, the relationship between sexual patterns and brain differentiation is much more ambiguous. We shall explore the possibility that human sex differences are caused by brain differences and hormonal stimulation a little later in the chapter.

ERRORS IN SEXUAL DIFFERENTIATION

With a process as complex as sexual differentiation, it is not surprising that biological mistakes occasionally arise. These inborn errors can occur at any point in the development process and can have grave effects on the individuals in whom they are expressed. A study of these errors is useful in understanding how sexuality is developed and controlled.

Chromosomal aberrations

The process of sexual differentiation may be impaired right from the beginning if the individual possesses a sex chromosome pattern that deviates from the regular XX or XY. Deviations include the addition of sex chromosomes (XXY, XYY, and so on) or the deletion of chromosomes (XO, with O indicating the absence of either an X or Y chromosome). Because no YO individuals have ever been discovered, we can assume that this particular arrangement is lethal. There are four clinical syndromes in which chromosomal deviations have been observed: Turner's syndrome, XXX females, Klinefelter's syndrome, and XYY males.

In **Turner's syndrome** (XO), an individual has only one sex chromosome. The missing chromosome could have been either an X or a Y. Such individuals are usually reared as females, have the genitals of a female, but never seem to reach physical or sexual maturity. They are usually short in stature (4½–5 feet tall) and display no breast or pubic hair development. The ovaries are absent or rudimentary, and it is this ovarian deficiency that is responsible for lack of puberty. Treatment consists of administrations of estrogen beginning at the time of puberty and continuing throughout much of the person's life. Although the hormonal treatment may allow the woman to develop normal secondary sexual characteristics, such as breasts, she will not be able to produce offspring because of the absent ovaries (see Fig. 5.5, left).

Individuals exhibiting an **XXX chromosomal pattern** are often called "super females" despite the fact that they are not usually any more feminine than normal XX females. The addition of the X chromosome does not appear to impair sexual differentiation, as these females have normal genitals and ovaries. However, it does have an effect on mental functioning, since mental retardation is often associated with this condition (see Fig. 5.5, right).

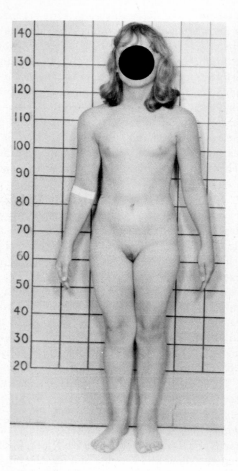
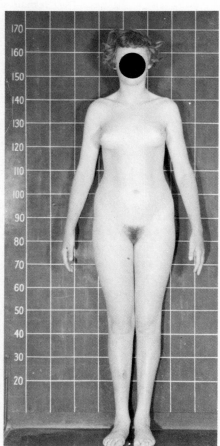

FIGURE 5.5

Two examples of sex chromosomal disorders in women: (Left) Turner's syndrome (XO) is represented here. Note the short stature and the lack of breast development. (Right) The sex chromosome constitution of this woman is XXX. There is normal feminine development, although mental retardation may sometimes be associated with this condition.

Individuals with **Klinefelter's syndrome** have a sex chromosome pattern of XXY or XXXY. They have a masculine body type despite the fact that the penis is small, the testes are rudimentary, and the breasts are developed (see Fig. 5.6, left). These males are usually tall and thin and are sexually inactive. Those with Klinefelter's syndrome are also at risk for a wide variety of other disorders, including severe mental retardation. On occasion, individuals with Klinefelter's syndrome also report gender identity disturbances and may be transsexuals or bisexuals. However, it is not the case that most transsexuals and bisexuals have Klinefelter's syndrome.

Controversy surrounds the fourth disorder, which is characterized by an **XYY chromosomal pattern.** It is quite clear that XYY individuals are men, are thoroughly masculine in appearance, and are usually over 6 feet tall (see Fig.

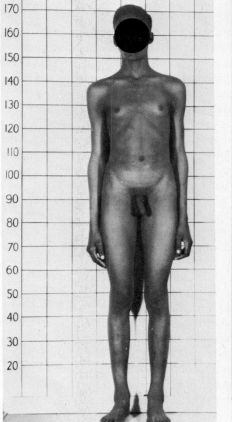 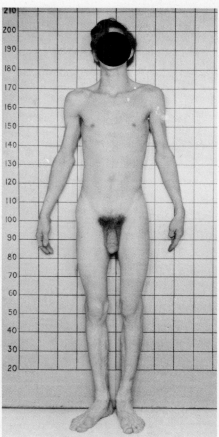

*FIGURE 5.6
Two examples of
sex chromosome
disorders in men:
(Left) This man
has Klinefelter's
syndrome (XXY).
(Right) This man
has a
chromosomal
constitution of
XYY.*

5.6, right). The controversy concerns how this genotype affects behavior. When it was discovered that the XYY genotype appeared more frequently in delinquents and criminals, some scientists suggested that the additional Y chromosome might contribute to antisocial or aggressive tendencies. Thus, XYY men came to be viewed as potentially dangerous and aggressive. Recent evidence counters this view, however. Although the incidence of the XYY condition is higher in prison populations than in normal populations, prisoners with the XYY condition have not generally committed violent crimes. Their higher representation in the prison population may be due to a lower level of intellectual functioning, which may get them into trouble with the law and make them less able to avoid arrest and prosecution (Witkin et al., 1976). The higher prison frequency of XYY syndrome is also not high enough to make it of any importance in understanding criminal behavior. Of 4293 criminals analyzed in 20 separate chromosome studies, only 61 men (less than 2 percent) were found to have the XYY genotype (Jarvik et al., 1973).

Inborn errors may also occur after the sex chromosomes have started the process of gonadal differentiation. Biological mistakes at this stage usually involve the development of both male and female structures in the same individual. This condition, referred to as **hermaphroditism**, can take two forms, depending on the affected structures.

A **true hermaphrodite** is an individual who has both ovaries and testes or a pair of combined gonads termed **ovotestes**. This male-female duality is often present in the external appearance, in that there are masculine genitals and feminine breasts. In some cases, the true hermaphrodite not only has a penis and scrotum but also a vagina. This condition is exceptionally rare—only 60 cases have been reported during this century.

A more common type is **pseudohermaphroditism**. A pseudohermaphrodite has sexual characteristics that are discrepant or mismatched. The discrepancy usually involves the gonads and the external genitals. Thus, individuals may have testes but have external genitals that resemble those of a female (clitoris and partial vagina). Or, conversely, individuals may have ovaries but have masculinized genitals (penis and partial scrotum). In some cases the genitals may be incompletely formed, making sex identification at birth difficult.

The occurrence of pseudohermaphroditism can be traced to the stage of sexual differentiation during which the external genitals are being formed. Under normal circumstances, the presence or absence of hormones from the newly formed gonads directs differentiation of the genitals. As we have seen, the presence of testosterone is necessary for the development of masculine genitals, while the absence of testosterone leads to feminine development. There are three abnormal circumstances, however, that can lead to a mismatch between gonads and genitals:

1. In **congenital adrenal hyperplasia** (CAH), the sexual discrepancy is such that a genetic female possesses ovaries and masculinized genitals. Sexual differentiation proceeds normally until the ovaries are developed. At this time another structure, the adrenal gland, begins to function abnormally and to produce large amounts of male hormones. These hormones act to masculinize the female's external genitals in much the way that testosterone from the fetal testes produces a penis and scrotum in males. Because of the appearance of the genitals at birth, such individuals are frequently identified and reared as males despite the fact that they are genetic females and have ovaries (see Fig. 5.7).

2. In **progestin-induced hermaphroditism**, genetic females also develop ovaries and have masculine genitals. In this case, however, the cause is hormones from a source different from the adrenal gland. For many years it was common practice to give pregnant women hormones called progestins in order to prevent miscarriage. Doctors unfortunately failed to realize that these pregnancy-maintaining hormones could have masculinizing side effects when given in high doses. When women took these substances in early pregnancy,

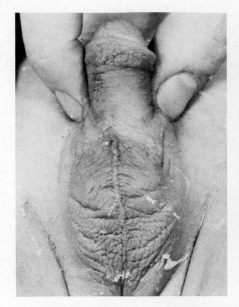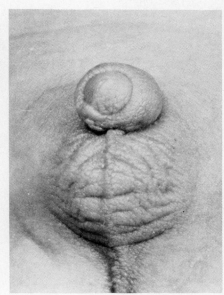

*FIGURE 5.7
Two examples of
penile develop-
ment in genetic
(XX) females born
with congenital
adrenal hyperpla-
sia (CAH).*

the hormones entered the bloodstream of the developing embryo. In genetic
males, this additional hormone apparently had no deleterious effects. But in
genetic females, it acted like testosterone and masculinized the genitals. At
birth these females were frequently identified and reared as males.

3. In ***testicular feminizing syndrome***, a genetic male has testes but his
external genitals are feminized. The cause is not the testes, which function
normally and secrete testosterone. Instead, the primordial genital tissue seems
to be insensitive to the circulating testosterone. The result is the development
of a clitoris and vagina rather than penis and scrotum. These genetic males are
frequently identified and reared as females. Later, at puberty, the small
amounts of estrogen produced by the testes are sufficient to cause the development of female secondary sex characteristics (breasts and so on) (see Fig. 5.8).

As we have seen, there are a number of ways in which pseudohermaphroditism can arise. However, what happens to the pseudohermaphrodite? Is this
individual destined to live his or her life in a mismatched state? In most cases,
the answer is no. If the condition is discovered at birth (through noticing the
incompletely formed genitals), sex correction surgery may be undertaken. This
involves altering the external genitals to conform with the gonads. Thus, a
genetic female with masculinized genitals would have those genitals altered to
resemble those of a female. Introduction of hormones at appropriate life stages
may be part of the treatment. If the condition is discovered later in life,
perhaps at puberty, sex correction surgery is not performed, since after the age
of 18 months sexual identity is thought to be so thoroughly established that

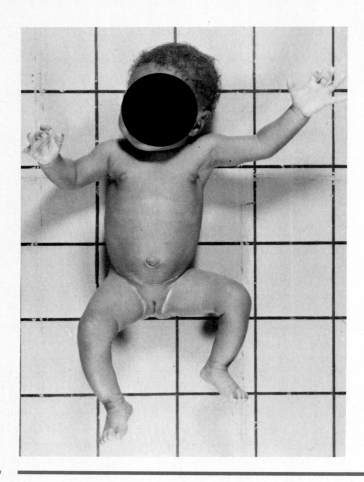

FIGURE 5.8
*An example of
feminine genital
appearance in a
genetic (XY)
male born with
testicular
feminizing
syndrome.*

attempts to reverse it are generally unsuccessful (Money, 1975). Instead, the individual may be given hormone treatments to facilitate the appearance of secondary sexual characteristics that are consistent with the external genitals.

SEX ASSIGNMENT
AND GENDER
IDENTITY

The presumed endpoint of the complex process of sexual differentiation is **sex assignment**. This determination usually takes place at birth when the physician examines the newborn's genitals and pronounces its sex. Although the genitals are the primary focus, the declaration "It's a boy" or "It's a girl" carries with it many additional assumptions about the physiology of the individual. If an infant has a penis and scrotum, he is assumed to have testes, an XY pair of chromosomes, and circulating levels of testosterone that will increase at puberty. If the infant has a clitoris and vagina, it is also assumed that she has ovaries, an XX pair of chromosomes, and circulating levels of estrogen that will change at puberty.

But the actual endpoint of sexual differentiation may occur later, when the individual has acquired a gender identity. The words *gender* and *sex* (referring to male versus female) are sometimes used in inconsistent and confusing ways. One useful clarification is to use *sex* to describe clear anatomical and physiological differences between males and females and to reserve *gender* for psychological variables, that is, masculinity and femininity (Stoller, 1968). In this regard, **gender identity** refers to our own personal view of being male or female, and **gender role** refers to the behavioral patterns we display as a function of our gender identity. This clarification is useful only if we recognize that sex and gender interact; that is, physiological and anatomical characteristics have an impact on and influence gender identity and gender role. The exact nature of this interaction is, as we will see in Chap. 9, difficult to characterize.

The distinction between sex and gender is important in another way. Sex is often viewed as representing two mutually exclusive categories, male and female. Gender, on the other hand, appears to represent a continuum, from extreme femininity to extreme masculinity. This is simply because anatomical differences tend to be much more distinct than behavioral differences. Gender can be used to emphasize the extent to which male and female behavior overlaps.

The process of sexual differentiation involves many different factors that, when taken together, can be used to define maleness and femaleness. Money and Ehrhardt (1972) have specified six such factors:

1   Chromosomal sex. *Females have an XX sex chromosome pair while males have an XY chromosomal pair.*
2   Gonadal sex. *Females have ovaries, males have testes.*
3   Hormonal sex. *Estrogen and progesterone levels are higher in females than in males; testosterone levels are higher in males than in females.*
4   Internal accessory organ sex. *Females have a uterus and fallopian tubes; males have vasa deferentia, seminal vesicles, a prostate gland, and so on.*
5   Genital sex. *The most common indicator of sex. Females have a clitoris and vagina; males have a penis and scrotum.*
6   Assigned gender. *The sex that a child is identified and reared as.*

For the sake of thoroughness, other investigators have proposed that additional factors be added to the list. The one that seems the most important and relevant is:

7   Gender identity. *The individual's own personal view of himself or herself as being masculine or feminine.*

These, then, are seven factors that interact to determine the maleness or femaleness of the individual. The first five are biological in origin, while the last two might be considered psychological in origin. For the majority of men and women, there is agreement across all seven of these variables. That is to say, most men have XY chromosomes, have testes that secrete testosterone, have male internal sex organs, have a penis and scrotum, are reared as men and act masculine, and feel that they are male. Most women, correspondingly, have

XX chromosomes, have ovaries that secrete estrogen and progesterone, have a uterus, fallopian tubes, clitoris, and vagina, are reared as women and act feminine, and feel that they are female. In some cases, however, there may be disagreement between two or more of the biological variables (as in pseudohermaphroditism) or between the biological and psychological variables (as in transsexualism). Thus, the determination of sex appears to be a complex psychobiological process, involving not only the genitals but all of the individual's biology and psychology.

THE BIOLOGICAL BASIS OF GENDER DIFFERENCES

Up to this point we have concentrated primarily on the biological events that underlie the development of distinct male and female anatomical structures. We are now ready to question the extent to which these early biological happenings affect an individual's psychology. How does sexual differentiation affect the acquisition of gender identity? Is it responsible for the observed differences in the behavior or men and women?

Nativists, scientists who emphasize the importance of biological variables, argue that there is a powerful link between the process of sexual differentiation and later behavior. They would suggest that the presence of testosterone during the prenatal period causes individuals to acquire a masculine gender identity and to behave in a manner characteristic of males. *Environmentalists*, on the other hand, argue that early experiences and environmental influences have more of an impact on gender identity and later behavioral differences between men and women. To them, rearing by the parents and early experiences with peers provide the foundation for masculinity and femininity. This is a controversy of some magnitude. We shall look first at its implications for gender identity and then at the explanations these two approaches provide for gender role behaviors, cognitive differences between the sexes, and the development of sexual orientation.

Biology and gender identity

One way to examine the nativist-environmentalist controversy with respect to gender identity is to look at case histories of individuals whose sex assignment and rearing has been at variance with their physiology and sexual anatomy. Perhaps the most illustrative case is that of a normal male infant whose penis was destroyed in a surgical accident. After much heartache and indecision, the parents decided to reassign the sex of the baby at 7 months of age and to raise him as a girl. Sex correction surgery was undertaken at that time, although the construction of an artificial vagina was put off until after puberty. What makes this case history so valuable is that the infant had an identical twin. Thus, the development of gender identity could be observed in two individuals with identical biological heritage but with different parental attitudes and rearing.

Immediately after the sex reassignment, the parents began to treat the twins differently. The girl was clothed in dresses, and her hair was allowed to grow long. The father, who ordinarily played vigorously with his son, was much more gentle with his "daughter." Within a short period of time, a difference in the behavior of the twins was noticed. The girl was neat, took pride in her appearance, and showed a preference for dolls. The boy was untidy, wore whatever was available, and preferred to play with trucks and cars. The girl did exhibit some tomboy traits, but they fell well within the realm of what society considers to be acceptable female behavior. The girl appeared to have an unambiguous sexual identity. This case study suggests that sexual identity is not necessarily predetermined by the genes or by physiology but rather can be markedly affected by rearing (Money and Ehrhardt, 1972). This conclusion is limited, however, by virtue of the fact that only one subject was studied and that this subject was only 5 years old at the time of the report.

Studies of patients with CAH pseudohermaphroditism also suggest that rearing may play a more important role than genes or physiology in the establishment and maintenance of gender identity. In all cases, these studies were of genetic (XX) females with ovaries whose genitals were partially or totally masculinized by the presence of androgens from an overactive adrenal gland. In some instances the children were reared as boys, and in others they were reared as girls. The majority of the children made a successful adjustment to the sex of rearing despite the fact that in some cases the gender was at variance with the internal sex organs (Money and Ehrhardt, 1972). Strife over gender identity occurred only in those children for whom the parents communicated uncertainty about the child's sex.

Studies of CAH patients who were not treated early in life are also informative. Hampson and Hampson (1961) studied 31 untreated females with CAH. They had masculinized genitals and had acquired secondary male sex characteristics early in life. Despite all this, they were raised as girls because the parents had been informed of the genetic sex of their offspring during early infancy. All but 5 of the girls developed an unambiguous female identity in spite of their contradictory appearance.

Further evidence for the importance of rearing comes from cases in which the individuals have unexpectedly become masculinized or feminized at puberty (by hormonal changes) and have developed secondary sexual characteristics in contrast to their gender identity. In these instances gender identity remains intact, although women may be disturbed by a change in voice and the growth of a beard and men by the development of breasts and the like. Such changes need to be corrected, but they do not result in an altered gender identity.

One interesting study, however, provides support for the nativist view that hormones play a pivotal role in gender identity. Imperato-McGinley and others (1974) described what appeared to be a shift from female to male gender at puberty in a group of interrelated individuals in the Dominican Republic. All of these individuals were pseudohermaphrodites and at birth had male sex chromosomes (XY), "profound ambiguity" of the external genitals, and normal testes. Most of these individuals were reared as girls. At puberty, however, an increase in testosterone from the testes led to a deepening of the voice, growth of a penis from what had been assumed to be a clitoris, erections, and enlargement and descent of the testes. Essentially, females appeared to be transformed into males as the result of the testosterone surge at puberty. Of 19 subjects unambiguously reared as females, 13 changed to a masculine gender identity at puberty. These individuals reported "realizing that they were different from other girls sometime between the ages of seven and twelve. Over a period of several years, they passed through no longer feeling like girls, to feeling like men, to a conscious awareness that they were indeed men." Although this study would seem to support the case for hormone control of gender identity, it is not clear that the subjects in the study were unambiguously reared as girls (Rubin, Reinisch, and Haskett, 1981). In contrast, 8 subjects with a similar type of pseudohermaphroditism identified and studied in the United States were unambiguously reared as females and continued to maintain their female identity despite pubertal masculinization (Walsh et al., 1974).

Another way to examine the relative contributions of biology and early experience to gender identity is to study transsexuals. Transsexuals (who will be discussed in Chap. 17) are individuals whose personal gender identity does not coincide with their anatomy and physiology. They report feeling that they are trapped in a body of the wrong sex. There is no evidence to support a physiological explanation, as these individuals are not hermaphroditic in any sense. In any case, hermaphrodites do not appear to suffer from problems associated with gender identity. A search for environmental factors that are consistently associated with transsexuality has yielded little. Although there is a tendency for the parents of transsexuals to have desired a child of the opposite sex, this pattern does not always predominate (Green, 1974). Our knowledge about the complex process of sexual differentiation, then, is not particularly helpful in explaining the gender identity disturbances experienced by transsexuals.

Biology and gender role behavior

The nativist-environmentalist controversy is also very much alive in the area of gender differences in behavior. By *gender differences* we mean consistent behavioral differences that can reliably separate males from females. The nature of these differences varies from culture to culture. In addition, there are some common beliefs in our society about the disparities between the sexes that cannot be verified by scientific fact. Nevertheless, men and women can be demonstrably differentiated from each other in several ways. First, women are physically weaker than men, although the differences in physical strength seem to be decreasing. (Perhaps the best evidence for this can be found in Olympic track and field records, where the existing discrepancies between the scores for men and women have consistently declined. Women also hold the speed record for swimming the English Channel round trip.) On the other hand, women are constitutionally stronger than men: They are less likely to die during the prenatal period or to succumb to childhood diseases, are more likely to recover from illnesses, and have a longer life expectancy.

Researchers who study behavioral gender differences in relation to hormonal effects typically focus on six broad categories of behavior typical of children and adolescents:

1   General activity. *Males are usually observed to be more active than females. They expend more physical energy in rough outdoor play.*

2   Social aggression. *Males are reported to be more aggressive than females, both physically and verbally.*

3   Parental role play. *Youngsters tend to select objects and play roles consistent with their same-sex parent. Boys, for example, tend to play with trucks and play the role of father. Girls, on the other hand, tend to play with dolls and to take on the role of mother.*

4   Preference for same-sex play partners. *During childhood, boys tend to play with boys, while girls associate with other girls. In addition, boys form large playgroups, while girls gather in small groups of two or three (Waldrop and Halvorson, 1975).*

5   Gender role labeling. *Children are often labeled by their peers on the basis of their play patterns and partners. Some children may be called sissies or tomboys if they engage in activities characteristic of the opposite sex.*

6   Dressing behavior. *Females tend to be more neatly attired than males and often adorn themselves with jewelry and makeup.*

These, then, are some of the more reliable differences between boys and girls. We should mention that these differences are not absolute. That is to say, not all boys are more aggressive, active, and so on than all girls. These statements are true only if we take the average of all males and compare it to the average for all females. This means that some girls will be more aggressive, active, and likely to play with boys than some boys, but these girls and boys will be in the minority.

The existence of apparent behavioral differences between the sexes requires some sort of explanation. To what extent can these differences be accounted for by biological factors, and to what extent can they be accounted for by experiential factors? Pure nativists, of course, argue that these differences are totally biologically determined, whereas pure environmentalists argue that these differences are shaped by society.

In recent years there has been some attempt to examine the contribution of prenatal hormones to the development of sex differences. Again, as in the study of gender identity, most of the data come from pseudohermaphrodites. Although such individuals make up less than 1 percent of the population, those cases that have been discovered have been studied quite extensively.

One of the earliest reports involved a comparison of CAH pseudohermaphroditic females with normal females matched on the basis of age and socioeconomic status (Ehrhardt et al., 1968; Ehrhardt and Baker, 1974). The researchers were interested in determining whether the CAH females had more masculine-like behaviors than did normal females. Although gender identity was not disturbed in the hormone-exposed girls, they did differ behaviorally from the control subjects. The pseudohermaphroditic females tended to be regarded by themselves and by their mothers as tomboys. They spent a lot of energy in athletic activities and often joined male playgroups. They also showed a preference for utilitarian as opposed to pretty clothes and were more interested in a career and less interested in marriage than were the normal females. There were no differences in terms of degree of homosexual or heterosexual interest, however. Because the hormone-exposed females tended to behave in a more masculine manner, Ehrhardt and Money concluded that hormones do play an important role in determining the behavioral differences between the sexes.

It would be a mistake to accept this conclusion without question, however, since the study was marred by a number of problems. For one thing, the interviewers knew which females were pseudohermaphrodites and which ones were normal. Thus, the possibility of unintentional bias in interpreting the answers or statements given during the interviews cannot be ruled out. Second, information was gleaned only from verbal reports of these girls and their mothers. There was no attempt to question other family members, teachers, or peers, or to actually observe the girls under everyday conditions. Finally, we cannot rule out the possible effects of early experience in the development of these changes. For example, the CAH females may have been treated differently by their parents than normal females because they were expected to display masculine behavior. Furthermore, the fact that the girls themselves knew of their condition could have influenced their behavior (Lips and Colwill, 1978).

A more recent study has overcome some of these objections (Reinisch, 1977). In this case, the behavior of females whose mothers had been given progestins during pregnancy was compared to that of their untreated sisters. Information was obtained by administering a personality test in which the testers had no knowledge of the purpose of the study or of the treatment category of the girls. As in the previous study, differences between the hormone-exposed girls and their unexposed sisters emerged. The progestin-exposed girls were found to be more independent, individualistic, self-assured, and self-sufficient than their sisters. As these differences were similar in some respects to those reported by Ehrhardt and others (1968), it is tempting to conclude that prenatal sex hormones can, in some way, influence or cause the development of more masculine types of behavior. However, this study, like its predecessor, does not rule out the possibility that parental or child expectations produced the differences. It should also be noted that the behavior of these girls still falls within the range of what is considered to be normal female behavior.

Biology and cognitive development

Prenatal sex hormones have been thought to affect two aspects of cognitive development: general level of intelligence and spatial versus verbal skills. Elevated intelligence has consistently been observed in CAH children, leading researchers to speculate that prenatal androgen facilitates intellectual development (Baker and Ehrhardt, 1974). Subsequent studies, however, have demonstrated that the normal siblings and parents of CAH children also show elevated intelligence. This may mean that there is an intellectual selection bias in families of CAH patients attending clinics.

It has generally been believed that women have better verbal skills, whereas men have better spatial skills (Maccoby and Jacklin, 1974). These particular differences, while typical of American men and women, are not universal, however. Female verbal superiority is not characteristic of German or Israeli women (Preston, 1962; Kugelmass and Lieblich, 1979). Nor is male superiority in spatial ability found in all cultures. Studies of Canadian Eskimos, for example, reveal no such differences (Berry, 1966; MacArthur, 1967). In general, there is little if any evidence to suggest that prenatal hormones play any role in the development of male and female differences in verbal and spatial skills (Baker and Ehrhardt, 1974; Yalom, Green, and Fish, 1973).

Biology and sexual orientation

Sexual orientation can be defined as sexual responsiveness to the same or opposite sex as revealed by dreams, erotic fantasies, and actual experiences (Ehrhardt and Meyer-Bahlburg, 1981). The process by which sexual orientation develops and the factors that might influence such orientation are largely a matter of speculation. Some researchers have argued that prenatal hormones might play a role, while others emphasize experience.

If prenatal hormones are involved, studies of pseudohermaphrodites might shed some light on the issue. Genetic females who are exposed to prenatal androgens ought to develop a homosexual orientation (i.e., prefer females). Studies of CAH females, however, have not provided support for this position. Most CAH women had a decidedly heterosexual orientation, although a few bisexual or homosexual individuals were also identified (Money and Schwartz, 1976; Ehrhardt et al., 1968). Researchers have also failed to find a homosexual orientation in genetic males with testicular feminizing syndrome (Masica, Money, and Ehrhardt, 1971). In general, then, sexual orientation seems to follow gender identity and thus appears to be based more on social learning than on hormones (Ehrhardt and Meyer-Bahlberg, 1981).

Hormones versus experience

As we have seen in this section, an accurate assessment of the contributions of hormones and experience to the development of behavior is extremely difficult to obtain. What might appear to be a biological (hormonal) effect can often be explained on the basis of experience. A final example can help to demonstrate this problem. As we have mentioned, American men seem to have a better spatial and mathematical ability than that of women. One might suppose that this difference is related to some biological factor in the brain or to brain differentiation that occurred during the prenatal period. However, it is also possible that this difference is culturally conditioned. The fact that men and women in some cultures show similar mathematical skills rather than differences argues strongly for the cultural explanation.

Let us consider how a sex difference in this trait could develop in societies such as our own. Men in this society might receive more encouragement for doing well in mathematics than do women. After all, math is a necessary skill in many "masculine" jobs such as science and engineering. Women who do well in mathematics, on the other hand, might be subjected to subtle forms of discrimination by teachers, parents, or peers who either hold to the stereotype that women are not good at math or who believe math skills are unimportant for women. As a result, many women may "learn" to perform poorly in mathematics.

The same arguments can be raised about the presumed higher levels of aggression in males. Which of these views—the biological or the environmental—is correct? Do biological factors such as the presence or absence of prenatal hormones explain these differences? Or is some sort of social conditioning a more useful explanation? At this point we really cannot say, although future research may provide us with a definitive answer. However, it is likely that we shall discover that *both* prenatal hormones and early experiences influence the development of behavioral differences between men and women.

Up to this point, we have examined the two sexes as if they were truly distinct—two separate entities formed prenatally and continuing that way throughout life. This approach follows our cultural tradition, in which men and women are viewed as being different from each other. But are they really that different? Should the sexes be viewed as opposite to each other? Researchers are beginning to discover that men and women are much more similar than is commonly thought. Consider the following points in support of this more contemporary outlook.

First, although there have been numerous attempts to uncover behavioral traits that differentiate men from women, only a few such traits apparently exist. Even some of these differences, such as the ones involving math and verbal skills, seem to be culturally determined. All in all, men and women are much more similar in their behavioral characteristics than they are different.

Second, studies of gender identity indicate that any individual is capable of assuming either a male or female gender identity, provided that such identification takes place prior to 18 months of age. This ability of the human organism to take on the "wrong" gender identity if forced to because of unusual biological events also argues for a basic similarity between men and women. But this view leads us to an interesting problem. If the sexes are so similar, why does transsexualism occur? Why do transsexuals feel so strongly that they are of the wrong sex? We cannot easily answer this question. Some studies suggest that transsexuals who undergo sex-change surgery may not, in fact, feel more content about their sexuality. Thus, the problem of the transsexual may involve more than gender identity.

Perhaps the most basic and already accepted difference between men and women lies in their anatomy and physiology. However, the more we learn about sexual anatomy, the more we find important similarities between men and women. For example, no one would dispute that the external genitals of men are different from the external genitals of women. Yet there are some interesting parallels between these structures. Consider the penis and the clitoris, which are derived prenatally from the same primordial genital tissue, the genital tubercle. Both of these structures have erectile tissue, and stimulation of both structures is the source of orgasm. Another similarity between men and women is found in an unexpected place, the sex hormones. As we have indicated, men have circulating levels of testosterone, while women have circulating levels of estrogens and progesterone. However, this is a simple view of a more complex process. Actually, men and women have both male and female hormones in their bodies. In females, small amounts of male hormones are normally produced by the adrenal glands. Although these hormones are present in small amounts compared to the levels of estrogen and progesterone, they are nonetheless there. Similarly, men produce small amounts of estrogens. Perhaps even more surprising is the finding that testosterone may be converted to estrogens in some organs, including the brain. In addition, the gonadotropins LH and FSH are identical in males and females (see Chap. 6). Finally, the sexual response cycle, which is described in detail in Chap. 11, is similar for men and women, although timed differently.

Without a doubt, then, there are many basic similarities between men and women. The differences have been emphasized, publicized, and heralded in the past. Perhaps it is now time to recognize that men and women are not really all that different from each other. (Although, as the French are fond of saying, *vive la difference!*)

SUMMARY

1 *Sexual differentiation* is the process by which an organism develops the anatomical and physiological characteristics of its sex. The physiological elements involved in sexual differentiation include the sex chromosomes, the gonads, the genitals, the connecting ducts, and the brain.

2 The *sex chromosomes* determine the genetic sex of an individual: XX indicates female, and XY indicates male. The *gonads* produce the sex hormones: *testosterone* in males and *estrogen* and *progesterone* in females. The gonads also produce the *gametes*: eggs and sperm.

3 The process of sexual differentiation begins during *prenatal development*. The generalized genital system first appears in the fifth or sixth week of embryonic development; it consists of three components: the *gonadal tissue*, the *rudimentary external genitals*, and the primitive ducts.

4 Differentiation of the gonads occurs in the seventh week in the male and in the eleventh week in the female. A substance called *H-Y antigen* is thought to be involved in this differentiation. Next, the ducts and external genitals develop. In males, testosterone influences the *Wolffian ducts* to develop into male reproductive structures. In females, the absence of testosterone causes the Wolffian ducts to regress, and the *Mullerian ducts* develop into female reproductive structures. The genitals are completely differentiated in both sexes by the end of 4 months.

5 During prenatal development in the male the testes must travel from the abdomen to the scrotum by means of the *inguinal canal*. Failure to do so creates a condition called *undescended testes*, or *cryptorchidism*.

6 Two main sexual differences in brain functioning are governed by changes during prenatal development: hormone cyclicity in the female, and any behavioral or personality differences that may exist between the sexes (at least in monkeys).

7 One type of error in sexual differentiation is chromosomal abnormality. Common aberrations of the sex chromosomes include *Turner's syndrome, XXX females, Klinefelter's syndrome*, and *XYY males*. Another type of error, which occurs during prenatal development, results in *hermaphroditism*, or the existence of male and female structures in the same individual. A *true hermaphro-*

dite has both ovaries and testes. A *pseudohermaphrodite* has gonads of one sex and external genitals of the other sex. There are three main types of pseudohermaphroditism: *congenital adrenal hyperplasia* (CAH), *progestin-induced hermaphroditism*, and *testicular feminizing syndrome*.

8   Among the factors that combine to define a person's maleness or femaleness are chromosomal sex, gonadal sex, hormonal sex, internal accessory organ sex, genital sex, assigned gender, and gender identity. *Gender identity* is one's own personal view of being male or female.

9   *Nativists* believe that gender identity and behavioral differences between the sexes are determined primarily by biological variables, whereas *environmentalists* believe they are determined primarily by early experiences and environmental influences. Studies of pseudohermaphroditic children indicate that labels of *male* and *female* play a greater role in a child's gender identity than does his or her biological sex. Although it is well established that human males and females behave differently in a number of different ways, research has not established how much of this difference is inborn and how much is learned.

10   *Sexual orientation* appears to be based more on social learning than on hormones.

11   Although there are obvious basic physical differences between males and females, close examination reveals many more similarities than differences.

ADDITIONAL READING

Bermant, Gordon, and Davidson, Julian. *Biological Bases of Sexual Behavior.* New York: Harper & Row, 1974.

> *Chapters cover evolutionary, environmental, neural, hormonal, and neuroendocrinological contributions to sexual differences and determination. The book does a good job of presenting technical information in a readable form.*

*   **Lips, Hilary, and Colwill, Nina Lee.** *The Psychology of Sex Differences.* Englewood Cliffs, N.J.: Prentice-Hall, 1978.

> *Well-presented and readable overview of sex differences. Includes chapters on research problems; sex differences in ability, aggression, and achievement; and the development of sex roles and gender identity.*

*   **Money, John, and Ehrhardt, Anke.** *Man and Woman, Boy and Girl,* Baltimore: Johns Hopkins University Press, 1972.

> *A very complete discussion of sexual differentiation and development from conception to maturity. Discusses both physiological and psychological aspects. Somewhat more technical than the aforementioned Lips and Colwill book.*

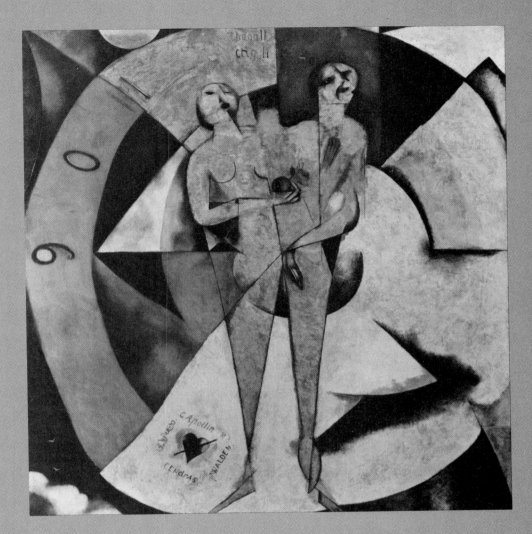

Hormones, reproduction, and human sexuality

6

chapter

6

Do fluctuations in women's hormones radically alter their moods at "that time of the month"?

Can men still respond sexually if their testes have been removed?

What causes the body to release egg cells or manufacture sperm?

Is there a deterioration in a woman's sexual responsivity if her ovaries are removed?

Does the administration of sex hormones alter sexual arousal?

Do men have a hormonal cycle similar to the female menstrual cycle?

Does female sexual interest change across the menstrual cycle?

These questions all concern processes within the human body that are significantly involved in reproduction and sexuality. Although most people are aware of the external factors (erotic movies, sensual caresses, and so on) that can stimulate sexual responsiveness, they may not be totally aware of how internal body factors can play a role in such responsiveness. Women, for example, may undergo regular changes in sexual interest, mood, and weight across the menstrual cycle, and men may have sexual desires that increase sharply at a certain time of day. The fact is that events within our bodies guide, control, and even alter our sexuality both over the course of a single day and over the course of our lives.

In this chapter we will look at the major physiological processes that are important determinants of sexuality. These processes include nervous system activity, which, among other things, allows us to perceive stimulating events in the environment and to respond to them, and hormone production, which influences both reproduction and sexual behavior.

THE BRAIN AND HORMONES

Hormones are substances produced by various **endocrine glands**, such as the pituitary, thyroid, testes, and ovaries. These chemicals are released directly into the bloodstream and move quickly to particular target cells or target tissues that may be quite distant from the gland. After being absorbed by the target cells, the hormones may direct the growth of these cells, control their metabolic activity, or regulate the synthesis of other hormones.

Three structures and the hormones they secrete have been identified as controlling elements in sexual behavior and reproduction: the hypothalamus, the pituitary, and the gonads (testes and ovaries). The **hypothalamus** is a small group of nerve cells located at the base of the forebrain. This small structure seems to be involved in the regulation of many biological motives, including hunger, thirst, and sexual behavior. It also exerts a powerful influence over the **pituitary**, a small pea-shaped structure lying just below the hypothalamus and above the soft palate of the mouth. The pituitary is often referred to as the "master gland" because it produces several different hormones that in turn stimulate the production of other hormones in various target tissues. Hormones that control the production of other hormones are referred to as *trophins*. The pituitary can be divided into three distinct lobes: anterior, intermediary, and posterior. It is primarily the **anterior pituitary** which affects sexual behavior. The **gonads**, or sex glands, not only secrete hormones (androgens such as testosterone from the testes and estrogens from the ovaries) but also produce the sex cells (sperm and eggs) that are necessary for reproduction.

To understand how the hypothalamus, pituitary, and gonads interact to control reproductive processes, we should recognize that these structures are all connected somewhat like an electrical circuit. In order to trace this circuit, we shall start at the hypothalamus, move to the other structures, and eventually return to the hypothalamus to complete the circuit (see Figs. 6.1 and 6.2). One of the primary functions of the hypothalamus in regulating reproduction is to produce and release a substance called **gonadotrophin-releasing hormone** (GnRH). GnRH travels a short distance from the hypothalamus to the pituitary, where it triggers or increases the production of two pituitary hormones: **follicle-stimulating hormone** (FSH) and **luteinizing hormone** (LH). The latter is sometimes termed **interstitial-cell-stimulating hormone** (ICSH) in reference to the cells it stimulates in men. For convenience, we shall use "LH" to refer to this hormone in both men and women.

FIGURE 6.1
The negative feedback loop for women, which depicts the relationship between brain hormones (GnRH, FSH, LH) and ovarian hormones (estrogen and progesterone).

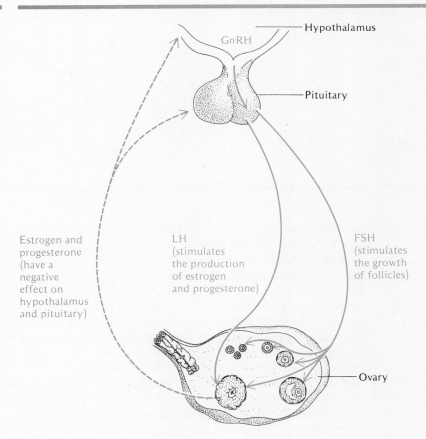

Hypothalamus

GnRH

Pituitary

Estrogen and progesterone (have a negative effect on hypothalamus and pituitary)

LH (stimulates the production of estrogen and progesterone)

FSH (stimulates the growth of follicles)

Ovary

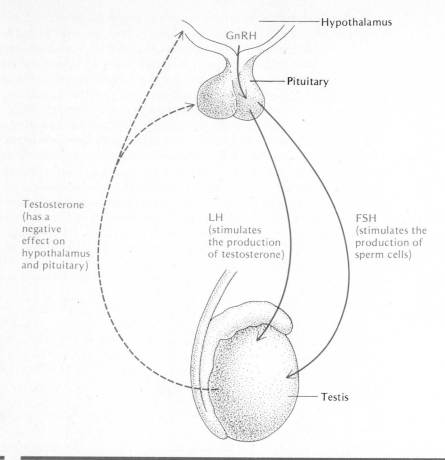

FIGURE 6.2
*The negative
feedback loop for
men, which
describes the
relationship
between brain
hormones (GnRH,
FSH, LH) and
testosterone.*

   The pituitary hormones, FSH and LH, are secreted into the bloodstream, where they travel to the gonads and stimulate the development of gametes and gonadal hormones. FSH is primarily responsible for the development of eggs and the manufacture of sperm, and LH is important in the production of the gonadal hormones, estrogens and testosterone. The gonadal hormones, in turn, move to specialized target cells throughout the body. **Estrogens** travel to the breast, where they facilitate growth and development, and to the vagina, where they maintain the elasticity of the vaginal walls. **Testosterone** moves to the hair follicles in the face, producing heavy growth. In addition, the gonadal hormones have a feedback effect on the hypothalamus. We use the word *feedback* in this case because the hypothalamus monitors the level of testosterone or estrogen in the blood and controls the production of GnRH accordingly. Thus, the gonadal hormones provide feedback, or information, to the hypothalamus. The nature of this feedback is essentially negative; that is, high levels of estrogen or testosterone will cause the hypothalamus to decrease its production or release of GnRH, ultimately acting as a brake on the production of gonadal hormones. Conversely, low blood levels of gonadal hormones will cause the hypothalamus to increase its production or release of GnRH, thereby increasing production of gonadal hormones. The ultimate result of such a system is that the levels of gonadal hormones are kept within an appropriate range.

The circuit that we have just described is called a **negative feedback loop**. It is not unlike the negative feedback loop involved in keeping the temperature constant in a hot-water heater. The hot-water tank contains a thermostat that controls the temperature of the water by turning a heating coil on and off. When the water temperature falls below a certain level, the thermostat turns the heating coil on; when the temperature rises above a certain level, the thermostat turns the heating coil off. The hypothalamic-pituitary-gonadal circuit works in a similar fashion. The hypothalamus is analogous to the thermostat, and the gonadal hormones are analogous to the water temperature. And, like the temperature of the water, the levels of the hormones are kept relatively constant.

*FEMALE HORMONE
CYCLES*

The negative feedback loop is only part of the story of hormonal changes in women. Superimposed on, and in conjunction with, the negative feedback loop are hormonal surges that fluctuate with the female menstrual cycle. A **menstrual cycle** is fairly unique among living organisms. Only the females of a few mammalian species, including some monkeys, apes, and humans, have a menstrual cycle. Other mammals have what is termed an **estrous cycle**. There are two important distinctions between menstrual and estrous cycles. First, with an estrous cycle there is no periodic bleeding—only an occasional slight spotting that occurs in association with ovulation. With a menstrual cycle, on the other hand, definite bleeding occurs that begins long after ovulation. Second, with the estrous cycle sexual activity is restricted to the ovulatory phase of the cycle. Thus, estrous females are sexually responsive to males only when they are "in heat." No such restriction is found in menstrual cycle females, who are capable of engaging in sexual activity throughout their cycle. This does not rule out the possibility, however, that there may be behavioral changes in sexual drive or desire that fluctuate with the menstrual cycle. We will examine this possibility later.

*The phases of the
menstrual cycle*

Biologically, the menstrual cycle can be divided into four phases, each with its associated hormonal, ovarian, and uterine changes. These separate stages of the cycle are: (1) the **follicular phase**, in which an egg matures within the ovary; (2) the **ovulatory phase**, in which an egg is released from the ovary and begins its journey down the fallopian tube; (3) the **luteal phase**, in which the empty follicle becomes a functioning corpus luteum and the uterus is prepared for the nourishment of a fertilized egg; and (4) the **menstrual phase**, in which the vascular lining of the uterus is shed through the cervix and vagina if the egg is not fertilized.

Follicular phase At the beginning of the follicular phase, estrogen levels are low. The hypothalamus responds to these low levels by releasing GnRH, which travels to the pituitary and stimulates the production of FSH. FSH, in turn, travels to the ovary, where it stimulates the growth of numerous follicles. LH, which is secreted in basal amounts by the pituitary, in turn stimulates the follicle to produce estrogen. Each follicle contains a potential ovum, or egg. Because of uneven growth, one follicle will mature more rapidly than the others and is destined to become the ovulatory follicle in this particular cycle, while the others will regress and deteriorate. As the designated follicle develops, it moves closer to the surface of the ovary and begins to produce high levels of estrogen. This increase in estrogen production has two main effects. First, the high levels of estrogen inhibit the production of FSH by the pituitary via the negative feedback loop. This decline in FSH leads to the total deterioration of the remaining follicles. Second, the high levels of estrogen stimulate the endometrium of the uterus to grow, thicken, and establish glands that will be used to secrete substances that will nourish a developing organism. Peak estrogen levels are reached about 2 days prior to ovulation.

Ovulation During the second phase, the follicle ruptures and releases the egg for its journey down the fallopian tube. Massive hormonal changes appear to trigger ovulation. In contrast to the typical inhibitory effect of gonadal hormones on the hypothalamus and pituitary, the high levels of estrogen now produce a brief positive effect, that is, a massive surge in LH production by the pituitary. It is this brief but dramatic 1–3-day increase in LH secretion that appears to trigger ovulation (Jaffe and Monroe, 1980). Thus, estrogen has an inhibitory effect on the hypothalamus and pituitary except at mid-cycle, where it exerts a positive influence.

Luteal phase During the luteal phase, significant changes occur in the empty follicle, which, although no longer possessing the egg, still has a major role to play in hormonal changes. As a result of the LH stimulation at mid-cycle, the empty follicle becomes a glandular mass of cells known as the **corpus luteum**, which means "yellow body," referring to the fact that the cells are yellowish in color. The corpus luteum begins to manufacture another hormone, **progesterone**. Progesterone, like all of the gonadal hormones, typically has a negative effect on the hypothalamus and pituitary. Thus, as the level of progesterone increases, it acts as a brake on the production of LH by the pituitary. Progesterone also stimulates the newly established glands in the endometrium to secrete substances that will nourish an embryo. The corpus luteum continues to produce estrogen and progesterone for about 12–14 days. If pregnancy does not occur, the corpus luteum deteriorates, and the levels of estrogen and progesterone drop rapidly. The actual demise of the corpus luteum is thought to be brought about by an interaction between estrogen and substances produced by the endometrium called **prostaglandins** (Cutter and Garcia, 1980; Yen, 1980). Prostaglandins are complex fatty acids that are found in many tissues, including the uterus, brain, and lung. They are implicated in a number of physiological processes. Particular prostaglandins, for example, are known to play a role in the onset of labor in pregnant women. The deterioration of the corpus luteum and the decline in estrogen and progesterone are associated with a failure to maintain the integrity of the uterine lining, which leads directly to the fourth phase, menstruation.

Menstrual phase **Menstruation,** which is apparently triggered by the rapidly dropping levels of estrogen and progesterone, involves the sloughing of the uterine lining through the cervix and vagina. Normally, the discharge for the entire duration of menstruation is only about 2 ounces (4 tablespoons). During the later part of the phase, the low levels of estrogen and progesterone cause an increase in the production of FSH, and the cycle begins anew.

Although we have just described the menstrual cycle from its biological beginning to end (from follicular development to menstruation), the majority of sex researchers use the onset of menstruation as the beginning of the menstrual cycle. This convention is based on the fact that menstruation is the most readily identifiable marker for the menstrual cycle. As a result, the first day of menstruation is considered to be the first day of the next cycle.

As we have indicated, most of the changes occurring during the menstrual cycle are related to changes in the levels of four hormones, two of which are produced by the pituitary as the result of stimulation from the hypothalamus (LH and FSH) and two of which are produced by the follicle within the ovary (estrogen and progesterone). Let's briefly review these changes by tracing the course of each hormone across the menstrual cycle (see Fig. 6.3). By convention we shall start with menstruation.

FSH During menstruation, FSH levels are rising in response to low levels of estrogen. During the follicular phase, FSH levels rise and then decline after the follicle starts producing estrogen. This is simply a manifestation of the negative feedback loop. Paradoxically, at ovulation, high levels of estrogen have a positive effect on FSH, causing a small temporary surge in FSH production. FSH levels are low during the luteal phase, when gonadal hormones are at high levels.

LH During the menstrual and follicular phases, LH levels are low but are sufficient to stimulate the production of estrogen by the growing follicles. Paradoxically, as ovulation approaches, high levels of estrogen cause a dramatic surge in LH, which triggers ovulation. Although the surge is only temporary, LH levels do not quite return to baseline. The LH surge changes the empty follicle to a corpus luteum and stimulates the production of progesterone. During the remainder of the luteal phase, LH levels decline to baseline as progesterone levels increase.

Estrogen Estrogen levels are low during the menstrual and early part of the follicular phases. As LH stimulates the follicles to produce estrogen, estrogen levels rise and reach a peak just prior to ovulation. By the time of ovulation, estrogen levels are declining. They plateau during the first two-thirds of the luteal phase but drop dramatically as the corpus luteum deteriorates.

Progesterone The level of progesterone is virtually zero during the men-

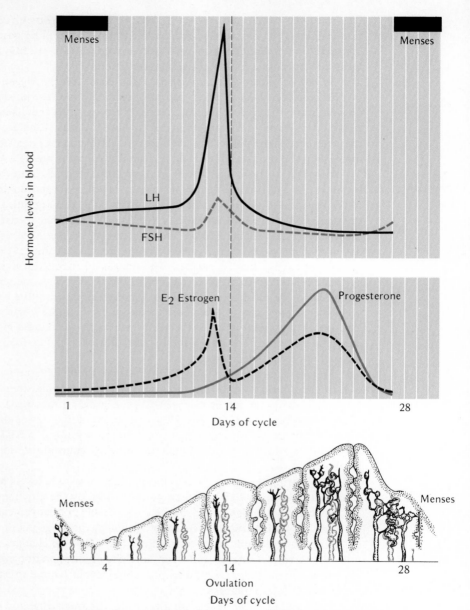

FIGURE 6.3
*Hormonal and
endometrial
changes across the
menstrual cycle.
The upper graph
shows the
fluctuations in LH,
FSH, estrogen, and
progesterone
across the 28-day
period in which
ovulation occurs
on day 14. The
lower figure traces
the changes in the
endometrial lining
of the uterus over
the same 28 days.*

strual, follicular, and ovulatory phases. During the luteal phase, progesterone increases dramatically as a function of the corpus luteum and declines just as dramatically as the corpus luteum degenerates.

Perhaps the most critical phase of the menstrual cycle is ovulation, for it is at this point, and for a short period of time prior to and after ovulation, that a woman can become pregnant. For pregnancy to occur, a live, active sperm must encounter and fertilize a live egg. A human egg cell lives for only 12–36 hours. A woman can get pregnant by having intercourse up to 48 hours prior to ovulation or within 36 hours following ovulation, since the sperm cells can live for nearly 48 hours in the female reproductive tract. The calculation of ovulation is important both for women who want to become pregnant and for those who wish to avoid pregnancy. Cycle length and other physiological processes can be used as guides to predict the time of ovulation.

Cycle length   The average length of the menstrual cycle is considered to be 28 days, although lengths of 20 or 40 days are not uncommon and fall within normal limits. The standard 28-day cycle is often used as a model, even though "the absolutely regular cycle of precisely 28 days is so rare as to be either a myth or a medical curiosity" (Israel, 1967).

Using a 28-day cycle, the timing of various menstrual phases can be described as follows. By convention, the first day of menstruation is considered day 1. Menstruation continues through day 4 or 5 (although 6–8 days is not unusual). The follicular phase extends from day 5 to day 13. Ovulation takes place on day 14, and the luteal phase starts on day 15 and continues to day 28. For cycles longer or shorter than 28 days, the change is reflected only in the follicular phase. If a cycle lasts 35 days, the follicular phase extends from day 5 to day 20. Ovulation occurs on day 21, and the luteal phase lasts the standard 14 days. If a cycle lasts only 20 days, the follicular phase is correspondingly shortened, and ovulation occurs on day 6.

With few exceptions, the luteal phase seems to be of constant length (14 days). Thus, one can always determine the day of ovulation in the *previous* cycle by counting backward 14 days from the first day of menstruation. This is not particularly helpful, however, if one wants to predict the day of ovulation in the current cycle. The only way in which women can count days and predict the day of ovulation with any certainty is if their cycles are extremely regular. To be regular, the cycle length should vary little if at all from month to month. If the length of the cycle varies, it is extremely difficult to make accurate predictions of when ovulation will occur.

Cervical mucus secretion   Given the massive changes in hormones that occur across the menstrual cycle, one might expect corresponding physical changes which could be used as indicators of a woman's phase in her cycle. Indeed, there are two measurable processes that are helpful in providing such information: cervical mucus secretion and basal body temperature.

The cervix contains glands that produce mucus throughout the menstrual cycle. The quality and quantity of the mucus have been found to vary with estrogen levels. During the early part of the follicular phase, the mucus is thick and alkaline, but at ovulation it becomes thinner, more elastic, and even more alkaline, in order to provide a supportive environment for sperm passing through the cervix. After ovulation, the mucus returns to its former, thickened state. A sample of mucus removed just prior to ovulation will dry in a fern-shaped pattern on a glass slide (see Fig. 6.4). This mucus can also be stretched into a stringy, thin thread between two slides. Neither of these features of ovulatory mucus is found in the mucus extracted during the luteal phase. Thus, both of these tests can be used to detect ovulation. Following a training session, any woman can perform these tests at home.

Basal body temperature A woman's basal body temperature also varies across the menstrual cycle. Providing that she measures her rectal temperature the first thing each morning, she should note the following pattern. Temperature is lower during the follicular phase and may take a dip on the day of ovulation. After ovulation, the temperature rises by as much as 0.4°F and stays at this level until the end of the luteal phase (see Fig. 6.5). The temperature increase appears to be directly related to the increased production of progesterone. Other variations in temperature caused by colds or emotional upset may make this method inaccurate for determining a woman's phase in her cycle, however.

Mittelschmerz There are some women who actually feel the rupture of the egg from the ovary at ovulation. These women experience a cramping pain (called **mittelschmerz**) that can be felt on one or both sides of the abdomen. The pain may be of brief duration or last as long as a day. Because of the similarity to gastric disturbance, it is not wise to rely on abdominal pain as an indicator of ovulation.

Anovulatory cycles In light of our discussion to this point, one might assume that each menstrual cycle is similar to the next. But this simply isn't the case. Not only is there variation in cycle length for the individual woman,

*FIGURE 6.4
Slides of cervical mucous showing (left) the fern pattern during ovulation (presumably an orientation of the mucous molecules, which provide pathways for sperm, and (right) the absence of the fern patterns during luteal phase.*

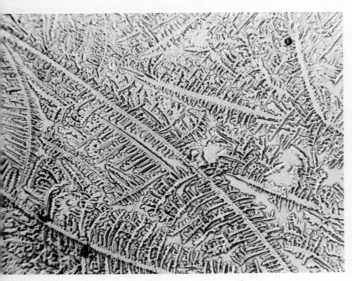
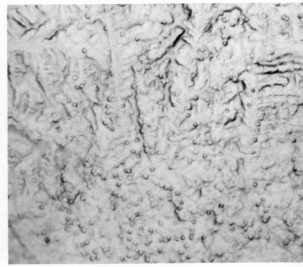

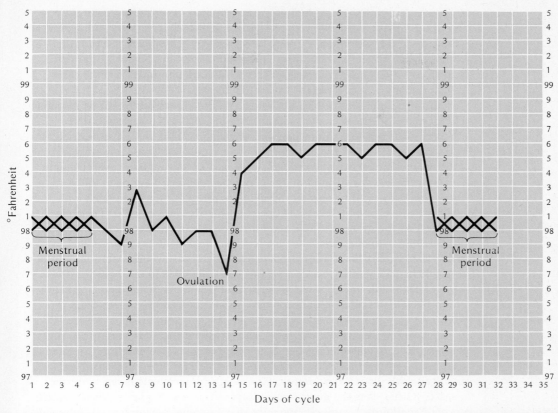

FIGURE 6.5

*Basal body
temperature
variation during a
typical menstrual
cycle. Basal body
temperature peaks
after ovulation
and remains
elevated until
menstruation.*

**Problems with
menstruation**

but the woman may not even release an egg in every cycle. Cycles in which no
egg is released are called **anovulatory cycles**. Except for the failure to release an
egg, these cycles resemble normal cycles in all respects. Anovulatory cycles are
common in young teenagers during the first few years of menstruation; they
occur once or twice a year in women between the ages of 20 and 40; and they
increase in incidence in older women approaching menopause.

The most common of all menstrual problems is **dysmenorrhea**, or painful
menstruation. The symptoms of dysmenorrhea can include painful abdominal
cramps, headache, lower back pain, nausea, and bloating. The symptoms are
strongest during the first few hours of menstrual flow and usually disappear by
the second day. Approximately 30–50 percent of all women of childbearing age
suffer from this condition. Because it is severe enough to entail bed rest for
some women, it results in the loss of 140 million working hours every year
(Marx, 1979).

Up until recently, the cause of painful menstruation was unknown, and the treatments were generally ineffective. Women experiencing painful menstruation either were given powerful painkillers such as codeine, which did not alleviate all the symptoms, or were put on a regimen of birth control pills—a rather drastic treatment involving hormonal manipulations for 21 days per month to solve a problem that lasts only 1–2 days a month. In some cases psychotherapy was tried, again with little success.

Evidence now suggests that a biochemical abnormality might be responsible for many of the cases of dysmenorrhea. It has often been noted that menstrual cramps feel somewhat similar to labor pains, which are caused by contractions of the uterus during the delivery process. These powerful labor contractions are produced by prostaglandins. Not surprisingly, prostaglandin levels in the menstrual fluid of dysmenorrheic women have been found to be three times higher than that in the menstrual fluid of normal women. In addition, prostaglandin levels decline from the first to second day of menstruation, just as the dysmenorrheic symptoms do (Chan and Dawood, as cited in Marx, 1979). Although the evidence linking prostaglandin secretion and dysmenorrhea is only correlational, treatment with prostaglandin synthesis inhibitors (substances that lower the levels of prostaglandins in the body) has been highly successful. In clinical trials of such drugs, women are reporting nearly complete relief of all symptoms (Chan and Dawood and Henzl, as cited in Marx, 1979).

Another problem, less common than dysmenorrhea but sometimes confused with it, is ***endometriosis***. As the name implies, the problem is related to the endometrium, the lining of the uterus, which becomes thickened and engorged with blood every month. However, endometriosis is not a uterine disease. Rather, it is the growth of endometrial tissue in places other than the uterus. Small growths of endometrium may be found on the ovaries, fallopian tubes, rectum, bladder, vagina, cervix, umbilicus, lymph glands, and other nearby abdominal organs. As the lining of the uterus grows and develops over the course of the menstrual cycle, so do these aberrantly located pieces of tissue. At menstruation, these pieces of tissue also "bleed." This condition occurs most commonly in women in their forties and in nulliparous (childless) women between 30 and 40. Symptoms include painful menstruation lasting a long time, painful defecation, painful intercourse (especially with deep penetration), and infertility (Deveraux, 1963; Karnaky, 1971). The cause of endometriosis is unknown, although it has been suggested that ***retrograde menstruation*** may occur; that is, menstrual fluid might be forced in the reverse direction up through the fallopian tubes and out into the abdomen. Some of this tissue may then adhere to other structures (Huff, 1979). Retrograde menstruation and the resulting endometriosis is known to occur in monkeys (McClure et al., 1971), but whether this unusual movement of menstrual tissue also occurs in humans remains unproven. If not treated, endometriosis may lead to permanent sterility. Treatment generally consists of hormone administration or surgery in severe cases.

A third menstrual problem is ***amenorrhea***, or the failure of menstruation to occur. The term **primary amenorrhea** is used if the woman has not menstruated prior to the age of 18. **Secondary amenorrhea** is applied to cases where menstruation has ceased for at least 1 year after menstrual flow has already occurred. Primary amenorrhea may be caused by excess androgens, anatomical defects, and genetic disorders. Secondary amenorrhea may be caused by pituitary failure, marked shifts in weight, birth control pills, or premature ovarian failure (better known as early menopause). It may also be associated with psychological disorders, such as depression or anxiety. A wide variety of treatments are available, depending on the nature of the disorder.

Hubert Humphrey's personal physician once said that it would be wrong for women to hold public office because "their raging hormones would interfere with their ability to carry out a job." In a *New York Times Magazine* article titled "Male Dominance? Yes, Alas. Sexist Plot? No," anthropologist Lionel Tiger (1970) argued that women's cognitive skills deteriorate during the premenstrual period, thereby placing them at a disadvantage in comparison to men. Others have suggested that women should not be airline pilots, apparently based on the limited observation by Whitehead (1934) that three crashes over an 8-month period involved women pilots who were menstruating at the time.

Given the major physiological changes that occur across the menstrual cycle, it is not unreasonable to assume that there are associated behavioral and emotional changes. Indeed, women do report alterations in mood at different points in their cycle but especially during the 3–4 days prior to menstruation, which have been characterized as a time of tension and irritability (McCance, Luff, and Widdowson, 1937; Ivey and Bardwick, 1968; Golub, 1976b). In 1931 R. T. Frank used the now popular term **premenstrual tension** to describe the syndrome of depression, anxiety, fatigue, irritability, headaches, and low self-esteem many women report experiencing just prior to menstruation.

What is the truth about premenstrual tension? Does it really occur? Are women really depressed? Is premenstrual tension caused by hormone changes? Does this depression and tension actually incapacitate women?

Let's start with the question of whether premenstrual tension really occurs. If we were to ask a random sample of women about the 3 or 4 days prior to menstruation, some women would report symptoms that resemble premenstrual tension, while others might not have any symptoms at all. In the McCance, Luff, and Widdowson (1937) study, data were obtained from 167 women for the duration of 4 cycles. Although no striking evidence of rhythmic and mood changes was found in individual subjects, such a pattern emerged when the data from all subjects were combined. In another study, Rees (1956) noted that 50 percent of her subjects did not report any significant premenstrual symptoms. And where mood changes have been found, their magnitude is actually rather small. Thus, women feel slightly more anxious or slightly more depressed (Golub, 1976b). It seems then that although premenstrual tension probably exists, it is by no means a universal or severe phenomenon.

For women who do exhibit premenstrual tension, it has generally been assumed that this is a period of depression, or a low point in the mood cycle, and that at other times they are in their "normal" mood. This assumption has been questioned by Hyde and Rosenberg (1976), who have suggested that women might be "normal" during the premenstrual period and have an elevated mood at other times in the cycle, especially at ovulation. In most previous studies of mood and the menstrual cycle, the researchers had relied on questionnaires emphasizing the negative aspects of the premenstrual period. Such an emphasis might have biased the interpretation of the results, especially because subjects were not asked to reveal their positive mood states. In 1973 Sommer attempted to correct this problem by asking her subjects to report on the positive as well as negative feelings that occurred across the cycle. She found a correlation between positive feelings and ovulation but no correlation between negative feelings and phases of the cycle. So the question becomes one of how mood changes from ovulation to the premenstrual period should be interpreted. Should the alterations be characterized as moving from feeling normal at ovulation to feeling depressed just prior to menstruation? Or should they be seen as moving from feeling unusually good at ovulation to feeling average during the premenstrual period?

Because mood shifts do occur in some women, we might next ask, "What is responsible for these mood alterations?" There are two likely sources: hormones and cultural training or experience. Let's examine the case for hormones first.

The hormones most commonly implicated in the menstrual cycle mood shifts are estrogen and progesterone. Their importance is derived from the fact that these two hormones undergo dramatic decreases in the days prior to menstruation. The exact relationship between hormones and mood fluctuations is unknown, although it has been suggested that mood shifts might be related to (1) the absolute level of estrogen in the body, (2) the absolute level of progesterone in the body, (3) the ratio of progesterone to estrogen in the body, (4) hypersensitive reaction to estrogen changes, and (5) withdrawal responses to the rapidly declining levels of progesterone and estrogen. Because much of the hormonal research is correlational, cause-and-effect inferences cannot be drawn.

Recent research in which women's hormonal states were manipulated with birth control pills does provide some suggestive evidence for a causal link between hormones and mood. Paige (1971) looked at mood alterations in women who took either no birth control pills, combination pills that provided an unchanging and high dose of estrogen and progesterone, or sequential pills that provided 15 days of estrogen followed by 5 days of progesterone, thereby mimicking the natural cycle but at higher hormone levels. Mood shifts were noted only for the no-pill and sequential-pill groups. The combination-pill group, which experienced no change in hormone levels, showed no fluctuations in mood.

Another possible source of menstrual mood shifts is cultural training and experience (Brooks, Ruble, and Clarke, 1977; Novell, 1965). It has been proposed that some menstrual mood shifts are related to expectations that women develop during their early cultural training. If women expect menstruation to be negative, based on conversations with their mothers and friends, then they might come to view menstruation as an unpleasant event and be much more sensitive to changes that occur just prior to menstruation. Indeed, it has been demonstrated that young adolescents have a negative view of menstruation (Clarke and Ruble, 1978).

Perhaps the best support for an experiential influence comes from a study conducted by Diana Ruble (1977). She suspected that women's reports of mood changes during the menstrual cycle might be related in part to these women's cultural beliefs about the kinds of symptoms that they should experience at different times in their cycles. Ruble selected a sample of female college students and obtained detailed menstrual histories from them. Based on an examination of their menstrual histories, Ruble then contacted the subjects approximately 7–10 days before their period was due and asked them to come into the laboratory. While in the lab, these women were told that it was possible with "new scientific techniques" to predict the phase of their menstrual cycle. The women were then hooked up to an EEG machine and were told that their brain waves would indicate their cycle phase. (This was a deception; EEG recordings actually have no relation to the menstrual cycle.) One-half of the women were then told that they were premenstrual (period due in 1–2 days), while the other half were told that they were intermenstrual (period due in 7–10 days). Thus, all that Ruble did was to tell some of the women that they were premenstrual even though they were not. All the women were then given a questionnaire to fill out. Interestingly, the women who *thought* they were premenstrual showed more symptoms on the questionnaire than did the intermenstrual women. Ruble suggests that learned associations or beliefs might make a woman exaggerate her symptoms because of her expectations.

Another question we raised at the beginning of this discussion was the extent to which menstrual events might lead to deterioration in performance. Although there may be mood changes from ovulation to the premenstrual phase, there is absolutely no evidence to support Tiger's view that there is any deterioration in performance. Researchers who have looked at test performance (Wickham, 1958), grade point average and exam performance (Bernstein, 1977), and perceptual-motor behavior (as reviewed in Sommer, 1973) have been unable to document any decline in performance in the days prior to menstruation. This also holds true for women between the ages of 30 and 40, in whom the premenstrual syndrome is most pronounced (Lloyd, 1963; Moos, 1969). Thus, there is no support for the position that female performance declines during the premenstrual period or that women are at a disadvantage in comparison to men. It is possible that women may develop coping strategies that allow them to deal with their mood shifts without affecting their performance. Thus, there is no reason why women should be barred from certain jobs because of their "raging hormones."

In general, the hormonal basis of male reproduction can be simply explained by the negative feedback loop between the gonads and the hypothalamus. This loop serves to maintain fairly constant levels of testosterone and sperm production. When testosterone levels rise to a certain point, the hypothalamus reduces its production or release of GnRH. When testosterone levels fall, the hypothalamus increases its production of LH and FSH by the pituitary and ultimately increases testosterone levels and sperm production.

Thus, men appear to maintain fairly constant levels of hormones. Nevertheless, male hormone levels do vary. Testosterone levels wax and wane across the day, being highest in the morning and lowest at night (Faiman and Winter, 1971). This is shown graphically in Fig. 6.6. Testosterone levels may also differ over a period of several days as a function of sexual interest and activity. For example, both the anticipation of sex and the act of sex can stimulate testosterone production. Fox (1972) found this out firsthand when he had his wife collect blood samples from him during intercourse, within 5 minutes after intercourse, and during control periods, for 45 consecutive days. The testosterone concentrations in the blood samples taken just before and after ejaculation were significantly higher than those in the control samples. Any major change in sexual activity over the long run can also alter hormone levels. Consider the sexually inactive man who suddenly becomes quite active. His testosterone levels will probably rise somewhat and be regulated at a higher level. Note that such changes are not cyclical. Thus, the typical view has been that the male hormone system exists in a steady state, perhaps gradually increasing or decreasing over long time periods upon which situational surges of testosterone are superimposed.

Within the last decade, however, researchers have become increasingly interested in the idea that men might have hormonal cycles that have the behavioral and emotional impact of female cycles. Unfortunately, this idea is much more difficult to test in men than in women. There are three frustrating problems that researchers have been unable to overcome in their search for

*FIGURE 6.6
The daily cycle of testosterone secretion in men. Testosterone levels are highest in the early morning and lowest in the late evening. (Faiman and Winter, 1971)*

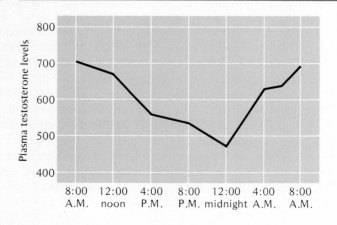

male hormone cycles. First, men have no major external referent comparable to menstruation as an indication of possible internal hormonal change. Without such an external referent, researchers would have to collect daily blood or urine samples from men, probably for many months, to establish that a hormone cycle exists. Second, it is possible that men have hormone cycles but that they are more subtle than female cycles. Thus, more sophisticated analyses of blood or urine samples might be required to detect these small changes. Finally, the measurement process itself might prove to be too difficult. As we have already indicated, brief situational factors can cause a temporary rise in testosterone. Depending on the state of the individual at blood drawing, cyclical changes may be obscured.

Given these problems, it is not surprising then that the issue of male cycles is still in question. While there is some evidence that testosterone levels increase and decrease over a monthly period (Luce, 1970), much more detailed data collection is necessary before it can be concluded that male hormone cycles exist. Evidence of cyclical mood shifts is also confusing and even contradictory. Hersey (1931) noticed that male industrial workers had emotional cycles lasting approximately 5 weeks. Hersey made no attempt to correlate these mood changes with hormonal state. In a subsequent study, Wessman and Ricks (1966) were unable to find any support for mood cycles in male Harvard students. Because of the scarcity of relevant studies, it is impossible to draw any conclusions about male cycles and their presumed effects at this time.

HORMONES AND
SEXUAL BEHAVIOR

In order to understand the connection between hormones and human sexuality, it is important to recognize that sexual behavior is controlled by a number of processes working together. The level of particular hormones is but one of these processes. Another is the totality of the individual's direct and indirect experiences with sex. Alternations in either or both of these factors can lead to changes in sexual behavior and sexual interest. Consider, for example, a man who suffers from inhibited sexual excitement. His inability to have an erection might be related to insufficient concentrations of testosterone, to some traumatic sexual experience, or to some combination of both.

Scientists have used at least three general approaches to examining the role of hormones in sexual behavior: (1) correlations of changes in sexual interest and responsivity with naturally occurring hormonal changes or cycles, (2) removal of sex hormones by means of removing the gonads and observation of the effect on sexual behavior, and (3) addition of externally injected sex hormones after removal of the gonads and observation of effects on sexual behavior.

Much of this work, of course, has been done with nonhuman subjects such as rats, cats, and monkeys. There are, after all, only a limited number of human subjects who have had their testes or ovaries removed, and such removal is generally prompted by medical problems such as cancer. Because of the relative scarcity of evidence for humans and because of possible sampling biases (is the sexual behavior of cancer patients the same as that of healthy individuals?), we must depend to some degree on studies of the rhesus monkey for information in this area. In addition to the similarities between the rhesus monkey and human reproductive systems, these two species have certain commonalities in their behavioral responses to hormonal manipulations. However, we recognize that the results from animal experiments can never serve as a real substitute for data on humans themselves.

*Sexual interest and
hormone cycles*

In general, the role of hormones in maintaining sexual behavior is of less importance in primates (monkeys, apes, and humans) than in other mammals (such as cats, rats, and dogs). This is especially true for female receptivity, which is measured as the willingness of the female to accept the male or (in humans) as sexual desire. The majority of female mammals exhibit the estrous cycle and are receptive to the amorous advances of males only during a few hours in their cycle. At all other times they will rebuff the sexual efforts of the male, even to the point of attack. This dramatic periodicity of sexual interest is in sharp contrast to the situation in monkeys, apes, and humans, in which the female can and does accept the male throughout her cycle. Thus, men and women may engage in sexual intercourse throughout the year and at any time during the woman's menstrual cycle. Any prohibitions of sex during the cycle are due to religious, societal, or personal reasons and are usually tied to menstruation (Ford and Beach, 1951; Mead, 1961).

Despite the continual receptivity of human females, it has been suggested that the *degree* of sexual interest might fluctuate with the hormonal changes that occur during their cycles. In addition, women might experience peaks or surges of desire correlated with ovulation. Unfortunately, the evidence for this idea is unclear. Early studies of sexual interest conducted by Davis (1929) and Terman (1938) indicated that women experience peaks of desire prior to and right after menstruation. These results are consistent with the finding of Kinsey and others (1953) that women experience their strongest feelings of arousal during the premenstrual period. Later research by Benedek (1952) and by Udry and Morris (1968) suggested that women experience peak desire right at mid-cycle, presumably at the time of ovulation (see Fig. 6.7). In 1977, however, Udry and Morris were unable to replicate their findings with another group of women.

The lack of consistency in these research findings may be related to the way in which the researchers measured sexual interest. In some of the studies women were merely asked to record their frequency of intercourse across the menstrual cycle. However, intercourse can be initiated by either the man or the woman. To get a more accurate picture of female sexual interest, perhaps we should look only at instances of female-initiated sexual activity. This reasoning was pursued by Adams, Gold, and Burt (1978), who examined female-initiated changes in sexual interest across the menstrual cycle. They also examined the influence of hormones on these changes by comparing women who used birth control pills with those who did not. The Pill provides a steady dose of hormones across the cycle. In the absence of hormonal birth control, hormones fluctuate in the normal manner. Adams and his co-workers

FIGURE 6.7
*Changes in sexual
interest across the
menstrual cycle.
The graph shows
the results of
questioning 40
women about
their frequency of
intercourse and
orgasm by reverse
day of menstrual
cycle. Note the
peak in
intercourse
frequency around
day 15,
presumably at
ovulation, and
another peak on
day 3 (3 days prior
to menstruation).
(Udry and Morris,
1968)*

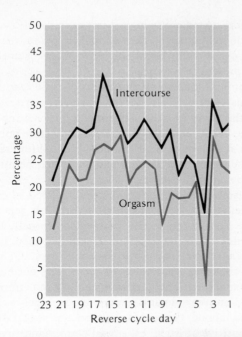

found that women did indeed experience a significant increase in sexual activity at the time of ovulation, but this was true only for the women who did not use the Pill. Pill users showed no significant changes in sexual activity across the cycle. This latter finding suggests that the increase in sexual activity at ovulation may be due to fluctuations in hormone levels.

We would have to conclude, then, that there may be a connection between sexual interest and the hormonal events of the menstrual cycle. Future studies will be needed to confirm this effect and to determine why the effect was not found in some studies. It may be, for example, that the effect is subtle and difficult to detect or it may be that experiential factors (such as the woman's mood on a particular day or her desire for a certain partner) obscure these hormonal effects. This latter explanation seems to apply to the rhesus monkey female. Although there is some trend for a mid-cycle increase in sexual behavior in the monkey (Herbert, 1968, 1970), this seems to be an oversimplification of the events. Such a fluctuation appears to be highly variable, is dependent on preferences for a particular partner, and is not stable from one cycle to the next (Michael and Welegalla, 1968).

*Effects of hormone
removal*

Perhaps the best way to assess the effects of sex hormones on sexual behavior is simply to eliminate them. In males, this can be accomplished through removing the glands that produce testosterone, the testes. This procedure has been loosely labeled ***castration***, but it is more properly called ***orchidectomy***. It should be noted that the adrenal gland produces a small amount of another androgen, **androstenedione**, which is not eliminated by castration. In females, the elimination of estrogen is accomplished by removing the ovaries in a procedure called **ovariectomy**. Small amounts of androstenedione from the adrenals also remain present in women.

Males General information about the effects of male castration has been available for thousands of years. Male slaves were often castrated so that they could be servants to the wives of their masters without creating any sexual problems. Such males, called **eunuchs**, were castrated before puberty. This procedure impaired sexual development and the potential for erections. Interestingly, eunuchs did develop both axillary and pubic hair because this hair growth is controlled by androstenedione.

Even with this historical information, the actual effects of castration have long been debated (Bremer, 1959; Tauber, 1940). While it is generally true that many men experience a decline in sexual desire and eventually become impotent following castration, this is by no means true for all men. In fact, some men continue to be sexually active for many years (Kinsey, 1953; Waxenberg, 1963). A complete elimination of testosterone, then, does not necessarily produce a total loss of sexual functioning. A man's ability to perform following castration may depend on psychological factors. If a man believes that castration will destroy his manhood, then he may experience sexual dysfunction. But if a man has a more positive attitude, his sexual performance may not be significantly impaired.

We should mention that castration or orchidectomy is distinctly different from *vasectomy*, a surgical procedure used as a form of permanent birth control in men (see Chap. 8). Vasectomy involves the severing of the tubes that carry sperm from the testes to the ejaculatory duct and has nothing to do with the testes, which continue to manufacture sperm and testosterone.

Like humans, castrated male monkeys exhibit a decline in sexual performance, and there is some individual difference in the rate at which the decline occurs (Phoenix, 1974; Phoenix, Slob, and Goy, 1973). Some monkeys show an immediate reduction in sexual activity, whereas others continue to mount and ejaculate for months—and, in a few cases, years—after castration. Castration in lower mammals such as rats, however, produces a more rapid and permanent decline in sexual behavior.

Females Ovariectomy does not appear to have as depressive an effect on sexual behavior in women as castration does on men. Although some women report a loss or decline in sexual functioning, women more commonly experience little, if any, change in their sexual behavior or desires. In a study of 39 ovariectomized women, 75 percent of whom were younger than 35, only 3 (7 percent) experienced a loss of sexual interest. Thirty-six (88 percent) indicated that sex was unchanged, and 2 (5 percent) reported an increase in sexual interest (Filler and Drezner, 1944). Thus it would appear that estrogen has no major effect on human female sexual behavior.

Estrogen levels decline naturally in all women at the time of menopause (see Chap. 14), thus providing another opportunity to examine the effects of estrogen on female sexual behavior. Masters and Johnson (1966) found that postmenopausal women were fully capable of attaining orgasm, although it was generally less intense, was shorter in duration, and took longer to achieve than for premenopausal women.

Recent research suggests that there is a relationship between the level of circulating androgens (testosterone and androstenedione) and sexual interest in women. Small amounts of testosterone are produced by the ovary. As early as 1959, Waxenberg and others demonstrated that sexual desire, sexual activity, and sexual responsiveness were either reduced or eliminated following removal of the adrenals in women who had previously had their ovaries removed. Persky and others (1978) subsequently demonstrated that intercourse frequency was related to a woman's testosterone level at her ovulatory peak.

In contrast to the human female, the rhesus female has been reported to show a sharp, dramatic decline in sexual behavior following ovariectomy and at the end of her offspring-bearing years. This decline ultimately leads to permanent nonreceptivity (Michael and Welgalla, 1968). Male interest in the female also declines following ovariectomy—males rarely ejaculate with females who have been ovariectomized for 3 months or longer (Michael et al., 1967).

More recent research, however, suggests that ovariectomy affects some but not all female patterns of sexual behavior in rhesus monkeys. The removal of the ovaries is associated with fewer female-initiated sexual encounters and with decreased attractiveness to the male (Johnson and Phoenix, 1976). On the other hand, females often continue to accept the advances of males—refusal occurs only if the female has also been adrenalectomized. Thus, as in the case of human females, androgens from the adrenal or ovary may also play a role in sexual behavior. In contrast to primates, ovariectomy in lower mammals such as rats leads to a rapid and permanent decline in sexual activity.

*Effects of hormone
replacement
therapy*

Another way to demonstrate the connection between hormones and sexual behavior is to determine whether externally administered sex hormones can restore sexual behavior after it has been lost through orchidectomy or ovariectomy. This procedure is called ***hormone replacement therapy***.

Males It is clear that injections of testosterone reverse most of the effects of castration (Gordon and Fields, 1943; Heller and Nelson, 1945). The most elegant demonstration of this fact comes from a recent experiment in which men suffering from gonadal failure were treated with testosterone (Davidson et al., 1979). The double-blind aspect of this study makes it unique. Subjects were told that they would receive monthly testosterone injections of varying amounts that would be unknown to them. The subjects were then given monthly injections that consisted of either a small dose, a moderate dose, or no testosterone at all. The medical personnel who interviewed the patients each month and gave them the injections were also blind to which type of injection the subjects received. The researchers noted a dramatic increase in the incidence of erections, masturbation, and intercourse in the months when the injections contained testosterone, whereas sexual activity remained at low levels in months in which the injections contained oil rather than testosterone.

By using the double-blind procedure, the researchers were able to rule out possible experimenter bias and the possibility that the changes in sexual behavior resulted from the fact that the subjects were receiving a psychological boost from the treatment.

Similar results have been reported for rhesus monkeys. The administration of testosterone to castrated male monkeys essentially restores sexual functioning. Males show a return of interest in females, and mounting behavior and ejaculations increase dramatically (Phoenix, 1978). Testosterone replacement therapy also restores sexual behavior in lower mammals such as rats.

Females As we have noted, ovariectomy and menopause do not typically lead to a loss of sexual functioning in the human female. Thus, it is not surprising that injections of estrogen have little effect on sexual behavior and sexual desire in women (Perloff, 1949; Sopchak and Sutherland, 1960). One report, however, has suggested that sexual desire may increase following injections of a combination of estrogen and progesterone (Bakke, 1965). In addition, injections of androgens have also been shown to increase female sexual desire and frequency of intercourse.

The effects of both ovariectomy and estrogen replacement therapy are somewhat different for the rhesus female. Estrogen replacement therapy restores the aspects of female sexual behavior decreased by ovary removal (Wallen and Goy, 1977; Michael et al., 1966). In addition, rhesus males respond to estrogen-treated females as if they were normal, intact females. At least for the rhesus female, then, estrogen may play some role in the expression of sexual activity. Estrogen replacement therapy in lower mammals such as rats is sufficient to restore all aspects of female sexual behavior that are lost through ovariectomy.

*Human sexual
behavior is
affected by a
number of diverse
factors, including
hormones and
experiences.*

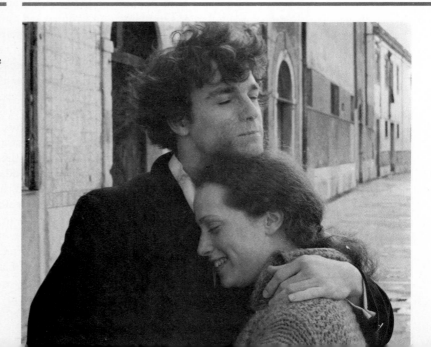

FIGURE 6.8
Role of hormones in regulating the sexual behavior of rats, monkeys, and humans.

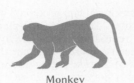 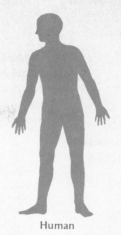

| Rat | | Monkey | | Human | |
Male	Female	Male	Female	Male	Female
Hormone removal (Orchidectomy in males; overiectomy in females)					
Rapid decline in sexual activity	Rapid decline in sexual activity	Fairly rapid decline although a few individuals will show sexual behavior for some months	Fairly rapid decline although some elements of sexual behavior remain	Generally declines although some individuals show sexual behavior for a long time (years)	No decline
Hormone replacement therapy (Testosterone in males; estrogen in females)					
Total restoration of sexual activity	Total restoration of sexual activity	Total restoration of sexual activity	Total restoration of sexual activity	Total restoration of sexual activiy	No effect

Conclusions

There are three general conclusions about the relationship between sex hormones and sexual behavior that can be drawn. First, the sex hormones, especially testosterone, do appear to play some role in the maintenance of human sexual behavior and desire. The presence of testosterone has been found to be important in both male and female sexual behavior. Second, the influence of the sex hormones on sexual behavior varies with the sex of the individual. Male sexual behavior seems to be much more affected by the sex hormones than female sexual behavior. Finally, human sexual behavior as a whole is less dependent on hormones than that of other animals. See Fig. 6.8 for a summary. Even a closely related species such as the rhesus monkey shows a greater reliance on hormones for the expression of sexual behavior. Lower mammals such as rats exhibit an almost total dependence on sex hormones for the maintenance of sexual activity.

As we indicated previously, human sexual behavior is controlled by a number of processes working together. The reduced role of hormones in human sexual behavior compared to that in other animals suggests that other factors, such as experience, are more important in humans. As we unlock the secrets of human sexual functioning, we will be able to more accurately predict the relative importance of and interactions between the hormones and experiences that form the basis for human sexual behavior.

SUMMARY

1   *Hormones* are chemicals produced by the *endocrine glands* that travel to specific target tissues. The endocrine glands that play the greatest role in sexual behavior and reproduction are the *hypothalamus*, the *anterior pituitary*, and the *gonads*. These structures interact through a *negative feedback loop* that keeps the levels of circulating hormones fairly constant. A key hormone in this feedback loop is *gonadotrophin-releasing hormone* (GnRH) from the hypothalamus.

2   Only humans, monkeys, and apes have a *menstrual cycle;* other mammals have an *estrous cycle,* in which the female is sexually receptive only during short periods of the cycle.

3   The four phases of the female menstrual cycle are (1) the *follicular phase,* (2) the *ovulatory phase,* (3) the *luteal phase,* and (4) the *menstrual phase.* The levels of *follicle-stimulating hormone* (FSH), *luteinizing hormone* (LH), *estrogen,* and *progesterone* vary within these four phases.

4   *Ovulation,* the release of an egg, occurs approximately mid-cycle. The time of ovulation can be calculated according to patterns in cycle length, changes in cervical mucus, changes in basal body temperature, and the occurrence of *mittelschmerz* (pain on ovulation). Cycles in which no egg is released are called *anovulatory cycles.*

5   The sloughing of the uterine lining in the fourth phase of the menstrual cycle is called *menstruation.* Many women experience physical problems with menstruation, including *dysmenorrhea* (painful menstruation), *endometriosis* (growth of endometrium on organs other than the uterus), and *amenorrhea* (lack of menstruation).

6   The term *premenstrual tension* is used to describe the syndrome of depression and irritability that some women experience just prior to menstruation. It has been debated whether premenstrual tension actually exists. If it does, hormones may be partly to blame, but research indicates that cultural expectations may also play a role. There is no support for the idea that women's performance deteriorates during menstruation.

7   Unlike women, men maintain fairly constant levels of hormones. However, testosterone levels may vary over the day or as a function of sexual activity and interest. Although it has been suggested that men may have long-term hormonal cycles, this hypothesis is difficult to prove scientifically.

8   There may be a connection between sexual interest and hormonal changes over the menstrual cycle, but if it exists, it is strongly subject to experiential factors.

9   The effects of sex hormones on sexual behavior have been studied in individuals whose gonads have been removed. In males who have undergone *castration* (*orchidectomy*), many experience a decline in sexual desire and eventually become impotent, but some remain sexually active. In women who have undergone *ovariectomy*, there is little effect on sexual behavior.

10 Another approach to studying the effects of hormones is *hormone replacement therapy* following removal of the gonads. In males, replacement of testosterone restores any reduced sexual activity, whereas in females, estrogen replacement has little effect on sexual behavior.

11 Human sexual behavior is less dependent on hormones than that of even closely related animal species such as the rhesus monkey.

ADDITIONAL READING

* Dalton, Katharina. The Menstrual Cycle. New York: Pantheon, 1969.
   A well-written and informative book by a leading authority in the field. Includes information on both the physiology and psychology of menstruation.

Weideger, Paula. Menstruation and Menopause: The Physiology and Psychology, the Myth and the Reality. New York: Knopf, 1976.
   Menstruation, menopause, and the myths and taboos surrounding them. The book is impressive in its detail and quite enjoyable.

Young, William (Ed.). Sex and Internal Secretions (3rd ed.). Baltimore: Williams & Wilkins, 1961.
   Articles on the influence of hormones on human sexual behavior. The book exemplifies the biopsychological approach to human sexual motivation.

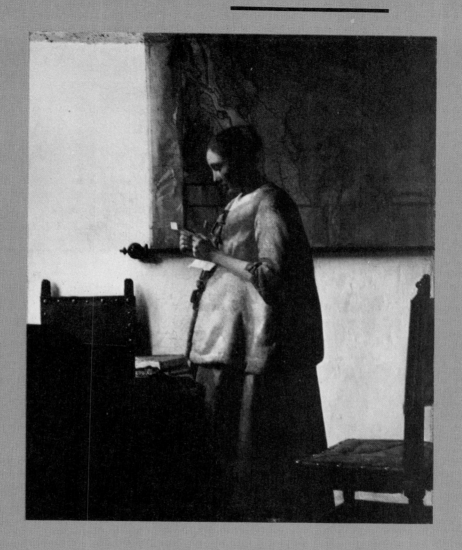

Conception,
pregnancy, and
childbirth

7

chapter

7

Until recently, pregnancy and childbirth, like sex, were not topics for open discussion. Curious adolescents either were rebuked or were given distorted information. Fathers were not allowed to participate in the births of their children. And even pregnant women themselves had to rely on less than totally adequate sources of information. As a result, a certain amount of mystery and mythology has come to surround the events of pregnancy and childbirth. Some of the more common myths include:

Pregnancy is a time of calm serenity. A woman looks more beautiful during pregnancy than at any other time.

Pregnancy is very much like an illness. Women feel poorly and must be cautious about what they do. They may have to stop playing sports or performing their job and may be confined to bed at certain times.

Sexual intercourse during pregnancy, especially during the last 3 months, is dangerous to the fetus.

Women who have given birth to a baby by cesarean section must have all of their subsequent babies delivered in the same way.

More reliable information about conception, pregnancy, and childbirth is necessary to dispel such myths and to equip people to deal effectively and realistically with these very basic processes of life.

Pregnancy can be a shared, rewarding experience for both mother- and father-to-be.

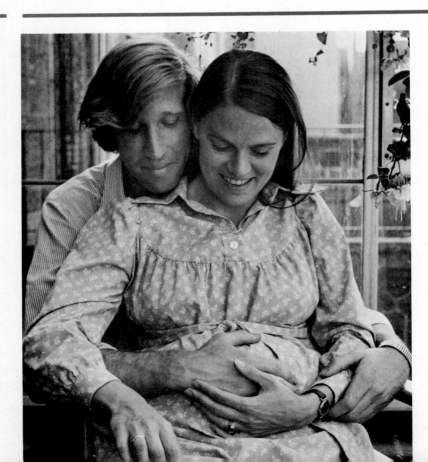

FIGURE 7.1
*The color line shows the
pathway along which
sperm travels to
meet the egg. Sperm
is released from the
testes, carried along
ducts through the
shaft of the penis,
and ejaculated into
the vagina. From
there, the sperm
swim through the
cervix, up the uterus,
and into the fallo-
pian tubes where
fertilization occurs
if an egg is present.
The black arrows show
the pathway of the
egg from the ovary
to the uterus.
Eggs are usually
released once per
month from the
ovary, enter the
fallopian tube, and
have a finite life of
about 2 days. If
fertilized, the egg
is then implanted
in the uterus.
Unfertilized eggs
pass through the
uterus and are
shed through the
vagina during
menstruation.*

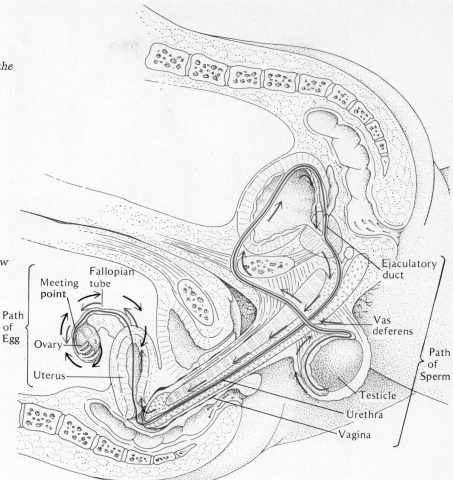

CONCEPTION

Conception, or ***fertilization***, is the process by which a sperm unites with an egg. Under normal circumstances, sperm are deposited in the woman's vagina during sexual intercourse (see Fig. 7.1). Millions of sperm enter the uterus through the cervix and swim up into the fallopian tubes. If an egg is present within the fallopian tubes, millions of sperm will surround it, and a single spermatozoa will penetrate the egg, causing it to subdivide. At this precise moment, conception has occurred. The egg immediately becomes impermeable to other sperm that may attempt to penetrate it (see Fig. 7.2).

Conceiving a baby is a complex event. It may not seem so to a woman

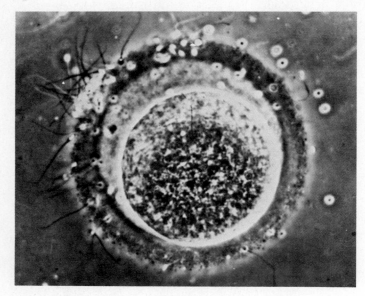

FIGURE 7.2
*Micrograph depict-
ing the union of
sperm and egg. Al-
though many
sperm (as shown
by small white cir-
cles) will surround
the egg, only one
will get through
and actually ferti-
lize the egg.*

with an unwanted pregnancy or to one who has conceived after only one act of intercourse, but it is true. The average fertile couple takes 4–6 months to achieve pregnancy (Macy and Faulkner, 1979), and it is not uncommon for couples to need 8 months.

Successful union of egg and sperm is essentially a problem of timing—one that is complicated by two factors. First, although men can deposit sperm into the woman's vagina at any time, the woman's ovaries usually release only one egg per month. Second, this single egg can only be fertilized during a short interval within that month (usually 12–24 hours). The objective for couples seeking to have children is to time intercourse so that it coincides with the release of the egg. There is some leeway, however, because sperm can live in the female reproductive tract for about 2 days while waiting for the egg. Thus, there is probably a 3-day period during each menstrual cycle in which conception can occur. However, given the difficulties in pinpointing ovulation (see Chaps. 6 and 8), it is not surprising that couples require several months to get the timing right.

The likelihood of conceiving a child is also affected by the age of the participants and their frequency of intercourse. In general, fertility is low in women during the early teenage years, increases to a peak at age 24, and then declines, with a rapid drop after the age of 30 (Behrman and Kistner, 1968). A similar peak is seen in males at age 25, followed by a pattern of decline (MacLeod and Gold, 1953). It should be kept in mind, however, that some of the effects attributed to aging may be related to the fact that frequency of intercourse also drops with age.

TABLE 7.1	Average frequency of intercourse	Number of cases	Conceptions in under 6 months (percent)
Percent of conceptions in less than 6 months for various rates of intercourse	less than 1 per week	24	16.7
	1 but less than 2 per week	109	32.1
	2 but less than 3 per week	123	46.3
	3 but less than 4 per week	100	51.0
	4 per week or more	72	83.3

Source: MacLeod and Gold (1953), p. 10.

As Table 7.1 shows, conception is best achieved when the frequency of intercourse is four or more times a week (MacLeod and Gold, 1953). Of course, a couple can still be successful with a substantially lower average frequency of intercourse, provided that they time their sexual activity with ovulation.

Infertility

Some couples experience difficulty in trying to conceive children. This was the case for Bill and Kathy (Chap. 1), who became frustrated and anxious when their attempts to create a baby failed. Approximately 25 percent of all couples are unable to achieve pregnancy even after a year of trying. Of these couples, 10 percent are probably sterile. While it is common to blame the wife for reproductive failure, this problem is more often the result of lowered fertility on the part of *both* partners. Some of the most common causes of infertility in women are:

1 *Developmental abnormalities—the failure of ovaries to develop, so that ovulation does not occur.*
2 *Diseases such as gonorrhea or endometriosis, which may permanently damage the fallopian tubes, ovaries, or uterus.*
3 *Surgery such as ovariectomy (removal of the ovaries) or hysterectomy (removal of the uterus or removal of the fallopian tubes).*
4 *Physical defects, such as blocked fallopian tubes, that prevent sperm from reaching the egg and block implantation.*
5 *Development of endocrine imbalances that may cause ovulation failure.*
6 *Abnormal or hostile cervical mucus, which may kill sperm.*
7 *Antibody reactions to sperm.*
8 *Poor general physical health, such as malnutrition.*
9 *Emotional problems—some of which may arise as a result of infertility.*
10 *Incomplete, inadequate, and mistimed sexual relations.*

The causes of infertility in men include:

1 *Impaired production of sperm as a result of testicular tumors, undescended testes, and other such problems.*
2 *Diseases such as gonorrhea or syphilis.*
3 *Surgery such as castration (removal of the testes) or vasectomy (cutting of the vas deferens, thereby preventing passage of sperm to the ejaculatory duct).*
4 *Low quantities of sperm or sperm with poor motility.*
5 *Interference with the passage of sperm through the genital ducts because of prostate enlargement or similar disorders.*

6   *Poor general physical health.*
7   *Emotional problems, some of which may arise as a result of infertility.*
8   *Incomplete, inadequate, and mistimed sexual relations.*

Before a couple becomes deeply frustrated by their failure to have children, they should seek medical help, in the form of a **fertility workup.** The purposes of the fertility workup are threefold: (1) to educate the couple about the timing of sexual relations, (2) to identify the causes of infertility, and (3) to provide some possible solutions.

At the beginning of the workup, couples are asked to describe their sexual relations in detail to rule out the possibility of mistiming or inadequate responses. Women are encouraged to keep a record of their daily basal body temperature so that they can learn to estimate the day of ovulation (see Chap. 6). They are also encouraged to use the missionary position (man on top) for maximal penetration with minimal sperm leakage. If a couple seem particularly frustrated about the situation, they may be urged to see a therapist to help reduce their anxieties.

Next, the husband and wife are evaluated on a variety of tests to measure their fertility. For the woman, these include the **Huehner test,** which examines the cervical mucus for the presence of sperm after intercourse, and the **Rubin test,** which determines whether the fallopian tubes are open. As a part of the Rubin test, carbon dioxide is passed through the uterus and into the fallopian tubes. If the tubes are open, the gas flows into the abdominal cavity. By examining pressure gauges, the physician can determine whether the tubes are open or closed. Although this procedure can be painful, it sometimes has the beneficial side effect of actually causing partially closed tubes to open. A newer, less painful procedure, called a **hysterosalpingogram,** involves the injection of radioactive dye through the cervix into the uterus and fallopian tubes. Using an X-ray machine, the physician can then determine whether the tubes are open.

For the man, fertility is assessed through examination of the semen for the quality and quantity of sperm. Of particular importance is sperm motility, since the sperm must travel long distances to reach the egg. Sheer number of sperm per volume of ejaculate is also important, although the cutoff point between fertility and infertility is not well established. In the past, some authorities used a value of 60 million sperm per milliliter of ejaculate as the cutoff point. Today, the cutoff may be closer to 10 million sperm per milliliter. Although males who fall below the 60 million range tend to have more difficulty achieving conception, they are clearly capable of impregnating a woman (Mastroianni, 1975).

After all test results have been obtained, possible solutions to the infertility problem are presented. In some cases, improved general health, better timing of sexual relations, or reduced anxiety may be all that is needed. In other cases, the problem may be much more complex.

If a woman fails to ovulate regularly, certain fertility drugs may be prescribed. The two most commonly used fertility drugs are **pergonal** and **clomi-**

phene citrate. Pergonal, which directly stimulates the ovaries, has the unwanted side effect of multiple births. This twinning, tripling, quadrupling, and quintupling with pergonal is probably the result of suppression of the negative feedback loop between the ovaries and the hypothalamus. Clomiphene, which has a lower probability of producing multiple offspring (twins at the most), acts by stimulating FSH, which in turn stimulates egg development. There is no disruption of the negative feedback loop with this drug. Even with the use of such drugs, fertility is not guaranteed. Of the women who take clomiphene, for example, 75 percent will probably ovulate. Of these, only about 40 percent will actually become pregnant. And of those who become pregnant, a certain percentage will miscarry (Rakoff, 1977).

If a man's sperm are of poor quality or quantity, artificial insemination by the husband (AIH) may be attempted. One of the advantages of AIH over natural intercourse is that the man's ejaculate can be divided into two portions. Only the first half of the ejaculate, which has a higher concentration of motile sperm, is used in the artificial insemination process.

If the husband is clearly infertile and his condition cannot be improved, the couple might want to consider artificial insemination by donor (AID). Sperm are obtained from a sperm bank donor who physically resembles the prospective father in hair color, eye color, general body build, and so on. Every year about 20,000 children are born through AID (Fleming, 1980). Despite AID's usefulness in achieving pregnancy, there are several potential problems associated with its use. First, the husband has to be psychologically prepared to accept a child whom he didn't father. This is not the same as adoption, in which case neither the father nor the mother is related to the child. Second, there may be numerous legal arguments over the status of a child produced by AID. In some states, for example, an AID-produced child is considered illegitimate and must be adopted by the husband. Also in question are the rights of the donor, if any, to the child(ren) he indirectly sires. As of now, the donor is uninformed about the use of his sperm. In the future, however, donors or their offspring may be able to demand such information in the same way that some adopted children demand information about their biological parents. One way of circumventing some of these problems is to mix some of the husband's ejaculate with the donor's output. If the husband has any sperm at all, there is at least some chance that the resulting child will be his. While the statistical likelihood may be minimal, the psychological benefits can be enormous.

Women can also serve as donors. Such female donors are called **surrogates** (Grobstein, 1979). When a couple cannot conceive because of the woman's infertility, the husband may contribute his sperm for artificial insemination of a woman surrogate, who will conceive the child, carry it to term, and then turn the baby over to the childless couple. Problems can also arise with this procedure. The surrogate may decide to keep "her" baby. In addition, the legal status of the child, the rights of the surrogate mother, and the rights of the adopting parents are still unclear.

Infertility can be a source of frustration and embarrassment for couples who desire to have children. Well-meaning parents and friends may constantly bring up the joys of parenthood. Fortunately, some of the problems that cause infertility can be identified through fertility workups and resolved with appropriate treatment. The chances for a successful pregnancy after medical consultation vary from 20 to 50 percent (about 1 out of 3). For the remainder, adoption is probably the only recourse. With the legalization of abortion, however, the pool of available infants has become smaller. Thus, a number of couples will remain childless despite their desire to have and raise children.

*Test-tube
babies*

In 1978 the world was rocked by the news of the birth of the first *test-tube baby*. This baby, Louise Brown, had been created by the union of the mother's egg and father's sperm outside the mother's body. Thirty-year-old Lesley Brown and her husband had tried for 9 years to have a child. When they had a fertility workup, it was discovered that Mrs. Brown had scarred and blocked fallopian tubes that prevented conception. Using techniques perfected by physicians Robert Edwards and Patrick Steptoe, some of Mrs. Brown's ova were extracted and were then fertilized by her husband's sperm in a culture plate. After the eggs started to divide, they were incubated. Finally, one of these masses of cells was inserted into Lesley Brown's uterus, where it implanted in the uterine wall. She had been given hormone injections so that her uterus would be ready to receive the embryo. Pregnancy and childbirth subsequently proceeded normally. At the end of 9 months, the healthy, 8-pound Louise was born.

The successful fertilization of an egg outside of a woman's body was a major scientific accomplishment based on extensive research by many scientists. Procedures had to be developed for transferring the ova from the woman to the culture medium, for growing or maintaining ova, for providing the necessary nutrition for the embryo prior to implantation, and for introducing the embryo into the uterus so that implantation could occur. This last procedure is particularly difficult, as it is often impossible to determine exactly when the woman's uterus is ready to receive the embryo. As a result, the success rate for this procedure is less than 10 percent. In fact, Lesley Brown was implanted 156 times before the procedure was finally successful.

Although the advent of the test-tube baby is a startling development and may provide hope for hundreds of childless couples, it will be years before this method can go into any widespread use. Its high cost, high failure rate, and other attendant problems present major stumbling blocks. To some, the tampering with the natural process of conception is both unethical and immoral. To others, it raises the possibility of genetic programming, in which the state or some other entity determines who breeds with whom. If these problems and objections can be overcome, test-tube conception may become a useful method for improving the fertility of childless couples.

PREGNANCY

Pregnancy is a time of great change both for the woman and for the growing organism within her. Major alterations in hormone levels, body shape, and psychological state are a necessary and natural consequence for the mother. These changes are brought about by an amazing process that transforms a single fertilized egg into a human infant.

The average length of pregnancy from conception to birth is approximately 9 months (280 days or 40 weeks). This timespan is usually referred to as *gestation*. The probable date of birth is usually estimated by adding 280 days to the first day of the last menstrual period. As many mothers will attest, these estimates are often inaccurate. Even under normal conditions, pregnancy may last longer than expected or may be foreshortened by a few days or weeks. As one might expect, the more regular a woman's menstrual cycle, the more accurate the estimate. Pregnancy is usually divided into three periods, or *trimesters*, each lasting about 3 months. Although there is no dramatic demarcation dividing these periods, there are sufficient changes between them to make the distinction useful.

Many women suspect that they are pregnant before the pregnancy is actually confirmed by medical tests. Their inkling is often based on several typical signs of pregnancy that appear soon after conception. The most common sign is a missed menstrual period. The blood-engorged uterine lining, which is ordinarily shed if the egg is not fertilized, remains to provide nourishment for the developing embryo. A missed period is not always indicative of pregnancy, but pregnancy is by far the most common reason for a missed period in women between the ages of 17 and 39. In addition, women generally experience enlargement and tenderness of the breasts, darkening of the pigmented area (areola) around the nipples, more frequent urination, and morning sickness.

The most uncomfortable of these signs is **morning sickness**, or nausea, which occurs in about 50 percent of all pregnant women. Actually, morning sickness can be felt at any time of the day and seems to be related to an empty stomach. Feelings of nausea are first noticed about 6 weeks after the last menstrual period, and they subside between the eighth and twelfth weeks. Possible causes of morning sickness range from physiological factors, such as hormones, to psychological factors, such as feelings of ambivalence about the coming baby. In the physiological realm, the hormone **human chorionic gona-dotropin** (HCG) is most often implicated because its increase and decrease seem to parallel the onset and subsequent decline of nausea. This hormone, which will be discussed later, begins to be secreted shortly after conception, reaches a peak at approximately 10 weeks from the last menstrual period, and then declines.

In the psychological realm, a woman's attitude toward pregnancy may affect the incidence and severity of nausea. In one study, for example, Chertok (1963) interviewed pregnant women in their third month and divided them into three groups on the basis of their attitudes toward pregnancy: those with a positive attitude (the child was desired, and pregnancy was greeted with joy), those with a negative attitude (the child was unwanted, but the mother had to endure it), and those with an ambivalent attitude (the child was both wanted and unwanted). What Chertok discovered was that the majority of women who

experienced nausea and vomiting fell into the ambivalent group. Similarly,
Wolkind and Zajicek (1978) found that women who experienced little or no
nausea during pregnancy had high positive feelings in early pregnancy that
declined somewhat as birth approached. Nauseated women had less positive
feelings (ambivalence) in early pregnancy, but these feelings became somewhat
more positive as the birth approached. We must be cautious in interpreting
these findings, however, as it may be that the nausea made the women
ambivalent rather than the other way around.

Pregnancy tests Women seldom react to a missed period with indifference
or nonchalance. For the woman trying to become pregnant, it may be a happy
sign. For the woman who does not wish a child at this time, it is cause for
great concern. In either case, the woman should and usually does seek a
pregnancy test to confirm or deny her suspicions.

There are a number of chemical and physical tests for pregnancy that
cannot be performed until about 6–8 weeks after the last menstrual period.
The typical chemical tests for pregnancy are based on the presence of HCG in
the urine or blood of the presumably pregnant woman. These tests are 95–98
percent accurate if they are made at least 6 weeks after the last menstrual
period. A more recently developed test, **beta subunit HCG radioimmunoassay**,
can detect HCG in the blood as early as 8 days after conception. It is not
widely used, however, because it is expensive.

Several home preganancy test kits are now available in drugstores. One
should note, however, that these kits are not inexpensive, can be used only
once, have extensive instructions that must be followed meticulously, and
have an accuracy rate lower than that of lab tests. In addition, some women
may be lulled into thinking that these home kits can replace a visit to the
doctor.

There are also several physical tests that a doctor can conduct to confirm
pregnancy. The most common is the test for **Hegar's sign**, which is a change in
the consistency of the lower part of the uterus from a firm to a soft state that
is detectable via pelvic examination. This change is manifested as early as the
sixth week after the onset of the last menstrual period.

Prenatal care Once a woman is sure of her pregnancy, she should seek
medical care. Women often use the services of a physician (obstetrician) and
clinical programs that specialize in pregnancy and childbirth. Prenatal-care
programs provide information for the prospective mother, assess her general
health, monitor her weight gain, prepare for possible abnormalities during
delivery, and make an important contribution to the successful delivery of a
healthy baby. Some obstetricians feel so strong about prenatal care that they
refuse to attend the deliveries of women who have not been through their
prenatal program.

During the first prenatal visit, the woman provides a complete medical
history, including information about past menstrual cycles, previous pregnancies, any miscarriages, childhood diseases, hereditary conditions, and so on.
She also receives a thorough pelvic examination, and her pelvic girdle is

measured to make sure that a typical vaginal delivery is possible. Blood and urine samples are taken for additional tests. Subsequently, the woman sees her doctor approximately once a month during the first 6 or 7 months and then more often until the time of delivery.

Changes in the woman   In some respects, the first trimester has an enormous impact on the woman, while in other respects, it hardly affects her at all. Some of the most important changes that occur during this time involve hormonal developments that allow for the maintenance of pregnancy. A woman usually becomes pregnant mid-cycle, when estrogen levels are high and progesterone levels are rising. The secretion of these hormones is controlled by the corpus luteum. Whereas within a nonconception cycle the corpus luteum has a life span of about 12 days, in a conception cycle there is a mechanism that keeps the corpus luteum alive and functioning after the egg has implanted in the uterine wall. This mechanism seems to involve HCG. HCG is released by cells formed from the fertilized egg and stimulates the corpus luteum to continue its production of estrogen and progesterone. By the seventh to ninth week after the last menstrual period, the burden of producing these hormones shifts from the corpus luteum to the **placenta**, the blood-engorged mass of tissue that connects the growing offspring to the mother. Interestingly, HCG declines to lower levels coincident with this shift in responsibility (see Fig. 7.3).

Unlike estrogen and progesterone, which increase across pregnancy, the gonadotropins FSH and LH, produced by the pituitary, are uninvolved in pregnancy. FSH and LH remain at low levels throughout the 9-month period. On the other hand, the pituitary does produce another hormone, **prolactin**, which increases severalfold over the span of pregnancy and acts to stimulate breast development for the purpose of breast-feeding (Tolis, 1980).

Besides hormonal changes, women also undergo some physical changes in the first trimester. Most of these changes are the signs of pregnancy we have already noted: cessation of menstrual periods, enlargement and tenderness of

FIGURE 7.3
*Changes in the
levels of HCG
during pregnancy.
(Mishell, Wide,
and Gemzell,
1963)*

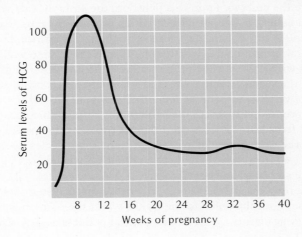

the breasts, increase in the size of the nipples, darkening of the areola, increased frequency of urination, and morning sickness. There is little in the way of overt body changes, as the growing organism is not yet big enough to produce a pronounced bulge in the abdomen.

Women do undergo changes in mood and anxiety during pregnancy. In particular, anxiety seems to rise during the first trimester. Much of this nervousness is simply related to the natural adjustment to being pregnant (Lubin, 1975). During the third month, a majority of women still find it difficult to believe that the fetus is really there. This is not surprising given that there is no movement of the organism or any substantial increase in the size of the abdomen. In addition, however, many women find it hard to imagine the fetus or to create a mental picture of it and do not think of it as a real individual (Macy and Faulkner, 1979). Although the majority of women react this way, about one-third of all pregnant women can and do think of the organism as their baby—a real entity—by the end of the third month.

Changes in the growing organism   Following fertilization, the egg travels down through the fallopian tube toward the uterus, growing and dividing as it moves along. Within about 36 hours after conception, the egg has divided into 2 cells, and at 60 hours a second division has lead to the formation of 4 cells. On the third day, the dividing cells have formed a ball of 16 cells. This ball is referred to as a **morula**, and this point in development is called the **morula stage**. At 96 hours, or on the fourth day, the morula changes into a hollow ball of cells called the **blastocyst**. The blastocyst continues to grow and float freely in the uterine cavity for about 2 days before **implantation** occurs. The beginning of implantation officially marks the onset of pregnancy.

Implantation is commonly thought of as a simple, rapidly occurring event. In reality, however, it is a complex process that begins at the end of the first week and continues through the second week after conception. As the blastocyst becomes attached to the endometrium, its outer cells form two membranes: the outer **chorion** (the source of HCG) and the inner **amnion**, which will encircle the embryo. From this point on, the embryo is surrounded by the amnion and bathed in amniotic fluid, which provides an aquatic environment for the organism until birth. As soon as the chorion is formed, it develops fingerlike projections, called **villi**, that push into the uterine wall. These projections, along with parts of the uterine wall, ultimately form the placenta.

During the second week of life, the embryo becomes organized into a disc consisting of three layers: the **endoderm**, the **mesoderm**, and the **ectoderm**. It is from these primordial layers that all the types of tissue that constitute the embryo and fetus arise. The ectoderm forms the nervous system, the sensory organs, and the skin. From the mesoderm come the muscles, skeleton, and circulatory, excretory, and reproductive systems. The endoderm gives rise to the digestive and respiratory systems.

In the third week of life, most of the major organ systems begin to develop. From the third week to the eighth week, the embryo is highly sensitive to drugs, viruses, and environmental pollutants. Any assault by these substances during this period can result in congenital defects, such as missing limbs, cleft palate, and other abnormalities.

The first major organ to form is the primitive nervous system, in the form of a **neural groove**, which will ultimately become the spinal cord and brain. Next come the rudimentary heart, blood vessels, gut, and muscles. The eyes begin to form at 21 days. A tube representing the fetal heart begins to pulsate on the twenty-fourth day.

During the fourth week, the embryo changes from a flattened disc to an enclosed cylinder curved like the letter C. Because of this curvature, the length of the embryo is usually measured from the top of the head (crown) to the rump—termed the **crown-to-rump** or **CR measurement**. By the end of the fourth week, there is a discernible head, which is quite large in proportion to the trunk, and a tail. At the end of this first month of development, the embryo has reached the size of 5 millimeters (0.2 inch) and has increased in mass about 7000 times. However, it looks little like a human being at this stage.

As the sixth week of development comes to a close, the embryo has a four-chambered heart that pumps blood, upper and lower limb buds, the beginnings of a nose and upper lip, and rudimentary ears and eyelids. At this point the embryo is 11–14 millimeters (about 0.5 inch) long (see Fig. 7.4).

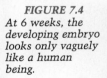

*FIGURE 7.4
At 6 weeks, the
developing embryo
looks only vaguely
like a human
being.*

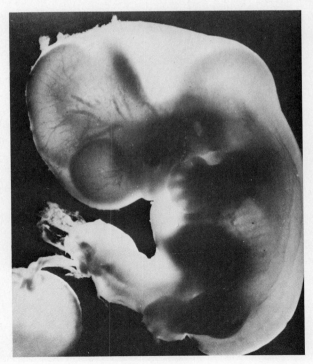

By the end of the eighth week, all of the major organ systems have begun development, and many are complete. Externally, the 31-millimeter (1.25-inch) embryo has a large head and brain, with discernible facial features. The limbs are formed, and fingers and toes are readily visible. The sex of the embryo is still unknown, because the genitals have not yet fully formed. It is at this point, when the embryo begins to resemble a human being, that it becomes a fetus. The characteristic posture of the fetus, persisting throughout most of pregnancy, is with the head bent forward, the arms folded against the chest, and the knees pulled up to the abdomen.

During the final 4 weeks of the first trimester, the fetus grows in size, reaching a length of 100 millimeters (4 inches) (see Fig. 7.5). At this point, the fetus weighs about 19 grams (0.6 ounce). During this time, facial features become more distinct, nails are formed, and the highly individualized lines on the surface of the hands and feet, which give rise to prints, develop. In addition, the kidneys and lungs begin to develop even though they are not used until birth. Finally, in the eleventh week, the sex of the fetus, as determined by the external genitals, emerges (see Chap. 5).

FIGURE 7.5
Human characteristics are readily apparent in this 12-week-old fetus, which is only 100 millimeters (4 inches) long and weighs about 19 grams (0.6 ounce).

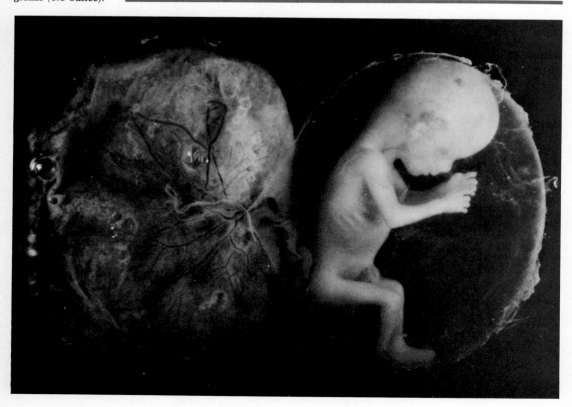

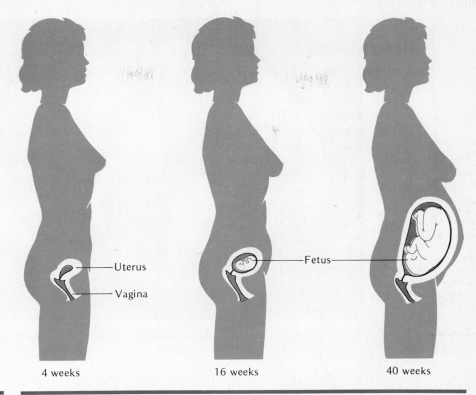

FIGURE 7.6
Growth of the
uterus during
pregnancy. Note
also the change in
the shape of the
abdomen and
breasts.

Uterus

Vagina

Fetus

4 weeks   16 weeks   40 weeks

**The second
trimester**

Changes in the woman The second trimester is generally considered to be a period of calm and tranquillity. The discomforts of the first trimester have passed, and the anxieties over delivery and birth are not yet present. Perhaps the most dramatic event during the second trimester is the mother's first detection of fetal movements *(quickening).* Such movements arise in the fourth month and continue throughout the rest of pregnancy. The quickening is an important event because it signifies to the mother that the fetus exists—that it is a real and living entity. From this point on, the fetus regularly moves, kicks, squirms, and even hiccups.

The primary hormonal events of the second trimester are the gradual increases in prolactin, estrogen, and progesterone. Physically, the woman's waistline expands rapidly, and maternity clothes may be needed as early as the fourth month (see Fig. 7.6). Women may also experience *edema*—swelling of the limbs, particularly the lower legs and ankles, as a result of water retention. In general, however, the mother is excited about the movements of the fetus and has few, if any, unpleasant symptoms during this period.

Changes in the fetus The primary changes in the fetus during the second trimester involve development of mobility, a small but substantial increase in

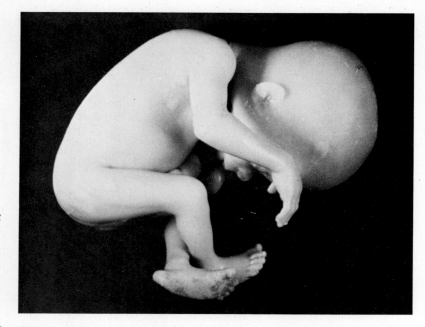

*FIGURE 7.7
By 20 weeks, the
fetus looks very
much like a young
baby. Because of
inadequate lung
development,
however, few of
these fetuses are
capable of living
outside the body
of the mother.*

size, and growth of a protective covering. The protective coating, called the
vernix caseosa, is oily, has a cheeselike texture, and probably serves to protect
the skin of the fetus from becoming irritated by constant contact with the
amniotic fluid. The growth of downy hair, **lanugo**, throughout the body of the
fetus may help to keep the vernix next to the skin. The fetus begins to move
its arms and kick its legs at the beginning of the fourth month, although such
movements are not detected by the mother until the fetus is several weeks
older. The fetus also possesses such reflexes as sucking and swallowing (see
Fig. 7.7). In the sixth month it responds to external sounds and to being
palpated through the mother's abdominal wall by increasing its heart rate.

At the end of the fifth month, at the rough midpoint of pregnancy, the
fetus has increased in size to 190 millimeters (7.6 inches) long and weighs 0.45
kilogram (1 pound). Nearly 90 percent of the total weight gain of the fetus
occurs between the beginning of the sixth month and birth. It is almost
impossible for a fetus to survive if it is expelled prior to the end of 6 months.

*The third
trimester*

Changes in the woman During the third trimester, the woman's abdomen
becomes increasingly large and rotund and she normally gains about 6.8–9
kilograms (15–20 pounds). Most women view the changes in their body shape
with mixed feelings. On the one hand, they may feel pride in the bulge because
it signifies pregnancy. On the other hand, the huge belly may be a source of
dismay for women who previously had a slim figure or for overweight women
who may resent a further increase in size. Nearly all women who are pregnant

with their first baby wonder whether their body will ever return to its prepregnancy shape. Wives may also be concerned about their attractiveness to their husbands.

As the fetus and uterus increase in size, there is growing stress on the mother's internal organs. The uterus may press on the lungs, causing shortness of breath, or on the stomach, producing indigestion. The heart is also strained as a result of the large increase—in some cases 40–50 percent—in blood volume. Not all of this blood volume increase is attributable to the growing fetus; some of it may serve to provide a cushion against blood loss (about 0.473–0.946 liters or 1–2 pints) during delivery.

Occasional painless uterine contractions, called **Braxton Hicks contractions**, may occur in the third trimester. These contractions have no direct relationship to the onset of labor; they are thought to strengthen the uterine muscles, thereby preparing them for labor.

Sometime during the third week prior to birth, the baby turns its head and enters the pelvic region. This movement, variously called **lightening, dropping,** or **engagement**, positions the baby for a head-first birth presentation.

In contrast to the calmness of the second trimester, the third trimester may be characterized by increased psychological stress. There is a rise in the frequency of mild emotional problems, especially in the last 6 weeks (Sherman, 1971). In addition, women may find horrible thoughts entering their dreams or fantasies (Macy and Faulkner, 1979). They may dream of accidents in which they are mutilated or give birth to a baby that is badly deformed or dead. But the most distressing dreams are those in which the mother behaves bizarrely toward the child, such as cooking and eating it. Despite the disturbing content of such dreams, they are common and quite normal in late pregnancy.

The third trimester is also a time for contemplation and reviewing of one's self-image (Macy and Faulkner, 1979). As pregnancy progresses, the woman may find herself recalling her past—brief reminiscences of interactions with her mother, events during courtship, perhaps an episode in school. According to psychologists, these are not random thoughts but rather are part of a process by which the woman reevaluates her self-image and adjusts it for the impending role of motherhood (Rubin, 1967).

Changes in the fetus The major development during the third trimester is fetal growth. The fetus actually doubles in size during the final 2 months, although its rate of growth slows down as birth approaches. At the end of the eighth month the fetus weighs, on the average, 2.38 kilograms (5.25 pounds). The average full-term fetus weighs in at 3.4 kilograms (7.5 pounds) and is 500 millimeters (20 inches) long.

At 8 months, the eyelids are open, and the testes of the male have descended into the scrotum. There is often considerable growth of scalp hair and fingernails. Most important, the central nervous system enlarges and expands, as evidenced by an increased rate of formation of brain cells and nerve connections.

Prior to the seventh month, the fetal lungs are not developed sufficiently to support life outside the body of the mother. During the last trimester, however, babies may be born early and survive. A baby born at the end of the seventh month has a 50 percent chance of survival; at the end of 8 months, a 90 percent chance of survival; and at the end of 9 months (normal term), a 99 percent chance of survival. Babies born during the seventh or eighth month are **premature** (if they weigh less than 2500 grams) and are considered to have a higher risk of encountering problems during development.

CONCERNS DURING PREGNANCY

Because pregnancy is a time of major physical and psychological change, the mother may develop some concerns about the effects of her behavior on the fetus and subsequently on the baby. The three most common areas of concern are weight gain and nutrition, sexual activity, and drugs and chemicals.

Weight gain and nutrition

Although thoughts about the ideal weight gain during pregnancy have fluctuated over the years, doctors currently recommend that women gain no more than 9–11 kilograms (19.9–24.3 pounds) during pregnancy. This figure is based on the assumption that the woman's weight is normal at the start. Slender women may be allowed to gain more, heavier women less. The newborn infant accounts for only about 3.4 kilograms (7.5 pounds) of this weight gain. The rest can be attributed to the placenta (about 0.45 kilogram or 1 pound), the amniotic fluid (about 0.95 kilograms or 2 pounds), enlargement of the uterus (0.9 kilogram or 2 pounds), enlargement of the breasts (about 0.68 kilogram or 1.5 pounds), and additional fat and water retained by the woman (about 2.37 kilograms or 5.2 pounds).

Some women mistakenly think that after becoming pregnant they need to eat for two. This kind of thinking can lead to excessive weight gain and perhaps to serious health problems. An increased weight gain over the recommended level in the third trimester may be associated with **toxemia**, a potentially life-threatening condition. Toxemia is characterized by edema, by a marked increase in blood pressure **(hypertension)**, and by the excretion of protein in the urine **(proteinuria)**. A woman with these symptoms is said to be in a state of **preeclampsia**. If these symptoms are not detected and treated in time, the woman may enter a state of **eclampsia**, which is characterized by convulsions and coma. While only 5 percent of women with toxemia go into the dangerous state of eclampsia, nearly 15 percent of those who do will die. The cause of toxemia is unknown, although it does occur most often in first pregnancies.

What a woman ingests during pregnancy is very important. In this period she has to satisfy the nutritional needs of both her own body and that of the child growing inside her. Thus, she should pay particular attention to protein, vitamins, and minerals (especially iron). If a woman's diet is nutritionally rich, she has an excellent chance of staying healthy and giving birth to a healthy child. The consequences of a poor diet have been demonstrated in a study comparing women on a nutritious diet to women on a poor diet. Mothers who followed a poor diet had four times as many health problems during pregnancy, seven times as many threatened or actual miscarriages, three times as many stillbirths, and longer labor than did mothers with nutritious diets (Newton, 1972).

*Sexual
activity*

Until recently, doctors took a restrictive view of intercourse during pregnancy. They routinely recommended that sexual activity cease at the end of the seventh month and be reinstated no earlier than 6 weeks after birth. Although most of this prohibition was directed toward sexual intercourse, other sexual activities leading to orgasm in the female were also considered to be dangerous. This restrictive medical view was based on the concerns that the woman or fetus might somehow develop an infection that would disrupt pregnancy and that sexual activity might prematurely induce labor and childbirth.

Today, most physicians see no reason to restrict sexual activity during late pregnancy, provided that there is no cervical dilation, bleeding, or rupture of the amniotic membrane surrounding the fetus. Sexual intercourse should also be limited if the woman feels pain, experiences bleeding or uterine cramps following intercourse, or is at high risk for miscarriage. High-risk women include those who are over 35, who have diseases such as diabetes, or who have a previous history of miscarriage or premature births. Women who fall into these categories should consult their doctor about sexual intercourse. Other forms of sexual activity (mutual masturbation, fellatio, cunnilingus, and so on) may be preferable and more appropriate, depending on the circumstances. One precaution should be noted, however. Husbands should avoid blowing air into the vagina during cunnilingus, as the increased carbon dioxide concentrations can be fatal to fetus and mother should the cervical plug be loose.

Sexual activity need not be limited for a long period of time after birth. Given the rapid recovery from the birth process, women may be able to enjoy sexual intercourse as early as a few weeks after birth and other forms of sexual activity as soon as desired. This is fortunate, as sexual responsiveness apparently does not wane through most of pregnancy. Women report that they continue to have intercourse at nearly their normal rate until the beginning or middle of the eighth month (Wagner and Solberg, 1974). A slight decrease can be detected for the seventh and eighth months, but it is not until the ninth month that substantial numbers of women refrain from intercourse.

Sexual intercourse may become more awkward as the woman's belly increases in size. This is especially true for the missionary (man-on-top) position, but most couples improvise quite readily and adopt other positions. Many find that a side-to-side orientation is more comfortable. The couple may also use the situation to explore other types of noncoital sexual activities. All in all, women may be surprised at their capacity to respond to and enjoy sex in the last trimester.

*Drugs and
chemicals*

It is becoming increasingly clear that a wide variety of drugs and chemicals can cross the placental barrier from the mother to the fetus and have a profound effect on the growing organism. A woman should be aware that certain prescription drugs, some over-the-counter drugs, various environmental pollutants, cigarette smoke, alcohol, and a variety of everyday cleaning substances may fall into this category. The extent of the damage may be subtle or may be so profound as to produce severe mental retardation or abnormal skeletal development. Substances that can alter structural development and produce congenital defects are called *teratogens.*

The devastating effects that drugs can have was dramatically demonstrated in the case of thalidomide, a mild tranquilizer that was prescribed for pregnant women back in the 1950s, primarily in Europe. If taken during the first trimester, this drug inhibited the growth of fetal limb buds. As a result, several thousand babies were born with flipperlike appendages in the place of arms or legs. Following this experience, some national governments moved to pass more stringent drug laws.

There are many other drugs and chemicals that are potentially dangerous to the fetus, including antihistamines; insulin; cortisone; antithyroid drugs; some local anesthetics such as lidocaine; antibiotics such as chloramphenicol, erythromycin, streptomycin, and tetracycline; quinine; narcotics such as heroin; and tranquilizers such as Valium, Librium, and reserpine. Pregnant women should be careful not to inhale cleaning products that contain benzene or carbon tetrachloride. Fortunately, most cleaning products now on the market no longer contain these substances. In addition, women must take care not to overdose with substances that are supposedly good for them, such as vitamins A, C, D, and K. All four of these vitamins are important for fetal development; however, excessive doses can damage the fetus.

Alcohol   It has long been established that alcoholic mothers produce babies that are also physically dependent on alcohol. Such babies may exhibit severe withdrawal symptoms within the first few days of life. A small percentage of alcoholic mothers give birth to babies with *fetal alcohol syndrome,* which is characterized by growth deficiencies, an abnormally small head, facial abnormalities, mental retardation, and severe learning disabilities (Streissguth et al., 1980). Even smaller doses of alcohol may have debilitating effects. Because the fetal liver cannot metabolize alcohol as rapidly as the adult liver, the alcohol remains in the fetus for a long period of time.

Smoking   Recent information about cigarette smoking suggests that it, too, has a hazardous effect on the fetus. The carbon monoxide gas in the cigarette smoke combines with the oxygen-carrying molecules in the fetal red blood cells and reduces the amount of oxygen that the fetus receives. Furthermore, nicotine rapidly constricts blood flow to the fetus, thereby further reducing the oxygen supply (Asmussen, 1978). As one scientist put it, "Cigarette smoking is equivalent to pinching the umbilical cord" (Witters and Jones-Witters, 1980, p. 164).

Statistics verify the effects of smoking on the fetus. Babies whose mothers smoked heavily during pregnancy are more likely to be premature or have a lower birth weight, to have more respiratory problems, and to experience more difficulty with childhood diseases than babies born to nonsmokers (Manning et al., 1975; Saxton, 1978). It is not even sufficient for the mother to be a nonsmoker, since she can inhale the carbon monoxide when someone else near her smokes. Recent evidence indicates that there is a greater mortality rate for newborn babies whose fathers consume more than 10 cigarettes a day, even when the mother is a nonsmoker.

Pseudocyesis, or false pregnancy, is a condition in which a woman may experience all or most of the signs of pregnancy without actually being pregnant. There may be failure to menstruate, morning sickness, detection of fetal movement, weight gain, enlargement of the abdomen, and breast tenderness with a milky secretion. False pregnancy is most likely to develop in women who either intensely desire pregnancy or intensely fear it. As a result, false pregnancy, sometimes called "hysterical pregnancy," is assumed to be psychological, an example of mind over body. In one typical case, reported by Yen and others (1976), a 16-year-old girl was supposed to be 38 weeks pregnant and had experienced all the typical symptoms. However, her physician was unable to feel the fetus by palpating her abdomen or to hear a fetal heartbeat with a stethoscope. A subsequent ultrasound examination revealed a normal, nonpregnant uterus. The enlargement of the abdomen appeared to be the result of intestinal gas, which was expelled soon after the girl was informed that she was not pregnant.

Another syndrome, somewhat related to false pregnancy, is *couvade*, or sympathetic pregnancy, which occurs in some tribal cultures. It also occurs infrequently in more advanced societies. In couvade the husband may develop symptoms similar to those exhibited by his pregnant wife. He may feel nauseated, develop a desire for unusual foods, or have a somewhat enlarged belly. In some cultures, men are expected to suffer the pains and moaning that accompany delivery, and they may retire to bed to thrash and moan for the duration of their wives' labor (Mead and Newton, 1967; Davenport, 1977).

COMPLICATIONS OF PREGNANCY

Not all pregnancies proceed smoothly or develop normally. Various pregnancy complications may arise spontaneously or because of certain attributes of the mother or father, such as age, physical health, and genetic constitution. Typical complications include genetically defective fetuses, miscarriage, ectopic pregnancy, and Rh incompatibility.

The most common genetic disorder is *Down's syndrome*, a condition involving certain physical abnormalities and mental retardation. The incidence of this disorder is 0.6 per 1000 births for women under 30, increases to 10 per 1000 births for women aged 40–45, and rises to 25 per 1000 births for women over 45. Thus, maternal age is thought to somehow play a role in the incidence of this particular disorder. Other common genetic disorders include Huntington's chorea, polycystic kidney disease, cystic fibrosis, sickle cell anemia, phenylketonuria, and hemophilia.

With modern technology the presence of Down's syndrome and many other disorders can be ascertained by the fourth month of pregnancy. Fetal cells can be extracted and examined through the process of *amniocentesis*. In this procedure, a long needle is inserted through the abdomen of the mother into the amniotic sac of the fetus. A small amount of amniotic fluid is withdrawn, and any fetal cells in the fluid are then examined for biochemical abnormalities and evidence of chromosomal damage. The procedure is not without risk, in that it may induce a spontaneous abortion or the woman may have to undergo the procedure again if the appropriate fetal cells were not obtained on the first try. However, these risks are quite small, and the potential reduction in anxiety of the parents may be extremely beneficial.

If a serious genetic disorder is found in the fetus, the pregnant woman and her partner are faced with the decision of whether or not to abort the fetus. The termination of a 4-month-old fetus is an emotionally and morally complex proposition. And if termination is chosen, aborting the fetus at this stage in development is not simple. Three chemicals that may be used for this purpose are hypertonic saline, prostaglandins, and urea. Fetal death is followed by a series of uterine contractions that cause expulsion of fetal tissue. Higher risks are involved in this kind of abortion than in abortions performed in the first trimester (see Chap. 8). Unfortunately, amniocentesis cannot be performed any earlier than the fourteenth week of gestation.

Miscarriage

In **miscarriage**, or **spontaneous abortion**, fetal death occurs spontaneously. It is estimated that nearly 10–15 percent of all pregnancies end in miscarriage, but this estimate may be low, since women can spontaneously abort without even knowing they were pregnant.

The actual cause of miscarriage cannot always be determined. In the majority of cases, there appears to be some abnormality in the sperm or egg that prevents full development of the embryo. As a result, the incompletely formed tissue dies by the second or third month and is expelled from the body. However, the occurrence of a miscarriage does not automatically mean that there is something wrong with the woman's eggs or the man's sperm. In most cases, the defective gamete is a chance event not likely to occur again. In a few cases, women may be prone to miscarriage. When a miscarriage occurs in three or more pregnancies in a row, the situation is called **habitual abortion**. Habitual aborters have a decreased likelihood of carrying a fetus to term.

*Ectopic
pregnancy*

Ectopic pregnancy is a condition in which the fertilized egg becomes implanted in an area other than the uterus. The most typical area is the fallopian tubes, so this condition is often referred to as **tubal pregnancy**. In an ectopic pregnancy, the fetus cannot be carried to term and must be surgically removed. The actual incidence of such pregnancies is difficult to establish, since in some cases the embryo may simply be absorbed into the woman's body without her having been aware of any pregnancy. The reported incidence ranges from 1 in 100 to 1 in 300 pregnancies.

The cause of ectopic pregnancy is assumed to be related to some impairment of the fallopian tube. There may be an obstruction, distortion, or tumor in the tube, or the tube may contain some endometrial tissue (endometriosis—see Chap. 6). Whatever the case, the fetus becomes attached to the wall of the tube. As it develops, it outgrows the space in the tube, leading to tubal abortion or tubal rupture. In a **tubal abortion**, the embryo is forced out the end of the fallopian tube and into the abdominal cavity. If this occurs early enough, the embryo may be resorbed by the woman's body. Otherwise, there is bleeding into the abdominal cavity. In a **tubal rupture**, the fallopian tube bursts or leaks. It is imperative that surgery be performed once a tubal pregnancy has been diagnosed because of the risk of death from bleeding. Surgery usually requires removal of the part of the tube containing the embryo. Once a woman has had an ectopic pregnancy, her chances of having another are increased. Thus, subsequent pregnancies should be monitored carefully by a physician.

*Rh
incompatibility*

Rh is a blood factor found in humans. Individuals may be positive or negative for the Rh factor, although the majority of people are Rh-positive. Rh incompatibility arises when a mother has Rh-negative blood and her fetus has Rh-positive blood (from an Rh-positive father). In such cases, the Rh-positive cells from the fetus can enter the mother's bloodstream during a delivery, an abortion, or a miscarriage and produce an antibody reaction in the mother. If an Rh-negative woman develops these antibodies, they will attack the blood cells of each subsequent Rh-positive fetus, possibly causing fetal death. Fortunately, there is now a vaccine that can be given to women within 36–72 hours after delivery, abortion, or miscarriage that will prevent this antibody reaction.

CHILDBIRTH

Childbirth, or **parturition**, is the culmination of 9 months of pregnancy. It is often greeted by the mother-to-be with a mixture of apprehension and excitement. Much of the apprehension, particularly in first-time parents, can be traced to concerns about pain during delivery, the potential effects of anesthesia, and the possibilities of a complicated delivery and birth defects. On the other hand, after 9 months of pregnancy the woman is usually eager to get on with it and is excited about the prospect of seeing her baby.

*The trigger for
childbirth*

The actual stimulus that triggers the process of expelling the fetus from the womb is unknown. Unlike other mammals, there appears to be no abrupt change in the levels of progesterone or estrogen in humans. In addition, the fetus itself does not seem to be responsible for the initiation of the birth process.

The most important structure in the onset of labor is the cervix. The cervix essentially acts like a plug, preventing the fetus from escaping from the uterus. The beginning of childbirth starts with the dilation, or opening, of the cervix, thus allowing movement of the fetus out of the uterus. Recent evidence suggests that rather than being a passive plug, the cervix actually prevents the fetus from being expelled (Seitchik, 1979). It does so by maintaining a stiff consistency until childbirth approaches. With the impending birth, the cervix becomes progressively softer and more compliant. The control systems that guide this change have not been identified, but prostaglandins (see Chap. 6) are thought to be involved.

*Stages of
childbirth*

The birth process is often referred to as **labor**, primarily because the woman must work hard and often experiences some discomfort while expelling the baby. Labor can be divided into three distinct stages.

Stage 1 The first stage of labor is generally the longest, lasting an average of 7–12 hours in **primiparas** (women giving birth to their first baby) and 5–7 hours in **multiparas** (women giving birth to a subsequent baby). The first stage begins with the expulsion of a mucus plug surrounding the cervix, usually followed swiftly by the rupture of the amniotic sac and the release of amniotic fluid ("the bag of waters") through the vagina. At the same time, the uterus begins the muscular contractions often referred to as labor pains.

Forceful uterine contractions are responsible for producing two changes in the cervix that are necessary for the successful delivery of the fetus: efface- ment and dilatation. **Effacement** is the extent to which the cervix is incorpo- rated into the lower part of the uterus and thins out. The cervix shortens from about 2 centimeters (about 0.8 inch) in width prior to labor to almost paper thinness. Effacement is generally more pronounced in primiparas than in mul- tiparas. **Dilatation** is the process by which the cervical opening undergoes expansion. Ultimately, the cervical opening must attain a width of 10 centime- ters (about 4 inches) before the fetus can be born.

The rate of uterine contractions varies over the course of the first stage of labor and is often divided into three substages: early first-stage labor, late first-stage labor, and transition. During early first-stage labor, contractions are about 15–20 minutes apart, and each contraction lasts about 1 minute. Al- though this is the longest substage, the woman usually tolerates it well and remains quite comfortable. In late first-stage labor, the cervix dilates 5–8 centimeters (about 2–3 inches), and the contractions are more closely spaced and of greater intensity. It is during the transition state that maximal cervical dilation is reached. This substage is considered to be the shortest and most demanding. Uterine contractions are frequent and very intense, causing some women to experience pain and exhaustion.

During the first stage of labor, the woman is encouraged to walk around or lie on her side rather than lie on her back, so as to remove the pressure of the fetus on the major veins and arteries in the abdomen. This reduces the strain on the heart and provides more oxygen to the uterus, thereby increasing the efficiency of the contractions. A woman usually enters the hospital after the first stage of labor is well underway and when the contractions are about 4–5 minutes apart.

Stage 2 The second stage of labor consists of the expulsion of the fetus through the cervical opening into the vagina and from there to the outside world (see Fig. 7.8). This stage is considerably shorter than the first. Primiparas require about 20 contractions over a 1-hour period to push out the baby, while multiparas require about 10 contractions over a 30-minute period.

Because the tissue around the vaginal opening may be ripped as the baby's head passes through, many obstetricians routinely make an incision that wid- ens the vaginal opening. This incision, called an **episiotomy**, is sutured at the end of labor (see Fig. 7.9). The episiotomy is not always necessary. It is usually performed because a cut is easier to repair than a tear. However, this procedure is becoming less routine, especially in cases where the parents have chosen natural childbirth.

Stage 3 The third stage of labor is delivery of the placenta. It is a very short stage, requiring only a few contractions and a few minutes. As the

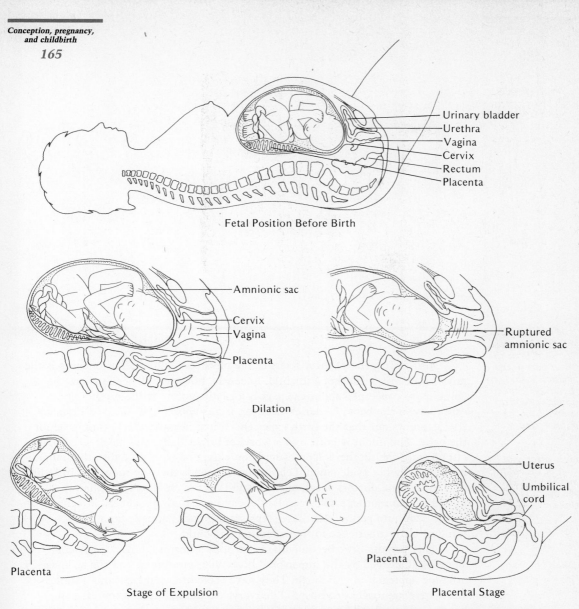

Fetal Position Before Birth

Amnionic sac

Cervix
Vagina

Placenta

Ruptured amnionic sac

Dilation

Uterus

Umbilical cord

Placenta

Placenta

Stage of Expulsion

Placental Stage

Urinary bladder
Urethra
Vagina
Cervix
Rectum
Placenta

FIGURE 7.8
The process of birth.

placenta is expelled, the blood vessels connecting it to the uterus contract and are sealed off naturally. If these blood vessels fail to close, however, the woman may have excessive blood loss and go into shock. Most physicians provide an injection of **oxytocin**, a hormone that facilitates uterine contractions and minimizes the risk of uterine hemorrhage. This is by far the most dangerous stage of labor—more complications or problems arise during this stage than during the other two stages combined.

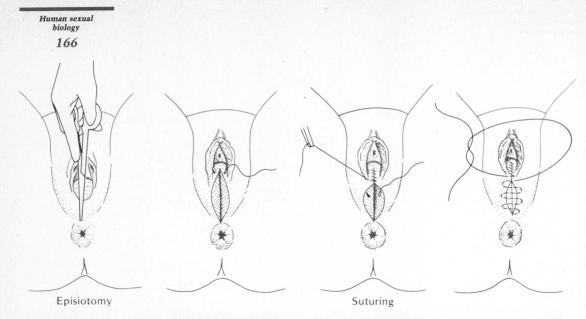

Episiotomy   Suturing

*FIGURE 7.9
An episiotomy.
The skin from the
lower part of the
vaginal opening to
the anus is cut to
provide a wider
opening for the
baby's head and
reduce the risk of
tearing. Immedi-
ately after expul-
sion of the infant
and the placenta,
the opening is su-
tured closed.*

During birth the primary focus of the physician and other attendants is the physical health of mother and child. Recently, however, physicians have become more concerned about the *psychological* comfort of the mother and especially of the baby. Frederick Leboyer, in his book *Birth Without Violence* (1975), points out that the birth experience must be particularly traumatic for the baby. The infant is born into a world of bright lights and harsh sounds, is cut off from the mother's blood supply quickly, and is subjected to the indignity of being held upside down. Leboyer recommends that the room be dimly lit, that nurses and doctors speak quietly, and that the child be immediately placed on the mother's abdomen while leaving the umbilical cord attached for a 4- to 5-minute period. All these steps are designed to make for a more tranquil birth experience for both mother and child.

Many parents have become dissatisfied with hospital births in general. They are disturbed by the impersonal hospital environment and the sickness-oriented approach to childbirth. They have therefore been exploring various alternative approaches to hospital delivery, including birthing centers and home births assisted by midwives. These alternatives are discussed in detail in Box 7.1.

*Problems in
childbirth*

The complex process of childbirth is, unsurprisingly, not trouble-free. Three of the most common problems are poor positioning of the fetus for delivery, adverse effects of anesthesia, and pain during labor.

Position of the fetus   Under normal conditions, the head of the fetus descends into the pelvis at the end of the third trimester. Such a head-first or **cephalic presentation** is characteristic of 96 percent of deliveries. However, in 3.5 percent of deliveries the buttocks are where the head should be, in what is called a **breech presentation.** In the remaining 0.5 percent of deliveries, the

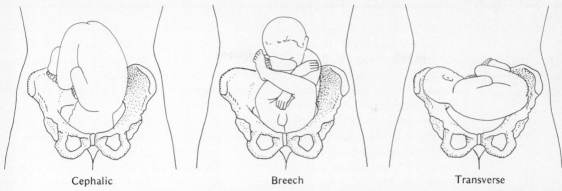

Cephalic	Breech	Transverse

FIGURE 7.10
Various presentations of the fetus prior to birth. Under normal circumstances, the fetus will be oriented in the cephalic (head-down) position, and birth will proceed smoothly. In the breech or traverse position, birth may be more difficult or require surgery.

baby is lying crosswise in the uterus, and an arm or leg may be where the head should be (**transverse or shoulder presentation**) (see Fig. 7.10). For both the breech and transverse presentations, the baby must be turned into the head-down position before it can be expelled from the uterus and delivered. Failure to do so may result in physical damage to the baby or may cause the baby to become dangerously entangled in the umbilical cord.

Under some conditions, it may not be possible to turn the baby in the uterus. In such cases, a **cesarean section** is usually performed. The cesarean section is a surgical procedure in which an incision is made into the abdominal and uterine walls. The baby is lifted out, and the uterine and abdominal walls are sutured closed. A cesarean section may be performed if the baby is too large or the mother's pelvis is too small, if there is excessive bleeding, if the cervix is not dilating properly, if some medical disorder prevents vaginal delivery, or if the baby is in the wrong presentation and if the umbilical cord is coming out first.

It has often been assumed that once a woman has had a cesarean section, any subsequent deliveries must also be cesarean. This is not true; a number of women who have needed a cesarean section for one delivery have had subsequent vaginal births. However, if the conditions that required this surgery in the first place are also present in later pregnancies (such as a too small pelvis), continued cesarean deliveries are indicated.

Effects of anesthesia A wide variety of drugs may be used during delivery. In the early part of labor, women may be given tranquilizers to relax them. It is during the second stage of labor, however, that women often require anesthesia. They may be given barbiturates, other general anesthetics such as halothane and methoxyflurane, or, most commonly, regional anesthetics (lidocaine, procaine, etc.) that serve to numb painful areas. The regional anesthetics may be administered in different areas for differential numbing: The **pudendal block** numbs the external genitals, while the **spinal, caudal,** or **epidural block** produces numbness in the entire birth area, from belly to thighs.

BOX 7.1

Alternatives to hospital delivery

We all know the stereotypical scenario of hospital childbirth. When the mother-to-be begins to feel labor pains, her anxious husband rushes her to the hospital, where she is wisked away to the delivery room. After hours of pacing up and down in the waiting room, the proud father is greeted with the news that he now has a bouncing boy or girl and that mother and child are doing fine. This basic series of events has remained relatively unchanged over the past several decades, although hospital equipment has become increasingly more sophisticated. The mother is given various anesthetics, and her physiological functioning is monitored; all the fetus' vital signs are detected through elaborate equipment. The delivery is performed in a brightly lit, highly impersonal hospital setting. Following delivery, the infant is quickly tested for normal signs and then is carried off to the nursery, while the mother is taken to a recovery room.

Until recently, this standard approach to delivery remained relatively unquestioned. But in recent years more and more couples have come to challenge the traditional scenario. They complain of the impersonality of hospital delivery and of the use of unnecessary procedures. As one registered nurse pointed out, "Just in case the woman tears, the hospital does an episiotomy; just in case she bleeds, they give her an intravenous solution during labor; just in case she may need a cesarean, they don't feed her" (Time, August 29, 1977, p. 66). In many hospitals, delivery is geared to the comfort and needs of the hospital staff, not of the mother and infant. This disturbs many parents-to-be. They would prefer that the father be present during the delivery, that a minimum of medical intervention be used, and that the baby be allowed to remain with them after delivery.

Prospective parents who feel this way about hospital births have two main alternatives: birth centers and home delivery. Birth centers are either private facilities or suites within a hospital that are designed to resemble ordinary bedrooms. Instead of being filled with imposing equipment, the rooms have a bed, comfortable furniture, and a homey atmosphere. The same room is used for both labor and delivery, and the father and other family members can be present throughout labor and delivery. The mother is attended to by a nurse-midwife or a physician, and should there by any complications, full hospital facilities are available nearby. However, complications are fairly rare in birth center deliveries because couples are carefully screened for high-risk factors. Such factors include maternal age, certain maternal diseases (diabetes, hypertension, etc.), past history of pregnancy and birth difficulties, and known problems with the present pregnancy.

Instead of treating birth as a medical problem, birth centers treat it as a natural process. The goal is to create a calm, confident, healthful atmosphere in which parents can experience an important event in their lives. Anesthesia is rarely used, and episiotomies are performed in only a small percentage of the deliveries. The rate of cesarean sections for birth center deliveries is lower than that of hospital deliveries, and forceps deliveries are rare. Thus, the birth experience is not interfered with except to provide for the mother and child's safety and comfort. Instead of being seen as a disease or aberration, birth is treated as "the most normal thing that can happen," as one birth center director described it (Norwood, 1978).

Home birth is another alternative that is gaining in popularity. Like birth centers, it offers a comfortable setting and costs much less than hospital delivery. In fact, a home birth supervised by a licensed nurse-midwife can cost as little as one-fifth of what a hospital birth costs. Sally Olds and her associates (1980) point out that home delivery is a warm, close, loving experience for which the parents have both responsibility and control. Home birth facilitates parent-child bonding by immediately incorporating the newborn into the household, and it contributes to the parents' self-esteem in that they can feel proud of carrying out the delivery on their own with minimum outside intervention. As with birth centers, however, couples must be carefully screened for factors that would make home delivery risky for either mother or infant.

With both types of alternative delivery, parents should go through extensive orientation and counseling to learn about the birth process, the measures they will need to take, possible complications, and postpartal care.

With careful screening and education of parents, alternative birth methods have proven to be quite safe. However, many medical organizations have actively opposed nonhospital deliveries and have fought such things as licensing of lay midwives. In a unique California case in which a lay midwife had been charged with murder because an infant she delivered had died of a rare complication, the judge dismissed the charges. In his decision, he pointed out, "Having a baby doesn't mean being sick, and the medical profession needs to recognize this. It's their obligation to work with parents who want alternative birth situations rather than saying, 'This is the way it is'" (Moramarco, 1979, p. 30).

Although births in special centers and at home are still a small proportion of all deliveries today, their number is increasing as more and more parents seek alternatives to the standard hospital approach. But those parents who choose an alternative method must realize that they will need a great deal of preparation and must work with qualified medical attendants to ensure the safety of their chosen method.

The primary advantage of anesthetics is that they reduce or eliminate the pain that many women experience during childbirth. On the other hand, recent evidence suggests that introduction of anesthetics during labor may adversely affect the fetus. It is well established that anesthetics introduced into the mother's body pass through the placenta and into the fetus. This is especially true for general anesthetics that put the woman to sleep during labor (barbiturates, chloroform, ether, and so on). Anesthesia initially depresses the fetal nervous system. At birth, babies whose mothers were anesthetized tend to have more sluggish respiration than do babies whose mothers received no anesthetic (Boston Women's Health Book Collective, 1976).

The effects of general anesthesia can be long term as well. Brackbill (1978) followed babies of mothers who did receive and babies of those who did not receive anesthesia and tested them at varying times after birth. She found that babies whose mothers had been heavily medicated were slower to sit, stand, and move about and cried longer even when comforted. Later studies have indicated that language development may also be slowed in such children.

Because of the potential dangers of anesthesia, it is wise for the pregnant woman to review with her physician the types of anesthetics and their uses. Because there are times when anesthetics are necessary, the woman should be prepared for this possibility and should be in agreement with her doctor about what types might be used.

Pain   The major reason for using anesthesia is to reduce or eliminate pain during delivery. As a result, it is commonly assumed that childbirth is extremely painful. Even the uterine contractions themselves are referred to as "labor pains." The particular view that childbirth is painful is common to Western women, who may say, "It is the most intense pain known to humanity; men know nothing like it." But in other societies, women do not necessarily report pain during delivery. This is especially true in societies that have couvade, where the father retires to a hut and moans for several days while the woman returns to work shortly after childbirth (Trethowan and Conlon, 1965). How, then, do we reconcile these opposing experiences? What differentiates the woman who has little pain from the one who is devastated during childbirth?

Although there are individual differences in pain tolerance levels, researchers suggest that the expectancy of pain, unfamiliarity with the experience, fear, and an inability to relax may substantially contribute to pain in the childbirth process. For first-time mothers particularly, the sensations that are felt during birth are foreign and very intense. It may be this very aspect of unfamiliarity that causes some women to label their labor contractions as painful. If familiarity is an important factor, one would expect that knowledge and rehearsal of childbirth might reduce the amount of pain that women experience. This seems to be the case. According to P. O. Davidson (1976), women who are informed about the specifics of the birth process are more tolerant of pain than are uninformed women. Mere information, however, does not eliminate pain altogether.

Fear may be another factor that contributes to the feeling of intense pain during labor. Fear leads to tension, which acts to increase the sensation of pain. The importance of fear in the pains of childbirth was recognized by an English physician, Grantly Dick-Read, early in this century. In his book *Childbirth Without Fear* (1944), Dick-Read attempted to educate women about childbirth and thus reduce their fear. Classes based on his method, which he called **natural childbirth**, emphasize demonstration and practice of relaxation, abdominal, and breathing exercises in addition to general education about labor and delivery.

It has long been known that feelings of pain can be obscured when people are relaxed and their attention is focused elsewhere. The ability to suppress pain is readily demonstrated in athletes who continue to compete despite serious injury. The same notion, that of diverting the woman's attention, can be used during labor to reduce the amount of pain experienced. This is essentially the basis of the **Lamaze method** of childbirth, which is becoming increasingly popular in this country.

The Lamaze method consists of extensive information sessions along with a training procedure that teaches women to dissociate the feelings of pain from uterine contractions and to focus their attention on specially designed breathing exercises. By using these breathing patterns, especially during the second stage of labor, the woman can work with the natural forces of the uterus to expel the baby. In this way the woman may not need any anesthetic. Nevertheless, the Lamaze method does not guarantee a pain-free childbirth, nor does it prohibit the use of anesthetics. Despite the training, some women may still need anesthetic relief from pain. Seitchik (1979) examined data provided by a San Antonio childbirth training association on 311 women of whom 180 were having their first child and all of whom had received Lamaze training. He noted that 17 required a cesarean section, 57 required local anesthesia (caudal block, etc.) during the birth process, 164 required anesthesia for the episiotomy, and 29 required total anesthesia during delivery.

Lamaze classes provide extensive information about the birth process, train women to breathe in ways to reduce labor pain, and promote a sense of sharing between husband and wife.

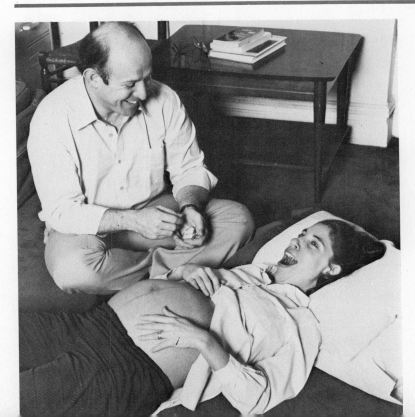

The Lamaze method allows and encourages the father-to-be to participate fully in the birthing process. He attends classes with the mother-to-be and practices with her at home. During delivery, he serves as a coach to ensure that she breathes correctly, and he provides much needed emotional support. Lamaze-trained men tend to be less anxious about birth, are more prepared for the sight of the baby following delivery, and feel a greater sense of participation than do waiting-room fathers. As the Lamaze method has increased in popularity, a number of hospitals have changed their policy and now allow the father in the delivery room.

Fathers and birth

For the most part, the father-to-be has been ignored as a factor of importance during a woman's pregnancy. He has been seen as a shadowy figure whose primary role is to cajole his wife through pregnancy, pace anxiously in the waiting room, and hand out cigars after the child has arrived. Yet men are both affected by and have a powerful effect on a woman's pregnancy, and this fact is finally being recognized.

Today fathers are playing an increasing role in the birthing and child-rearing processes.

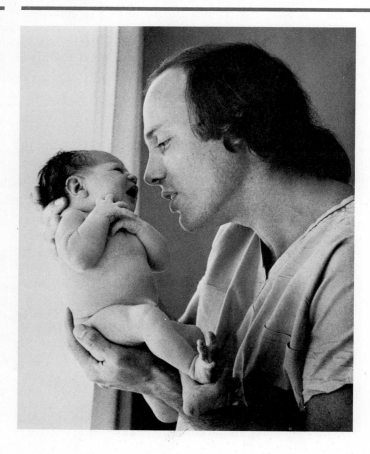

Men are deeply influenced by their wives' pregnancies, especially the first. Many men develop mood changes and erratic behavior while their wives are carrying babies (Lamb, 1976), and some men may become irritable or nervous, go on shopping sprees, or consume more alcohol than usual. Others seem to enjoy the experience and excitement of the impending birth.

Several researchers have found that the husband's personality is at least as important as the wife's in determining how the couple adjusts psychologically to pregnancy and childbirth. The more secure and emotionally supportive the husband is, the more successful the woman will be in dealing with these events. Thus, the father, albeit forgotten in the past, must today be acknowledged as important a force in pregnancy and childbirth as he is in child rearing.

THE AFTERMATH OF CHILDBIRTH

Shortly after childbirth, the new mother is faced with many new decisions and experiences. One of the decisions is whether to breast-feed or bottle-feed the new baby. The advantages and disadvantages of each feeding method are presented in Box 7.2. Many women must also cope with the onset of ***postpartum depression***. A short time after birth, the mother may develop feelings of sadness, may cry for no apparent reason, and may feel inadequate as a person and as a mother. Although this depression commonly lasts for only a few days to a week, in some women it may continue for months or a year. Such women may exhibit a slowness of drive, a sense of helplessness, a lack of humor, and a disinterest in sex.

There are a number of hypotheses that attempt to explain the occurrence of postpartum depression. Physiologists suggest that hormone changes that occur after birth may cause the depression. The hormone most likely to play such a role is progesterone, which decreases dramatically after the baby is born. Progesterone levels are also thought to be important in premenstrual tension. However, changes in the levels of progesterone are not a sufficient explanation, since adoptive mothers may also develop postpartum depression soon after they receive the child.

Psychologists suggest that the depression may be related to the adjustment a woman must make to the maternal role. It is quite a big step not only physically but psychologically to go from being pregnant to being a mother. Whatever the case may be, postpartum depression is usually temporary, and those who need help with it can also consult a therapist. Gordon, Kapostins, and Gordon (1965) developed a set of instructions to give to pregnant mothers that seem to reduce the amount of depression and disorientation that might develop after birth. These simple instructions include (1) get informed about motherhood, (2) make friends with other couples who are experiencing the same situation, (3) don't overload yourself with unimportant tasks, (4) don't move your residence soon after the baby arrives, and (5) get plenty of rest and sleep. All of these instructions emphasize being informed and allowing time for acquiring the new role of motherhood.

BOX 7.2

Breast versus bottle

Expectant parents have many decisions to make about the care and raising of their forthcoming child. One of the most fundamental decisions they face is feeding of the new baby: Should he or she be bottle-fed or breast-fed? For some, the decision is easy because, for medical reasons, the mother is unable to breast-feed. But for others, many other factors come into play. They must weigh the advantages and disadvantages of each method in terms of their particular situation. What are the facts about breast- and bottle-feeding, and what factors affect this choice?

The advantages of breast-feeding have become increasingly well known in recent years, leading to a major rise in the proportion of mothers choosing to breast-feed. Whereas in 1971 only 23 percent of mothers leaving the hospital were breast-feeding, in 1977 the figure had risen to 43 percent according to one study (Henig, 1979). The most obvious advantages of breast-feeding lie in the characteristics of breast milk when compared to cow's milk or to commercially prepared formula. Nutritionally, breast milk provides the combination and balance of nutrients the newborn infant needs. It has half the protein content of cow's milk, yet contains the specific amino acids the newborn requires and in the right proportion. Cow's milk, on the other hand, contains additional proteins that can be highly allergenic to infants. In addition, human milk contains important enzymes that help metabolize fat, fight harmful bacteria, and create an environment in the gut that is conducive to the growth of useful digestive bacteria.

Another major advantage of breast milk is that it arms the infant with immune protection not only by transferring antibodies from the mother but by directly supplying the baby with white blood cells that can destroy any bacteria they encounter. Because of the nutritional and immunological benefits of mother's milk, breast-fed infants are much less likely to suffer from respiratory infections, allergies, diarrhea, gastrointestinal infections, eczema, ear infections, and iron deficiency anemia.

The benefits of breast milk to the child are thought to show up later in life as well. For example, human milk is higher in cholesterol than is bottle milk, creating higher blood cholesterol levels in breast-fed infants. These higher levels may actually lead to reduced cholesterol levels in adulthood, since they teach the body how to better metabolize fats. According to researchers studying this effect, adults who were exclusively breast-fed for more than 2 months as infants have lower cholesterol levels than those with little or no breast-feeding, even if their fat intake is high. Thus, breast-feeding may indirectly protect against coronary artery disease (Marano, 1979). Furthermore, it has been suggested that breast-fed babies are less likely than bottle-fed babies to be fat. Not only do bottle-fed babies consume more calories in their milk, but they are often encouraged to overeat—to consume the entire formula. Because fat babies often grow up to be fat adults, breast-feeding may help to prevent obesity in adulthood.

In addition to the physiological benefits of breast-feeding, there are important psychological benefits to both infant and mother. Many psychologists have emphasized the importance of creating a strong bond between mother

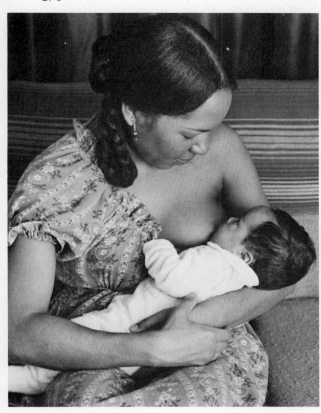

The decision of whether or not to breast-feed is an important one for new mothers.

and child in the sensitive period following birth. This bond is developed through close, intimate contact, in which the mother looks at, strokes, cuddles, and plays with this new individual who has come into her life. The strength of the initial bonding, or attachment, between mother and child can affect not only their relationship as the child is growing up but also the child's psychological, social, and intellectual development.

John Kennell is one physician who feels that breast-feeding is the most powerful way to create a strong mother-infant bond. According to him, breast-feeding "sets up and maintains many channels of communication be-

tween the two. Through it, mother and infant develop an 'interactional harmony' that locks them together. Breast-feeding continues the process begun in the sensitive period after birth" (Marano, 1979, p. 60). Another psychological benefit of breast-feeding is that it reduces stress for both the mother and child, thereby increasing the ability of both to cope with the outside world.

Given all these advantages of breast-feeding, why would any mother want to bottle-feed? As with all complex issues, there are additional factors that must be considered. For one thing, breast milk can be a carrier of unwanted chemicals. Certain environmental pollutants can become concentrated in breast milk, and the American Academy of Pediatrics has cautioned women in high-risk occupations or environments to have their breast milk analyzed before they begin nursing (Henig, 1979). Many drugs and medications can also be carried from mother to child via breast milk. Among drugs that can be harmful are narcotics, antithyroid compounds, anticoagulants, and cathartics. Other drugs may not be directly harmful but may set up allergies or sensitivities in later life.

But perhaps the major drawback to many new mothers is the commitment required by breast-feeding. It means stopping several times a day to sit for as long as a half hour feeding their babies. This is particularly difficult for the woman who wishes to return to work. Although a few places of employment have allowed women to nurse on the job, such situations are rare. Many breast-feeding women have learned to pump their milk by hand so the baby can be fed while they are away. Others have decided to mix breast-feeding with bottle-feeding in their child's diet.

In addition to the commitment required, breast-feeding has some other drawbacks. The mother has to be very careful about what she eats, what drugs she takes, and what and how much she drinks. If she goes too long without feeding her child, she can experience strong physical discomforts. If her baby refuses to be fed by anyone else, she is kept from going places the baby can't go. Some women experience anxiety because they don't know whether their infant is getting enough milk. And some have problems in getting their milk to flow. Many studies have shown that the delicate process of nursing can be hampered or interrupted not only by anxiety but also by such distractions as a tickle or a difficult mathematical problem to solve (Henig, 1979).

Advocates of bottle-feeding are also quick to point out that breast-feeding deprives the father of involvement in the feeding process. Bottle-feeding not only helps the father develop a bond with the child but also frees the mother from sole responsibility for the child's nourishment.

Bottle-feeding is particularly prevalent in low-income families. This may be partly because women in these families tend to have limited information on the benefits of breast-feeding and because hospital procedures tend to be geared toward separating mother and child during the first few days after birth. But preference for bottle-feeding at this socioeconomic level may also be a practical matter, since anyone in the family or even a neighbor or babysitter can feed the baby if the mother is too busy or working.

Even though the benefits of breast-feeding are becoming more obvious, it does not necessarily follow that children raised on the bottle are any less healthy or adjusted than in their breast-fed counterparts. Infant formulas are being developed that more closely mimic mother's milk, although it has yet to be matched exactly. As far as the connection between bottle-feeding and obesity is concerned, at least one study has found no significant differences in weight gain between breast-fed and bottle-fed babies (Trien, 1977). And mothers of bottle-fed babies resent the idea that they are thought to be any less attached to their babies than breast-feeding mothers are. Despite the evidence in support of breast-feeding, then, parents who choose bottle-feeding should not feel uncomfortable with their choice.

SUMMARY

1 *Conception* or *fertilization* is the process by which sperm and egg unite. Conceiving a child is a matter of timing, since the egg lives for only about 24 hours and the sperm live for only 2 days. Conception is also affected by the age of the participants and the frequency of intercourse.

2 Infertility can be caused by a number of factors in both husband and wife. A *fertility workup* is a medical procedure designed to identify the causes of a couple's infertility and to provide possible solutions. A woman's fertility may be tested via the *Huehner test* or the *Rubin test*. A man's fertility is tested through examination of the quality and quantity of his sperm.

3 Infertility in women is sometimes treated with fertility drugs such as *pergonal* and *clomiphene*. Infertility in men may lead to the use of artificial insemination either with a higher-quality portion of the husband's sperm (AIH) or with a donor's sperm (AID). In some cases of female infertility, the husband's sperm may be used to artificially inseminate a *surrogate* mother who goes through pregnancy for the couple.

4 Test-tube babies are children created by the union of the husband's sperm and mother's egg outside of the body. The fertilized egg is implanted in the mother's uterus, and pregnancy proceeds normally.

5 Pregnancy is usually divided into three periods, or *trimesters*. The average length of pregnancy is 280 days, referred to as *gestation.*

6 Signs of the onset of pregnancy include a missed menstrual period, enlargement and tenderness of the breasts, more frequent urination, and morning sickness. About 50 percent of pregnant women experience *morning sickness,* which may be caused by hormonal factors or psychological factors.

7 Most hospital pregnancy tests are based on the detection of *human chorionic gonadotropin* (HCG) in the mother's blood or urine. Another test for pregnany is examination of the uterus for *Hegar's sign.*

8 During the first trimester the major changes in the woman are hormonal and psychological. Estrogen and progesterone levels are high; these hormones are first produced by the corpus luteum and later by the *placenta.*

9 The first trimester sees the greatest changes in the growing organism. It goes from a ball of cells (*morula stage*) to a hollow ball (*blastocyst*), to an *embryo*, to a *fetus* in 8 short weeks. *Implantation* in the uterine wall occurs on about the sixth day after fertilization. At this point 2 membranes form around the embryo: the *amnion* and the *chorion*. The chorion sends out *villi* into the uterine tissue, ultimately leading to formation of the placenta. The embryo consists of 3 layers (*endoderm, mesoderm,* and *ectoderm*) that give rise to all the organs and tissues.

10 During the second trimester the woman is relatively calm and tranquil. *Quickening* (first detection of fetal movement) occurs. Levels of *prolactin* from the pituitary rise, and the woman may experience *edema* in the lower legs and ankles. During this time the fetus is increasing substantially in size, begins to move, and has reflexes such as sucking and swallowing.

11 During the third trimester the woman gains significant weight and girth, and there may be increased stress on her internal organs. She may experience *Braxton Hicks contractions,* have mild emotional problems, and have disturbing fantasies and dreams. Three weeks prior to birth she experiences *engagement* of the baby's head in the pelvic region. During this time the fetus is primarily growing; the central nervous system enlarges and expands, and the lungs go through final development so that the baby can survive outside the mother's body.

12 Major concerns during pregnancy include weight gain and nutrition, sexual activity, and drugs. Excess weight during pregnancy is associated with *toxemia* and *preeclampsia-eclampsia* in the mother. Sexual activity need not be restricted during pregnancy except in certain high-risk cases. The mother must be careful about the drugs and chemicals she uses during pregnancy, since many substances are *teratogens* that can produce congenital defects. Alcoholic mothers can produce babies with *fetal alcohol syndrome,* and women who smoke are more likely to have premature, low birth-weight, or ill babies.

13   Some women experience false pregnancy or *pseudocyesis*, which appears to be psychological in origin. Couvade or sympathetic pregnancy in the father is common in some cultures.

14   The major complications that can occur in pregnancy include genetic defects, miscarriage, ectopic pregnancy, and Rh incompatibility. The most common genetic disorder is *Down's syndrome*. Genetic disorders can be detected through *amniocentesis*. *Miscarriage* is spontaneous abortion, which occurs in 10–15 percent of all pregnancies. *Ectopic pregnancy* is pregnancy that occurs outside the uterus, resulting in *tubal abortion* or *tubal rupture*. *Rh incompatibility* occurs when a mother who is Rh-negative has a child who is Rh-positive; subsequent Rh-positive fetuses may be attacked by the mother's antibodies.

15   Childbirth is characterized by three stages of *labor*. In stage 1 the mucus plug surrounding the cervix is expelled; uterine contractions begin; cervical *effacement* occurs; and the cervical opening expands (*dilatation*). Contractions become more frequent and intense toward the end of this stage. Stage 2 consists of expulsion of the baby, which is sometimes assisted by an incision in the vaginal opening (*episiotomy*). Stage 3 is delivery of the placenta.

16   Problems in childbirth include poor positioning of the fetus for delivery (*breech* or *transverse* presentation instead of *cephalic* presentation), adverse effects of anesthesia, and pain during labor. Pain during labor can be reduced through reduction of the fear involved and through relaxation training (*Lamaze method*).

17   It is common for new mothers to experience *postpartum depression* for a short time after the birth of their babies. This depression may be caused in part by changes in hormone levels and in part by the psychological adjustments women must make to their new role.

ADDITIONAL READING

* **Flanagan, Geraldine.** *The First Nine Months of Life.* New York: Simon & Schuster, 1962.
    A detailed description of the infant's development in the uterus. Contains excellent photographs of different stages of fetal development.
Leboyer, Frederick. *Birth Without Violence.* New York: Knopf, 1975.
    Leboyer's explanation of his unique approach to birthing. Interesting, nontechnical, and well illustrated.
* **Macfarlane, Aidan.** *The Psychology of Childbirth.* Cambridge, MA: Harvard University Press, 1977.
    An excellent introduction to the psychological processes in both mother and child that accompany birth. Comprehensive, well written, and referenced.
* **McCauley, Carole S.** *Pregnancy After Thirty-Five.* New York: Simon & Schuster, 1976.
    A comprehensive guide to pregnancy in the older woman. Covers a wide range of topics including nutrition, genetic counseling, the role of the father, and more.

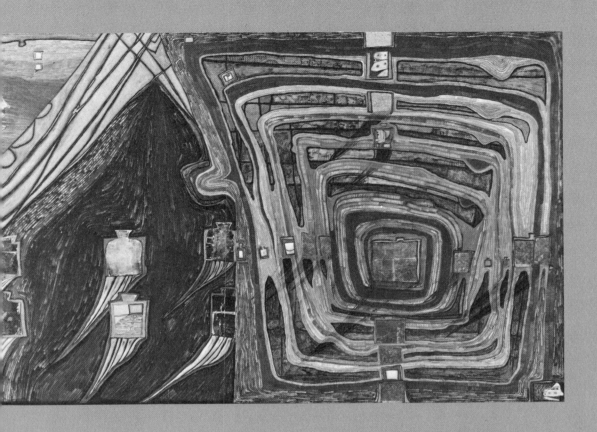

Birth control

8

chapter
8

Birth control is not a discovery of modern society. References to different techniques date back to 2700 B.C. The most common form of birth control in ancient times was the insertion of various substances into the vagina prior to intercourse. Animal excrement, especially elephant and crocodile dung, was popular as a form of birth control in India and Africa. Although excrement has no known spermicidal properties, it apparently formed a somewhat effective mechanical barrier that prevented sperm from passing through the cervix.

During the Greek and Roman periods, many physicians spent their time creating contraceptive concoctions for women. Some of these mixtures were quite elaborate. Rhazes of Baghdad, for example, recommended a paste of colocynth, pulp, pomegranate, elephant dung, animal earwax, and whitewash. These last two ingredients prevented the entire mixture from dissolving. The Achenese women of Sumatra came the closest to modern contraceptive technology. They inserted leaves containing tannic acid, a potent spermicide, into their vaginas before sexual intercourse.

A number of diaphragm-like devices were also developed early in history. Sumatran women took the head of the opium poppy, molded it into a small cap, and then placed it over the cervix. Pomegranates were hollowed out and also used in this manner. Hebrew women apparently inserted sponges into the vagina to soak up the seminal fluid.

A curette-like device (a scraper that can be inserted through the cervical opening into the uterus) was also invented by the Hebrews and was used for abortions. The curette could be used to scrape or sponge out the uterine contents. Given the rather unsanitary conditions under which abortions were performed in those days, it was probably a very dangerous procedure.

As people became more knowledgeable about the phases of a woman's menstrual cycle and pregnancy, another form of birth control developed: the rhythm method. Partners abstained from intercourse during the middle part of a woman's menstrual cycle, when the probability of becoming pregnant is greatest. This form of birth control was actively supported by some of the major religions and even today is still the only form of birth control approved for Roman Catholics.

It wasn't until the invention of vulcanized rubber in 1840 that birth control took a major step forward. Associated with this new technology was the development of the condom, the diaphragm, and the cervical cap, all made of rubber. The condom and diaphragm are still popular today. The cervical cap, which fits snugly over the cervix, can be worn for days or weeks at a time. The cap is popular in Europe but is generally unavailable in the United States. With continued improvement in rubber products, the modern versions of the condom, cap, and diaphragm are much more effective and reliable than their nineteenth-century predecessors.

Another significant step in contraceptive technology was taken when birth control pills were first placed on the market in 1960. The Pill separated the act of contraception from the actual act of intercourse. It eliminated the need to disrupt lovemaking to put on a condom. And yet the contraceptive action could simply be reversed by discontinuing the pills. To understand the impact of this form of birth control on women, one need only note that the Pill is the overwhelming choice of single women by a 5-to-1 margin. Indeed, approximately 20–40 percent of all women of childbearing age in developed countries have used oral contraceptives in recent years.

Today men and women have a number of birth control options, from hormonal manipulations via the Pill to calendar-counting rhythm methods. In spite of the advances in birth control technology and the variety and availability of birth control, myths still exist. Here are a few examples:

Douching or rinsing out the vagina with certain types of substances after intercourse can help prevent pregnancy.
Vasectomy (male sterilization) produces impotence and effeminate behavior in men.
If the man doesn't reach orgasm while his penis is inserted in the vagina, the woman cannot become pregnant.
A woman is still "safe" (unable to become pregnant) if she misses a birth control pill now and then.

In this chapter we will examine these and other issues by describing the most common methods of birth control—how they work, their possible side effects, their advantages and disadvantages. But first let us address some basic issues regarding contraception: why people use birth control, why people *don't* use birth control, and factors to consider in choosing a birth control method.

REASONS FOR CHOOSING BIRTH CONTROL

Physical concerns

Sexually active men and women may have a number of reasons for seeking and using birth control. These reasons include physical, psychological, and political concerns.

Despite the fact that modern medicine has made pregnancy and childbirth relatively safe, there are some women for whom these experiences can be risky and even dangerous. The incidence of spontaneous abortions and birth complications for women over the age of 40 and for young teenagers is significantly higher than for women in the age group in between. Women with certain types of diseases, such as diabetes, also face increased health risks during pregnancy, as do women who have had more than 3 or 4 children. Other women may use birth control because they are at high risk for having premature babies or children with birth defects. They include women over age 40, young teenagers, women who have had more than 4 children, and carriers of inheritable disorders, such as Huntington's chorea or sickle cell anemia.

In some instances, contraception can be used to facilitate the occurrence of pregnancy. Some women are infertile because they produce antibodies that inactivate and destroy their partner's sperm. Fertility can sometimes be restored if such women can keep sperm out of their body (vagina or mouth) long enough so that antibody levels decline. If the male partner uses a condom for a 3- to 6-month period prior to attempting conception, the chances for a successful fertilization may be dramatically increased (Hatcher et al., 1980).

There are many psychological reasons for using birth control. Couples may select birth control during their first few years of marriage in order to build their relationship with each other. The stresses of pregnancy and childbirth and the financial and psychological stresses of child rearing are put off to a time when the couple are better able to cope with them. There is also some evidence to suggest that contraception enhances sexual satisfaction in newly-weds by reducing the fear of pregnancy (Adams, 1966).

Married couples also use birth control to space their children and to limit family size. In the absence of birth control, a woman can become pregnant every year. In addition, accumulating evidence indicates that there may be some negative consequences to having large families. In particular, it has been found that adequacy of maternal care decreases as family size increases (Douglas and Blomfield, 1958), that achievement in school is not as satisfactory in children who come from large families (Douglas, 1964), and that the incidence of childhood accidents increases with increased family size (Meyer et al., 1963). The ability to control family size, then, may improve the quality of family life.

We should also note that some married couples use birth control to limit their family size to two: husband and wife. Today there is an increased desire among couples, especially those who both have careers, to remain childless. Whereas in previous decades childless couples were socially stigmatized, in recent years choosing not to have children has become more socially acceptable.

Many unmarried women who wish to be sexually active use birth control to prevent pregnancy. Although premarital sexual relationships are fairly common and accepted within large segments of our society, the pregnancies and children that can result from such relationships are not always so accepted.

Many women choose birth control because they are concerned with pursuing a career and other ambitions. The idea that women should spend their "best" adult years bearing children and taking care of them has come to be seriously questioned in recent years. In the more modern view, young women may be encouraged to pursue career goals and to put off childbearing to their late twenties or early thirties. In this way birth control allows career-oriented women who also want children to integrate child rearing with their career objectives.

With a burgeoning world population and decreasing resources, it is easy to understand how birth control has become a volatile political issue in many countries. A number of Americans use birth control because they are committed to Zero Population Growth (ZPG), a movement that became popular in the late 1960s. The goal of ZPG is to have birth rates level off so that they match death rates, keeping the population at a steady size.

Worldwide population has increased at alarming rates in this century. By the year 2000 the population of the world will be double what it was in 1960. Will there be enough food to feed all these people? Will there be adequate energy resources to supply all their needs? These are just a few of the concerns

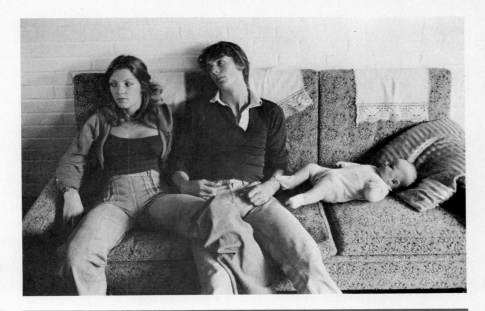

The birth of a child may have a disruptive effect on the aspirations and ambitions of young people.

of people who advocate ZPG. In their view, birth control is desirable not only for personal convenience but for the welfare of society.

REASONS FOR AVOIDING BIRTH CONTROL

Despite widespread availability and knowledge of birth control methods, there are still many individuals who do not use birth control even though they do not wish children. Why?

The most commonly given reason for not using physical forms of birth control is religious prohibition. Certain religions, such as Roman Catholicism, specifically forbid most forms of birth control on the grounds that they interfere with the normal and natural reproductive process and result in the destruction of life.

In addition, many people do not use specific types of birth control for medical reasons. Women who take the Pill, for instance, are subject to a number of side effects and may also be at risk for developing blood-clotting disorders. Nevertheless, there are several contraceptive techniques, such as the condom and the rhythm method, that carry virtually no health risk whatsoever. Thus, health concerns may dictate the *choice* of birth control method but cannot serve as an effective argument for avoiding birth control altogether.

Some people say that birth control techniques interfere with the natural flow of the sexual act. While this may be characteristic of devices such as condoms, diaphragms, and spermicidal chemicals, which must be used prior to lovemaking, it is hardly true of oral contraceptives or the IUD, which are not directly associated with the act itself. However, some people may reject the Pill or IUD as well on the grounds that they are too "planned" or "deliberate."

There are so many different birth control methods that a person may be overwhelmed by all of the possibilities. There are, however, a number of important factors to consider that may help an individual or couple choose the most suitable type of birth control. These factors include cost, availability, potential side effects, mechanism of action, timing, frequency of intercourse, and effectiveness. (See Table 8.1 for a summary of these factors.)

Cost may be an important factor for people who have little money. The rhythm method, for example, may cost nothing to use, whereas other methods may require $60–$100 a year or more to maintain. Availability refers to whether a doctor's prescription or treatment is necessary. This factor is also important from a cost perspective, since a visit to the doctor adds to the expense of the method. *Side effects* are those undesirable reactions that can be traced to the use of certain birth control techniques. For example, the Pill may cause weight gain and blood clotting; the IUD may cause heavier menstrual flow; and spermicides may cause an allergic response. In general, however, only a small percentage of users experience side effects.

The mechanism of action is how the birth control method works. Some techniques block conception by ensuring that the egg and sperm never meet (condom, diaphragm). The word *contraceptive* (from the Latin *contra*, meaning "against," and *ceptio*, meaning "union") is often applied to those techniques. Other methods interfere with the implantation of an already fertilized egg (IUD). Still others involve the termination of pregnancy after implantation has occurred (abortion). Because of the complex issues surrounding the ethics of some of these methods, individuals should be well informed about the way in which each method works so that they can choose one that is consistent with their moral beliefs.

Timing of birth control use is also significant for many people. As we have noted, some forms of birth control must be employed just prior to intercourse, while others are not directly related to the sex act at all. For those who find using contraceptive devices during lovemaking to be particularly disruptive, the Pill or IUD may be a reasonable solution.

Frequency of intercourse may be an additional consideration in the choice of method. For women who have intercourse only once or twice a month, for example, taking the Pill might be contraceptive "overkill." A sexually inactive woman may be subjecting her body to major hormonal shifts on a long-term basis just to be sure pregnancy does not occur on those one or two occasions each month that she has intercourse. Such a woman might be better off selecting another form of birth control, such as the diaphragm.

The standard procedure for determining the effectiveness of various methods of birth control is to select 100 women who use a particular method and calculate the incidence of pregnancy across a 1-year period. The failure rate is then calculated as the number of pregnancies per "100 women years," which refers to the number of women in the sample multiplied by the length of the study. The effectiveness rate is 100 minus the failure rate, or the number of women out of 100 who did *not* become pregnant that year.

There are actually two types of effectiveness rates: theoretical effectiveness (T.E.) and the actual use effectiveness (A.E.). The **theoretical effectiveness rate** is the effectiveness of the method when it is used perfectly, without error, and exactly according to instructions. Given human fallibility, however, the **actual use effectiveness rate** takes into account mistakes in using a method, such as forgetting to take a pill or using a condom with a hole in it. As might be expected, actual use rates are always less impressive than theoretical use rates, with the exception of sterilization and abortion, where both rates are virtually identical.

Sometimes unknowledgeable individuals can be misled by effectiveness rates. Counselors who favor certain forms of birth control, for example, may quote theoretical rates for their favorite method and actual use rates for all others (Hatcher et al., 1978). Table 8.1 contains failure rates for a number of birth control techniques.

In the remainder of this chapter we will discuss each of the most commonly used birth control methods in detail, indicating how the seven factors we have just discussed are involved in each. We have divided the methods into four categories: (1) those that employ hormonal manipulations, (2) those that involve chemical or mechanical barriers to the union of egg and sperm, (3) those that require special psychological control, and (4) those that involve surgery.

HORMONAL TYPES OF BIRTH CONTROL

One of the most popular birth control methods today is external administration of reproductive hormones. The rationale for using hormones is based on the female menstrual cycle. By keeping hormone levels constant or by changing them in abnormal ways, one can block ovulation or implantation. As we saw in Chap. 6, there are four hormones that regulate the menstrual cycle: FSH and LH from the pituitary and estrogen and progesterone from the ovary. Most birth control pills contain either estrogen, progesterone, or a combination of the two. Four types of hormonal birth control products currently in use are the combination pill (traditional Pill), the minipill, the shot, and the morning-after pill. Another hormonal approach currently being researched is discussed in Box 8.1.

The combination pill

The **combination pill** consists of both estrogen and progestin (synthetic progesterone) at doses higher than usual body levels. Currently there are more than 25 different brands of combination pills from which to choose (see Fig. 8.1, p. 189). These pills vary with respect to the ratio of estrogen to progestin and with respect to the relative potency of the hormones. Women who experience unpleasant side effects with one product may have no problems with another. It is not uncommon for women to switch brands, with medical consultation, during the first 6 months of pill use.

Women who use the combination pill are instructed to take one pill per day for 21 days and then stop for 7 days. At the end of the seventh day, the cycle is begun anew. During the 7-day period in which no pill is taken, the uterine lining is shed, and the woman experiences menstruation. For those women who suffer from dysmennorhea or heavy flow, such problems are markedly reduced during pill use.

TABLE 8.1

Comparison of
birth control methods

Method	Effectiveness	Cost	Medical services
Tubal ligation	Nearly 100%	Varies depending upon technique, and type of anesthesia	Hospitalization
Vasectomy	Nearly 100%	Ranges from $125–$300 for operation and follow-up	Minor surgery as an outpatient; follow-up necessary until no sperm are found
The Pill	T.E.: 99% A.E.: 90–96%	About $6 per month with prescription	Initial exam, instructions, regular checkups
Minipill	Slightly less effective than the Pill	About $6 per month with prescription	Examination and regular checkups
Intrauterine device (nonmedicated)	T.E. & A.E. the same: 94–99%	Cost of office visit and insertion	Examination, insertion, and regular checkups
Intrauterine device (medicated)	T.E. & A.E. the same: 96–99%	Cost of office visit and insertion; hormone IUDs replaced yearly	Examination, insertion, and regular checkups
Condoms	T.E.: 99% A.E.: 64–97%	$2 per package of three plain condoms	None
Diaphragm with jelly or cream	T.E.: 99% A.E.: 80–98%	Cost of examination, diaphragm $5–10, and cream $3–5 monthly	Initial examination, instructions, fit checked annually
Foams, creams, jellies, tablets	A.E.: 71–98% (Foam most effective)	About $5 for a can of foam (20 applications)	None
Rhythm method (cervical mucus)	A.E.: 74–99%	Possible cost for instruction	Careful instruction to learn method
Rhythm method (basal body temperature)	A.E.: 80–98%	Possible cost for instruction, ovulation thermometer $5–10	Careful instruction to learn method
Withdrawal (coitus interruptus)	15–30 pregnancies; ineffective	None	None
Douche	Ineffective	Cost of douch bag and douching substance	None

Action required at time of coitus	Common side effects	Risks
None	Recuperative period	Risk associated with any surgery, tubal pregnancy, if done improperly
None	Temporary scrotal swelling, soreness, discomfort	Risk associated with any surgical procedure
None	Irregular bleeding, vomiting, spotting, nausea, weight gain, headaches, impaired liver functioning	Circulatory disorders (blood clots, stroke, heart attack, high blood pressure, gall bladder disease)
None	Irregular periods, increased or decreased blood flow	None yet identified
None	Pain and bleeding on insertion, irregular or excessive bleeding, cramps, discomfort	Pelvic inflammatory disease, uterine perforation, miscarriage or tubal pregnancy, expulsion
None	Less pain on insertion, fewer cramps, less bleeding than nonmedicated IUDs	Hormone IUD believed to increase tubal pregnancy risk over non-medicated IUDs
Interruption of foreplay play when put on	None	None
May insert up to 6 hours prior to intercourse	Rare allergic reactions to jelly or cream, vaginal irritation	Vaginal or urinary infection
Insert not more than 10–15 minutes before coitus; tablets require waiting	Occasional irritation of vagina or penis	None
Coitus limited to 13–17 days	None	None
Coitus limited to 9–13 days	None	None
Interruption before ejaculation	None	None
Immediately after ejaculation	None	May destroy helpful, natural bacteria in vaginal area

BOX 8.1

Contraceptive peptides

One promising approach to developing the perfect contraceptive has focused on the brain hormones that ultimately control reproduction. In 1971, scientists succeeded in isolating luteinizing-hormone-releasing hormone (LHRH), a peptide produced by the hypothalamus. It is this peptide (small protein) that regulates the pituitary's production of LH and FSH, which in turn control the production of ovarian and testicular hormones. Thus, it seems logical that synthetic versions of LHRH that would be effective in controlling production of LH and FSH and thereby control of conception could be developed.

With this idea in mind, two main strategies are being explored. The first strategy is to create artificial peptides that mimic the effects of LHRH and to administer them in large enough doses so that they produce the paradoxical effect of inhibiting LH and FSH production. Such mimicking peptides—called agonists—are currently being developed, and a few are undergoing clinical trials in the United States with both women and men. In women, the peptides are being used either to inhibit ovulation or to induce premature menstruation. In men, they are being used to reduce sperm production.

The second strategy is to create antagonists for LHRH—compounds that block the natural action of the hormone. In animal experiments such antagonists have been shown to inhibit ovulation and to block sperm production. Human research using antagonist peptides has only just begun, however.

Agonist peptides have already been tested to some extent in Sweden, where they have been administered to both women and men in the form of a nasal spray used daily. Preliminary results with women have indicated that the peptide does inhibit ovulation, although there have been a few cases of "breakthrough" ovulation and of unexplained bleeding. When use of the nasal spray is discontinued, fertility returns to women after the next menstrual period and returns to men within about 6 weeks.

American studies of synthetic peptides are using compounds that must be injected, although forms that can be administered intravaginally and under the tongue are being developed. In research with men, care is being taken to determine whether the injections must be supplemented with testosterone in order to maintain secondary sexual characteristics and sex drive.

If such contraceptive peptides are developed, they would have several advantages. For one, both men and women could use them. For another, they would not have the general impact on the body that steroids do and thus should not have as many negative side effects (Miller, 1980). Thus, scientists expect peptide contraceptives to be safer than current oral contraceptives. However, it will still be a few years before researchers know for sure whether these artificial peptides can provide an effective, safe, and long-lasting method of birth control for both women and men.

The Pill is an extremely effective form of contraception. The theoretical failure rate is 0.34 pregnancies per 100 woman years, while the actual use failure rate is 4–10 pregnancies per 100 woman years. The majority of failures can be attributed to irregular patterns of pill taking. The combination pill can only be obtained through a doctor's prescription and costs less than $100 a year, excluding doctor's visits.

Mechanism of action The combination pill is an effective form of birth control because it keeps estrogen and progesterone levels artificially high, thereby blocking both ovulation and implantation. Estrogen acts to block ovulation by suppressing FSH and LH secretion from the pituitary. As a result, there is no ripening of a follicle and no mid-cycle surge of LH to trigger ovulation. Progestin keeps the cervical mucus in a thick, acidic state, which is inhospitable to sperm, and it prevents the implantation of fertilized eggs in the uterine wall. It may also retard the movement of an egg down the fallopian tube, and there is some evidence to suggest that progestin also has an antiovu-

FIGURE 8.1
There are many different brands of birth control pills. Most of these are packaged in special cases to simplify pill counting.

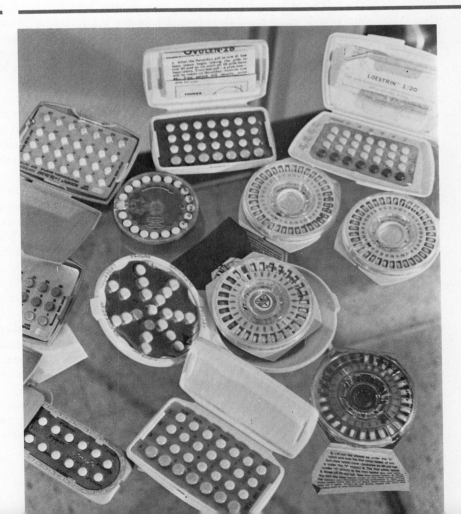

latory effect. Hormonally, the Pill appears to produce a condition similar to pregnancy, so it is not surprising that many of the side effects of the Pill mimic the symptoms of pregnancy.

Side effects   Within recent years there has been considerable controversy over the potential and actual side effects of the Pill. While some media reports have exaggerated the dangers without providing substantial scientific evidence, there are indeed some well-documented risks.

Thromboembolic (blood-clotting) disorders occur with slightly higher frequency in Pill users than in nonusers. The clots typically form in the legs (a condition called *phlebitis*) and may then travel to the lungs, heart, or brain, possibly causing heart attack or stroke. The chance of death from such disorders is about 4 per 100,000 women on the Pill and only 0.4 per 100,000 women who are nonusers. The rate is even higher for women over age 40 and for women who smoke. For nonsmoking women under 40, however, the chances of dying from pregnancy or childbirth (4 per 100,000 women) are about the same as for using the Pill. In any case, all Pill users are instructed to watch for the following signs and to report any such symptoms to their doctor immediately: *a*bdominal pain, *c*hest pain, *h*eadaches, *e*ye problems (blurred vision), and *s*evere leg pains. These symptoms can easily be remembered by the acronym ACHES, which is made up of the first letter of each. Any one or a combination of these symptoms may indicate the presence of a blood-clotting disorder.

In the past several years there have been rumored connections between the incidence of cancer (especially of the cervix, uterus, and breast) and the use of oral contraceptives. Currently there is no definitive evidence to suggest that taking birth control pills increases one's chances of getting cancer. Researchers have found, however, that birth control pills may aggravate existing cancer (World Health Organization, 1978).

The Pill has also been associated with a number of less serious symptoms. There may be an increase in blood pressure, and certain diseases such as asthma and epilepsy are worsened by Pill use. About 5 percent of women who use oral contraceptives develop painful headaches. In addition, hormones may produce **cloasma** (darkened spots on the face) and may increase the incidence of or susceptibility to vaginal infections. Other symptoms, such as nausea, water retention, weight gain, acne, irritability, and depression usually disappear within the first 2 months and can be minimized by switching to a different brand of birth control pill.

Because of possible side effects, the following women should not use oral contraceptives: (1) women with a history of heart or liver ailments, (2) women with a history of blood-clotting disorders, (3) women with cancer, (4) women over age 40, (5) women who have any unusual or abnormal vaginal bleeding, and (6) women who smoke.

Advantages and disadvantages   There are several advantages to using the Pill over other forms of contraception. First, it does not interfere with the spontaneity of lovemaking. Second, Pill users report fewer problems with menstruation and may experience an increase in sexual desire. Third, the Pill reduces any problems with dysmennorhea or heavy flow, and it regularizes irregular cycles.

Among the disadvantages to using the Pill are the unwanted side effects and the risks we have already mentioned. Although many of the side effects can usually be reduced by switching brands, some of the effects persist in a few women. A second problem is our lack of knowledge about the long-term effects of Pill use. Such questions as the length of time a woman can safely use the Pill and the effects of the Pill on the aging process remain to be answered. Finally, a woman must develop some kind of regimen to remind herself to take her pills. Skipping pills is one of the major causes of contraceptive failure. If one pill is missed, the woman should take the pill when she remembers and should take her regular pill at the usual time the next day. If a woman forgets her pill for 2 days in a row, she should take 2 pills for 2 days and use an alternate method of contraception until that month's supply of pills is exhausted. If a woman misses her pills for 3 days, she should throw away the remaining pills for that month and start a new package of pills on the next Sunday, whether or not she is bleeding, and should use an alternate form of contraception through the first 2 weeks of the next package of pills. A woman who frequently forgets to take her pills should seriously question whether this is a suitable form of contraception for her.

The minipill   The **minipill**, which first appeared on the market in 1973, contains the same progestin found in the combination pill but at considerably lower doses. It does not contain any estrogen. The trade-name products include Micronor and Nor-Q-D, both of which contain 0.35 milligram progestin, and Ovrette, which contains 0.75 milligram progestin. Because the combination pills contain anywhere from 0.5 to 10 milligrams of progestin, we can see that the minipill is exactly that—a minidose of hormone. As in the combination pill, the progestin acts to maintain hostile chemical conditions in the cervical mucus, inhibits implantation of fertilized eggs, retards the movement of the egg through the fallopian tube, and may inhibit ovulation.

Women who use the minipill are instructed to take one pill starting on the first day of their menstrual period and to continue to take a pill a day thereafter. The effectiveness rates are slightly worse than those for the combination pill. The theoretical failure rate is 1.25 pregnancies per 100 woman years, and the actual failure rate is about the same—5–10 pregnancies per 100 woman years. The slight difference can be attributed to the use of lower doses of hormone and to a necessary adjustment period—most pregnancies occur in the first 6 months of pill use. It is usually recommended that women use a backup form of contraception during this early period. As is the case with the combination pill, the minipill can only be obtained through a doctor's prescription and costs less than $100 a year.

Although the minipill eliminates the side effects caused by the estrogen contained in the combination pill, it does not eliminate side effects altogether. Some women report an increased tendency toward vaginitis, weight gain, and acne. In addition, some women may experience less frequent menstrual bleeding and may have spotting between periods. Some women have very few cycles (perhaps only one or two a year) while taking the minipill. There is also a slight increase in the risk of ectopic pregnancy (see Chap. 7). The minipill is still too new to determine whether there is an increased risk of thromboembolic disorders as there is with the combination pill.

Because the minipill has fewer and less severe side effects than the combination pill, it may be safely used by teenagers and women over 40. The pill-taking regimen is also easier to remember, since there are no pauses in pill taking and there is no counting of days. Instead, a woman simply takes one pill a day for as long as she wishes to use the method. The main disadvantages are the possible side effects and the increased irregularity of the menstrual cycle, which makes it difficult to determine whether a woman is pregnant or merely irregular.

*The
shot*

The shot is a long-lasting injection of progestin that has a contraceptive effect. One brand, Depo Provera, is currently available in 64 countries and has been considered for approval in the United States. Depo Provera, which provides 150 milligrams of progestin, must be injected once every 3 months. The theoretical failure rate is similar to that for the combination pill. Actual use failure rates are not available. The shot can only be prescribed by a doctor.

The side effects are similar to those described for the minipill, except that the menstrual bleeding may be even more irregular. Even after use has been discontinued, some women may not regain their periods for quite some time and fertility may be impaired. In addition, injections of this substance have been shown to produce cancer in dogs (Rinehart & Winter, 1975). The advantages are similar to those of the Pill, with the additional advantage that women do not have to remember to take a pill every day (although they do need to remember to visit their doctors four times a year). The disadvantages are probably more severe than those of the minipill, with the additional problem that if side effects develop, they may take several months to subside. Thus, unlike with the Pill, the action of the hormone cannot be stopped quickly.

*The morning-after
pill*

Unlike the other hormonal forms of contraception, the ***morning-after pill*** is taken postcoitally (after intercourse). Following unprotected mid-cycle intercourse, a woman may take pills containing high levels of estrogen to prevent the implantation of the fertilized egg on the uterine wall. This is an emergency form of birth control, often used with rape victims, and should never be considered a major method of contraception.

The most commonly used morning-after pill is ***diethylstilbestrol*** (DES). Women must take one 25-milligram pill twice a day for 5 days to ensure effective contraceptive action. The timing between intercourse and treatment is critical. The pill-taking regimen must begin no later than 72 hours after intercourse and preferably no later than 24 hours after. No effectiveness rates are available. However, recent reports indicate that among 5593 women who were treated with DES, only 26 became pregnant. Without DES, approximately 1100 of the women would have been expected to become pregnant (Hatcher et al., 1978). Failures are probably caused by too much time passing before treatment is begun. The morning-after pill is available only through a doctor's prescription, and the cost includes both the medical exam and the price of the pills.

There are several significant side effects to the use of morning-after pills. High levels of estrogen can and often do produce severe nausea, vomiting, headaches, and breast tenderness. The greatest risk of DES treatment, however, has been found to be not to the woman but to her potential offspring. In the 1950s and 1960s DES was commonly given to pregnant women in the first or second trimester to prevent miscarriage. Studies have revealed that female offspring of these mothers have an increased chance of developing precancerous vaginal conditions in their early teens or twenties and that male offspring show decreases in sperm volume, motility, and density and an increase in growths within the epididymis (Herbst et al., 1972, 1973, 1974). Large doses of DES may also produce skull, skeletal, and limb deformities in offspring. For these reasons, DES treatment should be considered only as an emergency form of birth control, and women who undergo DES treatment and still become pregnant should seriously consider obtaining a therapeutic abortion.

MECHANICAL AND CHEMICAL FORMS OF BIRTH CONTROL

A number of birth control techniques mechanically or chemically prevent pregnancy. The four that we will discuss in this section are the IUD, the diaphragm, the condom, and spermicidal foam. Some more experimental methods are presented in Box 8.2.

The intrauterine device (IUD)

The **intrauterine device** (IUD) is a small object inserted through the cervix into the uterus. Each IUD has one or two strings that extend from the uterus through the cervix into the vagina, helping the woman to determine whether the IUD is in place. The four most commonly used IUDs are the Lippes Loop, Saf-T-Coil, Copper-7, and Progestasert T, several of which are shown in Fig. 8.2. This last brand has an additional contraceptive component, progestin, and must be replaced every year. There are no data on the longevity of other devices, but most doctors suggest that they be replaced every 3–5 years. The theoretical effectiveness is 1–5 pregnancies per 100 woman years, while the actual use rate is 5–10 pregnancies per 100 woman years. The most common cause of failure is expulsion of the IUD by the uterus—a problem that is more common for women who have never had any children.

The IUD must be inserted by a doctor in a procedure that can be performed during an office visit (see Fig. 8.3). The IUD insertion procedure can be painful, although anesthesia of the cervix can be used to reduce this problem. The cost of an IUD, including the insertion, runs slightly more than a year's supply of birth control pills. During the first few days of wearing an IUD, the woman may experience cramps and vaginal bleeding.

The IUD acts primarily to prevent the implantation of the fertilized egg in the endometrium of the uterus. It does so by causing local inflammatory reactions that make the endometrium unsuitable for implantation by changing the speed of movement of the egg or by mechanically dislodging the egg from

BOX 8.2

Rings, caps, sponges, and tampons

As research continues in the effort to find the ideal method of birth control, many avenues are being pursued. One area currently being explored is improvement of mechanical-chemical methods. Among the devices being tested are vaginal rings, cervical caps, vaginal sponges, and contraceptive tampons.

Vaginal rings are pliable plastic rings that release hormones to be absorbed by the vaginal lining. These hormones inhibit ovulation, fertilization, or implantation. One version, which can be inserted by the woman herself, can be used for up to 2 years. It must be taken out during each menstrual period and reinserted afterward, however. Clinical trials being conducted by Daniel Mishell and others indicate that this method is as effective as the combination pill yet has fewer side effects because estrogen is not involved (Abrams, 1980).

The cervical cap is a rubber or plastic device that fits over the cervix. It blocks sperm from getting into the uterus, but it has a one-way valve that allows menstrual material to flow out. Like a diaphragm, the cervical cap must be fitted to each woman. Fitting is done by taking an impression of the cervix and using the impression to make the cap—a process that takes only a short time during an office visit. If properly fitted, the cap will rarely be dislodged. Suction from cervical fluid holds the cap in place. Each cap also has a marker that the woman can use to feel if the cap is properly positioned. A form of the cervical cap has been used in Europe for many years, but the latest version has only recently started to be tested in the United States.

Several types of vaginal sponges are currently being tested. These sponges are designed to block the cervix, to absorb semen, and in some cases to release a spermicide. One type is a small, cup-shaped piece of material that is inserted by the woman prior to intercourse; it provides contraceptive protection for up to 2 days. Another type, shaped like a cylinder, can be worn for as long as a month at a time (between menstrual periods) but must be removed or replaced within 2 days after intercourse. Some sponges are being designed to be reusable—they can simply be washed out; they do not contain a spermicide, however. With all types, the woman first moistens the sponge and then places it high in her vagina, where it expands to cover the cervix. Scientists studying the sponge method are optimistic about its effectiveness.

One laboratory is studying the feasibility of contraceptive tampons. The tiny tampon is inserted before intercourse, and during intercourse it releases a spermicide. After intercourse, it quickly absorbs both the spermicide and the semen. Supposedly, the tampon is effective for up to 72 hours. According to the developers, this technique is not only comfortable and convenient but gives minimal irritation to the vagina.

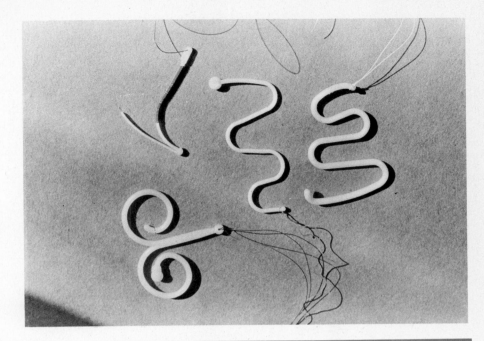

FIGURE 8.2
Different types of intrauterine devices (IUDs). Copper 7 (upper left), Saf-T-Coil (lower left), and Lippes Loop (two on the upper right).

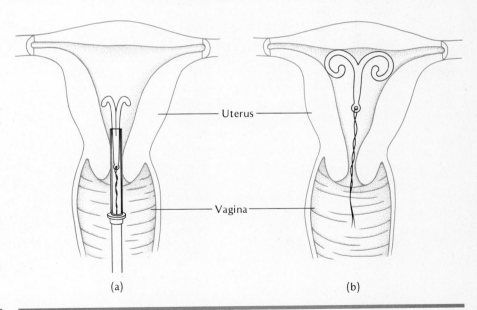

Uterus

Vagina

(a)   (b)

FIGURE 8.3
Insertion and placement of IUD into the uterus. Insertion (a) can be performed in a doctor's office. Following placement (b), the strings extending into the vagina can be used to determine that the IUD remains in place.

FIGURE 8.4
*(Top) The dia-
phragm consists of
a plastic dome
that covers the
cervix when
inserted into the
vagina. To be
effective, the
diaphragm must
be used with
spermicidal cream
or jelly. (Bottom)
Inserting the
diaphragm.*

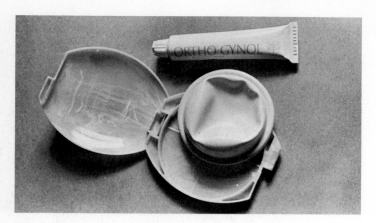

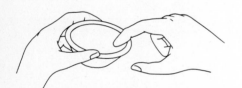

Place spermicide in dome and rub on
dome and rim.

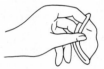

Fold diaphragm.

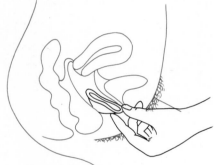

Insert it into
the vagina.

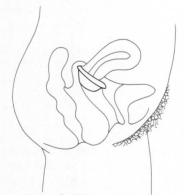

Guide it until it
covers cervix.

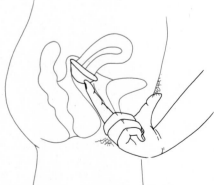

Use your finger to check that the cervix
is under dome of the diaphragm.

the uterine wall. There is also a possibility that the IUD immobilizes sperm that travel into the uterus, thereby preventing fertilization.

One of the most common side effects associated with the IUD is more painful menstruation with heavier bleeding. There is also a slight risk of uterine perforation when the IUD is inserted and a slight possibility of developing an infection of the uterus and fallopian tubes. This kind of infection, called **pelvic inflammatory disease** (PID), may lead to sterility. Women who plan to have children might therefore want to select another form of birth control.

The advantages of the IUD over other forms of birth control include the absence of major hormonal manipulations, no interference with the spontaneous flow of lovemaking, and little to remember. Once it has been inserted, the woman need only check periodically to make sure it is in place. Thus, this form of reversible birth control requires the least amount of effort for the user. However, women who have not yet had children or who have unusual vaginal bleeding may wish to consider other forms of birth control.

The diaphragm

The **diaphragm** is a dome-shaped latex cup that is covered with spermicidal jelly or cream and inserted into the vagina prior to intercourse. The flexible rim of the diaphragm makes its insertion and positioning against the cervix a relatively easy task (see Fig. 8.4). Following intercourse, the diaphragm must be left in place for at least 6 hours. If further acts of intercourse are desired during this time, additional spermicide must be applied.

The diaphragm acts primarily as a chemical barrier to the passage of sperm. It works because the spermicidal cream inactivates and destroys the sperm before they can travel through the cervix. The main function of the diaphragm is to hold the spermicide in close contact with the cervix. Because the diaphragm can move during intercourse, when used alone it is much less effective in preventing pregnancy.

Despite a theoretical rate indicating that the diaphragm is highly effective (3 pregnancies per 100 woman years), the actual use effectiveness ranges from 3 to 17 pregnancies per 100 woman years, depending on the study cited. Contraceptive failure can be traced to three common errors: The woman may fail to use the spermicidal cream with the diaphragm; she may remove the diaphragm before the 6-hour period has ended; or she may have multiple sessions of lovemaking without applying additional spermicide. Masters and Johnson also found a high incidence of dislodged diaphragms in couples that used the woman-above position with vigorous thrusting (Johnson and Masters, 1963).

Diaphragms can only be obtained with a doctor's prescription. It is the responsibility of the doctor to ensure that the device fits properly (they come in different sizes) and to instruct the woman in proper procedures for insertion and removal. Women must be refitted if they experience a substantial change in weight (either gain or loss) and if they give birth to a baby. The diaphragm costs somewhat less than the Pill.

Although the diaphragm lost favor after the development of the Pill, it is now becoming popular once again. Women are turning to the diaphragm because it produces no hormonal changes and has few if any side effects. It can be inserted several hours before intercourse, so lovemaking need not be disrupted. In addition, for those couples whose enjoyment of sex is diminished by menstruation, the diaphragm can be used to catch the menstrual flow.

On the negative side, the diaphragm may be perceived as somewhat messy to use. Women who are uncomfortable touching their genitals or who find the small leakage of spermicide from the vagina unpleasant should probably not use this method. The spermicidal jelly or cream may produce an allergic reaction in some men or women, and it may interfere with oral sex if the partner does not like the smell or taste of the substance used. A few women are unable to use the diaphragm because of anatomical variations that prevent a satisfactory fit.

The **condom** (Fig. 8.5) is the oldest and most common form of contraception used by men. It consists of a thin sheath of material that fits tightly over an erect penis. Condoms are made either of latex or of membrane from lamb intestines; they come rolled up in small packets. They may or may not be lubricated, and some are equipped with a nipplelike tip that collects the semen. There are also color and shape variations, and some have texturing designed to enhance sensation in the partner. When using a condom with a plain end, the man must leave a space about ½ inch at the tip to serve as a collection place for sperm.

Although the theoretical failure rate is low (3 percent), the actual failure rate is considerably higher (15–20 pregnancies per 100 woman years). Contraceptive failure can be attributed to a number of human errors. To be used properly, the condom must be unrolled onto the erect penis before the penis has been inserted—*not* just before ejaculation. As was mentioned in Chap. 4, the small amount of Cowper's gland fluid that is released by the penis during

FIGURE 8.5
(Left) The condom comes in different shapes and colors, with or without lubrication. (Right) The correct positioning of the condom on the penis.

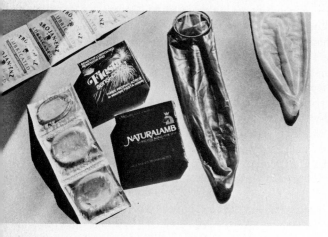
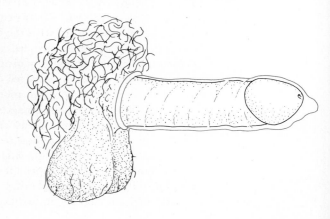

arousal can contain sperm. Thus, one possible error is penetrating the vagina and then withdrawing to put on a condom before continuing. Another error is failure to leave space for the semen in the plain-end condoms, which may cause the condom to burst or the semen to ooze up around the penile shaft and out into the vagina. Accidental spills may also occur if the condom slips off the penis after ejaculation but before the penis is withdrawn from the vagina. Thus, when using a condom a man should remove his penis from the vagina before the erection subsides and should hold the rim of the condom against the root of his penis as he withdraws. Another common error is lubricating condoms with petroleum jelly such as Vaseline. Although Vaseline has good lubricating properties, it is corrosive to rubber products and can weaken the strength of the condom or actually put holes in it. If external lubrication is desired, K-Y jelly, contraceptive chemicals, unscented coconut oil, or saliva can be used safely. In fact, the combination of condom and spermicidal foam is highly effective in preventing pregnancy, with an actual failure rate of around 3 pregnancies per 100 woman years. Finally, because condoms deteriorate with age and heat, they should not be kept for longer than 2 years, and they should not be stored in a man's wallet because of the exposure to body heat.

Among the advantages of the condom over other methods are that it does not involve any major bodily changes, it may reduce premature ejaculation, it can effectively prevent the spread of venereal diseases, and it is readily available and can be purchased in any drugstore for minimal cost. One significant disadvantage is that a few men are unable to maintain an erection when using a condom, presumably because of the partial loss of sensation from the penis. A second disadvantage is that donning the condom can disrupt the spontaneity of lovemaking. Couples who are most successful in using the condom have learned to incorporate the act of putting it on into their lovemaking behavior.

Spermicidal foam

Spermicidal foam (see Fig. 8.6) is a substance that is inserted into the vagina just prior to intercourse. It consists of an inert base that adheres to the cervix and a spermicidal chemical that kills sperm before they reach the cervix. Spermicidal products such as Emko and Delfen should not be confused with the wide variety of vaginal deodorants now available; products such as Summer's Eve have no contraceptive action whatsoever. We should also caution that spermicidal creams meant to be used with a diaphragm should never be used alone, as they do not stick to the cervical surface as well as foam. Although the theoretical failure rate for foam is low (3 pregnancies per 100 woman years), the actual failure rate ranges from 3 to 29 pregnancies per 100 woman years, depending on which study is quoted. Typical errors in the use of foam include using too little foam, not being aware that the foam can is empty, not shaking the foam can vigorously enough, and douching (rinsing out the vagina) too soon after intercourse.

In recent years a new spermicidal product called the Encare Oval has been marketed in the United States. It is not really a spermicidal foam, although it is classified as such. Instead, it is a small oval object that effervesces when placed in the deep recesses of the vagina. Women must wait 10 minutes for the

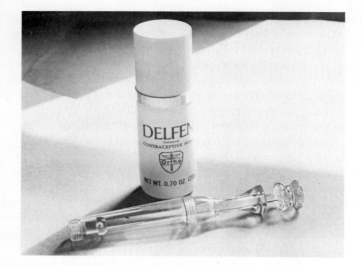

effervescing action to be completed before they engage in intercourse. However, the Encare Oval can be inserted up to 2 hours prior to intercourse, whereas foam must be used just before intercourse. The Encare Oval has a lower theoretical failure rate (1 pregnancy per 100 woman years) than spermicidal foam. Data are not yet available on the actual failure rate. All spermicidal foam products and the Encare Oval are available for purchase in any drugstore and are generally quite inexpensive.

There are few side effects with this method aside from the possible irritation or allergy that can affect the man or woman. The Encare Oval produces a sensation of heat during the effervescing process that some women find pleasant and others find unpleasant.

The main advantage of spermicidal foam is that it is a temporary form of birth control that involves no hormonal manipulations and has few side effects in addition to being easily available and inexpensive. From a negative standpoint, foam may be perceived as messy, entails handling of the genitals, which may make some individuals uncomfortable, and results in a small vaginal discharge for about a day after use. It is somewhat disruptive to the spontaneity of lovemaking (less so for the Encare Oval) and may have an unpleasant taste to some people, thereby interfering with the pleasures of oral sex.

Douching   We mention douching here not because it is a contraceptive method but because so many people erroneously think it is. **Douching** usually refers to rinsing or cleansing of the vaginal canal. It is currently popular to douche to remove possible vaginal odors and discharges and to change the pH value of the vagina. The possible therapeutic benefits of this practice are seriously questioned by most physicians, and in fact some douches may actually create chemical imbalances in the vagina that enhance the development of infection.

Some people assume that if they use the proper substances, douching can be a form of contraception. This notion is further enhanced by a folklore of suggested douching regimens. Acidic substances are often recommended because sperm are particularly sensitive to them. But in the absence of anything else, common folklore would have us believe the absurd idea that shaking a Coke bottle and inserting it into the vagina is an effective method of birth control.

Douching has two serious flaws when used as a contraceptive method. First, it occurs after intercourse has taken place. Even if the woman were an Olympic speedster, in the race between her and the sperm, the odds would greatly favor the sperm. Douching might kill some of the sperm by the time a woman has rushed to cleanse her vagina, but it certainly wouldn't kill all of them. Second, and most important, because douching chemicals are being propelled toward the cervix, they might actually force additional sperm into the uterus. Thus, douching should not be thought of as a form of birth control. It is not even a suitable backup method, and those who use it as such may actually be increasing their chances of becoming pregnant.

There are several techniques that require a special type of control from the participants. Both of the techniques discussed here, the rhythm method and coitus interruptus, require unusual degrees of self-restraint.

The **rhythm method** if based on accurately calculating the day of ovulation and then abstaining from intercourse for several days before and after that point. There are three techniques that can be used to predict the day of ovulation: the calendar method, the basal body temperature method, and the cervical secretion method.

Prior to using the **calendar method**, the woman must formulate her menstrual calendar, a record of the length of her menstrual cycles over the previous 8-month period. She then must examine the length of her longest and shortest cycle and then determine on which days abstinence should begin and end. To find the first day of abstinence, the woman should subtract 18 days from the length of her shortest cycle. The last day of abstinence is calculated by subtracting 11 days from the length of her longest cycle. Let's suppose that after careful record keeping a woman determines her shortest cycle to be 27 days and her longest cycle to be 40 days. To practice the calendar method correctly, she would begin abstinence on day 9 and end on day 29—a 20-day period. Thus, the rhythm method can be particularly frustrating for a woman with an irregular cycle. Consider another case in which the cycles are more regular: 28 days for the shortest cycle and 31 days for the longest cycle. Abstinence would start on day 10 and end on day 20—a 10-day period, which might be more tolerable.

The second technique involves measuring **basal body temperature**. As we saw in Chap. 6, body temperature increases at ovulation and remains elevated during the luteal phase of the menstrual cycle. The only difficult part of this technique is obtaining an accurate basal temperature measure. Women must take their temperature in the morning immediately upon awakening—before they go to the bathroom, drink coffee, or change clothes. In addition, because body temperature is sensitive to many environmental factors, women must make adjustments for possible elevations in temperature as a result of colds or infections, use of an electric blanket, or irregular sleeping hours. To ensure effective birth control, abstinence must begin on day 3 and continue until body temperature has increased 0.6–0.8°F and has remained elevated for 3 consecutive days. An abstinence period of 10 or more days is common with this technique. This time period can be shortened by using the calendar method to determine the day of onset and the temperature method to determine the day of ending the abstinence.

The third technique is the **cervical mucus secretion method**, which is also referred to as "natural birth control" or the **Billings method**. This technique is based on the fact that the cervical mucus undergoes visible and dramatic changes at ovulation (see Chap. 6). Both prior to and after ovulation, the cervical secretion is yellow-white and viscous. During ovulation, however, the mucus becomes a clear, sticky discharge that is amazingly elastic and that resembles raw egg whites. A drop of this clear mucus can be pulled between two glass slides into a thin strand that measures 6 centimeters or more.

Because the vagina can contain substances in addition to cervical mucus, women who use this method must be able to distinguish it from semen, spermicide, lubrication, or discharges caused by infections. Women who douche should not rely on the Billings method, as douching washes away the very secretions that should be examined. The Billings method also makes use of *mittelschmerz*—the mid-cycle abdominal pain associated with ovulation—as a marker. Not all women experience mittelschmerz, so it is helpful only to those who do.

Like the basal body temperature method, the Billings method is useful in determining only when ovulation *has* occurred and not when it *will* occur. It is not sufficient to begin abstinence on the day when cervical secretions change because sperm can live in the reproductive tract 2 to 3 days. A woman would have to be able to predict what the cervical secretions are going to look like 2–3 days after intercourse, which is not possible. Thus, it is recommended that abstinence begin on day 3 of the menstrual cycle or be determined by the calendar method and continue for 3 days after the appearance of the egg-white-like mucus.

The effectiveness of the rhythm method varies depending on which technique is used. Consistent users of the calendar method have a failure rate of 15 pregnancies per 100 woman years, while all users have a considerably higher failure rate (25 pregnancies per 100 woman years). Much of the difficulty can be traced to irregular cycles (which are unfortunately typical of 92 percent of the female population) and to taking chances during the abstinence period. Very low rates have been reported for couples using the Billings method (2–3 pregnancies per 100 woman years).

The rhythm method is medically safe to use and is readily available without major cost. On the other hand, it is generally associated with high failure rates, may involve handling of the genitals (the Billings method), takes a long time to implement, and can be frustrating if it is the only method used. Furthermore, it does require an understanding of the biology of reproduction, the scrupulous maintenance of menstrual charts, and abstinence from intercourse for fairly long periods of time. It is not recommended for women with very irregular cycles.

Many couples use a modified version of the rhythm method in conjunction with another form of birth control. Abstinence is replaced by protected intercourse with condoms, diaphragms, or spermicidal foam. The rhythm method is used not only as a form of birth control but as a technique to facilitate the occurrence of pregnancy, as we saw in Chap. 6.

Coitus interruptus, or **withdrawal**, is perhaps the oldest form of birth control known to humankind. It is also the least effective. As the name implies, coitus interruptus involves withdrawing the penis from the vagina just prior to ejaculation. Thus, ejaculation occurs away from the genital area of the female. The failure rate for this form of birth control is quite high. The theoretical rate is estimated to be about 15 pregnancies per 100 woman years, while the actual use failure rate is about 25–30 pregnancies. This high failure rate can be attributed to two factors. First, failure may be traced to the inability of the man to withdraw before ejaculation occurs. And, as mentioned previously, even if the man consistently withdraws prior to ejaculation, the small amount of Cowper's gland fluid released by the penis during arousal can contain sperm, so the woman can still become pregnant. There are no known medical side effects. Nonetheless, sex may become so focused on the timing and withdrawal that it produces a phenomenon called *spectatoring*. During spectatoring the partners become more involved in the mechanics than the joys of sex. This may alter expectations and make sex less pleasurable. Despite the drawbacks, coitus interruptus continues to be an attractive technique for some because it is available at any time for no cost.

Coitus interruptus

A number of birth control techniques involve minor and even major surgery. These include abortion and the more permanent form of birth control produced by sterilization.

The act and even the word *abortion* evokes a variety of reactions. These reactions stem from several ethical and moral dilemmas. Is abortion the same as murder? Is there a point in development when an embryo becomes a human being, or is it a human being from the point of conception? What rights do women have to control the fate of their own bodies? What rights do potential fathers have when abortion is being considered? What rights do embryos have, or, at least, who represents the unborn organism? These are but a few of the problems surrounding the abortion issue, and they have been with the human race for a long time. They are currently unresolved in our society today as witnessed by the intense and bitter disputes between pro-life and pro-choice groups.

METHODS INVOLVING SURGICAL PROCEDURES
Abortion

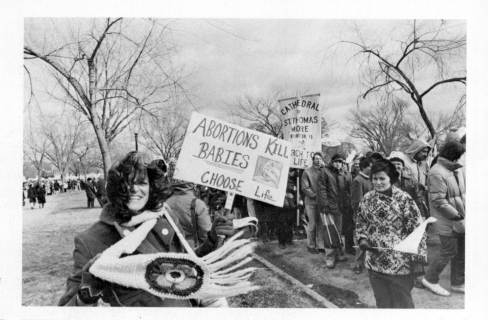

*People have very
strong feelings
about abortion, as
typified in these
pictures.*

As a form of birth control, **_abortion_** refers to surgical procedures in which
the already implanted embryo or fetus is removed from the uterus. The current
legal restraints surrounding abortion can be summarized as follows: (1) Prior to
the end of the first 3 months of pregnancy, the decision to abort the embryo is
left to the woman and her physician; (2) prior to the end of the second
trimester, the state can regulate the abortion decision in ways that will favor a
woman's health; (3) during the third trimester, the state can regulate and even
prohibit all abortions except those needed to save the life of the woman; and
(4) neither a parent nor a spouse can exercise veto power over the woman's
wish to have an abortion.

Although abortion is a fairly simple operation if done early enough in
gestation, it is not a simple process for the woman on whom it is performed.
She is faced with a decision that has moral and psychological repercussions as
well as possible physical ones. The decision requires considerable thought,
adequate support from professionals, family, and friends, and suitable reference
sources. The woman is likely to experience at least some doubts and anxieties
through the decision-making process.

The first step in the decision-making process is the pregnancy test. It is
important that a woman have a pregnancy test as soon as possible after a
missed period. This will provide her with an ample amount of time in which
to make a decision. With a confirmation of pregnancy, the woman may need to
examine her life situation, feelings about pregnancy, reactions to abortion,
moral convictions, feelings toward her partner, and her life plans, all in a

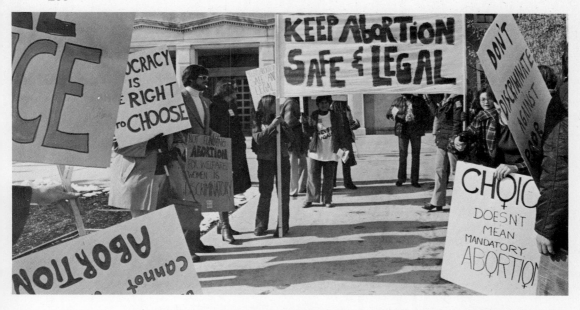

nonjudgmental atmosphere. Some women may need counseling, while others may be able to make a decision rather quickly.

The actual abortion procedure used depends on the age of the embryo or fetus. Because age is sometimes difficult to determine, it is usually calculated in terms of weeks since the last menstrual period (LMP). Within the first trimester, abortion is usually performed with the vacuum curettage method or with the more traditional dilatation and curettage method.

The ***vacuum curettage method*** can be performed in a doctor's office and generally takes about 10 minutes. It involves two steps. First, the cervix is locally anesthetized and a speculum is inserted to widen or dilate the cervical opening. Next, a vacuum curette (hollow plastic rod) is inserted into the uterus and the contents are sucked out, with suction provided by a syringe, foot pump, or electrical vacuum pump (see Fig. 8.7). This method empties the uterus in a short time and requires minimal cervical dilation. If the abortion is performed early enough (4–8 weeks LMP), dilation and anesthesia may not be necessary. In such cases the method is referred to as ***menstrual extraction***.

The traditional ***dilatation and curettage*** (D and C) requires a sharp metal curette in place of the vacuum curette. This curette is used to scrape out the contents of the uterus. The D and C is considered to be inferior to the vacuum method because it requires general anesthesia, is associated with increased blood loss, and is less effective in removing all of the uterine contents.

In the early part of the second trimester, the most commonly used abortion method is ***dilatation and evacuation*** (D and E), which is a combination of the vacuum and D and C methods. At this stage more dilation of the cervical

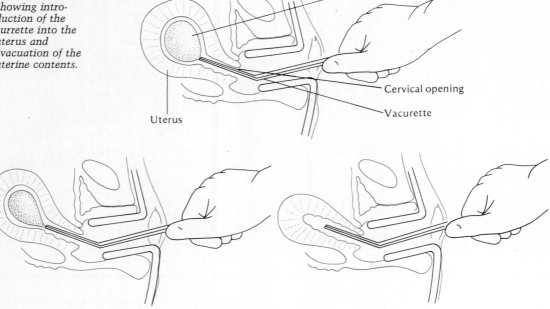

opening is required, and patients are often given *oxytocin*, which promotes uterine contractions and restricts blood loss as indicated in Chap. 7.

Physicians occasionally use a procedure called *hysterotomy* for fetuses 16–24 weeks old. This procedure is major abdominal surgery in which the fetus is excised from the uterus and removed through an incision in the abdominal wall. Because of the increased risks that are associated with major surgery, hysterotomy is used primarily when other methods cannot be employed.

During the late part of the second trimester surgical procedures such as D and E become more difficult to use. Instead, abortion is typically performed by inducing labor and causing miscarriage. The induction of labor is usually produced by the injection of toxic substances into the amniotic fluid surrounding the fetus. The most commonly used substances are a hypertonic saline solution (concentrated salt solution) and prostaglandins. Abortions in the second trimester are usually performed because of genetic defects in the offspring. *Amniocentesis* is the procedure used to detect these defects, and it cannot be carried out until the fourth month of pregnancy (see Chap. 7).

Abortion is a highly effective form of birth control. It is available to most women during the first trimester and requires the skills of a physician. As the fetus grows older, it becomes increasingly more difficult for the woman to obtain an abortion, and the costs and risks rise accordingly.

Any type of surgery entails some health risks, and it is no different for abortion. Excessive bleeding, infection, uterine perforation, retained fetal tissue, and other such complications arise in 13 percent of all abortions (Meeker and Gray, 1975). There is also the possibility of dying from the complications of an abortion, although this is quite rare today. The risk of complication or death is lowest for vacuum suction and highest for hysterotomy.

There has been considerable concern about the possible psychological effects of abortion. Stories and first-hand accounts published in magazines and books seem to emphasize the traumatic nature of abortion. Nevertheless, documented evidence suggests that the abortion experience is more balanced (Osofsky and Osofsky, 1972). Most women seem to be relieved and content after their abortion experience. Only 10 percent of women undergoing abortion develop psychological problems, and many of them have had a previous history of such problems. In addition, women who are able to obtain an abortion are better adjusted than those who are denied treatment, and the children who are born under the latter circumstances tend to be more disturbed than other children. Thus, psychological problems may more typically result from failure rather than success in obtaining an abortion.

Because of the risks involved, abortion should never be considered a primary form of birth control but should only be used as a possible backup method in the case of contraceptive failure.

Sterilization　　The term **sterilization** has come to carry negative, emotion-laden connotations. Historically, sterilization has been viewed with a great deal of suspicion, fueled in part by stories (some true, some false) of involuntary sterilization programs directed against such groups as the retarded, the insane, and the poor. Furthermore, there are many misconceptions about sterilization. Some think it is a form of castration (removal of the testes), which it is not. Others assume that it will permanently change their sexual behavior and desire. Still others are put off by the permanency of sterilization. Nevertheless, as indicated in Fig. 8.8, sterilization has become increasingly popular as a form of birth control and, in fact, is a very common form of birth control for married couples over age 30 (Presser and Bumpas, 1972; Hulka, 1977).

Sterilization procedures involve blocking off or surgically removing part of the reproductive system of the male or female in such a way as to prevent the union of sperm and egg. Because the procedures are different for men and women, we will discuss them separately.

Sterilization in the male　　The standard sterilization procedure used for men is **vasectomy**. This minor surgical procedure can be performed under local anesthesia in a doctor's office. The method consists of making two incisions in the scrotum, cutting the two vasa deferentia, and tying off the ends (see Fig. 8.9). The cutting of the vasa deferentia has no effect on the functioning of the testes, which continue to manufacture sperm and produce testosterone. The surgery only prevents sperm from being transported to the ejaculatory duct. Even the semen looks pretty much the same after surgery except that it contains no sperm. After all, semen consists primarily of secretions from the

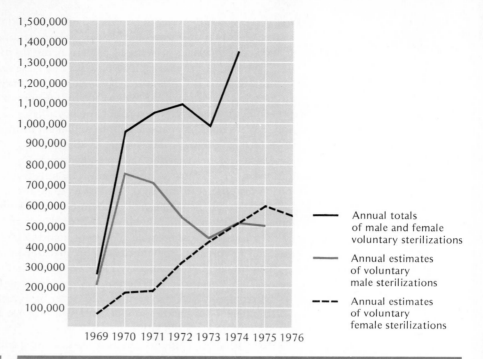

FIGURE 8.8

Sterilization for men and women between 1969 and 1976. (Hatcher, et al., 1980)

seminal vesicles, Cowper's glands, and prostate, all of which empty their contents into the ejaculatory duct and not into the vas deferens. The vasectomy, then, does not decrease sexual drive, nor does it impair sexual response, lead to the development of female characteristics such as breasts or a high-pitched voice, or result in any substantial decrease in the amount of semen produced.

There are relatively few possible side effects to vasectomy, the primary one being development of an infection in the vas deferens. Some psychological complications may arise. One study indicated that of 1000 men who underwent vasectomy, 1.5 percent reported decreased sexual pleasure. This percentage is rather small, however, especially when compared to 73 percent who reported increased sexual pleasure (Simon Population Trust, 1969). Some men may develop antibodies to their own sperm, but the consequences of this reaction are not known (Henry et al., 1972; *Population Reports*, 1975).

All in all, vasectomy is an extremely effective form of permanent birth control. It involves no major hormonal shifts, does not interfere with the spontaneity of lovemaking, and does not involve any daily or monthly preparation. The failure rate is close to zero. Pregnancies, when they do occur, develop within the first 2 months after surgery. This may happen because some sperm continue to survive in the ejaculatory duct for a period of time or because the end of the vas deferens has grown back together. As a result, couples are

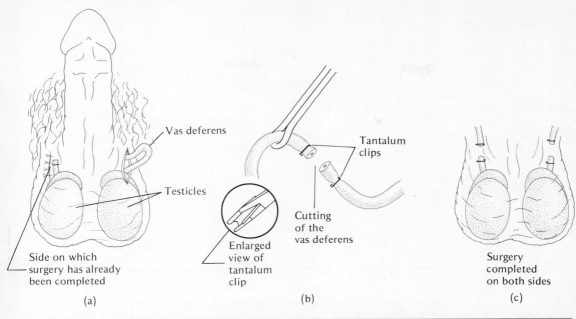

Vas deferens

Testicles

Side on which
surgery has already
been completed

(a)

Enlarged
view of
tantalum
clip

Tantalum
clips

Cutting
of the
vas deferens

(b)

Surgery
completed
on both sides

(c)

FIGURE 8.9

*Vasectomy.
Following
injection of a local
anesthetic, (a) an
incision is made
near the vas
deferens, and the
tube is pulled
through the
opening. (b)The
vas is cut and
clips are applied to
each end. (c) After
surgery, sperm are
unable to travel
from the testes to
the penis.*

advised to use another form of contraception until a semen analysis indicates an absence of sperm.

The main disadvantage of vasectomy for some is its relative permanence. We use the word *relative* because vasectomies can sometimes be reversed. The success of reversal depends on the extent to which the severed ends of the vas deferens can be reconnected. For those men who have developed antibodies to their own sperm, however, even successful reconnection will not be sufficient to restore fertility. It would be misleading, then, to suggest that vasectomies are generally reversible, since it is extremely difficult to predict reversibility on an individual basis. A vasectomy can be obtained following discussions with a physician about the procedures involved, the alternative birth control methods, and the irreversibility.

Sterilization in the female Sterilization in women is a more complicated process than it is in men. The reproductive organs are not so readily accessible, so major surgery is required. The object of the surgery—to block union of egg and sperm—is the same, however. The usual procedure in women is to tie off the fallopian tubes. There are a number of different sterilization methods, depending on the manner in which the tubes are tied and the way in which the tubes are reached. In the traditional **tubal ligation,** a section of the tube is removed, and the remaining ends are tied off. In more recently developed methods, electrical coagulation (burning), elastic bands, rings, and clips may be used to close the tubes.

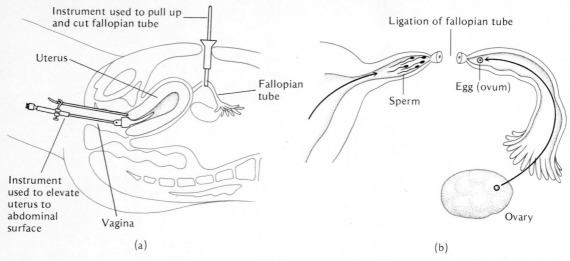

Instrument used to pull up and cut fallopian tube

Uterus

Fallopian tube

Instrument used to elevate uterus to abdominal surface

Vagina

(a)

Ligation of fallopian tube

Sperm

Egg (ovum)

Ovary

(b)

*FIGURE 8.10
Minilaparatomy.
Under general
anesthesia, (a) a
small incision is
made in the lower
abdomen, and the
fallopian tubes are
located. They are
then cut and
clipped. (b) After
surgery, the sperm
cannot reach the
egg.*

Tubal ligation can be performed by either a vaginal or abdominal route. Vaginal ligation can be performed by ***culpotomy***, a surgical incision made in the vagina just behind the cervix. Following the incision, the tubes are pulled out, tied, and pushed back into the abdominal cavity, and the incision is sutured closed. The two most widely used abdominal approaches are minilaparotomy and laparoscopic tubal sterilization. The ***minilaparotomy*** involves inserting an instrument into the uterus via the cervix so that the uterus and tubes may be elevated to the top of the abdominal cavity. A small abdominal incision is then made directly over the elevated uterus. The tubes are located and either tied, cauterized, or clipped (see Fig. 8.10). In recent years, ***laparoscopic tubal sterilization***, also known as Band-Aid sterilization, has become quite popular. A laparoscope is a thin rodlike viewing instrument with a light at one end that can be inserted into the abdomen and used to locate the fallopian tubes. A small incision is made in the navel to accommodate the laparoscope. After the tubes are located, they are usually cauterized or clipped.

All of these procedures are nearly 100 percent effective in preventing pregnancy, with the few failures attributed to the regrowth of the damaged ends of the tubes. The complication rate for vaginal tubal ligation is nearly twice that for the abdominal methods. Sterilization may be obtained after detailed counsel with a physician in which the risks and permanence of sterilization and the virtues of other birth control methods are discussed. The cost varies from $300 to $700 or more.

***BIRTH CONTROL
IN THE FUTURE***

Despite the plethora of birth control methods currently available, none of them is really 100 percent satisfactory. Thus, the search for newer and better forms of contraception continues. With respect to hormonal forms of contra-

BOX 8.3

A male pill?

American scientists have been working for years to develop a safe and effective oral contraceptive for men. Their research has focused primarily on the use of synthetic or natural male hormones to affect sperm production. Although they have made great progress in this direction in recent years, such a male pill is still a bit in the future.

Meanwhile, however, the Chinese have announced development of a male pill that is already being used by thousands of Chinese men. This chemical, called gossypol, is not a hormone at all but an extract from cottonseed. According to a report in a Chinese medical journal, the idea for the pill began back in the 1950s when it was noted that infertility was high in localized populations where food was often cooked in crude cottonseed oil. Research later revealed that the active agent that seemed to affect fertility was gossypol, a compound known to be toxic to animals who ate contaminated feed.

The Chinese proceeded to purify gossypol and to use it in a series of animal studies. They found that rats given small daily doses became infertile. Apparently, the compound affected various precursor stages of sperm, thereby causing the sperm themselves to be malformed. Rats who stayed on gossypol had a gradually reduced sperm count until they eventually produced no sperm at all. However, testosterone production and sex drive appeared to be unaffected (Science, June 1979).

In 1972 the Chinese began clinical trials with humans. Thousands of men took a daily pill for 2 months and then maintenance pills twice a week for up to 2 years. The Chinese medical journal reported that in more than 2000 men followed over 2 years, the gossypol was 99.89 percent effective, based on monitoring of sperm counts. The men suffered a few side effects, including an initial weakness, when they began taking the pill. Some complained of bloating and gastrointestinal discomfort, and a few were found to have lowered serum potassium. However, they apparently maintained normal sex lives, and their testosterone level was normal. In those who stopped taking the pill, sperm production returned to normal within about 3 months. However, there are no data available on their subsequent fertility or possible side effects on subsequent offspring.

American scientists are somewhat cautious about the Chinese studies with gossypol, and this compound is not yet being studied in the United States. Many interested researchers are concerned about the drug's possible toxicity over the long run and have adopted a wait-and-see attitude (Fortino, 1979).

One problem the Chinese have run into with their male pill is the reluctance of men to take it—they still want women to be responsible for contraception. The same problem will confront American pharmaceutical companies when they finally develop a marketable male pill. According to Ashton Barfield of the Population Council's Center for Biomedical Research, "A lot of men in our culture confuse fertility with libido, which is the amount or frequency of sexual desire. With many of the potential male contraceptives, there is no physiological reason why potency or libido would be lowered (Schultz, 1980, p. 44). Nevertheless, there are obviously psychological reasons why men would balk at using oral contraceptives, and until these psychological matters are dealt with, companies that want to market a male pill may have more trouble selling it than they've had developing it.

ception, drug companies are already testing the use of plastic capsule implants that might last for several months or a year. The small capsules would be inserted under the skin and would provide a steady dose of hormone, obviating the need for a pill. Another idea under consideration is injecting semen into women in an effort to produce antibodies to sperm. Such antibodies would kill the sperm as they made their way through the female reproductive tract. At issue is whether this effect could be successfully reversed.

Some of the other experimental approaches to birth control were presented in Boxes 8.1 and 8.2. Among the stranger ideas that have also been proposed is that women's mouth odor may be used to determine ovulation. Researchers have discovered that the concentrations of certain volatile sulfur compounds found in the mouth vary cyclically. Whether these cyclic variations are tied to the hormonal changes that occur across the menstrual cycle has not been determined, however.

Despite improvements in the quality of condoms and the increase in effectiveness of various spermicidal foams, they are probably not the harbingers of the ultimate method of birth control that everyone is searching for. One of the greatest hopes may lie with the development of readily reversible sterilization procedures already being developed for both men and women.

There is some concern that most of the birth control methods already in existence are available for females and not for males. Why hasn't research developed something for men that is comparable to the Pill or IUD in women? There are several reasons why women have been emphasized in recent years. First, the woman may have a stronger desire to control conception, since it is she who bears the immediate consequence of failure. Second, from a physiological standpoint, it is much simpler to prevent a single egg from being fertilized every month than it is to prevent several hundred million sperm from swimming up the female reproductive tract every time intercourse occurs. Finally, there are more steps in the reproductive process of the female that can be disrupted than there are in the male. Nevertheless, some research is being conducted to develop a male contraceptive pill, and one such pill has achieved success in China, as Box 8.3 explains.

The ideal birth control technique of the future will be one that does not disrupt the act of lovemaking, does not interfere with internal body functioning, is readily reversible, and is simple and inexpensive to use. Whether this goal will be reached in the near future is uncertain. Nevertheless, even with present contraceptive technology we have come a long way from our ancestors and their practice of using elephant dung to prevent conception.

SUMMARY

1   People have physical, psychological, and political reasons for wanting to prevent conception. Among the reasons are desires to space children in a family or to put off childbearing until the couple or woman has achieved other goals. People also have reasons for avoiding contraceptive methods, including religious, health, and psychological reasons.

2   Choice of a birth control method should be based on seven factors: cost of the method, availability (whether or not medical prescription or treatment is necessary), possible undesirable *side effects*, mechanism of action, timing of use of the method, frequency of intercourse, and effectiveness. The *theoretical effectiveness rate*, expressed in number of pregnancies per 100 woman years, indicates the effectiveness of the method when used perfectly. The *actual use effectiveness rate* takes into account mistakes in using the method.

3   Hormonal types of birth control include the combination pill, the minipill, the shot, and the morning-after pill. The *combination pill*, which consists of estrogen and progestin, is taken for 21 days and stopped for 7 days. This method works by manipulating hormone levels so that ovulation and implantation are prevented. Effectiveness is quite high. Possible side effects include blood-clotting disorders, increased blood pressure, headaches, and *cloasma* (darkened spots on the face). Women who suffer from various contraindicated conditions and women who smoke are advised not to use the Pill. One of the disadvantages of this method is that women must remember to take their pills regularly.

4   The *minipill* contains only small amounts of progestin. The woman takes a pill each day for as long as she wants to use the method. The failure rate is only slightly higher than that for the combination pill. Possible side effects of the minipill are vaginitis, weight gain, acne, less menstrual bleeding, and infrequent periods. The way the *shot* works is similar to the minipill, but it needs only to be administered every 3 months.

5   The *morning-after pill* is taken following unprotected intercourse. It acts to prevent implantation. The most commonly used type is *diethylstilbestrol* (DES). The effectiveness rate is quite high. Not only are side effects strong, but use of DES can increase the chances of offspring developing problems if the woman does become pregnant.

6   Mechanical forms of birth control include the IUD, the diaphragm, and the condom. The *intrauterine device* (IUD) is a small object inserted into the vagina that acts to prevent implantation. It must be inserted by a physician. Possible side effects include increased menstrual bleeding, painful menstruation, uterine perforation upon insertion, and *pelvic inflammatory disease* (PID).

7   The *diaphragm* is a latex cup that is covered with spermicidal cream and placed over the cervix. It acts primarily as a chemical barrier to the sperm. A diaphragm must be properly fitted by a physician. The actual use effectiveness is lower than the theoretical effectiveness for this method because women sometimes use it incorrectly.

8   The *condom* is a rubber sheath placed over the erect penis that prevents sperm from being ejaculated into the vagina. The actual failure rate with this method is quite high despite a low theoretical rate because men make mistakes in using the method.

9   *Spermicidal foam* is a chemical inserted into the vagina just prior to intercourse that acts to kill sperm before they reach the cervix. A similar chemical method is the Encare Oval, a small object that effervesces when placed in the vagina. *Douching* (cleansing of the vagina) is *not* a method of birth control and may in fact actually increase a woman's chances of becoming pregnant.

10   The *rhythm method* of birth control is based on accurately calculating the day of ovulation and then abstaining from intercourse during the woman's

fertile period. Three techniques that can be used to predict the day of ovulation are the *calendar method*, the *basal body temperature method*, and the *cervical mucus secretion method (Billings method)*. The failure rate for the rhythm method is fairly high because of the difficulty in pinpointing ovulation and because of couples taking chances during the abstinence period.

11   *Coitus interruptus*, or *withdrawal*, is removal of the penis from the vagina prior to ejaculation. The failure rate for this method is quite high, since men are asked to exhibit a high level of self-control and since sperm can still enter the female system from the penis prior to ejaculation.

12   *Abortion* is the use of surgical procedures to remove the embryo or fetus from the uterus early in gestation. Methods used during the first trimester include *vacuum curettage* and *dilatation and curettage* (D and C). The method used most commonly early in the second trimester is *dilatation and evacuation* (D and E). Late in the second trimester *hysterotomy* or *induced miscarriage* may be necessary. The risks of abortion include excessive bleeding, infection, uterine perforation, retained fetal tissue, and possible psychological problems in a few women.

13   *Sterilization* procedures include *vasectomy* (cutting and tying of the vasa deferentia) in males and *tubal ligation* (cutting or clipping of the fallopian tubes) in females. Vasectomy is a minor surgical procedure that can be done in a doctor's office, while tubal ligation requires hospitalization and anesthesia. Both methods are highly effective. Vasectomy may be reversible in individual cases.

**ADDITIONAL
READING**

Fleishman, N., and Dixon, P. L. *Vasectomy, Sex, and Parenthood.* Garden City, NY: Doubleday, 1973.
> *A complete and positive presentation of vasectomy. Discusses physiological, psychological, and family aspects of the procedure.*

* **Montreal Health Press.** *Birth Control Handbook* (12th ed.). Montreal: Montreal Health Press, 1974.
> *Clear, concise, and accurate information on birth control geared for the lay reader. An excellent guide.*

* **Shapiro, Howard.** *The Birth Control Book.* New York: St. Martin's Press, 1977.
> *A clear overview of mechanical, hormonal, and surgical forms of birth control. Written in question-and-answer format and easy-to-read, nontechnical language.*

*Human sexuality
across the life span*

three

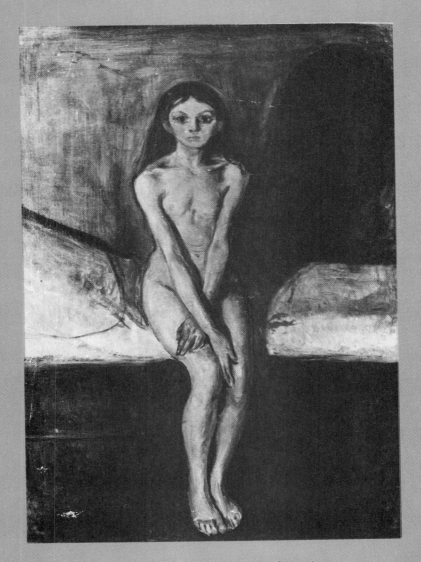

*Sexuality in
the early years*

——

9

chapter
9

True or false:

The occurrence of erections in male infants is unnatural and should be suppressed.
Genital touching between children leads to early promiscuity.
Masturbation occurs only in infants who are reared with minimal maternal contact.

These are all commonly held beliefs in our society, and they are all false. Myths such as these have arisen because Western culture has tended to ignore or deny the existence of infantile sexual responsivity (Martinson, 1980). Sexuality is a characteristic that people tend to attribute to individuals *after* they have reached puberty. It is as if some switch is turned on that miraculously transforms the sexless child into a sexually motivated teenager. This view is strongly reinforced by the fact that the human body becomes obviously more sexual at puberty, with females developing breasts, males experiencing an increase in the size of the penis, and other such changes.

The denial of sexuality in infants and children, however, goes against actual fact. Researchers of child development have discovered that elements of sexual behavior are present in some form throughout early life. Newborn male infants, for example, exhibit erections, and young children fondle both their

Gender role behaviors are established in early childhood and are probably influenced by child-rearing practices.

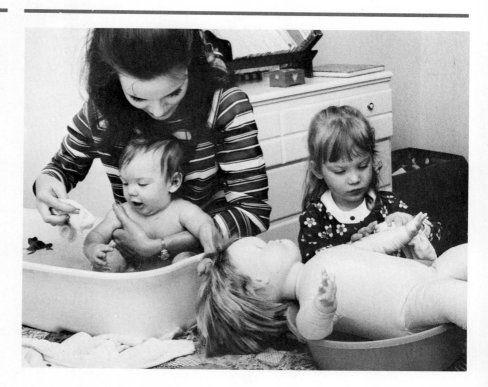

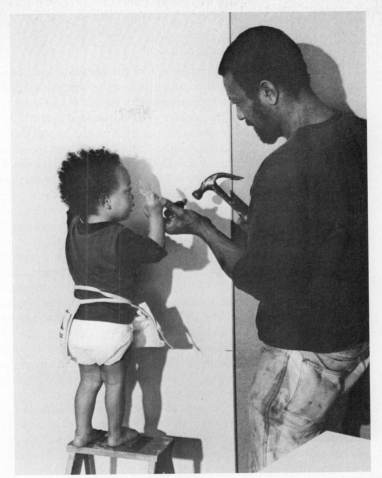

*Fathers may play
an important role
in shaping the
gender role
behavior of their
children, especially
their sons.*

own genitals and those of their peers. We are not saying that these behaviors have the same significance for children as they have for adults; we are only pointing out that they exist.

Another aspect of sexuality that develops early in life is our awareness of masculinity and femininity. We learn not only our *gender identity* (see Chap. 5) but our **gender role**—the constellation of behaviors that are more characteristic of our particular sex. Most people would agree that gender-role development begins early in life and spans a major part of childhood. Many disagree, however, on whether gender roles are biologically inborn or culturally imposed.

Sexuality is a complex phenomenon that develops and changes throughout life. In this chapter, we are concerned with the development and changes in sexual responsiveness and gender role that occur in infancy, childhood, and adolescence. In the following chapters, we will focus on various issues about sexuality that arise in the early, middle, and late adult years. Thus, we will be examining sexuality across the entire life span.

Intrinsic theories

If sexuality unfolds gradually across the life span, what factors play a pivotal role in guiding or directing this development during early life? A number of theories have been proposed to answer this question. Most of these theories can be divided into two types: intrinsic and extrinsic.

Intrinsic theories are those that emphasize the importance of characteristics within the individual that bring about sexual development. These theories include physiological theory and Freud's theory of psychosexual development.

Physiological theory   Physiological theory assumes that sexuality develops as a result of hormonal and neural stimulation. During prenatal life, hormonal events guide the development of male or female genitals and may cause certain alterations in parts of the brain, thereby molding later gender-role behavior patterns. During infancy and childhood, sexuality is assumed to be latent or quiescent because of the low levels of hormone production by the sex glands (Money, 1973; Martinson, 1980). Presumably, then, children do not desire each other sexually. With the onset of puberty, however, the sex glands are stimulated into greater activity by the hypothalamus; hormone levels increase; and sexual desires and behaviors emerge. After puberty, sexual urges are controlled more by social factors (such as attraction) than by hormones. This theory tends to attribute sexual dysfunctions, such as failure to obtain erections or excessive sexual desire, to hormone malfunction. Such dysfunctions are explained in terms of hormone levels being too high, too low, or imbalanced with respect to one another.

The most basic objection to the physiological or hormonal theory of sexual development is that it is too restrictive. It tends to emphasize sexual behavior and desire as it occurs in the adult without studying the antecedents of such behavior in children. What about the self-stimulation, erection, and genital fondling that occur during childhood? If they are not the precursors of adult sexuality, what are they? How can these behaviors be reconciled with the relative inactivity of the sex hormones during this period?

Freud's theory of psychosexual development   The first recognition of childhood sexuality can be traced to Sigmund Freud, who early in this century suggested that sexuality begins at birth and not at puberty. As cited in Kirkendall and Rubin (1977), in continuing the work of her father, Anna Freud wrote:

> The sexual instincts of man do not suddenly awaken between the thirteenth and fifteenth year, i.e., at puberty but operate from the outset of the child's development, change gradually from one form to another, until at last adult sexual life is achieved as the final result from this long series of developments. (p. 142)

In order to explore sexuality in children, Freud entertained a very broad view of the term. He expanded *sexuality* to encompass many semierotic, pleasurable, and stimulatory behaviors prevalent in childhood. He considered sucking, masturbation, exhibitionism, looking at the genitals of others, excretion, retention of feces, rocking, and pinching all to be elements of sexuality. There are two reasons why Freud developed such a broad view of sexuality.

First, he noted that children seemed to derive a great deal of pleasure from such activities, and, second, he found that these patterns reappeared in other forms as a part of adult sexual behavior. For example, he related sucking behavior to kissing, anal retention to anal stimulation, and so on.

The basic element of Freud's developmental theory was the force he called *libido*, or life energy. He believed that the libido controlled important behaviors throughout life. Freud postulated that beginning in infancy different parts of the body progressively become the focus of libidinal energy. He suggested that children go through a sequence of *psychosexual stages* that are invariant, although the age at which a child enters a particular stage may vary. Freud assumed that normal psychosexual development is dependent on passing through each stage and successfully resolving the conflicts inherent in each one. Failure to resolve the conflicts in any of the stages could lead to *fixation* in a particular stage or could result in *regression* back to that stage later in life. This would be the basis for abnormal psychological and sexual adjustment in adulthood.

The stages Freud proposed are as follows:

1. *The oral stage.* During the first year of life, sexual energy is focused on the mouth. The infant sucks at the breast and receives immediate gratification in the form of food and contact from the mother. Infants who are undersatisfied or overindulged may become fixated in this stage and develop an oral personality as adults. Such individuals might be characterized as craving food or love and as searching for a kind of trust and relatedness they can never obtain.

2. *The anal stage.* In the second to fourth years of life, libidinal energy becomes focused on the organs and activities of elimination. Not surprisingly, this shift is associated with a critical event: toilet training. For perhaps the first time in its life, an infant is subjected to the demands of the parents. Freud noted that toilet training may induce strong feelings of either pleasure or anxiety in the child. If the child learns to cope and adjust to the pressures of such training, he or she will move on to the next psychosexual stage. If not, fixation at the anal stage will occur. Freud suggested that two personality types may result from fixation in or regression to this stage. The "anal retentive" person is generally excessively neat, is stingy, and may be compulsive about cleanliness. Conversely, the "anal expulsive" person is typically sloppy and dirty and may be disorganized and pushy.

3. *The phallic stage.* Freud's views about this stage were and continue to be very controversial. Between the ages of 4 and 6, the child's attention is directed to the genitals and the pleasures of masturbation. Boys discover that they have a penis; both boys and girls discover that they are different from each other. More important, however, Freud argued that children begin to have sexual longings like those that are attributed only to adults. These longings lead to several important conflicts.

The nature of the conflict in the male child is relatively straight-forward. During this stage, the boy develops a preoccupation with his penis, and at the same time his powerful love for his mother takes on sexual overtones; that is, he wishes to possess her sexually. This desire brings him into competition with his father for the affection of his mother. The boy begins to think of ways to eliminate his father as a rival for his mother's affections. But soon he becomes fearful of his father and of the possibility of losing his penis through retaliation. This conflict of wanting to possess the mother and eliminate the father is termed the **Oedipus complex**. The name comes from the tragic myth of the Greek king Oedipus, who unknowingly killed his father and married his mother.

Ultimately, the conflict associated with the Oedipus complex must be resolved. Freud suggested that this resolution depends on a process of **identification**, in which the boy eliminates guilt feelings by striving to be exactly like his father. By identifying with his father and adopting his father's mannerisms and actions, the boy relieves his anxiety and develops traits that will allow him to successfully compete for the attentions of women later in life. It is in this manner that a developing boy takes on the characteristics and attitudes of the male sex. Thus, for Freud, the key to gender-role development was the process of identification.

Freud faced a more difficult task in explaining the behavior of girls during the phallic stage. After all, if development were to proceed the same as for boys, girls would develop an identification with their fathers. But girls do not develop a masculine orientation, so they must not experience the same Oedipal conflicts. Neither could Freud invoke a simple reversal of the process, whereby the girl eventually identifies with her mother, since both boys and girls are initially attached to the mother. So, Freud ultimately proposed a number of different hypotheses to explain the source of female conflict in the phallic stage. In his most widely discussed view, he suggested that a girl becomes angry with her mother because she does not satisfy her needs and because she blames her mother for her lack of a penis. This **penis envy** causes the girl to become attracted to her father. Freud called this conflict the **Electra complex**. Unfortunately, Freud had a difficult time explaining how the girl ultimately returns her attentions to and identifies with the mother. Freud's solution was to say that the girl remained in this conflict (mother-hate, father-love) for a long time and only broke away from it partially. This conclusion is generally consistent with Freud's Victorian prejudice that women are somehow different and less successfully adjusted to life than are men.

Freud considered the phallic stage to be an important step in psychosexual development. Successful resolution of the conflicts present at this stage means that boys will develop a masculine orientation and girls a feminine orientation. According to Freud, fixation in or regression to the phallic stage results in an adult personality characterized by gender-identity problems. In his view, adult sexual problems occur because of unresolved conflicts from the phallic stage.

4. **The latent stage**. From age 6 until puberty, the child remains in a latent stage with regard to psychosexual development. During this time, libidinal energy is not localized in a particular body area. Freud suggested that this is a

quiet phase for the preadolescent, with little of the sexual upheavals that
marked the earlier stages.

5. *The genital stage.* The genital stage represents the culmination of psychosexual development. Libidinal energy resurfaces and is directed toward
sexual pleasure with others. In contrast to the rather selfish sexuality of the
phallic stage, the adolescent in the genital stage becomes prepared to establish
a meaningful sexual relationship with an individual of the opposite sex. Gratification is now centered on the genital area and seeks expression through the
act of sexual intercourse.

When Freud first presented his theory of psychosexual development, it was
so startling that he was ridiculed and scorned by his colleagues and by Victorian society in general. It was not until years later that his theory was embraced
by the scientific community. Today, the pendulum has swung back once again,
and Freudian theory is less popular. Nevertheless, Freud has left us with a
heritage that we can draw on and utilize. He was the first to suggest that
sexuality begins in infancy and to propose that identification accounts for the
development of gender identity. Both of these notions are still considered valid
and useful today.

However, the utility of Freud's stages, their conflicts, and their contribution to personality development have not been established. Opponents of
Freudian theory note that his ideas are so vague that his hypotheses cannot be
readily developed and tested scientifically (Chodoff, 1966). One might ask, for
example, "What is libido, and how can it be measured?" In addition, Freud
developed his theory from his observation of patients who suffered from a
variety of neurotic disorders. These patients were primarily adults from the
upper socioeconomic class of Vienna; he did not base his ideas on observations
of large numbers of normal children. Thus, his hypotheses about sexual activity in children are not necessarily supported. For example, subsequent case
histories of large numbers of children have indicated that sexual urges do not
seem to be submerged during preadolescence. Therefore, it is unlikely that a
latency period actually exists.

Freud's particular views were also shaped by the conventional mores of his
day. Living in the Victorian period in Vienna, Freud was under the influence of
a sexually repressive society that maintained a strong double standard for men
and women and that generally viewed women as inferior to men. It is not
surprising, therefore, to see these prejudices reflected in Freud's writings.
Today many feminists reject Freud's theory outright on the grounds that it
condones sexual inequality and contributes to the spread of sexual prejudice.
They note that perhaps Freud was right in identifying female envy of males.
However, they say that the envy is not of the penis per se but of the power and
privileges the male enjoys because of his gender role.

*Extrinsic
theories*

Extrinsic theories of sexual development focus on factors outside the
individual that shape both social behaviors and sexual patterns. These theories
all invoke learning as the mechanism by which children acquire gender roles
and sexual behaviors.

Conditioning theory   Early in this century Ivan Pavlov (1927) demonstrated that a dog could learn to associate the action of salivation, which normally occurs in response to food, with a neutral stimulus, such as a bell. This type of learning has come to be called **classical conditioning**. In classical conditioning, a person or animal learns to associate a particular response (particularly an emotion or a physiological behavior, such as fear or thirst) with a stimulus that does not usually bring about that response.

Some years after Pavlov's research, B. F. Skinner (1938) helped popularize another form of learning called **operant conditioning**. The basic idea of operant conditioning is that responses that are rewarded tend to be repeated, whereas responses that are punished tend not to be repeated. To put it simply, people tend to behave in ways that are rewarding or reinforcing. Behavioral psychologists have identified many principles of operant conditioning that play a role in the way human beings acquire everything from language to personalities.

According to learning theory, gender roles develop because boys and girls are conditioned differently. Young boys, for example, receive reinforcement (in the form of approval) from their parents for wearing pants, playing aggressively, and doing other things the parents consider appropriate for little boys. Furthermore, boys are punished if they act like "sissies" or engage in female play activities. Girls, on the other hand, are rewarded for being quiet, compliant, and agreeable and are scolded when they are aggressive or assertive. In general, parents treat male and female children differently and have different expectations about their behavior (Block, 1978; Block, Block, and Harrington, 1974).

Some sexual patterns can also be explained in terms of conditioning theory. For example, if an individual always plays a certain type of music during sexual encounters, through classical conditioning processes, the music alone may come to elicit arousal and erotic thoughts. Similarly, children may learn to associate sex with "bad," or they may be punished for sexual behaviors, such as touching themselves or "playing doctor" with other children. This type of learning can make it difficult for individuals to enjoy sexual encounters as adults. In fact, some sexual dysfunctions can be traced back to such conditioning in childhood, and therapy often consists in helping the person "unlearn" inappropriate associations or responses.

Although conditioning theory is intuitively appealing, it can be criticized on the grounds that (1) it oversimplifies sexual development and the building of new patterns from old, (2) it ignores the role of hormones, and (3) it cannot readily account for all the social and emotional components of sexuality.

Imitation and observation   Many learning theorists emphasize the importance of imitation and observation in the development of sexuality. This approach is particularly applicable to the development of gender roles but is not too relevant to direct sexual behavior, since such behavior is generally hidden from children in our society.

One of the major proponents of this view, Albert Bandura (1962; Bandura, Ross, and Ross, 1963), has conducted many studies showing that children are excellent imitators. In a famous series of experiments, he showed children a film in which an adult model repeatedly hit a balloonlike toy called a Bobo doll. When these children were later placed in a room containing a Bobo doll, many approached it and started hitting it as the model had done. Learning theorists suggest that a similar process is at work in the acquisition of gender-role characteristics. Children observe individuals around them and imitate their actions. In early childhood, the important models are parents and siblings. Later, children begin to model their behaviors after other important adults and after peers they admire.

We have all seen examples of such gender-role imitation in children. Picture, for example, a young girl attired in her mother's dress, hemline dragging on the ground, with high heels that can barely be moved by such tiny feet. Strands of jewelry hang down below her waist, and her cheeks and lips are ruby red. There seems to be no question that this girl is imitating and emulating her mother. Similarly, boys will imitate their fathers by attempting to use a hammer and nails before they have the dexterity to do so or by trying to shave (with razor sans blade) long before whiskers begin to grace their chins.

Conditioning is often a part of the observation and imitation process. For one thing, parents reward children for imitating the *right* models, and they discourage children from imitating the *wrong* ones (little boys are punished if they try to dress up like mommy). For another thing, children may see others rewarded for behaving in certain ways and punished for behaving in other ways. So without actually having performed these behaviors themselves, they learn what is "appropriate" and "inappropriate" behavior for someone of their sex.

Cognitive learning or self-socialization Cognitive-learning theorists suggest that children progressively take on gender-role characteristics as their mental abilities develop (Kohlberg, 1966). The key is recognizing that children only come gradually to understand the concept of gender and gender roles. The influence of training and reinforcement, therefore, is limited by the concepts and beliefs that a child has at a given age.

Initially, children have a very rudimentary notion of gender and gender roles. This notion becomes refined as the child's mental capabilities expand. Thus, boys come to believe that they are boys, develop a desire to do things that boys do, and find it satisfying to do so. The same sequence of events occurs in girls. This process can be contrasted with conditioning theory, according to which reward is the key element. Given the variety of responses that young boys might make in a given situation, a boy finds that when he behaves like other boys, he is rewarded. This reward increases the likelihood that the boy will behave in this manner again. Thus a gender role is acquired.

One of the strengths of cognitive theory is that it emphasizes the thoughts and concepts that children have in their heads as being important in the development of gender role. This theory does not explain the many sex differences that occur in the first few years of life before the concept of gender is fully formed in the child's mind.

Social scripts Some theorists have emphasized the important role that society plays in governing the development of gender roles and sexual behavior. They have observed that individuals in a variety of societies follow a fairly orderly progression in acquiring gender roles and in achieving active sexual status. This progression, they argue, calls for some implicit plan of action. John Gagnon (1977) calls this mechanism guiding people's actions a **social script**. According to Gagnon, "Scripts are the plans that people may have in their heads for what they are doing and what they are going to do, as well as being devices for remembering what they have done in the past" (p. 6).

Just like scripts in a play, social scripts specify the whos, whats, whens, wheres, and whys in a person's life. Sexuality, then, is a process that unfolds and develops on a cognitive level. Although each person draws on a generalized cultural script that incorporates the expectations of society, each script is also highly individualized. Thus, different people, even within the same culture or subculture, have somewhat different sexual scripts.

According to Gagnon (1977), the components of a sexual script might include the following:

1 The who. *About whom do we fantasize, or with whom would we prefer to have sex?*
2 The what. *With what types of acts would we be comfortable, and would these preferences change as a function of the particular partner?*
3 The when. *Is sex appropriate for us only at a given age or only at a certain time (such as after the children are in bed)?*
4 The where. *What is the appropriate environment for sexual activity? (the shower? the bedroom? the kitchen table? sand dunes?)*
5 The why. *What are our reasons for engaging in sexual activities? Do we do them for fun? to express love? for procreation?*

Gagnon's notion of scripts is interesting because it combines societal and personal values with the processes of thinking, evaluating, and remembering. Learning to apply and manipulate a sexual script, however, may be more an accumulation of indirect hints from the social world than the result of direct thought processes.

None of the theories we have described here, taken alone, is totally satisfactory in explaining sexual development. Each theory seems to be too restrictive and narrow in focus to adequately characterize the development of sexuality and gender roles. There is nothing, however, to prevent us from assuming that all these theories contribute to understanding certain aspects of sexual development. We should, therefore, look to the future for a synthesis that will integrate these viewpoints in a meaningful way. Until then, what we have are some pieces of the puzzle but no real knowledge of how they all fit together—and whether they're all here.

AREAS OF STUDY
IN SEXUAL
DEVELOPMENT

Researchers who study the development of sexuality from infancy to adolescence tend to focus on three facets of sexuality: (1) *sexual behavior*, (2) *sexual awareness*, and (3) *gender roles and gender differences*. Each of these areas of study has its own unique set of methodological and theoretical prob-

*Sexual
behavior*

lems. And each carries with it certain issues that may obscure or confuse the findings.

It is extremely difficult to measure and record sexual activity in infants and children. For parental, social, ethical, and religious reasons, the direct observation of childhood patterns of sexuality is rare. As a result, the study of sexual behavior in childhood is typically based on verbal reports from three sources: parents, children themselves, and adults who recall activities from their childhood.

Each of these three sources contains potential biases. The parents, depending on their moral and religious views, may report certain behaviors and ignore others in their own children. The children, on the other hand, may be too naive to understand the questions posed by the researchers. In addition, there may be ethical concerns about posing sexual questions to children. How does one ask a child if he has erections or masturbates? Even adult retrospective reports may be biased, particularly by a faulty memory. It is often difficult to recall one's sexual activities during childhood, let alone infancy. For example, can you remember your sexual activities at age 5? at age 1? And if you can, would you tell a stranger about these activities? Guilt, embarrassment, and even wish fulfillment can alter an adult's self-report. Thus, in the absence of direct measurement, the sex researcher must deal with inherent biases in the information that is gathered.

*Sexual
awareness*

We use the term *sexual awareness* here to refer to the child's knowledge of reproduction and intercourse. There are fewer methodological problems involved in studying sexual awareness than in studying sexual behavior, as researchers can rely on questionnaires specially developed to assess children's knowledge. Furthermore, because the researchers are careful not to provide the children with answers, they cannot be accused of "unauthorized" sex education. The biggest difficulty that may arise in this type of research is trying to interpret some of the children's more creative responses. Errors in interpretation may lead the researcher to believe that the child is more or less sexually aware than the child actually is.

*Gender roles
and gender
differences*

Researchers are particularly concerned with how gender roles arise and how they are learned. **Sex-role typing** is the process by which children acquire the values, motives, and behaviors thought to be appropriate for males or females in a particular culture. Because the notion of gender roles and gender differences is a sensitive issue, the study of these topics is fraught with controversy.

Perhaps one of the most sensitive theoretical and political issues concerning gender differences is the source of these apparent variations. Some people argue that gender differences are biologically determined, while others claim that they develop through cultural influences. Is it the case, for example, that women are more nurturant than men because of some biological drive or hormonal influence, or does our culture merely expect women to be more nurturant and reward them for such behavior? A logical answer is that both biological heritage and cultural experiences interact to shape and control such behavior. There is no simple method for separating their relative contributions.

Taking a side on this particular issue can lead us to define our expectations of society and behavior in specific ways. If we assume that our biological heritage is responsible for gender differences and gender roles, then we view such differences as unchanging and enduring. If, on the other hand, we assume that cultural experiences are responsible, then we view these same differences as being flexible and capable of alteration. Thus, depending on our orientation, the disparities between men and women are either something we have to live with or something we have to change in order to eliminate all sexual inequalities.

Both these approaches are based on an implicit assumption that may be erroneous: the idea that there is something wrong with the existence of gender differences. Why is that? Essentially, the basic problem stems from the tendency of people to apply value judgments to these differences, especially when such differences directly concern human activities. Yes, men sometimes differ from women, but perhaps these differences should not be interpreted as making them in some way better or worse than women. Unfortunately, the behavioral disparities between men and women have become a political issue.

As this discussion indicates, people tend to focus primarily on the differences between men and women rather than on their similarities. Perhaps this is because differences tend to be intrinsically more interesting than similarities. As a result, however, we may erroneously assume that differences are *more numerous* than similarities or that such differences are *more important* than the similarities. The truth is, however, that men and women, boys and girls share an overwhelming commonality of behaviors (Maccoby and Jacklin, 1974); and the more gender differences are studied, the fewer are found to be genuine. For example, it has indeed been found that boys tend to be more aggressive than girls, and that girls have greater verbal ability than do boys. But there is no evidence that boys are more independent, ambitious, or achievement-oriented than girls or that girls are more nurturant or sociable than boys (Maccoby and Jacklin, 1974).

The traditional view of gender roles has given rise to the concepts of masculinity and femininity, each supposedly representing the epitome of conformance to one's gender role. These terms not only continue to promote the idea that the two sexes are very distinct from each other in behavior and personality but also imply that sexuality falls on a continuum, with the two terms at opposite ends. Many psychologists believe, however, that masculinity and femininity are not mutually exclusive. Rather, each person possesses both masculine and feminine traits to differing degrees (Bem, 1974; Rossi, 1969). Some have even suggested that the highly masculine male and the highly feminine female are greatly hampered by their extreme sex-role orientations. Sandra Bem, for example, has promoted the idea that a balance of masculine and feminine traits, or **androgyny**, is the most desirable orientation (see Box 9.1).

BOX 9.1

Androgyny

"I have come to believe that we need a new standard of psychological health for the two sexes, one that removes the burden of stereotypes and allows people to feel free to express the best traits of men and women (p. 60). These are the words of Sandra Bem (1975), a psychologist who has argued that men and women should break free from the traditional sex-role behaviors of the past and move toward a repertoire of behaviors that combines the best of both feminine and masculine traits.

Bem refers to this combining of traits as androgyny, from the Greek andro, meaning "male," and gyne, meaning "female." It is her contention that individuals who most closely conform to the traditional stereotypes for their sex—"masculine" men and "feminine" women—are not only highly restricted in their behaviors but also more prone to anxiety, low self-esteem, low self-acceptance, and lower intelligence, spatial ability, and creativity than are individuals who are not as sex-typed. Androgynous individuals, in contrast, "are not limited by labels. They are able to do whatever they want, both in their behavior and their feelings" (p. 60).

In order to prove her conjectures, Bem first developed the Bem Sex Role Inventory (BSRI), a test to determine people's degree of masculinity and femininity. The inventory consists of a list of 60 carefully chosen personality characteristics: 20 traditionally masculine traits ("ambitious," "self-reliant," "assertive"), 20 traditionally feminine traits ("affectionate," "gentle," "understanding"), and 20 neutral traits ("truthful," "friendly," "likable"). These traits are listed in random order

on the inventory. The respondents are asked to indicate how accurately each word describes them by rating it from 1 ("never or almost never true") to 7 ("always or almost always true"). The answers are then tallied to produce a masculinity score and a femininity score for each person. If the two scores are approximately equal, the individual is considered to be androgynous.

When Bem and her associates administered the BSRI to students at Stanford University in the early 1970s, they found that about 50 percent fell into the traditional sex roles, 35 percent were androgynous, and 15 percent were cross sex-typed (masculine females and feminine males).

Bem was then ready to test her hypothesis that sex-typed people are more restricted in their behaviors, whereas androgynous people are more adaptable. She and her associates devised a series of experiments to examine how people act in various situations. They predicted that sex-typed people would do well only when the behavior called for was appropriate to their sex, whereas androgynous people would do well regardless of the masculinity or femininity of the behavior required. For example, in one experiment each subject was left alone in a room with a kitten and was observed through a one-way mirror. As the researchers expected, men who had scored high in masculinity and low in femininity on the BSRI were much less likely than the other subjects to play with the kitten; playing with small, cuddly things is seen as a "feminine" behavior. Highly masculine men were also the least likely to play with a 6-month-old baby. Similarly, in tests of "masculine" behaviors, women who scored high in femininity and low in masculinity were the least successful of all groups. They showed the most conformity in tests of independence, and they found it difficult to assert themselves when the situation required them to do so.

In analyzing these results, Bem concluded that the masculine men were independent and assertive when they needed to be but "lacked the ability to express warmth, playfulness, and concern—important human, if traditionally feminine, traits." Similarly, feminine women did feminine things well but "weren't independent in judgment or assertive of their own preferences." Androgynous individuals, on the other hand, "could be independent and assertive when they needed to be, and warm and responsive in appropriate situations. It didn't matter, in other words, whether a behavior was stereotypically masculine or feminine; they did equally well on both" (Bem, 1975, p. 62).

In further studies, Bem and her associates found that sex-typed individuals not only stuck to their own sex's stereotyped behaviors but would actually make a point of avoiding opposite-sex behaviors. Even when offered pay for performing a simple opposite-sex behavior (preparing a baby bottle for males, oiling a hinge for females), highly masculine males and highly feminine females chose to perform a same-sex task.

Bem finds such results distressing. "In a modern complex society like ours," she says, "an adult has to be assertive, independent and self-reliant, but traditional femininity makes many women unable to behave in these ways. On the other hand, an adult must also be able to relate to other people, to be sensitive to their needs and concerned about their welfare, as well as to be able to depend on them for emotional support. But traditional masculinity keeps men from responding in such supposedly feminine ways." Thus, traditional sex roles actually hamper both sexes in their ability to get along in the world. And as far as Bem is concerned, an androgynous approach is the answer. Androgyny "greatly expands the range of behaviors open to everyone, permitting people to cope more effectively with diverse situations" (p. 62).

Subsequent research into androgyny versus traditional roles has to some extent substantiated Bem's assertions. Studies have found that androgynous individuals tend to make good parents because they can be both authoritarian and loving and that they tend to be more successful in business than conventionally masculine individuals.

Recently, however, Bem's approach has been subject to some criticism. Faye Crosby and Linda Nyquist have pointed out that the flexibility characteristic of androgyny may not be a positive trait if it means that a person switches personalities from situation to situation. In fact, such fluctuation would be considered a disorder by many psychologists (Rubenstein, 1980). Other researchers, Warren Jones and his associates (reported in Human Behavior, November 1978), have suggested that it is not androgyny that provides psychological adjustment as much as the preponderance of masculine traits in those who do well in androgyny studies. After giving the BSRI to over 1400 students at the University of Tulsa, they concluded that androgy-

*nous men are actually more limited
and restricted, less effective and more
vulnerable to influence, less sure of
themselves, and perhaps less well-
adjusted. Androgynous women, on the
other hand, were less conventional,
more outgoing, more politically aware,
more creative, and less shy, sensitive to
criticism, and awkward than feminine
females. Jones and his associates therefore surmised that androgyny is more*
*adaptive for females than for males and
that masculine traits continue to be
more valued than feminine ones.*

*Thus, the value of androgyny is far
from being proved. If nothing else,
however, Bem has drawn attention to
the fact that all people have both masculine and feminine traits to some degree and that the more one set of traits
is denied, the more restricted a person
will be in his or her behavior.*

**STAGES OF
SEXUAL
DEVELOPMENT**

There is a growing body of evidence to support Freud's idea that children are
more sexual than they have been given credit for being. Children do experience
sexual arousal, masturbate, and engage in rudimentary sexual actions at quite
early stages. In this section we will look at the four basic stages of childhood
to see how sexuality develops. In particular, we will examine hormonal and
physical changes, sexual behavior, sexual awareness, and gender-role development.

**Sexuality in
the infant**

It is difficult to think of an infant under the age of 2 as a sexually
responsive organism. But as we shall see, even newborn infants show signs of
sexual activity.

Hormonal events   In the first months of life, sex hormones coursing
through the bloodstream are at a high level compared to that of later infancy
and childhood. Testosterone levels are high for both male and female infants at
birth. In males, the slightly higher testosterone levels reach a peak at 2 months
and then gradually decline to childhood levels by 1 year. In females, however,
the testosterone levels decline to the level found in older infants and children
by 2 weeks of life (Forest, Saez, and Bertrand, 1973; Forest, et al., 1974). There
is a small increase in FSH and LH during the first year, with boys showing
higher concentrations of LH and girls showing higher levels of FSH. There are
no studies of estrogen levels in infants (Higham, 1980). Contrary to belief,
then, this is not a period of hormonal quiescence.

Sexual behavior   The most obvious manifestation of sexuality in infants is
the appearance of erections in males and vaginal lubrication in females. Both
erection and lubrication can occur very early in life. Halverson (1940) found
that 7 of 9 male infants, age 3–23 weeks, that he studied experienced daily
erections, with the number of erections ranging from 5 to 40 per infant.
Vaginal lubrication is more difficult to detect but probably occurs within the
first 6 weeks of life (Martinson, 1973, 1976).

Pelvic thrusts are also common in both sexes during the first year of life.
Lewis and Kagan (1965) suggested that pelvic thrusts in the 8- to 10-month-old

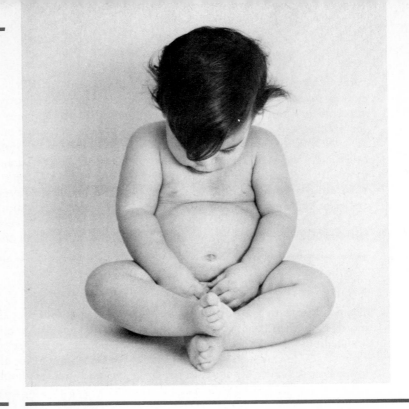

Even at a very young age, children often play with their genitals.

infant may be a sign of affection from the infant to the caregiver (typically the mother). Such thrusting usually reaches a peak during the first year of life and declines as the infant becomes more mobile.

Infants are quite responsive to genital stimulation by others. This form of contact can attract the baby's attention or can pacify a baby who is restless and cranky (Sears, Maccoby, and Levin, 1957). In fact, mothers in some cultures routinely use genital stimulation to soothe their infants (Kardiner, 1939).

It is difficult to determine whether infants experience orgasm. However, Kinsey (1953) recorded data on both a male and a female infant who showed orgasmlike responses as early as 6 months of age. In the case of the male, the orgasm consisted of a series of jerky body spasms following self-stimulation of the penis. The female infant appeared to rub her legs together, grunted, became red in the face, and spasmed in the same way the male did. Whether orgasm actually occurred cannot be completely substantiated, however.

It isn't until the period between the sixth and twelfth months of life for boys and somewhat later for girls that infants discover and begin to manipulate their genitals (Spitz, 1945; Galenson, 1975). René Spitz observed that genital stimulation was much more common among home-reared children, for whom the quantity and quality of maternal care was high, than among institutionally reared children, for whom contact with caretakers was minimal. Genital stimulation was also lower in those home-reared babies who had low maternal contact or who experienced high tension in the mother-infant relationship.

Spitz has argued that genital self-stimulation is a natural part of development and reflects a nurturant relationship between mother and infant.

There has been some concern over whether genital self-stimulation in infancy should be called masturbation. Much of the early genital self-stimulation resembles the spontaneous play activity that a baby might direct toward any part of its body, such as its fingers and toes, and it does not have the purposiveness implied by masturbation. Nor is it clear that such stimulation has the erotic implication for infants that it has for adults. Thus, Spitz (1949) and others have suggested that this stimulation be termed *genital play* rather than masturbation. Others have argued that the occurrence of orgasm in 6-month-old babies proves that this stimulation can be purposefully directed and may be erotic (Bakwin, 1973; Kleeman, 1965).

Infant-infant contact is quite rare, not only because infants do not get around too easily but because even in the presence of each other they tend not to interact very much. It isn't until about 2 years of age that children begin to exchange hugs, kisses, and touches.

Sexual awareness Although infants can't tell us whether or not they know about reproduction and intercourse, it's fairly safe to assume that they are rather ignorant in these areas.

Gender roles and gender differences Although male and female infants are overwhelming in their similarities, there are a few differences that can be discerned shortly after birth. Males tend to be slightly longer and heavier than females, and they may also be stronger and have a more mature muscular development (Jacklin, Snow, and Maccoby, 1980). Girls, on the other hand, are physically and neurologically more developed at birth and are less vulnerable to disease, malnutrition, and hereditary defects (Maccoby and Jacklin, 1974). Contrary to popular opinion, there is little evidence to suggest that male infants are more active than female infants (Jacklin and Maccoby, 1978) or that solitary play patterns vary as a function of sex. As early as age 2, however, boys are more likely to play with trucks and cars and girls to play with dolls and cuddly toys, even when a variety of toys are available (Smith and Daglish, 1977).

Male and female infants apparently make different demands on their parents and respond differently to demands made on them. Studies show that male infants typically display stronger resistance to training and are more likely to pressure parents to fulfill their needs. By 10 months of age, boys demand more attention from their mothers than do girls; they are also more persistent in trying to get their mother's attention (Martin, 1980). The character of mother-infant interactions also varies. Boys primarily seek to have their immediate needs satisfied, while girls share more kinds of activities with their mothers (Edwards and Whiting, 1977). In times of family stress, the relationship between parents and their sons may be more tense than the relationship between parents and their daughters (Hetherington, Cox, and Cox, 1976). Finally, even from a very young age, boys tend to be more mischievous (to handle forbidden objects and the like) than girls, thus sorely testing their parents' patience.

*Sexuality in
the child*

By the time children reach the age of 3, they are aware of and routinely manipulate elements of their environment. They are capable of expressing their wants and desires and of asking an infinite variety of complex and unanswerable questions. The childhood years of 3–7 also mark the beginning of sex play and sexual awareness.

Hormonal events   Childhood is a period of hormonal quiescence. Estrogen, testosterone, FSH, and LH circulate through the bloodstream in small amounts. Nevertheless, sexual activity continues and increases in frequency.

Sexual behavior   During the early part of childhood, there is a marked increase in sexual interest. About 5 percent of boys between the ages of 3 and 5 have actually masturbated and not simply fondled their genitals (Kinsey et al., 1953). There are no adequate figures for the incidence of female masturbation, but it is probably lower than that for males. Children learn quickly that masturbatory activities are to be conducted in private. Not all touching of the genitals during this period is sexual in nature. For example, boys may grab their penis when they are learning to walk. Such stimulation may serve as a source of security during awkward moments. Similarly, girls may touch their genitals in times of stress, using them as a kind of security blanket.

Children seem to discover each other during this period of life. They may kiss, cuddle, and tickle each other. It is not unusual for children to develop attachments to each other and to show grief upon separation, as when one child's family moves away. The game of "show"—exhibiting one's genitals to a child of the opposite sex—is quite common, as is genital touching and fondling of oneself (Kinsey, Pomeroy, and Martin, 1948).

The young child is often curious about activities normally performed in private. For example, children may be intrigued by the bathroom and like to

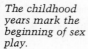

*The childhood
years mark the
beginning of sex
play.*

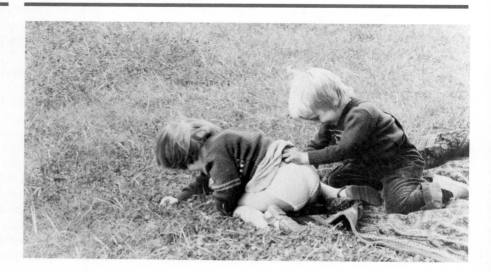

watch others use the toilet (Martinson, 1980). Or they may be curious about their parents' bodies and interested in the clothes their parents put on or take off.

After the age of 5, casual sex play and games of "show" decline. The child—especially girls—becomes more modest. On the other hand, remaining sex games become more sophisticated. The childhood game of "doctor" provides a rationale for permitting examination of the genitals. Romances between boys and girls may occur, although the boy is likely to be teased by his peers. Despite the fact that there are some heterosexual interactions as a result of such "romances" and of playing doctor, *isosexual* (same-sex) play is far more common during this period (Comfort, 1963; Martinson, 1973).

Sexual awareness One of the most elaborate studies of sexual awareness in young children was conducted by Kreitler and Kreitler (1974). Their subjects were 4½–5 years old and came from either a predominantly Eastern (Arabian, Indian, etc.) or Western cultural background. The Kreitlers noted that by the age of 5 many children had acquired knowledge about the location and function of the sex organs. In general, boys seem to be better informed and have more exacting knowledge about the organs of the opposite sex than do girls. Eastern children as a whole tend to be less well informed than Western children.

By age 5 children have also developed concepts about the creation and birth of babies. When asked, "How does a baby come into the world?" nearly 90 percent of both Eastern and Western children mentioned the enlarged belly of the mother. Much more creative and unusual answers were obtained when the children were asked, "What must the mother do in order to get a baby?" The most common answer, at least for Western children, was that the baby was formed from the food the mother eats. They emphasized the amount rather than the kind of food as being the key factor. Another popular view was that no creation was necessary because the baby had been in the mother's body even when she was a young girl. Supporters of this view stressed the importance of the type of food the mother ate in helping the baby grow. Finally, a view that was popular primarily with the Eastern children was that the mother had to first swallow the baby before it could be born. When asked how the baby was born, the majority of children suggested that the mother's belly was cut open and the baby was removed.

Although children have a general knowledge of gender differences and the creation of babies, they do not seem to understand the role of the father in reproduction. When asked, "What should the father do to make the baby appear?" most children suggested that the father should earn money and help the mother *after* the baby was born. Undoubtedly, the fact that the mother's body changes during pregnancy while the father's does not contributes to this rather one-sided view of reproduction.

Gender roles and gender differences During the preschool years, children tend to choose same-sex playmates (Strayer, 1977). This tendency to respond differently and more positively to same-sex partners is apparent by 3 years of age (Jacklin and Maccoby, 1978). In elementary school the same-sex preference persists, but girls' playgroups become smaller (2–3 individuals), whereas boys continue to interact in large playgroups (Waldrop and Halverson, 1975).

The nature of play also differs between boys and girls. When given an opportunity to play freely and without adult interference, all-girl groups tended to organize their play activities by establishing a set of rules. These rules concerned who went first, who played with what for how long, and so on. In contrast, the all-boy groups tended to engage in a lot of rough-and-tumble play and wrestling (Maccoby, 1980). However, boys and girls were equally active in terms of the amount of time they spent in play.

Boys tend to be more aggressive in their play than girls (Whiting and Edwards, 1973). This finding is one of the most well-established differences between the sexes. Not only is this tendency apparent in all cultures that have been studied, but it is a difference that persists into adulthood (Whiting and Whiting, 1975; Edwards and Whiting, 1977).

During the early phases of childhood, children develop concepts of their own gender identity. By age 3, children know enough to label themselves as boys or girls, but they seldom understand that they share this identity with other boys or girls. In addition, the 3-year-old has no sense of the permanency of the label *male* or *female* (Thompson, 1975). Emmerich and others (1976) discovered that children had little doubt that an individual's gender would change if that person's hairstyle, clothing, or activities were altered to conform to those of the opposite sex. Despite the fact that children tend to show a preference for playing with members of the same sex, the idea of gender permanence is not generally achieved until around age 7.

*Sexuality in
preadolescence*

Preadolescence (ages 8–11) begins with childhood and ends with puberty. Freud assumed this to be a latency period, in which sexual urges lie dormant. But as we shall see, sexual interest and activity are quite high in the preadolescent.

Hormonal events Between the ages of 6 and 10, gonadotropin levels (especially of FSH) rise gradually in both boys and girls. Dramatic increases in FSH and LH concentrations occur just after age 10 and signal the onset of puberty.

Sexual behavior Children often become knowledgeable about masturbation during preadolescence. In Kinsey's surveys (Kinsey et al., 1948, 1953), over 20 percent of boys and 12 percent of girls had discovered masturbation by the age of 12. A more recent survey (Hunt, 1974) suggests that children begin masturbating at earlier ages. Sixty-three percent of boys and 33 percent of girls in Hunt's survey had masturbated to orgasm by the age of 12. Boys generally start to masturbate earlier than girls. In addition, boys generally learn about masturbation from other, usually older, boys, while girls are more likely to learn from accidental self-discovery. As part of the phenomenon of boys teaching other boys to masturbate, occasionally a number of boys will masturbate together. No such comparable phenomenon has been reported among girls.

Although preadolescents don't usually go out on dates per se, they often attend mixed parties at which kissing games may be played. Events seldom progress beyond this stage, however, and it is uncommon for preadolescents to engage in sexual intercourse. During the early part of this developmental period, in fact, sex play continues to be more prevalent with same-sex rather than opposite-sex partners (Comfort, 1963). This is especially true for males. In a study of children aged 4–14, Elias and Gebhard (1969) noted that 52 percent of males had engaged in some form of homosexual play as opposed to only 34 percent who had engaged in heterosexual play. The figures were 35 percent and 37 percent, respectively, for females. Such sex play typically involves genital fondling and, much less frequently, oral, anal, or vaginal insertions (Broderick, 1966). By the end of preadolescence, interest has usually shifted from members of the same sex to members of the opposite sex.

Sexual awareness By the time children have reached preadolescence, they are quite knowledgeable about sexual matters. In fact, the age at which a child obtains such knowledge has been steadily declining. In a sample of subjects questioned between 1940 and 1960, more than 50 percent of males and females had learned about coitus between the ages of 10 and 13. In contrast, over half of a sampling of subjects questioned in 1975 knew about intercourse by the end of their tenth year (Gebhard, 1977). The difference was even greater in knowledge of pregnancy. The earlier subjects understood the rudiments of pregnancy by age 10, but the later subjects had this information by age 6.

The potential sources of knowledge vary greatly depending on the child's sex and socioeconomic status. The primary source of information for children of blue-collar workers is the peer group (friends and schoolmates), whereas the primary source for children of white-collar workers tends to be the mother. In general, the father appears to provide little in the way of sex education for children in either social class (Elias and Gebhard, 1969; Gebhard, 1977).

It is during preadolescence that many children learn about the sex act—the actual insertion of the male's penis into the female's vagina. Such a notion is often shocking to preadolescents, and many cannot envision their parents doing such a thing. Despite learning about the nature of the sex act, Western children have little, if any, opportunity to actually observe sexual intercourse. In other cultures, however, such observation may be only mildly prohibited or may even be encouraged. Among the Melanesians, for example, children share the bedroom with their parents. They are told not to look during intercourse, but furtive glances are typical (Brecher and Brecher, 1966). Alorese parents tell their children about the sexual act at age 5 and give them instructions in sex. Both Pukapukan and Lesu children are allowed to watch intercourse, but the latter are forbidden to watch their mothers engaging in sexual activity.

Gender roles and gender differences During preadolescence, gender roles become well established. Sex-role typing is generally much more rigorous for boys than for girls. By the age of 4, most boys have developed a masculine orientation that has been shaped by parents and peers. As boys grow older, there is very little parental tolerance of feminine traits, especially by fathers. Boys are not supposed to be "sissies." Sex-role typing is much more flexible for girls. Girls can get away with being tomboys, and during much of preadolescence girls often display a masculine orientation. This orientation begins at around age 4 or 5 and lasts until age 10. Girls show a preference for male toys and say they want to grow up to be a daddy (Ward, 1973). Perhaps this orientation arises from the girls' realization that boys have more privileges and prestige than do girls (Hetherington and Parke, 1979). Ultimately, however, most girls return to a feminine orientation. Thus, in preadolescence both boys and girls must undergo the pleasures and pains of growing up, but boys have the added burden of learning to suppress any girlish behaviors they may possess (Emmerich, 1959).

The adolescent is faced with two major life changes. One is the onset of puberty, which changes the individual forever, both physically and emotionally. The other is the entry into high school, with its associated social and academic pressures. Adolescence is often characterized as a period of upheaval, since it serves as a crossroads between childhood and adulthood.

Physical changes A number of biological changes occur before and during adolescence that transform the child into a sexually mature individual. Some of these changes are internal and may go unrecognized, while others are quite obvious. There is also considerable variation in the age at which both males and females enter puberty, as shown in Figs. 9.1(a) and 9.1(b).

The word *puberty* refers to the development of pubic hair. More generally, however, **puberty** is used to describe the many physical changes that occur in the process of sexual maturation. It is a curious fact that the onset of puberty and the time necessary for full maturation differ in boys and girls. Girls enter puberty earlier and become sexually mature more rapidly than boys. This means that girls become interested in boys sooner than boys become interested in girls—which makes for some awkward encounters. It also means that for about a year girls are taller than boys of the same age.

The onset of puberty in females is triggered by a complex set of hormonal changes. As FSH and LH concentrations gradually increase in preadolescence, the hypothalamus becomes sensitive to the small circulating levels of estrogen. This causes further increases in FSH and LH, which in turn increase the amount of estrogen in the bloodstream. It is this estrogen increase that is associated with the physical changes that begin to occur at puberty. These physical changes, such as the development of breasts and pubic hair, are referred to as **secondary sexual characteristics**—"secondary" in that the gonads and genitals, which were formed prenatally, are primary.

The development of secondary sexual characteristics in the female follows a typical pattern. The onset of puberty usually begins at about age 10 or 11 and is associated with the appearance of pubic hair. Under the stimulation of estrogen, the breasts begin to develop. Starting as a small bump of tissue just off center of the nipple, the breast gradually expands to form a conical shape. At the same time, modifications occur in the pelvic girdle, and the body forms more contours as the result of deposition of fat in the hips, thighs, and buttocks. The clitoris increases in length, and the labia become thicker. The uterus grows and expands, nearly doubling in size by age 17.

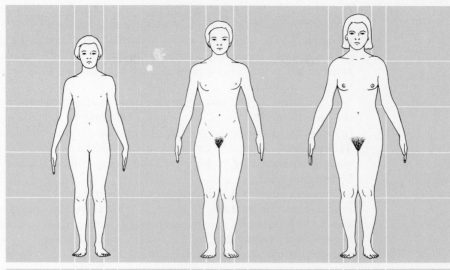

FIGURE 9.1(a)
Normal variation
in the maturation
of three girls aged
12.75 years. The
girl on the left has
not yet reached
puberty; the girl in
the middle is part
way through
puberty; and the
girl on the right
has finished her
development.

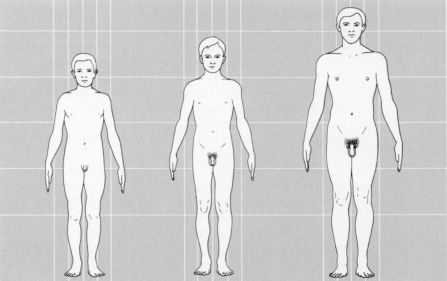

FIGURE 9.1(b)
Normal variation
in the maturation
of three boys aged
14.75 years. The
boy on the left has
not yet reached
puberty; the boy
in the middle is
part way through
puberty; and the
boy on the right
has finished his
development.

From J. M. Tanner, "Growing Up." Copyright © by Scientific American, Inc. All rights reserved.

At around age 12 or 13, the female will experience her first menstruation. This first menstrual period is called **menarche**. Some societies treat menarche as a major event, while others consider it to be minor. Furthermore, menarche can have negative or positive connotations, depending on cultural traditions. In American society, menarche has major significance, with slightly negative connotations.

Although the average age of menarche is 12, there is considerable variation, with normal onset as early as age 8 or as late as 17. The average age of
menarche in the United States and other industrialized countries has dropped
only slightly in the last 150 years (Bullough, 1981). This decrease may be
attributable to improved nutrition, social conditions, and public health over
the century and a half.

In the majority of cases, the first menstruation does not necessarily mean
the girl is capable of having children. There may be a sterility period of 12–18
months during which the girl menstruates but does not ovulate (Marshall and
Tanner, 1969). Even after ovulation, there may be decreased fertility because of
uterine immaturity. Despite these facts, many young teenagers can and do
become pregnant.

During puberty, a girl undergoes a spurt in height that is controlled by
growth hormone from the pituitary. It is estrogen, however, that ultimately
acts as a brake to this growth and prevents further skeletal development. This
is one of the reasons that men are taller, on the average, than women. Height
changes little for women after about age 17 or 18.

The same process that underlies the onset of puberty in females underlies
its onset in males. During childhood, FSH and LH levels are low. Just prior to
puberty, the hypothalamus becomes sensitive to the levels of testosterone in
the body, and the levels of FSH, LH, and testosterone increase. The increasing
levels of testosterone are responsible for the development of secondary sexual
characteristics in males.

Male puberty begins around age 12 or 13. Even though it seems like
females develop much more rapidly than males, puberty begins only 6 months
later in boys. The discrepancy arises because growth spurts occur at the beginning of puberty for girls while they occur in the middle of adolescence for boys
(Tanner, 1975) (see Fig. 9.2).

The first overt sign of puberty in males is the acceleration in the growth of
the testes and scrotum at around 10½. This growth is followed by the appearance of some pubic hair. A year later, the penis begins to show further development, and the boy starts his growth spurt.

Instead of showing differential fat deposition like girls, boys undergo a
marked increase in muscular strength. The seminal vesicles and prostate gland
enlarge, and, within another year, the boy will experience his first ejaculation.
One-third of all males show a distinct enlargement of the breasts in the middle
phase; this breast tissue regresses within a year.

Toward the end of adolescence, both axillary and facial hair make their
appearance. Facial hair begins at the corners of the upper lip, spreads across the
lip to form a mustache, and then progresses to form a beard. Finally, the voice
deepens, and the hairline begins to recede (Marshall and Tanner, 1970). Facial
and chest hair continue to develop beyond age 20. Major changes in height occur
at around age 14 or 15, and total growth slows down considerably by age 20.

A common but temporary problem among adolescents is acne. This skin
problem can have profound psychological effects on teenagers, who may think

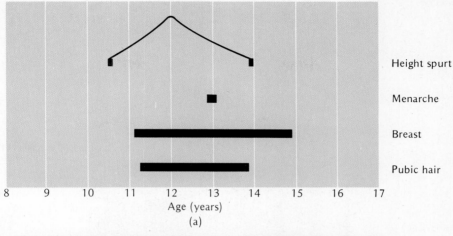

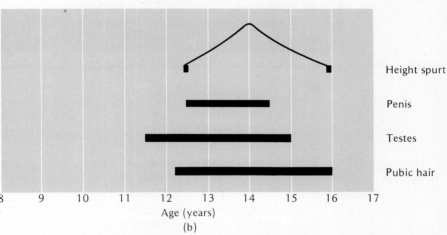

*FIGURE 9.2
Sequence of events
of puberty at
various ages for
girls (a) and boys
(b). The hump in
the bar labeled
"Height spurt"
represents how
fast this growth
occurs. The bar
represents the
beginning and
completion of the
events of puberty
for the average
child.*

From J. M. Tanner, "Growing Up." Copyright © by Scientific American, Inc. All rights reserved.

of themselves as disfigured and unattractive. Acne is related to hormonal changes. Good skin care and the use of special soaps can alleviate the problem somewhat until the hormonal system becomes regulated.

Sexual behavior   There is a marked surge of interest in sexual behavior during adolescence. Masturbation, for example, increases dramatically in males. Over 68 percent experience their first ejaculation through masturbation, while others achieve ejaculation through nocturnal emission or heterosexual activity. By age 15, 82 percent of all males are experienced in masturbating to ejaculation (Kinsey et al., 1948, 1953). Males usually reach their peak in terms of orgasmic frequency about 2 years after the onset of puberty; that is, the number of orgasmic experiences a male can have on a given day is highest during the teenage years.

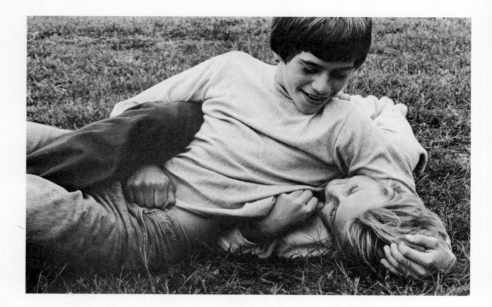

*Interest in the
opposite sex
increases
markedly during
puberty.*

Female masturbation to orgasm is less common in adolescence. By age 13, only 33 percent of all females had masturbated, according to Hunt's research. Females show a general increase in orgasmic frequency, reaching their peak in the mid-twenties and thirties.

There are wide discrepancies in data on the extent of sexual intercourse in adolescence. Depending on the study cited, anywhere from 9 to 44 percent of males and 7 to 30 percent of females have engaged in heterosexual intercourse by the age of 15 (Sorenson, 1973; Miller and Simon, 1974; Vener and Stewart, 1974). The percentage reaches 81 percent for males and 69 percent for females by age 25 (Hunt, 1974). Males and females are likely to react differently to their first intercourse. Sorenson (1973) found that girls tend to attach less significance to this event but are more likely to have a negative reaction, such as guilt or sorrow. Males, on the other hand, are more likely to experience feelings of joy and maturity.

With the increasing permissiveness accorded to sexual behavior in recent years, many people are concerned that sexual behavior among adolescents has become excessive and impersonal. Is sex for its own sake becoming the norm? Morton Hunt (1974) suggests this is not the case. Although adolescents and young adults seem to engage in sexual intercourse more frequently today than in previous generations, individuals still tend to have few partners prior to marriage. According to Hunt's research 54 percent of young, sexually active females have had sex with only one partner, and for half of these that partner is their fiancé. Young males then tend to have had sex with about 6 different partners prior to marriage.

Sexual awareness Adolescents face the difficult task of connecting their incomplete mechanical knowledge of sex with its emotional and social aspects. Subjects in the Kinsey sample, for example, learned about fertilization and prostitution in early adolescence but did not learn about venereal disease, abortion, condoms, or homosexuality until 1 or 2 years later, on the average. The major source of the adolescent's information was the same-sex peer group. More recent evidence suggests that the age at which such information is acquired has decreased by several years for the current generation (Gebhard, 1977). Although the peer group is still pivotal in the dissemination of information, sex education classes and more explicit treatment of sex in the media have also contributed.

Gender roles and gender differences One of the most obvious differences between the sexes that arises during adolescence is strength. During puberty, males show a marked increase in the size and number of muscle cells, thereby contributing to their greater strength. Not as obvious are differences in academic performance, both in terms of grades and achievement tests. During early elementary school years, girls outstrip boys in classroom performance. By the time of adolescence, this trend is reversing, and during the college years, the proportion of female underachievers exceeds the proportion of male underachievers (Ralph, Goldberg, and Passow, 1966).

In high school, girls do better on verbal tasks than on spatial tasks, while the reverse is true for males. Males achieve higher grades in geometry, where spatial skills are important. There is no differential performance in algebra, however, where word problems are common (Fennema, 1974). It has been suggested that boys are more skillful at spatial problems because of exposure to certain kinds of toys. Whatever the case, the differences in spatial abilities between men and women have been shrinking steadily over the last decade or more (Flanagan, 1978).

Females react differently to success or failure than males do. Dweck and Goetz (1977) found that when girls had difficulty carrying out a particular task, they were likely to associate their failure with a lack of the necessary ability. In contrast, boys were more likely to attribute their failure to factors other than ability, such as motivation. Boys, therefore, were less affected by teacher evaluations of their performance. Girls may also have difficulty dealing with success. They often conceal their academic ability, especially from males, perhaps because they feel they will appear less "feminine" in males' eyes. Matina Horner (1972) noted that females are much more likely than males to lie about their grades, reporting them as lower than they are, most likely for the same reason that they conceal their academic skills.

As we have seen in this chapter, sexuality is not something that emerges at puberty along with pubic hair, breasts, or a deep voice. Instead, sexuality has its start in infancy and gradually develops over childhood and adolescence, ultimately emerging in the form of adult behavior patterns. This developmental sequence is complex and is influenced by a wide range of factors, including hormones, parents, peers, media, and culture.

SUMMARY

1   *Intrinsic theories* of sexual development emphasize the importance of characteristics within the individual that bring about sexual development. Such theories include physiological theory and Freud's theory.

2   *Physiological theory* assumes that sexuality develops as a result of hormonal and neural stimulation. The main objection to this theory is that it emphasizes sexual behavior beginning with puberty and thus ignores the antecedents of such behavior in children.

3   According to Freud's *theory of psychosexual development*, sexuality begins at birth. Freud suggested that children pass through a sequence of *psychosexual stages* in which sexual energy, or *libido*, becomes focused on different parts of the body. At each stage the child must resolve specific conflicts; failure to resolve the conflict at a certain stage could result in adult *fixation* in or *regression* to that stage.

4   Freud's stages of psychosexual development are (1) the *oral stage*, in which sexual energy is focused on the mouth; (2) the *anal stage*, in which sexual energy is focused on the organs of elimination and deals with the issue of toilet training; (3) the *phallic stage*, in which energy becomes focused on the genitals and the boy must resolve the *Oedipus complex* and the girl, the *Electra complex*; (4) the *latent stage*, in which sexuality becomes dormant; and (5) the *genital stage*, in which libidinal energy becomes directed toward heterosexual relationships.

5   *Extrinsic theories* of sexual development focus on factors outside the individual that shape social behaviors and sexual patterns. These include conditioning theory, theories based on imitation, and the theory of social scripts.

6   There are two main types of conditioning. In *classical conditioning*, a person learns to associate a particular response with a stimulus that does not usually elicit that response. In *operant conditioning*, a person learns to do things that are rewarded and to not do things that are punished. According to conditioning theory, sexuality and gender roles develop through both these types of learning.

7   Other learning theorists suggest that the main way children learn gender roles is by observation of role models and imitation of their behavior. This is opposed to Freud's theory, which emphasizes the importance of the child's *identification* with the same-sex parent in the development of gender roles.

8   According to Gagnon, the development of gender roles and sexuality is governed by *social scripts* that specify the who, what, when, where, and why of sexual behaviors.

9   Researchers who study sexual development focus on three main areas: (1) *sexual behavior*, based on verbal reports of children, parents, and adults who recall childhood experiences; (2) *sexual awareness*, or the child's knowledge of reproduction and intercourse; and (3) *gender roles and gender differences*.

10   There is a great deal of disagreement as to whether *gender roles*—the constellation of behaviors that are characteristic of each sex—are biologically or culturally determined. Not only is it likely that both forces contribute to gender roles, but it turns out that the sexes are not that different in their behaviors. Bem has suggested that the best adjusted individuals are those who have a balance of traditionally male and female traits, or those who display *androgyny*.

11   Sexuality in infancy is evidenced by erections in males, vaginal lubrication in females, pelvic thrusts in the first year of life, genital play, and responsiveness to genital stimulation by others. Male and female infants display certain behavioral differences from birth, but these differences are minor compared to the overwhelming similarities.

12   Between the ages of 3 and 7, children show an increase in sexual interest by playing sex games such as "show" and "doctor" with their peers and by expressing curiosity about activities normally performed in private. Five-year-olds have a beginning awareness of gender differences and of the creation of babies but have little conception of the father's role. Preschoolers tend to choose same-sex playmates, and boys tend to be more aggressive in their play than girls.

13   In *preadolescence* (ages 8–11) sex play is primarily same-sex, and masturbation may be discovered. Most preadolescents are quite knowledgeable about sexual matters, deriving most of their information from peers or their mothers. Gender roles become well established during this period, as boys are discouraged from being "sissies" and girls may go through a tomboy period that usually ends with a return to a feminine orientation. *Sex-role typing* is much more flexible for girls than for boys.

14   *Puberty* refers to the many physical changes that occur in the process of sexual maturation. The onset of puberty in females is triggered by an increase in estrogen that leads to the development of such *secondary sexual characteristics* as breasts, pubic hair, and modification of body contours. The average age of first menstruation, or *menarche*, is 12. Male puberty, which begins about 6 months later than female puberty, is triggered by increased levels of testosterone that lead to the development of such secondary sexual characteristics as pubic hair; enlargement of the testes, scrotum, and penis; increased muscular strength; facial and chest hair; and a deepening voice. Because the growth spurt happens earlier in girls than in boys, early adolescence can produce awkward encounters between females who are rapidly becoming women and males who are still boys.

15   During adolescence, masturbation increases dramatically in males, and females begin to show interest in self-stimulation. For many, the first sexual intercourse occurs by the age of 15 or earlier. Although adolescents appear to be engaging in intercourse more frequently today than in the past, they tend to limit their sexual behavior to only a few partners.

16   Gender differences that emerge in adolescence include better verbal abilities in girls and better spatial abilities in boys. These differences have become smaller in recent years, however.

**ADDITIONAL
READING**

Bernstein, Anne. How children learn about sex and birth. *Psychology Today*, January 1976, p. 35.

> *A well-written article that discusses the types of sexual knowledge children can absorb and utilize at different ages.*

* **Chafetz, Janet S.** *Masculine/Feminine or Human? An Overview of the Sociology of Sex Roles*. Itasca, IL: F. E. Peacock, 1974.

> *A readable introduction to the sociological view of how sex roles are acquired and maintained.*

Gordon, Sol. *The Sexual Adolescent.* North Scituate, MA: Duxbury, 1973.

A good discussion of adolescent sexuality. Originally written for professionals and parents.

Tanner, J. M. *Growth at Adolescence* (2nd ed.). Oxford: Blackwell Scientific Publications, 1962.

An excellent discussion of the changes that occur at puberty. Considered to be a classic in the field.

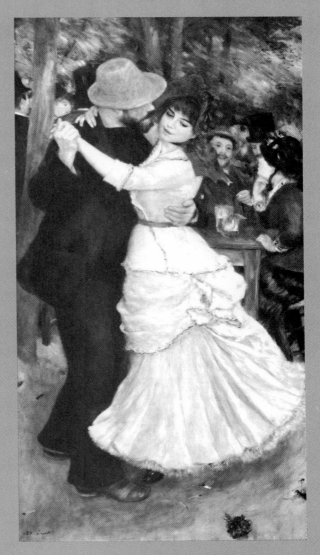

From attraction to love: Emotional attachment and human sexuality

I feel wide open to new people and new experiences, which I wasn't before. Not that I sleep around—I have to really feel something about a man. I have to be totally absorbed by him. But it can happen fast. Just last week I looked into someone's eyes in a bookstore, and I knew at once I wanted to know that person. . . .

This statement by a 26-year-old woman was included in Morton Hunt's book *Sexual Behavior in the Seventies* (1974) as an example of a contemporary attitude toward sexual behavior. This woman, let's call her Joanne, holds what most of us would consider a reasonable, if somewhat liberal, approach to current sexual attitudes and conduct. On closer examination, however, there are some interesting aspects to Joanne's statement. First, her openness to sexual encounters is modified by her requirement that she "really feel something about a man." Second, she refers to the necessity for a deep relationship in her desire to be "totally absorbed" by a man. Finally, she mentions that she can be immediately attracted to a man, even a complete stranger.

Joanne's statement raises many of the issues we face in trying to understand the nature of attraction, attachment, love, and intimacy, of which sexuality is but a part. The statement also raises questions about the sequence of events in the development of deep relationships. How does a person move from a state of noninvolvement to interest in another person, to emotional attachment, and perhaps to sexual encounter? How is an individual moved from glances and eye contact in a bookstore through a complex chain of events that could result in direct sexual expression? At what points are various go, no-go decisions made? And why do some people immediately lead our thoughts to a possible sexual encounter, while others seem to turn us off from the start? These and similar questions are some of the concerns of this chapter.

ATTRACTION

Let us assume that Joanne was in that store looking for books—not romance. How can we explain the movement of Joanne's attention from books to a stranger's eyes? And what was there about that particular set of eyes that both attracted her attention and led her to contemplate a sexual encounter?

These questions lead us into the vague area of **attraction:** the study of why people like each other. As an area of psychological investigation, it is concerned with more than just the momentary experience of noticing someone who looks good to us. Such a momentary attraction may have the potential for initiating an encounter, but the continuation of the interaction depends on many other factors as well. During both the initial encounter and the developing relationship, many aspects of the individuals and their environment come into play in determining how well the couple will "hit it off." Most of us can remember experiences of initial attraction changing to disinterest or even to revulsion. Or we may have been disinterested at first and only gradually developed an important relationship. Researchers interested in attraction have studied many diverse aspects of this elusive phenomenon and have arrived at a few conclusions about how interpersonal attraction works.

The factors that are particularly valuable to our study of sexual behavior include physical attributes, proximity (physical closeness), similarity and complementarity, reinforcement, and reciprocity.

The first thing we are likely to notice about another person is his or her appearance, or physical attractiveness. We do not easily admit to being attracted by physical attributes. Homilies such as "Beauty is only skin deep" and "You can't judge a book by its cover" are often quoted to remind us that physical beauty should not be our main criterion in assessing others. Nevertheless, study after study has shown that physical attractiveness is the most important factor in determining whether we will go beyond the cover of the book and explore the pages, that is, whether we will initiate an encounter with a person.

One well-known study that revealed the importance of physical attributes in attraction was conducted by Walster and her associates (1966). In this study, college freshmen were paired for blind dates for a dance. At the dance, observers rated the physical attractiveness of each student, and the students were previously rated for intelligence, personality, and social skills. After the dance, the students were asked to fill out questionnaires indicating how much they liked their dates and whether they wanted to go out with them again. The researchers found that regardless of a date's personality, intelligence, and social skills, it was his or her physical attractiveness that determined the extent to which he or she was liked and would be desired for a second date.

What is there about physical attractiveness that makes it so desirable? It may seem obvious that we should like attractive people, but *why* is this the case? There is no simple answer to this question. What researchers have found is that people attribute a variety of positive qualities to attractive individuals about whom they have no other knowledge. In one study, for example, when photographs of very attractive, average, and unattractive people were presented to subjects, they indicated that the attractive people would have more socially desirable personality traits, would have better occupational success, and would make better marriage partners (Dion, Berscheid, and Walster, 1972). On the basis of these findings, the researchers concluded that there is a "what is beautiful is good" stereotype operating in our society. Other studies have produced similar results. Researchers have also found that attractive people are thought to be kinder, warmer, more interesting, stronger, more poised, more sociable, sexier, and more outgoing than less attractive people. This view is even held by children as young as 4 years of age (Dion and Berscheid, 1972).

What characteristics make a person attractive? For some people, faces are most important; for others, it's physique that counts. The notion that people have specific preferences—that Tom is a "leg man" or that Sue goes for redheads—is another stereotype about initial attraction that has been investigated. For example, Wiggins and others (1968) showed men silhouetted figures of women who varied in size of buttocks, legs, and breasts. Two silhouettes were presented at a time, and the subjects selected the one from each pair that they liked the best. The results showed that men did indeed fall into prefer-

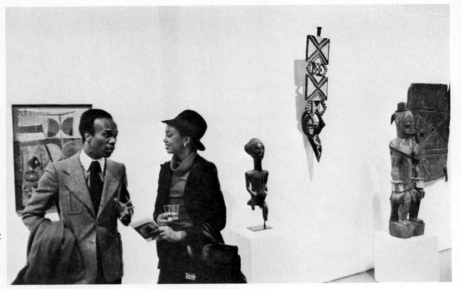

The attraction of one person to another seems to just happen. Yet it is an extraordinarily complex process to understand.

ence groups—there were leg men, breast men, and buttocks men. Furthermore, Wiggins suggested that there were different personality types associated with these preference groups. Those who favored large breasts, for example, were sports minded, dated frequently, and were more likely to read *Playboy*. Those who favored small breasts were, on the average, more submissive, religious, and depressed.

Studies of women's preferences have produced less clear-cut differences. Women do show a slight preference for a V-shaped male figure, that is, a large chest tapering into a small waist. No correlation has been found between women's personalities and such a preference, however (Beck, Ward-Hull, and McLear, 1976). One interesting, if informal, survey of women's preferences was conducted by the *Village Voice*, a Greenwich Village newspaper. Readers were asked to rate which part of a man's body is most sexually attractive to women. The men who responded thought that women would look for a muscular chest, arms, and shoulders first, then a large penis, and tallness third. However, the women said the first thing they looked for was "small and sexy" buttocks, followed by slimness, lack of a protruding stomach, and expressive eyes.

Thus, we might say that Joanne was attracted by an important feature (the man's eyes) but not the prime one (buttocks) in her bookstore encounter. Had the man been leaving the bookstore, she might have been more (or less) attracted by his prime feature. Interestingly enough, women in the *Village Voice* survey did not rank highly the muscular build that men think is so important and that many spend so much time trying to enhance through exercise.

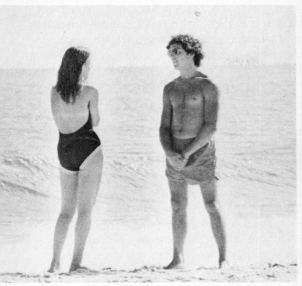 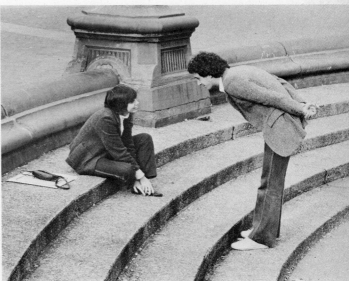

Sexual releasers We have been discussing physical attributes, but there are other aspects of a person that may also be used to elicit attraction. In other species, stimuli such as odors, sounds, or specific body postures (called visual displays) serve as attractants. Such attractants are called **sexual releasers**—stimuli that elicit instinctual chains of sexual behavior. Could there be such sexual releasers at work in the attraction process in humans? When boy meets girl, could they be sampling a wide array of sounds, odors, body movements, and facial expressions, built into the species, that trigger various instinctual chains of sexual behavior? For example, could lipstick be the human equivalent of the sex-releasing visual display of some monkeys who have rumps that turn bright red? It has also been suggested that perfumes are used to *hide* our natural odors so that we do not turn each other on in inappropriate places, like theaters and buses. Several popular books, such as Desmond Morris's *The Naked Ape*, have covered this subject. But while such speculations are interesting, there is no actual evidence that such sexual releasers exist in humans. The most accurate summary of our current state of knowledge about the function of sexual releasers in humans has been provided by Gagnon (1977):

> *The sexuality and the reproductive behavior of human beings is characterized by open genetic programs; that is, there is no evidence that one set of stimuli either from the world outside, or from inside the organism, will automatically and invariably produce sexual activity. . . . In the intact human organism, sexual conduct is determined by the learning history of the organism, in interaction with the changing demands of the environment. (p. 125)*

Attractiveness and self-esteem We have seen how important physical attractiveness is in judging others. But it is also important in judging ourselves. It is no surprise that self-esteem is strongly related to one's self-image of attractiveness. If a person feels attractive, he or she will function in a more self-assured manner and will tend to do well in social situations. In turn, this self-assurance will increase the person's attractiveness in the eyes of others. Thus, believing that one is attractive can be a self-fulfilling prophecy. One answer, then, to our question of why physical beauty plays such a dominant role in our assessment of others is that people who are physically beautiful may make an effort to live up to the social stereotype, making into reality the belief that "what is beautiful is good." Furthermore, merely associating with "beautiful people" can be enhancing to a person's self-esteem, so attraction to such people can provide rewards other than aesthetic ones.

Proximity

According to the principle of proximity, the closer people are to each other physically, the more likely they are to like each other. Sociologists have long recognized that all levels of relationship, including marriage, are enhanced as distance is reduced. For example, a college student living in a dorm is more likely to be best friends with the student in the room next door than one on the next floor. And marrying the boy or girl next door is not as much a fairytale as many people think. Thus, Joanne is actually more likely to develop a relationship with a co-worker or a neighbor than with a stranger glimpsed across an aisle in a bookstore.

An important aspect of the proximity effect is familiarity. Those whom we see at school, at work, or in the neighborhood on a regular basis become familiar figures in our lives. And rather than breeding contempt, it seems that such familiarity breeds liking. To examine this effect in the laboratory, Robert Zajonc (1971) had subjects look at a series of pictures of people in which some of the pictures were shown more frequently than others. When the subjects were later asked how much they liked each of the people in the pictures, their positive judgments were directly related to the number of times they had seen each picture; that is, the more often they had seen a person, the greater was their liking for that person. People we encounter in our routine lives tend to benefit from this familiarity effect.

*Similarity and
complementarity*

If you were to subscribe to a computer dating service, you would be asked not only to describe your ideal date but also to provide a great deal of information about yourself. Why the emphasis on you? Shouldn't the data on your requirements for a partner be enough? The fact is that those who program such computers have found that matching people on similar characteristics—including background, race, social class, religion, even hair color—is more likely to lead to positive results. The computer is told to search out those potential dates who most resemble you as well as meet your stated requirements.

Social psychologists would generally agree with the computer dating services that similarity is a fundamental factor in attraction. Experimental studies have supported the similarity hypothesis by showing that subjects expect to like people described as being similar to themselves (Byrne, 1971). Furthermore, husbands and wives generally have similar racial, educational, religious, social, and economic backgrounds. They also show more similarities in subtle factors, such as personalities and attitudes, than would be expected from purely chance matches. These findings suggest that similarity probably plays a key role in a married couple's initial attraction and in the eventual development of their relationship.

Additional social psychological research has suggested, however, that the relationship between similarity and attraction may be more complicated than originally thought. Similarity may be of prime importance in forming the first impression and helping the initial encounter (the couple has more to talk about, similar experiences, and so on), but after this initial stage other factors may become more important in continuing the relationship. Here is where the idea of opposites attracting comes in.

When people quote the old cliche "Opposites attract," they are really speaking of complementarity. Complementarity is not so much the opposition of characteristics as it is the matching of one person's strengths, weaknesses, and needs with another person's in such a way that these characteristics balance each other. Thus, a relationship in which one parnter is dominant and one is submissive can meet the needs of both. Complementarity may not always seem so beneficial, however. In Neil Simon's *The Odd Couple*, the neat-sloppy complementarity of the main characters, Felix and Oscar, seems to be a source of conflict rather than benefit. However, fighting does not necessarily mean that the relationship does not function in some positive way for the participants.

It would appear that similarity, differences, and complementarity are all important in attraction, and the importance of each seems to vary with the stage of the relationship. Similarity helps a relationship in its initial stages by providing a common ground for communication and shared activities. Differences may be necessary for the initial attraction to move to a deeper level—after all, it could be awfully boring to be in a relationship with someone who is too similar to oneself. Finally, complementarity is valuable as the relationship becomes more stable and one partner's weaknesses and strengths come to be balanced by complementary traits in the other person.

Reinforcing capacity

The seeking of **rewards** or **reinforcers** is important in all aspects of interaction and certainly has an important place in the understanding of attraction. We are attracted to people who can supply us with rewards. But what makes another person reinforcing? There is a large body of psychological research demonstrating the power of social reinforcers in maintaining and modifying behavior. **Social reinforcers** are interpersonal cues that signal the feelings of one person toward another. *Positive* social reinforcers include praise, smiles, pats on the back, nods, and other gestures of approval. *Negative* social reinforcers include criticism, frowns, head shaking, saying no, and other signs of disapproval.

The relationship of social reinforcers to attraction has been verified by a number of social psychological studies (Byrne, 1969; Homans, 1961). These studies show that when a person is in a position where his or her praise is important, any praise that person gives us will increase our liking for him or her. If, however, we perceive the person to have ulterior motives for praising us (such as trying to sell us a new car), we may actually like him or her less. This is called the "apple polisher" effect (Jones, 1964).

In an interesting series of experiments, Aronson and Linder (1965) demonstrated that we are most attracted to people whose evaluations of us become more positive over time than to people who praise or reinforce us consistently. Four experimental situations were created. In the first one, the subjects were deliberately allowed to overhear another subject (actually a confederate of the experimenters) say nice things about them. In the second condition, the subjects overheard the confederate make critical comments about them. In the third condition, the confederate started out praising the subject but ended with criticism. And in the fourth, the evaluation started out critically but ended with praise. Later the subjects were asked to indicate how much they liked the confederate. The results showed that the confederate was most liked in the fourth condition, when evaluations went from criticism to praise, and was least liked in the third condition.

Aronson (1972) concluded from this and similar research that the relative balance of reinforcers given and received is a major factor in the initiation and maintenance of relationships. According to his **gain-loss theory** of interpersonal attraction, we get more out of a relationship if we experience *increasing* rewards from our partner than if our partner rewards us in a constant, invariant manner. Conversely, if our partner gives us fewer rewards over time, it is likely to have a greater impact than if he or she has given us few rewards all along. Aronson suggests that if a friendship or relationship is to be kept alive, the partners need to be open and honest with each other and share negative feelings rather than to try to be "nice" all the time. Such honesty allows for a "zigzagging" of sentiment that keeps the partners at high levels of rewarding each other in order to make up for criticisms and to maintain each other's esteem.

*Reciprocity
of feelings*

We tend to like people who like us. Conversely, when people think we like them, they tend to like us. This tendency is referred to as **reciprocity**. Reciprocity seems easily explainable in terms of social reinforcement and helps account for how relationships grow and develop. But there seems to be one exception to the rule of reciprocity: How can it explain the fact that people are often attracted to those who play hard-to-get? It is commonly believed that men and women are constantly falling in love with someone who is aloof and doesn't return their positive feelings. In an interesting series of studies, Walster and her associates (1973) studied this phenomenon.

The researchers wanted to study the imbalanced, nonreciprocal relationship of a hard-to-get, elusive woman and the men who are attracted to her. By interviewing male college students, they did find that the elusive woman was considered very attractive. However, their attempts to directly measure such attraction provided confusing results. After conducting some additional interviews, the researchers proposed a new hypothesis: The hard-to-get woman is attractive only if she is hard for *other* men to get but not for the subject making the rating; that is, the man is attracted to a woman who has a *reputation* for being hard-to-get but who is accessible to the subject and will not reject him. Walster and her associates tested this idea by using a computer dating situation. Each subject was told that certain of the computer-selected women had chosen his file and had rejected all other men's files presented to them, that other women had accepted many of the files offered to them, and that a third group had generally rejected all men. Nearly all of the subjects wanted dates with the selectively hard-to-get women and rated them (presumably on the basis of their folders) as most attractive. The women who supposedly rejected most of the dates—the truly hard-to-get women—were rarely chosen for dates.

Thus, it would appear that the reciprocity principle holds true even in cases that seem to be an exception to it; that is, men have to feel that their positive feelings will be reciprocated before they will admit to being attracted to a potential dating partner.

COURTSHIP
AND DATING

There is a period between the onset of attraction and the formation of more permanent affectional bonds when the goal is to get to know the other person better. In our society, the terms *courtship* and *dating* have been applied to this period.

Most societies have a period similar to our courtship. Although the nature of the relationship and the time allotted for it vary from culture to culture, the particular period in which strangers come to know each other as potential partners and future mates is typically given formal status in societies all over the world.

Anthropologists indicate that no human society tolerates totally promiscuous mating. On the surface, some societies seem to have very few rules, but in all cases clear boundaries regarding the number and nature of sexual partners that members are allowed are set. Issues of family relationships, inheritance, and genetic lineage are concerns in all cultures and are guarded by the rules of mating. This helps explain why families are often involved in courtship and marriage arrangements. Not infrequently, it is the kinship group that arranges marriages rather than the actual participants.

Courtship patterns in the United States are most remarkable for their differences from other patterns that sociologists, historians, and anthropologists have described. The main difference is in the amount of control the participants are given. In the United States, they have control over both the selection of their partner and how they spend their time together, whereas in other cultures control is more formal and courtship is often family-arranged.

In the 1940s, 1950s, and 1960s, sociologists were quite interested in studying dating, and several classic studies analyzing the dating practices of American youth were conducted. In recent years, however, such investigations have

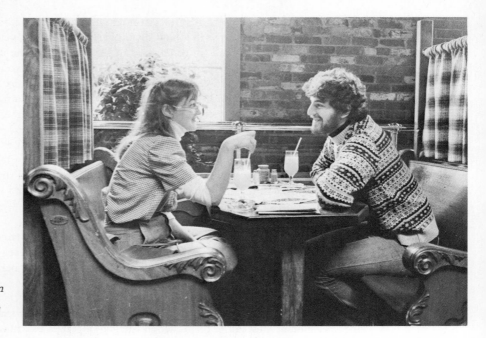

*Dating has its
many forms and
stages, but it is an
important part of
developing sexual
relationships.*

declined. The 1970s saw a change in the nature of dating, so that the idea of formal dating no longer had much meaning. People today do not necessarily think of time spent together as being a date. Despite the informality, however, the courtship pattern is there and is just as important as ever in providing the setting for the activities that may proceed to deeper relationships and possible pair bonding. Because these initial stages are so important, we will describe current patterns in some detail.

*Patterns
and stages
of dating*

Dating emerges as a natural extension of the friendship groups of the preadolescent. The early teenage years provide a bridge from same-sex friendships to experiments in developing relationships with the opposite sex. Early "dates" tend to be informal arrangements, often negotiated by friends, among adolescents who already know each other. They are most likely to go to movies and dances and to be part of a small group of couples rather than to be alone. These early encounters provide experience in being in the presence of members of the opposite sex under conditions that are less anxiety-provoking than would occur in a one-to-one situation. Through such preliminary dating, young people learn behaviors appropriate to developing heterosexual relationships.

Reiss (1972) has described a sequence of stages that dating couples can go through: casual, regular, steady, and exclusive. Couples who date with reasonable frequency move rather quickly to the final stage.

Casual dating involves little commitment and appears to function primarily as a means of recreation. Reiss feels that casual dating is strictly American, since most other cultures reserve dating for more serious mate selection rather than for "fun." In our culture it is considered appropriate to date someone occasionally with no future commitment or necessity for deepening the relationship. Such dating partners may refer to each other as "just friends" or may say they just enjoy each other's company.

It is expected that couples who are more interested in each other after some trial dates will move to more *regular dating* During this stage, the individuals see each other more frequently but may still see others as well. At this point, the couple share a moderate degree of interpersonal involvement and commitment.

A deeper stage of commitment is the "going steady" or *steady dating* stage. Despite the implication of total commitment, going steady can include a range of other relationships. For example, a college student might go steady with one person at school and another in his or her hometown, or a student may go with one person during the school year and another during summer vacation. Thus, the designation *going steady* appears to indicate a strong commitment but not necessarily an exclusive arrangement.

Exclusive dating does entail total involvement with one person only. Reiss (1972) divides exclusive dating into two subtypes: engaged and nonengaged. The engaged couple have made a commitment to formal marriage. While the engagement may be broken before the legal bond occurs, at the time of the agreement each partner is stating to the other and to the community that they intend to form a marital union. In becoming engaged, the couple have announced their unavailability for courtship interaction with others. The engagement also has legal status, and, though rare today, a breach of contract suit can be brought against a partner who backs out of the engagement. The nonengaged, exclusive dating pattern has all the features of the engaged arrangement but with no commitment to marriage. This pattern has been on the rise with the increased acceptance of couples living together without benefit of marriage.

College dating

Most of the direct research on dating has come from the college campus. Early studies by Waller (1937) at Pennsylvania State University are considered classics and are still cited in descriptions of college dating patterns. Waller found a dating system in which men and women paired off according to the advantages each could offer to the other. The males were valued for their potential status, cars, fraternity memberships, and so on. Women were valued for their attractiveness, clothing, dancing ability, and sorority membership. Family status and wealth were important issues for both sexes. In this system, those who rated highest in the various criteria went out with those who also rated highly. The "best" dated the "best," and everyone else was arranged in rank order below them. Waller referred to this as the "rating and dating" complex and described it as an informal class-caste system.

The decade of the 1950s found students rejecting this class system. During this period, interpersonal qualities and personality became the dominant crite-

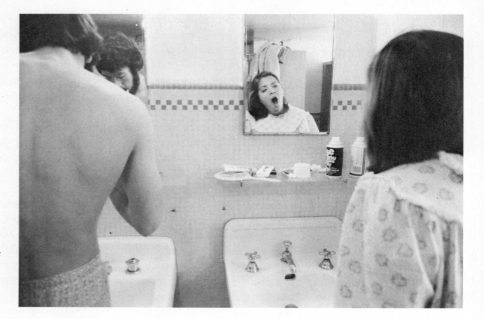

*Living in a coed
dormitory can
ease the process of
forming
relationships for
males and
females.*

ria for selecting a potential date. This trend continued into the 1960s, with
even greater emphasis on the person's individual qualities. Students described
the ideal date as someone possessing qualities they would like to find in a
potential marriage partner. Thus, students were dating people as a part of a
mate selection process. The 1970s proved confusing for researchers interested
in dating-courtship patterns. Dating was not conducted in quite the same way
as in previous decades, and there was an increase in experimentation with
variations on the traditional approaches and a reduced emphasis on mate
selection. Today there is some indication that this experimentation is giving
way, and there is a return to a more traditional mate selection process similar
to that of the 1950s.

The nature of contemporary college life has made many of the more
formal aspects of dating unnecessary. Mixed-sex dormitories and lack of room
visitation restrictions have helped reduce the need for formal dating as a means
of providing a setting for young people to get to know potential sexual partners. And the informal patterns developed on campus seem to have been
exported to outside communities. As college students have migrated to cities
after graduation, they have brought with them the style of college heterosexual
life. Singles bars and other common meeting grounds provide the opportunity
for mixing, meeting, and matching without the necessity of formal arrangements. In these settings, people can come together to form relationships with
little or no commitment.

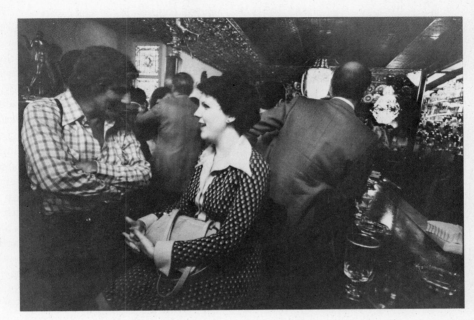

*The singles' bar as
a place to meet
potential sexual
partners has
become a fixture
in most urban
centers.*

*Courtship
sex roles*

The idea that one person of the dating couple (usually the man) seduces the other is part of our folklore of courtship and dating. It was thought in Victorian times that women had to be subtly manipulated into sexual encounters, and it seems that this idea lingers today. Peplau, Rubin, and Hill (1977), in a long-term study of 231 couples from four colleges in the Boston area, found that males typically exercised positive control, urging sexual contact. Females, on the other hand, exercised negative control, generally holding the relationship back from further sexual activity. The researchers felt that these were the socially expected roles and that the men and women were acting out of tradition.

The view of the seducing male and the resisting female is changing, albeit slowly. Another, related stereotype, the scheming female who entraps a naive male, is also weakening. Neither of these sexual scripts is conducive to people developing open and sharing relationships. In fact, such scripts can create paranoia and defensiveness in partners. These scripts also tend to be self-fulfilling. Men feel they *should* be seducing their dates even when they might prefer not to, and women feel they *should* get commitments and trade-offs for any sexual concessions they make. The peer group exerts extra pressure by reinforcing these scripts.

Many couples today see themselves as more equal in their power and in decision making about the direction and speed of the developing relationship. By moving away from the seduction scenario, modern couples are avoiding the feelings of victimization and guilt this script produces. It is still true that one partner may pressure the other, and there will always be differences and conflicts over decisions about sexual interaction. But it seems that responsibility for the decisions will be shared more equally and realistically in the future and not be based on sex-role-determined scripts.

The special problem of shyness

In an attempt to understand relationships and how they are initiated, developed, and deepened, we must look at those people who would like to experience deep relationships but who are prevented from doing so because of shyness. This is no minor problem in our society. Philip Zimbardo (1978) found that over 40 percent of his sample of college students considered themselves to be currently shy and that 80 percent said they had been shy at some time in their lives. Most important, though, was a smaller group that labeled themselves as shy to the point where it seriously interfered with their lives.

Shyness shows itself in many ways. Reluctance to speak is a common characteristic. And when shy people do speak, it is often very softly. Eye contact is another problem; shy people are reluctant to look at others. In addition, blushing is a frequent visible sign of the person's shyness and embarrassment.

All of these signs demonstrate the intense self-consciousness and self-preoccupation so basic to shyness. For shy people, interacting with individuals of the opposite sex is a highly anxiety-producing experience, and many never become involved in dating at all. If a shy person is able to enter into dating situations, he or she is plagued by shyness at every turn. Should an encounter proceed to something more directly sexual, such as petting, the situation dramatically worsens. As Zimbardo (1978) has said, ". . . shy men and women have fewer sexual experiences and enjoy them less" (p. 92).

Shyness is a complex problem, and no simplistic solution can or should be prescribed. In Chap. 15 we will see how important it is for people to reduce their performance anxiety in sexual situations. For the shy person, all situations arouse anxiety and self-consciousness, and any treatment approach must focus on helping the shy person away from this tense state.

FORMING ATTACHMENTS

The courtship-dating period provides couples the opportunity to develop emotional attachments. If conditions prove favorable, one of the outcomes of dating is the deepening of the relationship and the formation of an emotional bond. What is the nature of this bond and what is its basis in human behavior?

Affectional bonding

We can observe behaviors in many animal species that make us suspect we are not the only animals that form strong affectional bonds and feel deep attachments to one another. If such behavior is part of animal behavior generally, it raises some interesting questions about the functions and necessity of affectional bonding in humans.

In the 1950s and 1960s Harry Harlow conducted some pioneer research with monkeys which shed some light on the development of affectional bonds. Through a series of experiments, Harlow found that monkeys have very basic affectional needs that are met through maternal caretaking in infancy and through complex social interactions with other animals during adulthood (Harlow and Harlow, 1965). He showed that monkeys raised without mothers, with cloth or wire mothers, with unfriendly mothers, and so on developed into neurotic adults with distorted affectional and sexual responses.

Harlow discovered the importance of affection to monkeys by depriving them of it. Obviously, it would not be ethical to conduct similar studies with humans. But some researchers, notably Spitz (1946) and Bowlby (1960), have contributed to our knowledge of the need for affection in humans by studying children raised in foundling homes, orphanages, and prison nurseries. Because the quality and quantity of maternal care was low in these settings, children raised in them are said to have suffered from ***maternal deprivation.*** Even though physical care was adequate for most of these children, the researchers found them to be impaired by the lack of mothering. There were particularly dire effects if the child had lost its mother after a strong relationship had developed. Sometimes the child would go into a life-threatening syndrome that Spitz called ***anaclitic*** (loss of love) ***depression.***

The main conclusion from these kinds of studies is that from birth humans have a basic need for affection that, if not met, can affect later development in important ways. Parents are now encouraged to hold, stroke, fondle, and breast-feed their infants much more than parents of earlier generations were. However, older children also tend to be deprived of affectional interaction in our society. We rarely touch children, and we teach them early and firmly not to touch each other or themselves. In effect, we forbid the tactile behaviors that children need if they are to grow up with adequately functioning affectional systems. Masters and Johnson (1974) suggest that this early deprivation does indeed result in an inability to relate to adult sexual encounters on an appropriate sensual level. The possibility exists that humans, deprived of early and appropriate affectional interactions, respond in a manner similar to that of Harlow's monkeys by showing disturbances in their adult affectional and sexual responsiveness.

*From attachment
to deeper
relationships*

How does attachment between two people develop? How does a relationship deepen to the levels of more intense involvement? In reviewing the available research in this area, George Levinger (1980) found that there had been few studies directed toward understanding the development of closeness among dating couples. On the basis of his own research and the work of others, he was able to arrive at a few insights about the development of closeness:

1   *Over a 6-month period, approximately 60 percent of attached pairs became closer, while the rest stayed the same or deteriorated.*
2   *Couples who were unequally involved at the beginning of the relationship were less likely to proceed to a deeper relationship.*
3   *There was no single route that couples took in developing their relationships.*
4   *The amount of involvement at the beginning of the relationship was the best predictor of later involvement. (p. 522)*

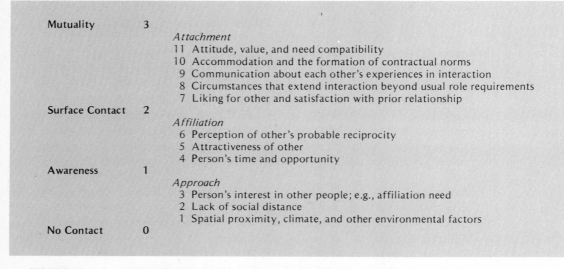

Mutuality	3	
		Attachment
		11 Attitude, value, and need compatibility
		10 Accommodation and the formation of contractual norms
		9 Communication about each other's experiences in interaction
		8 Circumstances that extend interaction beyond usual role requirements
		7 Liking for other and satisfaction with prior relationship
Surface Contact	2	
		Affiliation
		6 Perception of other's probable reciprocity
		5 Attractiveness of other
		4 Person's time and opportunity
Awareness	1	
		Approach
		3 Person's interest in other people; e.g., affiliation need
		2 Lack of social distance
		1 Spatial proximity, climate, and other environmental factors
No Contact	0	

FIGURE 10.1
Levels of relatedness in ascending order of depth. (Based on Levinger and Snoek, 1972)

To emphasize the dynamic, changing nature of relationships, Levinger developed a model of how relationships develop, deepen, or deteriorate. Figure 10.1 shows how couples might move from initial attraction through various stages of interaction to different outcomes. This model is just one possible approach, however. Psychologists still have a long way to go in explaining the process by which relationships develop.

LOVE

At some point in the continuum of mutual involvement between two people, they may describe themselves as being "in love." Love is a very special state about which much has been written and little is known. Psychologists have tended to ignore it as a topic of study until recently.[1] The investigator who wishes to study love is in a difficult position—that of trying to study a highly individualistic, indescribable feeling state that is probably the most important thing that can happen to a person. A few researchers have focused on the physiological correlates of this emotion (see Box 10.1), but such studies fail to explain the whys of love—why we fall in love with one person and not another, why some people fall in love quickly and others fall slowly, why some love is obsessive and some quiet, and so on. Despite the problems that love poses for researchers, it occupies too important a place in human sexual behavior to simply ignore. So in this section we will try to summarize some of the research that has provided a few insights into what we call love.

[1]Two important recent contributions to our understanding of love are Dorothy Tennov's *Love and Limerence* (1979), describing her research on passionate love, and Nathaniel Branden's *The Psychology of Romantic Love* (1980), which relates love to self-esteem.

Liking versus loving

In pursuing the elusive concept of love, we may start by trying to distinguish it from other positive interpersonal feelings. For the social psychologist, positive feelings toward another person that are reasonably stable over time are referred to as *liking*. Zick Rubin (1970) felt that the differences between liking and loving could be studied directly and would contribute to our understanding of love. As the result of some preliminary research, Rubin developed two scales: a Liking Scale and a Loving Scale. The Liking Scale contains statements that reflect respect, confidence, perceived similarity, and favorable evaluations. The Loving Scale contains statements that reflect feelings of absorption, attachment, affiliation, dependency, and a predisposition to help. These two scales have been used in several studies both to validate the difference and to further explore the relationship between liking and loving (Rubin, 1975). One interesting finding is that people have only slightly stronger liking for lovers than for friends but a great deal more loving for lovers than for friends.

Stages in the development of love

Is there a natural sequence of events in the progression toward love after a relationship begins? Levinger and Snoek (1972) were interested in this question as part of their study of the development of relationships. They hypothesized that there are natural stages in the deepening of relationships. Figure 10.2

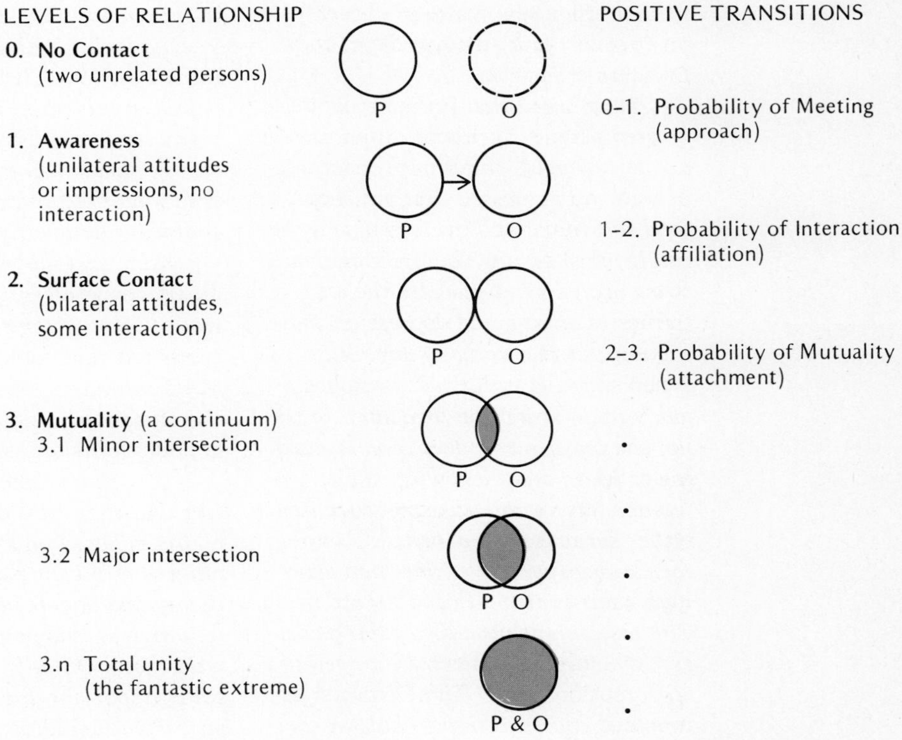
LEVELS OF RELATIONSHIP
0. No Contact (two unrelated persons)
P
O
1. Awareness (unilateral attitudes or impressions, no interaction)
P
O
2. Surface Contact (bilateral attitudes, some interaction)
P
O
3. Mutuality (a continuum)
3.1 Minor intersection
P
O
3.2 Major intersection
P
O
3.n Total unity (the fantastic extreme)
P & O
POSITIVE TRANSITIONS
0–1. Probability of Meeting (approach)
1–2. Probability of Interaction (affiliation)
2–3. Probability of Mutuality (attachment)

FIGURE 10.2 Stages in the deepening of a relationship. (Levinger and Snoek, 1972)

BOX 10.1

The
chemistry
of love

Scientists have known for awhile that body chemistry can influence the experience of love. Experiments have shown, for example, that people with increased epinephrine in their body may label the accompanying sensations as "love," given the right circumstances. But is the opposite true—can love affect body chemistry?

According to New York City psychoanalysts Donald F. Klein and Michael K. Liebowitz, it can for at least some people. They have identified a condition they call hysteroid dysphoria, in which the person experiences wide mood swings as a result of variations in production of a "love chemical." Klein and Liebowitz, of the New York State Psychiatric Institute, observed this condition in several patients, mostly women, they saw while in clinical practice at the Institutes' Depression Evaluation Service.

They noted that unlike most depressed people, hysteroid dysphorics do not lose weight, suffer from insomnia, or wake up depressed. Rather, they tend to overeat and oversleep, and they can be cheered up. The main characteristics of this syndrome are the extremes of elation and depression that accompany the woman's love life. When she falls in love, she reaches a giddy high; when the love affair breaks up, she crashes to a deep low. According to Klein and Liebowitz, such women have a roller coaster love life either because they choose the wrong men or because they drive men away with their continual need for attention. The researchers described their patients as "love junkies" in constant need of an "emotional fix." These women use romance and attention to bolster their

self-esteem and to provide energy, but they are extremely sensitive to rejection.

Most psychoanalysts would approach women with this problem by having them talk it out in therapy. But Klein and Liebowitz went beyond psychotherapy to try to find a biochemical cause that could be treated with drugs. They suggested that when a person is in love, the brain emits an amphetamine-like chemical, phenylethylamine, that helps create the giddy feeling or euphoria of being in love. But when a person is rejected or the love affair ends, the brain stops producing this chemical, and the subsequent crash in mood is not unlike amphetamine withdrawal. The researchers further suggested that hysteroid dysphorics are individuals in whom the control mechanism for release of phenylethylamine is genetically or otherwise impaired or unstable. They noted that many hysteroid dysphorics in the withdrawal phase turn to chocolate to help ease their depression—and chocolate contains phenylethylamine.

Klein and Liebowitz found that ordinary mood-elevating drugs did not work with their hysteroid dysphoric patients but that some responded well to MAO inhibitors—antidepressant drugs that apparently inhibit the breakdown of phenylethylamine.

These researchers emphasize the fact that their idea of hysteroid dysphoria is based on a very small sampling of clinical cases and that their theory and conclusions are still quite tentative at this point. Nevertheless, writer Jane O'Reilly (1980) has raised some important questions about their approach, including:

To what extent can this condition be seen as an extreme extension of traits that have been culturally rewarded in women?

Is the drug therapy designed more to help the therapist than the patient by removing the more disturbing symptoms?

If a patient has a history of oral dependence (the researchers said many hysteroid dysphorics had histories of alcohol and drug abuse as well as overeating), is it wise to offer an oral drug?

Could hypersensitivity to rejection be accounted for to some extent by aspects of the sexual revolution (such as confusing sex with love)?

Thus, although the idea of a love chemical is intriguing, it is still a long way from being substantiated, and its possible implications are yet to be explored.

presents their model of this sequence. Using P to indicate the Person and O to indicate the Other, Levinger and Snoek postulated three levels of interaction: unilateral awareness of the other, surface contact, and mutuality. The increasing overlap of the P and the O indicates the increasing degree of interaction. Movement along the sequence may differ from one relationship to another. Relationships could move through the stages in order; they could stop at a particular stage and stay there; or they could dissolve completely at any stage. Within each of the major stages are substages representing finer degrees of movement.

Level 1—awareness—is the stage of potential approach. For Joanne, the attraction in the bookstore provided awareness and proximity. Suppose she approached the man and, after talking books for a few minutes, asked him if he would like to join her for coffee. Similar attraction and affiliation needs in the man might cause him to move the relationship to the next level of surface contact by accepting the invitation. At this stage of superficial contact and interaction, the pair would be able to test their initial perceptions of each other. The coffee date would provide the opportunity to explore their potential mutuality. This would put them in a level 2 relationship. At this point, the pair could stop and go their separate ways or move on to the next level, depending on what each found in the other. If they were to move on to a level 3 relationship, we would see the beginnings of attachment. It is in level 3 that interdependence begins to develop. Issues of trust, accommodating to the needs of the other, self-revelation, and the forming of a sense of unity are central at this stage. The couple begins to speak in terms of "we" and "us" rather than "I" and "me." It is this sense of unity that we associate with people in a deep relationship.

In understanding this model proposed by Levinger and Snoek, it might be useful for you to think about one of your own deep relationships and how it moved along the dimensions they have outlined. You may realize from your own experience how very complex relationships are in their development. Even if you feel that you fell in love rather suddenly, closer inspection might reveal that there were indeed several levels to your relationship. The development of openness, trust, and sensitivity to one another's needs usually takes time and requires at least some approximation to the stages Levinger and Snoek have described.

One interesting aspect of the relationship sequence is how one's perceptions of the other change with each level. At the initial stage, physical qualities are dominant. Joanne's attraction to the stranger's eyes is consistent with level 1 interaction. For a couple at level 2, different qualities become important. Here Joanne might find the man's similar views on politics and current events to be appealing. At level 3, Joanne might say that her partner's most attractive qualities are his openness, honesty, and intuitive knowledge of her. At this point, she probably would not mention his eyes (or even other parts of his anatomy that she may have come to know).

*Love
and sex*

Sexual intercourse can occur without emotional involvement, and love can be maintained without sexual intercourse. Given these facts, how important is love in determining human sexual behavior? In Chap. 1, we quoted Ingrid Bengis as saying that "sex deepened love and love deepened sex." Most of us would agree with her appraisal. We *feel* that emotional involvement has extraordinary importance for sexual behavior. Is there any basis for this feeling that love and sex are so important to each other?

The social sciences have provided few answers to this question. However, if nothing else, the widespread belief in the importance of this connection has served as a self-fulfilling prophecy; that is, it has created the conditions under which there is true enhancement of the total experience. Our own view, expressed throughout this book, is that sexual behavior can only be understood as an expression of the whole person, including the person's emotions, intellect, and body. Love as a concept includes the idea of a totality, and although it may continue to present difficulties in our attempts to study it, the topic can never be dismissed as unimportant. It is, in fact, at the core of our understanding of sexual behavior.

*Types
of love*

In the study of any phenomenon, science often begins by recognizing the variations of that phenomenon and attempting to classify them. Love has not been excluded from this process, and the result has been some interesting attempts at classifying love into various types.

Passionate versus companionate love Frequently love is divided into two types: **passionate** and **companionate**. According to Walster and Walster (1978), passionate love encompasses extremes of feeling, such as elation, anxiety, relief, altruism, possessiveness, and jealousy. (Jealousy is an elusive emotion to study; see Box 10.2.) Companionate love, on the other hand, is far less emotional. It is typified by affection and attachment, with little in the way of extreme feelings. Companionate love sounds a lot like our earlier description of liking. Walster and Walster point out that there is only a slight difference in depth between liking and companionate love. They note that people experiencing companionate love have difficulty deciding whether they are in love or "in like." For those who experience passionate love, there is little doubt about the emotion they are feeling.

BOX 10.2

Love and jealousy

What is jealousy? One particularly telling description of this often elusive emotion was offered by Judith Viorst in her book Yes Married *(1972): "No matter how perfect—or practically perfect —a wife may be, she always has to watch out for the Other Woman. The Other Woman, according to my definition, is anyone able to charm my husband, amuse my husband, attract my husband, or occupy his wholehearted interest for more than 30 seconds straight."*

Jealousy is a feeling of hurt and anxiety that accompanies real or imagined involvement of one's partner with someone else. What produces such jealous feelings? Fear of being abandoned? A blow to one's self-esteem? A threat against one's keeping a piece of "personal property"? A feeling of battered pride? Social psychologists are interested in determining what jealousy is and what causes it. They are also interested in discovering who is most likely to get jealous, how people respond to jealousy, and whether there are sex differences in jealous behavior.

One of the problems psychologists encounter when trying to study jealousy is in designing appropriate research. It is difficult—and some would say unethical—to try to induce jealousy in an experimental setting. It is also difficult to go into the field and look for jealous people to observe. As a result, most studies have been based on questionnaires designed specifically to get at people's experiences with jealousy and their attitudes toward that emotion. Although much of current jealousy research has been based on such questionnaires, it must be kept in mind that self-reports are subject to a

certain amount of unreliability; that is, people may deny that they are jealous for various reasons, or they may respond in a way they think they are supposed to respond rather than record their true feelings.

Nevertheless, self-reports continue to be our main source of information on jealousy. Elliot Aronson and Ayala Pines designed the Sexual Jealousy Inventory, which contains 200 questions covering many aspects of this emotion, and they have been administering this inventory to various individuals since 1979. Gregory White has conducted extensive research on jealousy through the use of a 35-page Relationships Questionnaire that he initially administered to 150 couples. He has been able to correlate the answers to questions about jealousy with answers to questions about numerous other personality traits, attitudes, and behaviors. A third approach was developed by Robert Bringle, who constructed a 20-item Self-Report Jealousy Scale to examine the role of jealousy in social, family, and work situations.

Although all these researchers have used only small samples to date, they have drawn a few tentative conclusions based on their findings thus far. They are in general agreement, for example, on the type of people who tend to be jealous. The Aronson-Pines and White research both indicate that jealous people tend to feel insecure in their relationships and to have a negative self-image or low self-esteem. In White's study, for example, people who responded that their self-esteem depended greatly on what their partners thought of them usually scored high on inventory items indicating jealousy

(Adams, 1980a). On the other hand, people who scored low on jealousy items tended to agree with statements such as "I find that I am pretty happy with myself regardless of what my partner thinks." Apparently, people who feel inadequate live in constant fear that someone will come along whom the partner will like better.

Aronson and Pines have also identified some other characteristics of the jealous person. They suggest, for example, that jealous people are basically unhappy; that is, those who say they are dissatisfied with their lives are most likely to be prone to jealousy. The researchers have also found that people who cheat on their partners are likely to be jealous—perhaps because they suspect their partner of doing the same thing they are. It has also been found that people who have been in relationships a short time are more likely to be jealous than those who have been with their partners 9 or more years.

Are there sex differences in jealousy? None of the researchers found any significant differences in propensity to jealousy; that is, contrary to popular belief, women are not more jealous than men. However, research has shown some differences in how men and women experience and respond to jealousy. Aronson and Pines found that women scored higher than men in the intensity of jealousy they would feel if their partner had an affair. Women also indicated they suffered more from the pangs of jealousy, with such physical reactions as nausea and headaches and such emotional reactions as humiliation and confusion. Clanton and Smith (1977) had earlier pointed out that jealous men are more likely to react with

rage and violence, followed by despondency, whereas women are more likely to accept their jealousy and blame themselves for their partner's behavior. Jeff Bryson (1977) has suggested that both men and women respond to jealousy either by trying to protect their own egos (attack the partner, try to get even) or by trying to improve the relationship (talk it out, win back the partner through self-improvement).

The main sex difference in jealousy seems to be in behavior following the precipitating incident. It seems that women who have suffered jealousy tend to make every effort to patch things up, whereas men are more likely to give up on the relationship and start looking for a new partner. This conclusion is borne out by recent experimental findings and by Kinsey's 30-year-old research, which showed that more than 50 percent of divorced men gave infidelity of their partner as the major cause of their marriage breakup, whereas only 27 percent of divorced women cited such a reason.

Another sex difference that White explored was in the proclivity to induce jealousy in one's partner. He found that women are much more likely than men to try to make their partner jealous. Methods used to produce jealousy included talking about an attractive person, flirting with another, dating someone else, and fabricating another partner. Why do people want to make their partner jealous? Most commonly, men and women want to see whether their partner still cares. Many want to get the partner to pay more attention to them. And some act out of anger or a desire to punish the partner.

Once psychologists have learned

more about jealousy, will they be able to provide guidelines for eliminating this negative emotion? Aronson and Pines doubt it. "America is a paired, family-oriented society. It is a society that emphasizes ownership and private property. It is characterized by competition and by a strong desire to have a perfect relationship. All these aspects of contemporary American society tend to aggravate the feeling and expression of jealousy" (quoted in Adams, 1980a, p. 106).

According to these researchers, then, jealousy is likely in our society. Nevertheless, there are things that individuals can do to deal with their jealous feelings. Walster and Walster (1978) have summarized psychologists' basic advice to those trying to control their jealousy: (1) Try to find out exactly what is making you jealous—try to pinpoint the exact situations that create jealous feelings. Make an effort to understand what you feel in these situations and why you feel that way. (2) Try to put your jealous feelings in perspective. Determine which elements are irrational (are you being unreasonable or childish?) and which are rational (you're justified in being unhappy if he spends three nights a week with another woman). (3) Negotiate a "contract." Work with your partner to achieve a balance between security and freedom in your relationship, and lay down some ground rules regarding interactions with other people.

Styles of loving Another classification scheme involves a more detailed typology in which the loving style is the defining feature. To arrive at this typology, Lee (1974) studied love as it is depicted historically in literature and interviewed lovers in Canada, England, and the United States. Lee suggested that people's loving styles are important determinants of what happens in a relationship and that the high failure rate of love relationships is a result of stylistic differences between the partners, creating incompatibility in the relationship.

Lee's six basic styles of loving are:

1. **Eros**—the love of beauty. The erotic lover is attracted to the physical appearance of the loved one. He or she may experience sudden attractions, "chemical" reactions, and extreme physiological arousal in the presence of the love object. Erotic lovers, more than any other type, are likely to experience love at first sight. They are also likely to want to introduce sex early in the relationship. There is a tendency for erotic love to flame and then die when the initial attraction wears off.

2. **Ludis**—playful love. To the ludic lover, the "game" of love involves various maneuvers to win the lover. Emotional attachments are less important than skillful manipulation to win "prizes." The so-called Don Juan syndrome would be an example of the ludic style. In today's context, individuals who are more concerned with "scoring" than with deep relationships would be classified as ludic lovers.

3. **Storge** (stor-gay)—peaceful love. Storgic love is quiet and affectionate. This love grows slowly, almost imperceptibly, with time. The storgic lover

may not notice at what point friendship turns to love. This is the kind of love that might develop in a couple who have known each other for a long time, perhaps since childhood. In societies where marriages are arranged between strangers, love is expected to grow slowly over the years after the marriage ceremony. In our society, where romantic, intense involvements are the ideal, this practical, slow-growing love is often given lower status. An advantage of this style, as Lee points out, is that "there is a lack of ecstasy but also a lack of despair."

4. *Mania*—obsessive love. This is a favorite style in Western literature. The manic lover scales the heights of joy only to be plunged to the depths of despair. Manic lovers are completely involved with the attention and affection of the loved one, as if nothing else exists. As you can imagine, these are difficult lovers to relate to. Their perception of a slight from their lover is the occasion for tragic overresponse. They are likely to be possessive and jealous, and they can be insatiable in their need for affection. The result is that they are unhappy most of the time, despite brief periods of elation.

5. *Pragma*—practical love. Pragmatic lovers look for partners who fit a mental list of requirements. Once they have made a match, emotional love may grow as the relationship develops. For this reason, there is a strong storgic component in pragmatic love.

6. *Agape* (ah-ga-pay)—altruistic love. This type of love involves always giving and never asking anything in return. Not surprisingly, Lee found few such unselfish lovers in his survey.

Lee found that people may also have mixed styles of loving. The most common combinations were storgic-erotic, ludic-erotic, and storgic-ludic.

There are other typologies in the psychological literature but none as detailed as Lee's. Reiss (1967), for example, mentioned four types, (1) romantic, (2) romantic-rational, (3) sexual-romantic, and (4) combined. The overlap with Lee's types can easily be seen.

The value of such systems is that they point out that there are different needs and approaches in deep relationships. When two people have different styles, the fact that they love each other may not help them develop or maintain a deep relationship if their styles clash. For example, it would seem that an erotic lover trying to relate to a pragmatic lover would be doomed to failure. What such systems do not stress enough is the adaptability of people's behavior. Most people are more flexible than such typologies suggest and can modify their behavior to the styles and needs of others. Thus, relationships are in reality changing, dynamic, mutual experiences rather than the match or clash of highly stylized, predetermined patterns. In fact, most psychologists would consider such inflexibility to be maladaptive. We would argue that the ideal is not to find the person who has a style of loving perfectly matched to one's own but rather to help people change, grow, and develop flexibility so that eventually they can exist in a give-and-take arrangement with another person. This is the basis of a truly satisfying relationship.

When a relationship is maintained and deepened, it is likely to do so because it has met the deeper psychological needs of the individuals involved. While these needs may vary from person to person, a few seem to be basic to most people: the desire for security, the yearning to be understood, the need to have someone take care of one, the desire for excitement, and the need for sex (Walster and Walster, 1978).

If love is to survive the initial levels of attraction and proceed to deeper levels, it will probably be by satisfying several such needs in both partners. Joanne may get excited by eyes across a room, but if she is to go past a first encounter and superficial dating, the relationship will have to satisfy more basic psychological needs.

For every joyful song about falling in love there are several blues numbers about the loss of love. Most people who have gone through the breaking-up process describe it as being among the most disruptive experiences of their lives.

Love relationships are difficult to establish, requiring as they do the adaptation of two people to each other's needs. And they are even more difficult to maintain over long periods of time. The result is that love affairs often do break up, with much pain for both people concerned.

Why do loving couples break up? One reason is that people change as a part of adult development, which may mean that they will outgrow their relationships. Habituation to one's partner is another factor. In this case the loss of novelty and excitement and the resulting boredom are what kills the relationship. A third reason is that people's role demands change as they move through the various stages of their lives. Partners whose roles mesh well at one stage may not have complementary roles at a later stage.

One of the few direct investigations of the breaking up of relationships was conducted by Hill, Rubin, and Peplau (1976). Of the 231 couples they had followed in their study of dating, 103 had split up by the end of the 2-year period. The researchers studied this group further to see whether they could shed some light on the factors that contribute to the ending of relationships. Hill and his associates found that the less intimate and less attached couples were more likely to break up. Using the Rubin scales, they learned that a high love score was a better predictor of staying together than a high liking score. Interestingly, having sexual intercourse and living together did not correlate with the continuation of the relationships. Thus, the common assumption that such behaviors contribute to the success of a relationship was not supported by this research.

Equality of involvement was found to be another important factor. Of those couples who rated themselves as equally involved, only 23 percent had broken up. Of those couples in which there were clear imbalances in the degree of involvement, 53 percent had broken up.

The similarity of the partners was also correlated with the breakup statistics. The more similar a couple was in age, scholastic aptitude test scores, educational goals, and physical attractiveness, the less likely they were to break up. This finding supports our earlier discussion of the importance of similarity in forming and maintaining relationships.

Hill and his associates also studied the circumstances surrounding a couple's breaking up. They found that the most likely time for college couples to break up was at the beginning of the school year, during vacation period, and at the end of the year. It is at these times that partners are more likely to be separated from each other and to meet new partners. Furthermore, it is easier to call it quits at these times because the partners can attribute the breakup to having to be apart rather than being forced to look at the failings of the relationship.

Breaking up is not the only way that love affairs end. If we think of a love affair as passionate love, then another way for it to end is to evolve into some other kind of relationship. Walster and Walster (1978) note that as passion dies it may be replaced by companionate love. They cite the work of Cimbalo, Faling, and Mousaw (1976), who measured the change in a couple's scores on the Rubin Love Scale over the years of marriage. They found that the longer a couple had been married, the lower they scored (see Table 10.1).

TABLE 10.1	Years married	Passionate love score
The relationship of passionate love scores to number of years of marriage	0–3	98.40
	4–6	88.90
	7–9	85.20
	10–17	84.04

Source: Cimbalo, Faling, and Mousaw (1976), pp. 1292–1294.

Breaking up may be appropriate for some couples, but the evolution into companionate love may be appropriate for others. While we do not hear many popular songs about evolving into companionate love, this may in fact be the most common pattern of all.

Finally, we should note that many relationships end without an actual breakup. Both in and out of marriage, couples may continue a relationship long after all feelings of love have gone. This seems the saddest development of them all.

SUMMARY

1 Researchers have found that the most important factor in *attraction*—why people like each other—is physical attributes. Physically attractive people are imbued with a variety of positive traits by sole virtue of their appearance.

2 Although *sexual releasers*—stimuli that elicit instinctual chains of behavior—are important in the attraction process in other animals, their role in human behavior is unclear.

3 A second major factor in attraction is proximity—the closer people are physically, the more likely they are to like each other. A related factor is

familiarity, in that the more exposure people have to each other, the more likely they are to like each other.

4   A third fundamental factor in attraction is similarity. The more people have in common, the more likely it is that they will form a relationship. Whether or not the relationship continues may depend on the couple's complementarity—the matching of one person's strengths, weaknesses, and needs with the other's in a way that achieves a balanced relationship.

5   Another factor in attraction is a person's ability to *reinforce* or *reward* the other. According to Aronson's *gain-loss theory*, people are most attracted to those who give them *increasing* rewards over time.

6   A related concept is *reciprocity*—people tend to like those who like them. Researchers have found that this principle even holds true for supposedly "hard-to-get" women—a man likes a woman who is hard to get only if she is aloof to other men but responds positively to him.

7   The terms *courtship* and *dating* are applied to that period between initial attraction and more permanent bonding when a couple are trying to get to know one another better. Reiss has suggested that in the United States couples go through a sequence of dating stages: *casual dating*, in which there is little commitment; *regular dating*, in which the couple are more involved but may still date others; *steady dating*, in which there is strong commitment but other alliances may still occur; and *exclusive dating*, which may take the form of engagement or living together.

8   Most studies of dating have focused on college students. On campus the traditional, formal approach to dating of the fifties has given way to a more informal pattern for providing men and women with the opportunities to get to know potential sexual partners.

9   One script of traditional dating that appears to be weakening is the idea that the male must try to get his date into bed and the female must hold back, trading her sexual favors for promises of commitment.

10   Individuals who suffer from shyness have particular difficulty in developing relationships, and those who date are considerably anxious and self-conscious.

11   Studies with primates and with infants suffering from *maternal deprivation* lend credence to the idea that humans have a basic need for affection and for strong attachments to other human beings. One of the functions of dating and courtship is to foster such attachments in couples.

12   Love is a difficult topic for research. Rubin was able to develop scales that measure the degree of liking and loving in dating couples and in friends. Levinger and Snoek hypothesized a series of stages by which couples fall in love: from awareness of the other, to surface contact, to mutuality.

13   Some researchers have classified love into various types. Walster and Walster distinguished between *passionate love* and *companionate love.* Lee identified six styles of loving: (1) *eros* (love of beauty); (2) *ludis* (playful love); (3) *storge* (peaceful love); (4) *mania* (obsessive love); (5) *pragma* (practical love); and (6) *agape* (altruistic love). The point of these various classifications is that people have different needs and approaches in deep relationships. For love to survive, each partner must fulfill many of the other's basic needs and must be flexible in adapting to the other's style.

14   Relationships break up when people outgrow each other, become

bored with each other, change roles, or find other partners they consider more suitable to their needs. Passionate love relationships may also end when they turn into companionate relationships.

**ADDITIONAL
READING**

Cook, Martin, and Wilson, Glenn (Eds.). *Love and Attraction.* New York: Pergamon Press, 1979.

Proceedings of the International Conference on Love and Attraction. The book has many well-written articles on a variety of topics in this area.

* **Peele, Stanton, and Brodsky, Archie.** *Love and Addiction.* New York: Taplinger, 1975.

An interesting view of how, for some people, love for another person can be much like an addiction.

Walster, Elaine, and Walster, William. *A New Look at Love.* Reading, MA: Addison-Wesley, 1978.

An excellent book on passionate and companionate love. Spans the range from research findings to practical advice. Well written and fun to read.

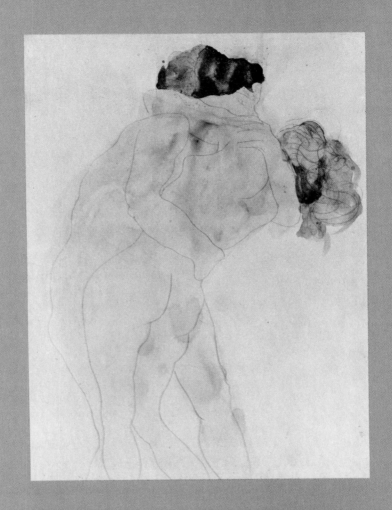

Sexual arousal
and sexual acts

11

chapter
11

We all tend to have high expectations of our sexual encounters, whether they be with a partner after many years of intimacy or as a result of a "one-night stand." On an ideal level, we may visualize sexual actions as beautiful and moving experiences that can cement relationships and provide the fullest range of emotional commitment and satisfaction. And, at the very least, we expect sex to be fun and enjoyable and to provide physical release. In many instances, however, our sexual experiences may not live up to such expectations, and we feel somehow let down. Such letdowns occur simply because sexual experiences are not automatically fulfilling. Good sexual experiences take knowledge and practice—two elements not easily found in our society. However, sexual experiences can become positive and extremely satisfying if we do have the necessary knowledge and, most important, if we can become aware of our partner's desires and pleasures through the opening of mutual avenues of communication.

It is not surprising that there are numerous books that attempt to educate us about sexual acts and behaviors. Some of these books, like *The Joy of Sex* (Comfort, 1972), provide a pictorial guide to sexual positions and expressions, while others, like *The Sensuous Woman* (J, 1969), concentrate on techniques of sexual arousal. Such books can be invaluable both to the sexually inexperienced who do not wish to fumble through their first sexual encounter and to the sexually experienced who wish to inject some variety into their sexual activities.

For the most part, however, people in our society receive very little information about sexual arousal and sexual acts prior to their first experiences with these activities. Parents are often reluctant to teach their children about such things, and sex education classes in school tend to be concerned with reproduction and contraception rather than with sexual techniques. In fact, the teaching of such techniques is seen as encouraging sexual experimentation and thus has generally been suppressed. As a result, young people often get most of their information about the nature of sexual contact from their peers or from their own initial experiences with sex. Unfortunately, these early experiences, whether good or bad, may serve as models for all subsequent sexual encounters.

Ignorance of sexual arousal and activity sometimes has profound consequences. In the early part of this century, for example, it was not uncommon for women to consider sex as something to be endured as part of their marriage vows—a view that severely affected their sexual responsiveness. We would like to think that such attitudes are rare today, but that may not be the case. In the early 1970s, Shere Hite (1976) set out to discover how women viewed their own sexuality. She first developed an elaborate questionnaire about sexual behavior and then distributed it to women all over the country. As the answers came back, it became clear that while many of the respondents were enthusiastic about their sex lives, others thought sex was boring, unpleasant, or just not for them. Here are a few of the statements from women who found their sex lives unsatisfactory or unfulfilling:

> *I have been divorced one and a half years and in that time, I haven't had much sex. At this point in my life it's just not really important and I can't find men that turn me on enough to want to have sexual relations with them anyway. Sex plays a very small part in my life and I really don't seem to miss it. (p. 360)*

> *I used to have desires for sex but never reached the heights of passion I desired. A mental block formed somewhere during the last few years and I just gave up. (p. 361)*

On the other hand, here are some statements from women who enjoyed sex:

> *My husband is the best lover I ever had and I hope we have sex till we're a hundred and ten years old . . . (p. 141)*

> *Sex is beautiful because such a complete contact with another person makes me feel my being is not solely confined to my own body. It is one of the most direct ways to get beyond the barriers between "them" and "me." (p. 299)*

> *Sex is a form of communication without words based on bodily responses, and is the ultimate in human closeness where a person can express and understand more than the mind can conceive of. It brings me closer in spirit to others in ten minutes than I can get in ten years to people I do not share sex with. (p. 300)*

One should keep in mind the sampling biases that exist in this informal kind of survey, of course. Although Hite sent out over 100,000 questionnaires, she received only 3,000 replies. Of these, 37 percent of the replies came from readers of *Oui* magazine; approximately another third came from women in the women's movement; and the remaining third came from readers of the *Village Voice*. It is likely that the sexual attitudes of these women differ from the attitudes of all women in the United States. Nonetheless, even with this bias, it is clear that for some women sex is not a particularly fulfilling experience.

How do we account for the fact that some find sex objectionable while others find it rewarding? Some of the dissatisfaction undoubtedly comes from ignorance and misinformation. But it is also a result of poor communication. A couple's pattern of sexual interaction is established early in their relationship, and whether or not the pattern produces enjoyment for both partners, it may persist throughout their relationship. This is particularly true when partners fail to communicate. Thus, two individuals may be conjoined in the act of sexual intercourse but, because of insensitivity or ignorance, may be far away from each other emotionally. The keys to enjoyable and fulfilling sexual experiences are thus *knowledge* about the particulars of sexual intimacy, *communication* between partners during sex, and *practice* of sexual techniques.

Before proceeding with our discussion of sexual interaction, we should point out that sexual activities need not be stereotyped into a single script, that is, intercourse. In reality, there is no single universally used sex act.

Rather, individuals have a wide variety of choices in their sexual encounters. As a result, we will use the phrase *sexual acts* in recognition of the fact that sexual interactions may take many different forms.

Prior to 1966, little was known about the physiological responses that occur during sexual acts. Most of the research effort was directed toward studying sexual behavior in animals or gathering data on sexual attitudes and practices through the use of questionnaires. The direct study of various sex acts was considered taboo, and even Alfred Kinsey, who merely reported on verbal statements about people's sexual attitudes and practices, was subjected to a great deal of persecution.

In 1966, however, the situation changed dramatically with the publication of William Masters and Virginia Johnson's *Human Sexual Response* (1966), a book on their research of behavioral and physiological changes associated with sexual arousal and orgasm. This book, which had a profound impact on the whole field of sexology, contains data on 382 women and 312 men observed in approximately 10,000 occurrences of sexual intercourse.

In 1954 Masters began his ground-breaking work in human sexual behavior by interviewing male and female prostitutes. They provided extensive information on techniques for maintaining and increasing sexual arousal. Masters also established a laboratory for observing and recording sexual behavior. Rooms in the lab were equipped with one-way windows and with a variety of recording instruments. An electrocardiograph (EKG) machine was used to measure changes in heart rate during sexual intercourse; an electromyograph (EMG) machine measured changes in muscular contractions in various parts of the body during intercourse; and a pH meter monitored the acidity of the vagina.

Masters decided not to rely on prostitutes in his physiological research, as the "normalcy" of their sexual arousal and responsiveness was questionable, and many also had pelvic disorders (typically chronic pelvic congestion from repeated arousal without orgasm) that might affect his results. Instead, Masters recruited subjects from the medical school and university community by placing local advertisements, putting up bulletin-board notices, and using word of mouth. Subjects were initially screened through detailed interviews, and those with emotional problems were excluded.

Despite the care that Masters and his research assistant Virginia Johnson used in selecting their subjects, their sample was still not representative of all sexually mature people (see Chap. 3 for a discussion of sampling procedures). Essentially, Masters and Johnson used a subset of people who were willing to engage in sexual activity while being monitored by machines and observers. Clearly, this is not a typical characteristic of all sexually mature people. The issue, then, is the extent to which the sexual response of these subjects is representative of the larger population, which includes many people who would not engage in sex under these circumstances.

The researchers have tried to minimize this problem by suggesting that the processes they were studying are so basic as to be the same in all people. Indeed, this point of view is readily accepted in the study of heart function, digestion, or kidney function, where the basic mechanism of action seems to be the same in all healthy individuals. Whether or not this is a compelling argument for behavioral sex research is still being debated.

Whatever the case, as the result of their research Masters and Johnson divided the **human sexual response** into four stages: (1) **excitement**, (2) **plateau**, (3) **orgasm**, and (4) **resolution**. These stages should not be considered as distinct divisions but rather as phases that gradually unfold from one to the next along a continuum.

Masters and Johnson have described the differences between these four stages in terms of two major physiological processes: **vasocongestion**, or the buildup of blood and fluid in particular areas of the body, and **myotonia**, or muscle contractions. Both of these processes change dramatically in the course of the sexual response cycle.

*Excitement
stage*

The excitement stage usually begins with physical contact or exposure to erotic visual stimulation. A kiss, a caress, a touching of hands, a view of erotic art may be sufficient to trigger sexual excitement. Even books, fantasies, or sexy clothes may initiate excitement. The stimulation must continue, however, if the excitement stage is to become fully developed. The quality of the stimulation is also important. If the stimulation is suitable to the individual, the intensity of sexual excitement accelerates quickly. But if the stimulation is sporadic or somewhat objectionable, the excitement may be drawn out or even extinguished. The excitement stage and the resolution stage consume the greatest portions of time during the sexual response cycle.

Excitement in males   During the excitement phase, the penis becomes erect as the result of blood engorgement (vasocongestion) of the corpus spongiosum and the corpora cavernosa (Fig. 11.1). Erection can occur through direct stimulation of the penis by hand or mouth; by stimulation of other body parts, such as the neck, lips, or inner thighs; or by erotic thoughts.

Although penile erection is the primary manifestation of the excitement stage in men, other changes also occur. Heart rate and blood pressure begin to increase. The nipples may become erect, and the skin of the upper body may start to redden and flush. Men tend to become excited more rapidly than women and often move from the excitement stage to the plateau stage faster than women.

Excitement in females   A number of changes occur in women during the excitement stage of the human sexual response. First, the vaginal barrel becomes lubricated. This lubrication begins within 10–30 seconds of the onset of sexual arousal and can be attributed to a vasocongestive reaction in the walls of the vagina. As fluid builds up in the arteries of the vaginal wall, it flows through the mucosa (a semipermeable membrane) and appears on the vaginal surface. These glistening drops, which adhere to the surface, give the vaginal barrel the appearance of sweating. The presence of this lubrication does not necessarily signal that the woman is ready for penile penetration, however.

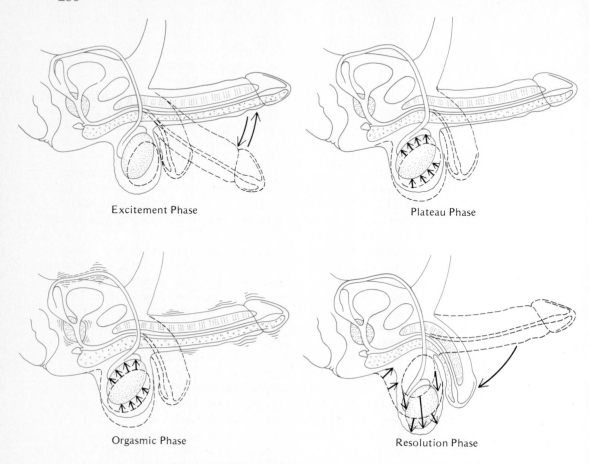

Excitement Phase

Plateau Phase

Orgasmic Phase

Resolution Phase

FIGURE 11.1
Stages in the erection of the penis. Excitement phase —penis becomes erect. Plateau phase—testes increase in size and move closer to the body. Cowper's gland fluid appears at the tip of the penis. Orgasmic phase—penile contractions and expulsion of semen occur. Resolution phase—penis gradually becomes flaccid.

As the excitement stage continues, the shaft of the clitoris thickens, and the head of the clitoris enlarges. The outer lips flatten to expose the inner lips, which swell and spread apart. The inner two-thirds of the vaginal canal involuntarily expand, creating a ballooning effect, while the cervix and uterus are drawn up into the body, producing a tenting effect in the immediate area (Fig. 11.2). This tenting response enlarges the opening in the cervix, facilitating the passage of sperm into the uterus. Overall, the space within the vagina increases considerably, not only in length (ballooning from 8–9 centimeters to 11–12 centimeters) but also in width (tenting from 3–4 centimeters to 6–7 centimeters). The color of the vaginal wall changes from purplish-red to dark purple as the vasocongestive and expanding processes of the vagina continue.

Other signs of heightened arousal are also present during this first phase. The woman's nipples become erect as a result of muscular contraction (myoto-

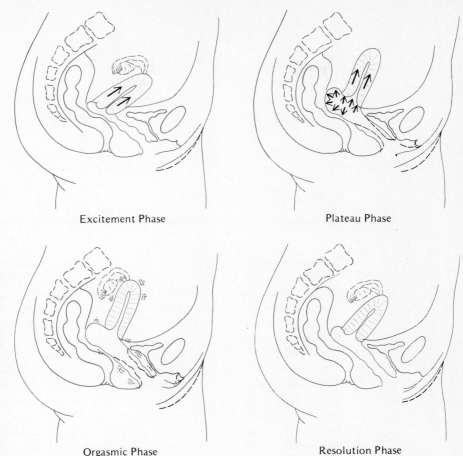

FIGURE 11.2 Changes in the sex organs of the female during sexual arousal. Excitement phase—major and minor lips increase in size; vaginal barrel lengthens. Plateau phase—beginning of the orgasmic platform with full vaginal expansion. Orgasmic phase—uterine, vaginal, and clitoral contractions occur. Resolution phase—reduction in vasocongestion.

Excitement Phase

Plateau Phase

Orgasmic Phase

Resolution Phase

nia) of the area surrounding them. This nipple erection may be obscured, however, by a vasocongestive reaction in the breasts, causing them to swell and enlarge (Fig. 11.3). Women also characteristically experience an increase in blood pressure and heart rate during this stage.

Plateau stage

During the plateau stage there is a continuation of both vasocongestive reactions and muscular contractions. If effective stimulation is maintained, sexual tensions will intensify to the point of orgasm. If stimulation is not adequate, sexual tension will decline, and the individual will enter a prolonged resolution stage. The duration of the plateau phase varies as a function of both the quality of the stimulation and the individual's desire to achieve increasing levels of sexual tension.

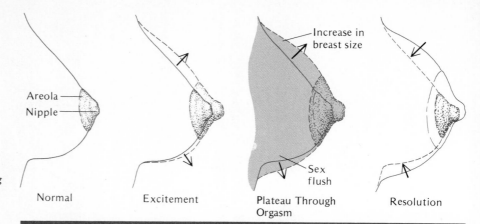

Areola
Nipple

Increase in breast size

Sex flush

Normal   Excitement   Plateau Through Orgasm   Resolution

Plateau in males   During the plateau stage, vasocongestive reactions reach a peak. The coronal ridge of the penis swells and expands. The testes become sufficiently blood-engorged that they appear to be 50 percent larger, and they are drawn up close to the body, a response predictive of impending ejaculation.

The man may or may not develop a **sex flush**. The flush arises from the stomach area and spreads over the chest and into the neck and face. It may also appear on the thighs, shoulders, and forearms. When fully developed, the sex flush resembles a measleslike rash. Masters and Johnson noted that the sex flush appeared in 25 percent of all acts of intercourse and that it was not associated with particular men or situations. Although the flush may develop during the excitement phase, it more commonly arises after the plateau stage has been reached. The flush reaches its full development during the plateau and disappears rapidly during the resolution phase. It initially fades from the shoulder and thigh areas, then from the chest and stomach region, and finally from the head and face. During the plateau stage heart rate and blood pressure continue to increase.

Plateau in females   One of the major events of the plateau stage in women is the development of the **orgasmic platform**: a swelling and thickening of the tissues surrounding the outer third of the vagina. As a result of this swelling, the vaginal barrel acts to grip the penis. Vaginal lubrication, which reached peak production in the excitement stage, now declines somewhat.

Surprisingly, the clitoris retracts at this point and is shielded from direct stimulation. The clitoris appears to withdraw within the body because the shaft becomes 50 percent shorter, and the head of the clitoris, the glans, becomes tucked into or hooded by the folds of the clitoris (Fig. 11.4). However, the retracted clitoris can continue to be stimulated by pressure on the labial folds or even by pressure on the mons pubis region.

Although the female sex flush may develop during the late part of the excitement stage, it more commonly occurs in the plateau stage. The flush

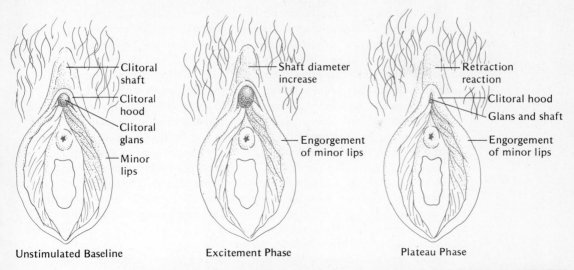

Clitoral shaft
Clitoral hood
Clitoral glans
Minor lips

Unstimulated Baseline

Shaft diameter increase
Engorgement of minor lips

Excitement Phase

Retraction reaction
Clitoral hood
Glans and shaft
Engorgement of minor lips

Plateau Phase

FIGURE 11.4
Changes in the shape and position of the clitoris during sexual arousal.

begins on the abdomen, spreads rapidly over the breasts from the upper to the undersurface areas, then moves to the shoulders, back, thighs, neck, and face. The extent of the measleslike rash seems to be related to the strength of the impending orgasmic experience. After orgasm, the flush disappears rapidly in the reverse order in which it developed. Masters and Johnson noted the appearance of a sex flush in 75 percent of all women some of the time. However, their figure may be slightly higher than one might expect to find in the general population, because a sex flush may be more typical of sexually experienced women with a prior history of orgasmic responding.

During the last part of the plateau stage, the inner lips are transformed from a bright red to a deep wine color in multiparous (one or more children) women or from a pink to a bright red color in nulliparous (no children) women. This change indicates that orgasm is imminent. Heart rate and blood pressure continue to increase during this stage.

Orgasmic stage

Orgasm consists of a short but intensely and explosively pleasurable period when the sexual tension produced by vasocongestion and muscular contraction is released. The source or subjective focus of the pleasure resides in the pelvic region. In males, it is concentrated in the penis, the prostate, the seminal vesicles, and occasionally the testes. In females, the focus of sensation seems to be concentrated in the clitoris, vagina, and uterus. Female orgasmic response is much more variable in both intensity and duration than the male response.

Orgasm in males   Male orgasm consists of a series of rhythmic penile contractions, initially occurring about 0.8 seconds apart, that serve to forcibly expel semen. After the first three or four major contractions, minor contractions continue for several seconds, but they are less intense, and the interval between them becomes longer.

Ejaculation, subjectively and physiologically, occurs in two phases. During the first phase, **emission,** the vas deferens, seminal vesicles, and prostate contract and force the semen into the base of the urethra. This creates the sensation of "coming" or "ejaculatory inevitability," and, indeed, the process cannot be stopped at this point. During the second phase, **expulsion,** the urethral bulb and the penis contract, expelling the semen with great force.

The man also undergoes a sharp increase in heart rate, blood pressure, and breathing rate, which subside fairly quickly. In addition, other male structures may undergo muscular contraction: The face may be distorted into a grimace, and the muscles of the arms, back, legs, feet, or hands may become rigid.

Orgasm in females   The female also experiences a series of rhythmic contractions at about 0.8-second intervals during orgasm. The number of contractions seems to be related to the intensity of the response. A mild orgasm may contain only 3 or 4 contractions, while an intense orgasm may involve 12 or more contractions. These contractions are usually felt in the vagina but may be generalized to the entire genital region.

It has generally been assumed that women experience orgasm but not ejaculation. Recent evidence, however, indicates that some women may actually expel a clear fluid through the urethra at orgasm (Belzer, 1981; Sevely and Bennett, 1978). This fluid is not urine and may come from a system of glands and ducts that surround the female urethra (Addiego et al., 1981). Women who do experience some form of ejaculation tend to have stronger pubococcygeal muscle contractions and stronger uterine contractions than nonejaculators.

It can sometimes be difficult for a woman to determine whether she has had an orgasm. Unlike men, whose production of semen is a visible sign of orgasm, most women do not have tangible evidence for this experience. Some women probably mistake a spreading feeling of warmth for orgasm. But orgasm is more than a pleasant feeling. Once a woman has experienced orgasm, she is unlikely to fail to recognize it on subsequent occasions. But the woman who has never experienced orgasm may have difficulty identifying exactly what it is. It is for this reason that many sex therapists recommend that women clients attempt to learn about the sensations of orgasm through masturbation.

Prior to the work of Masters and Johnson, female orgasm was thought to be of two types: clitoral and vaginal. This distinction was first developed by Sigmund Freud, who argued that clitoral orgasm resulted from stimulation of the clitoris and was therefore an infantile form of sexual response. He believed that mature sexual response was developed only when the woman could achieve orgasm through vaginal stimulation, presumably by the penis. Masters and Johnson have clearly demonstrated that this is a mistaken view of the female sexual response, however. They have noted that all orgasms are physiologically the same. In most instances orgasm develops from clitoral stimulation, either directly or through thrusting motions of the penis that exert enough pressure to pull on the inner lips, thereby pulling on the hood and stimulating the clitoris. Although it is possible for a woman to reach orgasm through stimulation of the breasts or even through fantasizing, stimulation of the vagina alone does not appear to produce orgasm. For most women to experience orgasm through penile thrusting, then, enough indirect stimulation of the clitoris must occur. For some women, direct clitoral contact is necessary for orgasm.

Today considerable attention is being focused on the female orgasm. Some of this attention has created pressure on women to have orgasms and on men to ensure that their female partners have them. The general dictum seems to be that women should have orgasms with every sexual encounter and that failure to have such orgasms is a reflection on their own femininity or on their partner's ability. As a result, some woman may be put into the position of "faking" orgasms. Such faking creates deception in the relationship, which may have negative consequences. It might be better to recognize that not all women will, or necessarily want to, have orgasms with every sexual act. Furthermore, if a woman wants to experience orgasm and feels she is not getting the appropriate kind or amount of stimulation, the best way for her to deal with the situation is to communicate her desires to her partner. This solution would seem preferable to faking the experience and then dealing with any ensuing frustration. Despite the attention that female orgasm has received, it is up to each individual woman to determine her orgasmic needs and not be swayed by popular opinion or partner pressure. This should also be true for men.

*Resolution
stage*

During the resolution stage, the body returns to its previous, unaroused state. Through a reversal of the arousal process, tension is gradually lost. Thus, from the peak of orgasm, individuals move back to plateau-stage levels of tension, then to the levels of tension characteristic of the excitement stage, and finally to the unstimulated stage. As a result, the resolution stage may last a considerable length of time.

Resolution in males One of the most obvious changes in the male during this final stage is the loss of erection, which occurs in two phases. First, it is lost as a result of the emptying of blood from the corpora cavernosa. Second, the enlarged penis returns to its unaroused size when fluid is drained from the corpus spongiosum.

At the same time, other physiological processes are returning to normal. The sex flush, if present, disappears, and heart rate, blood pressure, and breathing rate return to normal levels. Perspiration may appear on the body, particularly on the palms of the hands and the soles of the feet.

Men enter a ***refractory period*** following orgasm. During this period they are not responsive to sexual stimulation and cannot become sexually excited. In fact, attempts to produce arousal may lead to unpleasant sensations. Stimulation of the penis, for example, may be mildly painful. The length of the refractory period varies considerably (from 20 minutes to 24 hours) and is dramatically affected by age. Although teenagers may be capable of reaching a subsequent orgasm within a short period of time, young men may need a few hours before orgasm can be experienced again, and the older men grow, the longer the refractory period becomes. Men typically are not capable of multiple orgasms, that is, repeated orgasms within a short period of time, although there are some rare exceptions (Robbins and Jensen, 1978).

Resolution in females Following orgasm, women experience changes that are consistent with a decline in sexual tension. The breasts decrease in size, and, as a result, the nipples now appear erect. The sex flush, if present, fades, and blood pressure, heart rate, and breathing rate return to normal. The orgasmic platform relaxes and shrinks as the vasocongestive response fades. The ballooning and tenting responses of the vagina deteriorate, and both the vagina and uterus return to their original size and shape. Body perspiration, especially

*FIGURE 11.5
Changes in the
sexual arousal of
men and women
during the sexual
response cycle.
Some women may
show repeated
orgasms within a
short period of
time, as evidenced
by the multiple
peaks. (Masters
and Johnson, 1966)*

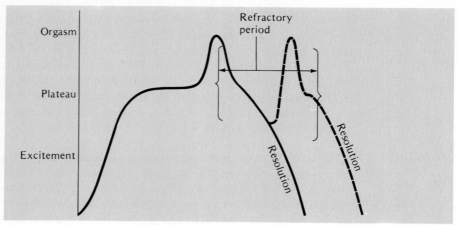

Male sexual response cycle

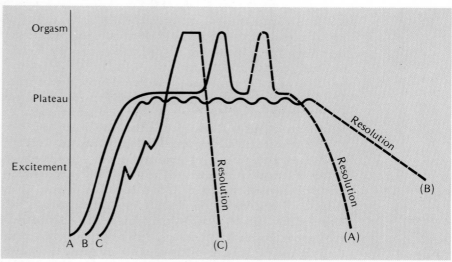

Female sexual response cycles

on the palms and soles, may be evident. The resolution stage generally lasts 15–30 minutes but may be longer, around 60 minutes, in women who have not reached orgasm during the response cycle.

In contrast to men, many women do not seem to have a refractory period but rather can be physiologically rearoused and can reach orgasm again within minutes of the first orgasm. In fact, it may be easier to reach orgasm the second time around, depending on the decline of sexual tension. If the tension has declined to plateau stage levels, rearousal may produce a second orgasm very quickly. If the tension has returned to excitement stage levels, more time may be required to reach a second orgasm.

The number of orgasms that may occur in a short period of time seems to be limited only by the woman's endurance and continued desire. With hand stimulation of the clitoris, some women may have from 5 to 20 orgasms in a single session. With a vibrator, the number of continuing orgasms can be numerous. Many women, however, are content with a single orgasmic experience, as additional orgasms may vary considerably in quality.

In summarizing Masters and Johnson's description of the human sexual response, we can see that sexual tension begins early in the excitement stage, builds to a peak in the plateau stage, is released dramatically during the orgasmic stage, and declines slowly during the resolution stage. We can also see that the sexual responses of men and women are quite similar. There is, for example, little difference between men and women in their reports of orgasm (Vance and Wagner, 1976). The primary differences between men and women arise during the excitement and resolution stages. During the excitement stage, men may become aroused more rapidly than women, while in the resolution phase, women do not enter a refractory period as men do and are thus capable of having multiple orgasms (Fig. 11.5).

SEXUAL INTERACTION

Now that we have examined the physiology of sexual acts, let us look more closely at the specifics of sexual arousal and then explore the most common types of sexual acts.

Sexual arousal and foreplay

Sexual arousal is an essential part of any sexual act. It develops through the interaction between partners prior to sexual climax. Such interaction is referred to as *foreplay*, or sex play. Although foreplay is an intensely personal experience that differs widely from one couple to another, research has uncovered a few general principles, which will be discussed in this section. According to the anonymous author of *The Sensuous Woman* (1969), the three most important ingredients of foreplay are (1) a good imagination, (2) sensitivity to the partner's needs and desires, and (3) willingness to experiment with new procedures or positions.

Typical problems with foreplay Given that men become sexually aroused more quickly than women, it is not surprising that both men and women may have to make adjustments to each other in order to enhance their experiences during sexual arousal. In the absence of such adjustments, men may be described by women as selfish—as satisfying their own needs and ignoring the needs of their partner. A man may not adequately prepare his partner for intercourse and may be too rough during penile penetration. In addition, some women indicate that men seem to be too inhibited verbally during intercourse. A man may maintain the "strong, silent approach" throughout the sexual encounter and may seem unable to let go during orgasm and express his reactions (DeMartino, 1970).

On the other hand, men argue that many women expect too much, that they expect the man to be something he is not. Such women seem to assume that men are quite experienced sexually and will automatically be aware of their needs. Furthermore, such women seem to make little effort to help when they feel their needs are not being satisfied. They may not tell the man when he makes a wrong move, mentally characterizing him as inept instead. Nor do they reward the man when he does provide pleasure (Hamilton, 1971).

Clearly these complaints do not necessarily apply to all or even many sexual relationships. But when they do, it is an indication of a lack of effective communication. As we have mentioned before, sex is not automatically wonderful. However, open lines of communication, both verbal and nonverbal, between the partners can go a long way toward achieving satisfying sex.

Touch and the erogenous zones   Touch is an important element in sexual arousal and foreplay. Not only are there various ways to stroke and caress the body, but there are a number of highly sensitive areas that, when stimulated, produce sexual excitement. These highly sensitive areas, which contain many nerve endings, are called **erogenous zones.**

The typical erogenous zones include the genitals, anus, breasts, lips, neck, ears, and inner thighs. But parts of the back, buttocks, palms, and feet can become erogenous zones through association with the sex act. For example, if light stroking of the inner arm becomes a frequent prelude to sex, the inner arm can be conditioned as an erogenous zone. After repeated pairings of this stroking of the inner arm with sexual intercourse, the mere caressing of the inner arm will come to induce sexual arousal if conditions are favorable. In addition, certain kinds of *fetishes* (sexual arousal by specific objects) can develop through this kind of conditioned association.

Although the kinds of touches and caresses that can enhance sexual arousal vary greatly from individual to individual, a few generalizations can be made on the basis of reports from many men and women.

Initial sexual excitement is usually brought about by a light, feathery stroke rather than by heavy pressure or squeezing (Eichenlaub, 1961; Masters and Johnson, 1966). In addition, it is usually more arousing if the initial stroking encompasses many or all of the erogenous zones and then becomes focused more specifically on the genitals as foreplay continues. Some women like to have the visible unclothed parts of their body stimulated first (neck, lips, ears, palms, and so on), then the breasts and inner thighs, followed by the genitals, while other women have different preferences. Because there is no set rule for the order in which erogenous zones should be stimulated, partners need to communicate their individual preferences.

After the initial period of sexual excitement, further arousal is produced by alternating between light, fingertip strokes and more intense palmar pressure. One must be particularly careful about sharp fingernails, which may irritate delicate tissues, and about too much palmar pressure, which may become painful. Each person should attend to the reactions of his or her partner to determine whether the stroking is having the desired effect.

Another stimulating tactile maneuver has been termed *advance and retreat* (Eichenlaub, 1961). Stimulation of an erogenous area, usually the breasts or genitals, is begun and then withdrawn in a seductive manner. Stimulation begins anew, reaches higher levels, and is withdrawn again. The art to this maneuver is timing. One must know when to retreat without frustrating the partner and how long to continue the advance and retreat until optimal sexual tension is reached. The advance-and-retreat method should ultimately be replaced by more directed stroking as foreplay continues.

Each of the various erogenous zones may respond to particular kinds of tactile contact. The lips, an important erogenous zone, are stimulated through kissing. Kisses may involve hard or soft pressure, depending on individual preferences, and the lips of the couple often move with each other in a circular or pulsing pattern. Initial kissing often leads to **French kissing**, also called deep kissing or tongue kissing, in which the lips are separated and the tongue darts back and forth into the mouth of the partner. French kissing is usually mutual; the partners move their tongues in and out of each other's mouth, now touching each other's tongue, now not, gyrating and swirling back and forth.

The neck and ears are also stimulated by kissing. The neck may be particularly sensitive to nibbles and light kissing. The ears respond to feathery kisses and to the tracing of the tongue along the rim of the outer ear and into the center of the ear. The same sensation can often be achieved using a fingertip stroke.

The breasts are an important erogenous zone for women. In some women, stimulation of the entire breast is pleasurable, while for others sexual excitation occurs primarily through stimulation of the nipples. Stimulation may commence with a light stroking of the entire breast, which should be accompanied by brief movements across the surface of the nipple. Stroking progresses to a gentle massaging of the breasts, interspersed with touching and rolling the nipple between the thumb and forefinger. Many women find it pleasurable to have their breasts kissed and their nipples sucked.

The nipples are also an erogenous zone in men. Men's nipples become erect when mild pressure is applied to them with thumb and forefinger. Besides tactile contact, kissing and sucking of nipples may enhance sexual excitement in men.

The genitals are perhaps the most sensitive erogenous zone. Tactile and oral contact in the genital areas can have a profound effect on sexual arousal. Because the genital structures of men and women are somewhat different, we shall consider them separately.

The major sensual center in women is the clitoris. Nevertheless, continuous direct stimulation of the head of the clitoris is usually unpleasant or painful. Instead, stroking should be directed to the shaft or glans of the clitoris. As sexual excitement peaks and the clitoris retracts, the partner may lose contact with the clitoris altogether. Fortunately, pressure applied to the mons pubis can maintain the sexual excitement. Important to clitoral stimulation is rhythmicity. For some women, this rhythm is provided by penile thrusts, which act to indirectly stimulate the clitoris and mons pubis. For other women, the rhythm can more readily be maintained through continued finger stroking. The clitoris can also be stroked by the tongue of the partner. Such contact is usually more gentle than that provided by fingers and has the added advantage of providing lubrication. In addition to clitoral stimulation, women may find vaginal stimulation by means of repeated finger insertions pleasant. Tactile contact of the anus may also be used to heighten sexual excitement, especially at orgasm.

The primary center of sexual sensations in men is the penis. The preferable tactile stimulation is for the partner to grasp the penis and then rhythmically move her hand up and down the shaft. The underside of the penis is particularly sensitive to pressure of this type. Intermittent contact with the glans and corona of the penis during this rhythmic activity also heightens and enhances sexual excitement. The penis can also be orally stimulated. The partner takes the penis into her mouth and moves her lips rhythmically up and down the penile shaft. She may also use her tongue to dart and swirl across the glans and coronal ridge. In addition to penile stimulation, light stroking of the scrotum and stimulation of the anus may be pleasurable for the man.

Other factors important to sexual arousal Besides touching and kissing, there are a number of other factors that may play a role in enhancing sexual arousal. For example, many women indicate that being talked to during sexual interaction is very important to them (Hamilton, 1971). Loving, endearing terms and expressions of delight in the woman's body can increase sexual excitement. Vulgar language may stimulate some women. Men, too, appreciate words of endearment, but they especially respond to comments about their bodies. Attention to and praise of the penis may alleviate any doubts a man may have about his sexual attractiveness.

Another factor that may affect sexual arousal is general grooming. Slovenliness in manner and dress seems to turn off most people. We are not suggesting that everyone should have just stepped out of the shower before having sex, but it is considered appropriate for people to pay a modicum of attention to the neatness and cleanliness of their bodies.

Another factor that is especially important to women is the amount of time spent in foreplay. In general, the longer the foreplay, the greater the likelihood that a woman will reach orgasm. Gebhard (1966) noted that only 40 percent of women nearly always reached orgasm if foreplay lasted 1–10 minutes. That percentage increased to 50 percent when foreplay lasted 15–20 minutes and could be extended to 60 percent when foreplay lasted more than

20 minutes. From the woman's point of view, then, the more foreplay the better. Gebhard (1966) also noted that the tendency to achieve orgasm was correlated with the duration of penile thrusting, or **intromission** Only 25 percent of women nearly always reached orgasm when intromission was less than a minute in length; 50 percent nearly always reached orgasm if intromission lasted 1–11 minutes; and the percentage rose to 65 percent when intromission was longer than 11 minutes. The time spent in foreplay and intromission, then, can greatly affect the woman's response.

Variations in approach and setting are further considerations in enhancing sexual arousal. Nothing can dull one's sex life more quickly than sexual routines. Sexual activities can become mechanical if they always occur in the same place, at the same time, in the same way. Both partners should strive to find new ways of arousing each other and to engage in sexual interaction when the desire is present, even if it is not the "usual" time of day for the couple. An interlude in a motel, in the woods, in the shower, or even in the back seat of a car can also do much to spice up a couple's sex life.

Before going on to examine particular sex acts, we should say something about the tempo of sexual arousal. We have already noted that men tend to become aroused more quickly than women. As a result, men may have to pace themselves during the initial phases of intercourse. Women can contribute to this pacing by engaging in "delaying tactics." Instead of throwing off all her clothes and jumping immediately into bed, for example, a woman could seductively take off her clothes or allow them to be removed a little at a time. This, of course, is but one of the delaying tactics that can be used to adjust the tempo.

*Types
of sexual
acts*

Human beings in many eras and many cultures have come up with every imaginable way of performing sexual acts. Sex may be conducted through genital-genital contact, oral-genital contact, or anal-genital contact. Partners may assume postures ranging from face-to-face to head-to-toe. Men and women may take turns in the "on top" position. This great variation in sexual patterns is nearly unique to the human species, as most animal sexual behavior follows rigid, unvarying patterns. This human "blessing" deserves to be fully explored by couples who wish to enrich their sex lives and avoid monotony.

Genital-genital sex   The most common type of sexual behavior between heterosexual partners is genital-genital contact, that is, the insertion of the penis into the vagina during the act of sexual intercourse. This is essentially all that happens in the sex act. But humans have raised this basic act to an art by varying the way they conduct it. Genital-genital sex can be achieved through several different physical positions. There are four primary positions from which all other positions are derived: (1) the man-on-top, male superior, or missionary position; (2) the woman-on-top or female superior position; (3) the rear-entry position; and (4) the side-to-side position.

For a number of decades, the most common genital-genital sexual position in Western culture was the **man-on-top** or male superior position. Kinsey noted that 70 percent of his sample used the man-on-top position regularly and even

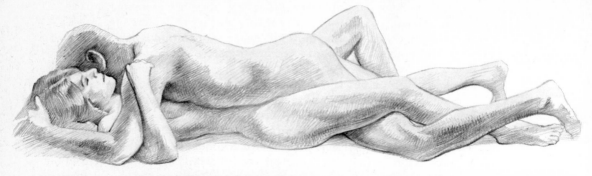

FIGURE 11.6

*The man-on-top
position of sexual
intercourse.*

exclusively. It was not necessarily the most common position among other peoples of the world, however (Ford and Beach, 1951). Because sexual knowledge has increased in the last decade or so, people of Western society now seem to exhibit more variety in their choice of sexual positions than they did at the time of Kinsey's research (Hunt, 1974). An even more recent survey of sexual preferences (Kahn, 1981) indicates that *both* men and women may prefer the woman-on-top to the man-on-top position. Note that Kahn measured sexual preferences and *not* sexual behavior. What people prefer may actually differ from what they do in practice.

As the name indicates, the man puts his body on top of the woman, resting his weight both on his arms, which are placed at her side, and on his legs, which are placed between her legs. The woman may straighten her legs next to the man's legs, may keep her knees flexed, may wrap her legs around the man's waist, or may hook her legs over his shoulders (Fig. 11.6).

The man-on-top position is particularly useful for conception, as deep penetration can be obtained and there is little leakage of semen from the vagina. Many people also find this position appealing because it involves face-to-face contact. However, this position is not satisfactory if the woman is in an advanced stage of pregnancy or if either partner is considerably overweight. Furthermore, this position is not recommended for men who experience premature ejaculation, as control may be more difficult in this situation.

The second most common position in Western culture was the **woman-on-top** or female superior position (Kinsey and Gebhard, 1953). Today, it may be the preferred position of both men and women (Kahn, 1981). This position may be accomplished by the woman straddling the man, inserting his penis into her vagina, and then sitting or lying on the man. In an interesting variant, the couple may start off with the man on top and then roll over (carefully). Most commonly, the woman orients her body so that face-to-face contact occurs (Fig. 11.7). In another variation, however, the woman faces the opposite direction, that is, a head-to-toe arrangement.

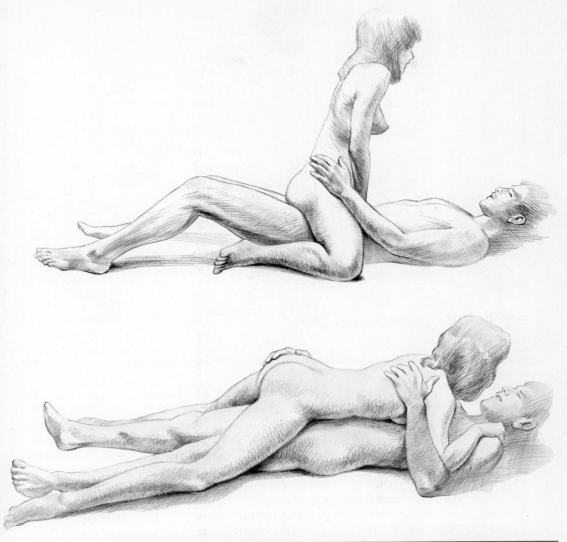

FIGURE 11.7
The woman-on-top
positions of sexual
intercourse.

The woman-on-top position is particularly useful for female orgasm, as the woman can control the extent and rhythmicity of the stimulation. In addition, the man's hands are free to caress the woman's body. This position is used for several types of sexual problems (see Chap. 15) and is often preferred during pregnancy. It is also the position of choice if the man is tired or needs to restrict movement due to health problems, as the woman assumes most of the responsibility for movement.

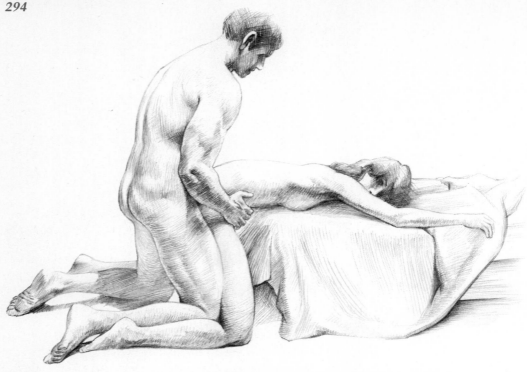

FIGURE 11.8
*The rear-entry po-
sition of sexual in-
tercourse.*

When using the **rear-entry position**, the man faces the woman's back. The woman may be kneeling or may be on all fours while the man enters her vagina from behind (Fig. 11.8). Because of the postural similarity to the way animals conduct intercourse, it is not surprising that the rear-entry position has also been called the *dog position*. The major disadvantage of this position is that face-to-face contact is eliminated. On the other hand, the man's hands are free to stimulate the clitoris and breasts of his partner. This position is often preferred during pregnancy.

In the **side-to-side position**, the man and woman face each other while lying on their sides. The man may place his legs between the woman's thighs or may have one leg between her thighs and one leg outside (Fig. 11.9). Because full penetration is often difficult to attain in this circumstance, this position is suitable for women in advanced stages of pregnancy. The side-to-side orientation usually leads to leisurely, prolonged intercourse.

An almost unlimited variety of other sexual positions can be derived from any of the four basic ones. The couple may vary their posture by standing or sitting rather than lying down. Slight variations of angles or limbs can change the sensation dramatically. In addition, different props or settings may be used. The couple may try the floor or a table instead of the bed, or they may have intercourse in a swimming pool or bathtub. The actual number of sexual

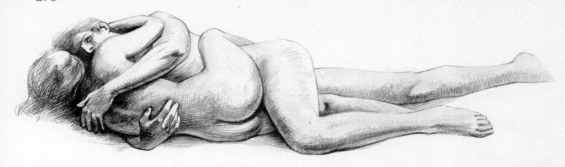

FIGURE 11.9
*The side-to-side
position of sexual
intercourse.*

positions and variations of settings appears to be limited only by the imaginations of the individuals involved.

Oral-genital sex One of the most significant changes in sexual awareness during the last decade has been the increased popularity of oral-genital or mouth-genital sex (Hunt, 1974). In Kahn's report on sexual preferences, both men and women rated oral-genital sex in which they were the receiver as their most preferred sexual activity (Kahn, 1981). There are two types of oral-genital stimulation, depending on the sex of the person whose genitals are being stimulated. These two types are called *cunnilingus* and *fellatio*.

Cunnilingus (Fig. 11.10) is stimulation of the woman's genitals by the partner's mouth. Most of this stimulation is directed to the clitoris. Cunnilingus usually involves a gentle sucking of the clitoris and inner lips, along with darting tongue strokes applied to the sides of the clitoris. From time to time the tongue may swirl across the sensitive clitoral head. The tongue can also be used to stimulate the opening of the vagina or can be inserted into the vagina directly. Sexual excitement may be heightened by the insertion of a finger into the vagina or anus. However, one should be careful not to follow anal insertion with vaginal insertion because of the possibility of infection.

Cunnilingus is viewed by many women as a highly pleasurable form of sexual intercourse. It provides more direct stimulation of the clitoris than penile thrusting does; it is more gentle than finger stimulation; and it provides lubrication. Some women indicate that they can reach orgasm only through oral-genital techniques. For other women, cunnilingus may produce qualitatively the most sensational orgasms (Hite, 1976).

Some partners may object to performing cunnilingus on the grounds that the genitals are dirty, are unclean, or carry bacteria. The truth is, however, that the vaginal area has fewer bacteria than might be found in the mouth. Thus, kissing may pose more of a health risk than cunnilingus. Negative attitudes about cunnilingus may stem from societal views about the genitals. Children who are taught that the genitals are dirty and not to be touched may carry these attitudes into their adult sexual relationships.

In all instances but one, cunnilingus is a perfectly harmless activity that brings much pleasure to the woman. The only potentially dangerous practice

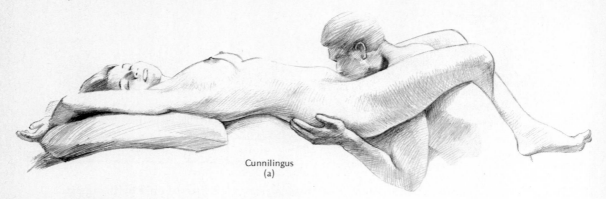

Cunnilingus
(a)

FIGURE 11.10
Oral-genital sex.

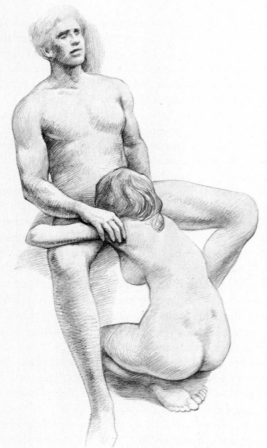

Fellatio
(b)

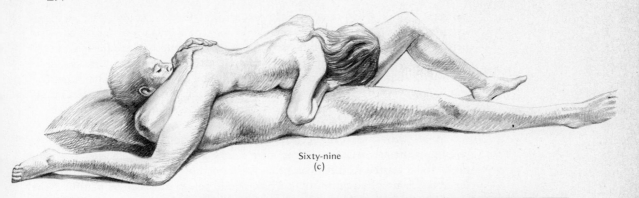

Sixty-nine
(c)

in cunnilingus is the technique of forcibly blowing air into the vagina. While normally harmless to the nonpregnant woman, this practice may force air into the enlarged uterine veins of a pregnant woman, producing an embolism with possibly fatal consequences (Sadock and Sadock, 1976).

Cunnilingus is popular among heterosexual couples, where it may be used in place of penile intercourse or in addition to it. It is even more popular among female-female couples, where it may be performed mutually.

Fellatio is stimulation of the man's penis by the partner's mouth (Fig. 11.10). Most commonly, the penis is taken into the mouth, and the lips move up and down the shaft, with the tongue licking and flicking across the glans and corona. These movements may be interspersed with sucking. As with cunnilingus in women, fellatio is viewed by men as a highly pleasurable experience.

Concerns about the "cleanliness" of the penis bother some people, but this is a moot point since, as we have noted, the mouth is more laden with bacteria than are the genitals. Others are bothered by choking sensations they experience when attempting to take the penis fully into their mouths. Individuals can learn to suppress this gag reflex or they may take only part of the penis into the mouth and stimulate the remaining area with their hands. Finally, some may be bothered about ingesting semen when ejaculation occurs. However, the amount of ejaculate is not very large, and its taste is usually inoffensive. Semen has been described as tasting like cooked egg white, with a salty aftertaste. Furthermore, not all oral-genital stimulation need end with the partner taking semen into the mouth. To dispel two interesting myths of the 1980s, semen is neither a magical health food with healing properties for a wide variety of ailments, nor is it highly fattening.

Fellatio is popular among heterosexual couples, where it is performed as an arousal technique or in place of penile insertion. It is also popular among male-male pairs and may be performed mutually.

The occurrence of fellatio and cunnilingus together is called *sixty-nine* (Fig. 11.10). The name is derived from the physical configuration that the partners assume when they perform mutual oral-genital sex (69). The partners usually lie on their sides. If the man is on top, the woman may feel choked by penile thrusts. If the woman is on top, she may have to balance herself precariously so that she can receive adequate stimulation to the clitoris.

Many couples report thoroughly enjoying the experience of sixty-nine. For some, however, the practice may be too distracting, since they are attempting to simultaneously stimulate and be stimulated. Such couples may prefer to engage in fellatio and cunnilingus sequentially.

Anal-genital sex   **Anal-genital sex** is the insertion of the penis into the rectum of the partner. Anal intercourse can be a pleasurable experience. One needs to be alerted to three potential problems, however. First, the anal sphincter muscles are often quite tight. Thus, penile penetration can be painful if the man does not proceed slowly and carefully. Second, there is a lack of lubrication in the anal area. Thus, a lubricant such as K-Y jelly must be used to facilitate penetration. Finally, the rectum does contain bacteria, so it is important that the penis not be inserted into the vagina after anal intercourse unless a condom is used. In fact, the penis should probably be cleansed directly after anal intercourse.

Anal intercourse is not as common as some of the other patterns of sexual behavior among heterosexual couples, although the incidence is increasing. Anal finger stimulation during genital-genital or oral-genital intercourse is far more typical. Among male homosexual pairs, however, anal intercourse is more frequent (see Chap. 13).

AUTOEROTICISM

An individual's sexual responsiveness is acquired primarily through learning. And a great part of this learning may come from the self-initiated experiences of sensuality through **masturbation**. We have seen that masturbation was viewed extremely negatively in the not-too-distant past. As a result, people were often inhibited in exploring their own sensuality. In recent years, however, our society has moved toward a much more positive view of masturbation. Today, for the most part, masturbation is considered to be a perfectly healthy and normal sexual outlet. In fact, this mode of sexual expression is now used in helping people learn about sexuality and is even used therapeutically for those with sexual dysfunctions.

Masturbation techniques

Learning to be sensual involves more than developing specific masturbation techniques. Setting is also important. The individual might want to be totally relaxed, to play enjoyable music, to recline on a comfortable couch or bed, and to get into the mood for sex. The person might start by gently stroking different parts of his or her body just to identify areas of pleasure. Some people like to rub cream or lotion all over their body. Whatever the case, the goal is to learn more about one's own body through exploration and touch.

Women usually masturbate by stimulating their genitals by hand or with a vibrator. Most women direct this stimulation to the clitoris and inner lips (Fig. 11.11). Direct stimulation of the glans of the clitoris is unusual. Most women rhythmically fingerstroke the side or shaft of the clitoris, occasionally

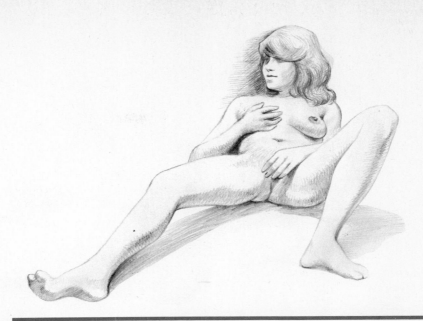

*FIGURE 11.11
Female masturba-
tion technique.*

making direct contact with the glans. In contrast to the stereotyped view that
women insert fingers or other objects into the vagina to achieve orgasm, Hite
(1976) found that only 20 percent of women used vaginal insertion alone to
produce orgasm. Some women use breast stimulation or thigh pressure from
crossed legs as techniques. Indeed, about 2 percent of Kinsey's (1953) female
sample were capable of using fantasy alone to produce orgasm.

Masturbation techniques are generally less variable in men than in
women. The standard technique is to grasp the penile shaft and move the hand
up and down in a rhythmic manner (Fig. 11.12). Both the amount of pressure
and the rate of movement may be increased as orgasm approaches. The stimulation is slowed or stopped at orgasm, since further stimulation is often unpleasant (Masters and Johnson, 1966). At the moment of orgasm, the man may
grip the penis tightly without using any movements (Sadock and Sadock,
1976). Male masturbation is usually accomplished in a short period of time—
on the order of a few minutes (Kinsey et al., 1948).

*Myths about
masturbation*

Masturbation has long been a subject of great concern to people in our
society. Instead of being dealt with in a forthright manner, however, masturbation has been shrouded in a cloak of guilt, shame, ignorance, and superstition.
Thus, it is not surprising that many people have negative attitudes toward
masturbation.

Over the years a number of myths about the evils of masturbation have
surfaced, most of which have absolutely no factual basis. Some of these myths
include the following:

1. *Masturbation occurs only in young people.* This is clearly false. Unmarried men between the ages of 26 and 30 have indicated that masturbation
accounts for 50 percent of their sexual activity (Kinsey, Pomeroy, and Martin,

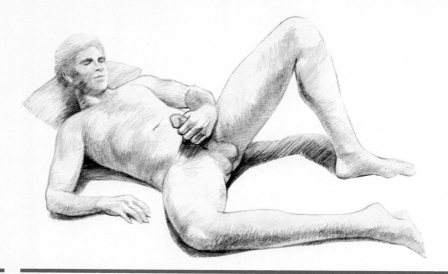

FIGURE 11.12
*Male masturba-
tion technique.*

1948). In women, masturbation rates increase through the thirties, reaching a peak in the forties.

2. *Masturbation leads to sexual frustration.* This is true only if the individual feels guilt or shame about the act. Masturbation can be a satisfactory substitute for sexual intercourse when it is not available, and it can be a sexual enhancer in both men and women who are totally functional and orgasmic. In addition, some women depend on masturbation during or after sexual intercourse in order to reach orgasm.

3. *Masturbation causes physical deterioration or severe fatigue.* There is absolutely no evidence to suggest that any part of the body deteriorates with masturbatory activity. One's eyesight does *not* decline; the penis does *not* become insensitive; warts do *not* appear; and hair does *not* grow on the palms. It is difficult to become sexually fatigued, since the body has its own inherent control system. Men, for example, have a refractory period during which any additional sexual stimulation is unpleasant. Once the body is sated by orgasm, further sexual activity is unlikely to occur.

4. *Masturbation produces asocial tendencies.* Although masturbation is a solitary event, there is no evidence to suggest that masturbation causes an individual to become withdrawn or removed from social contact. Most men and women seem to prefer social sexual activity to masturbation (Kinsey et al., 1948) and indicate that the sensations produced by intercourse are superior to those produced by masturbation.

Thus, masturbation is not an unhealthy, infantile, or shameful practice. Perfectly normal people masturbate regularly as a healthy sexual outlet. In cases where masturbation becomes excessive (as in disturbed schizophrenic patients), the masturbation is a result of the disorder, *not* the cause of it (Ellis, 1966). Masturbation may be used as a substitute for intercourse or during intercourse. In addition, when the sexual appetites of partners differ substantially, one partner may use masturbation to satisfy some of the sexual desire not resolved by the partner. Finally, masturbation may be used to learn about the kinds of stimulation each individual likes.

Fantasy

Fantasy refers to thoughts about people, situations, or events that have little or no basis in reality. Fantasy occurs in daydreams and in wanderings of the imagination, and it is also an important part of masturbation and other sexual activities.

In general, men fantasize more than women (Wilson, 1978). Over 72 percent of the men and 50 percent of the women from Kinsey's sample reported that they fantasized most of the time during masturbation. The types of fantasies varied considerably, but there were a few common elements. Common fantasies included having intercourse with a sex symbol (today's representatives might be Robert Redford, John Travolta, or Billy Dee Williams; Farrah Fawcett, Bo Derek, or Diana Ross), experiencing group sex, being forced or forcing someone to engage in sexual intercourse, and engaging in homosexual activity by heterosexuals and vice versa (although this last fantasy was less common).

Male fantasies differ somewhat from female fantasies. Males tend to fantasize situations in which they are strong and aggressive and in which the sex itself is impersonal. Their imagined partner may have a vividly fantasized body but no particular identity. Women, on the other hand, tend to be more romantic in their fantasies or to imagine being forced to have sex (Barclay, 1973; McCauley and Swann, 1978; Shope, 1975). These findings have led people to conclude that men are turned on by erotic, pornographic material, while women need romantic themes to enhance their sexual arousal. Recent work by Julia Heiman (1977) contests this idea. Heiman measured sexual arousal in college students who had listened to romantic or erotic audiotape descriptions of sexual encounters. Both men and women showed significantly higher levels of sexual arousal in response to the erotic tapes. Romantic tapes did not appear to have any enhancing effect on sexual arousal.

Fantasies often occur during sexual acts as well as during masturbation (see Box 11.1). This is especially true for couples in long-term relationships that have become somewhat monotonous. Through fantasy, individuals can introduce variety and novelty.

Female fantasies during sexual encounters have been studied in some detail. In one study of married women, 65 percent reported that they fantasized during sexual intercourse (Hariton, 1973). Not surprisingly, their fantasies were similar to the kinds evoked during masturbation. Fantasies often involved an imaginary lover, being forced to have sex, having sex in different places (woods, beach, and so on), engaging in forbidden acts, and observing oneself during sex. Additional evidence suggests that women who have fantasies may have better sexual relationships than women who do not fantasize (Hariton, 1973). Unfortunately, little is known about male fantasies during intercourse except that they do occur.

BOX 11.1

Sexual fantasies

Almost everyone has sexual fantasies—erotic reveries about making love with imagined or real partners. Such fantasies are most commonly used as a method of arousal during masturbation, but they may also be used to spice up intercourse with one's partner. Are such fantasies during sex healthy, or can they be harmful? Research seems to indicate that they can be both.

Erotic fantasy can enliven and enhance a sexual relationship in many ways. Sexual thoughts are physically arousing in both men and women and can bring almost immediate engorgement of sensitive tissues, making one more responsive to one's real partner. Imagined scenes can also help to release inhibitions or to trigger sexual feelings in a person who feels slightly uncomfortable or tense, perhaps after the stresses of the day. A woman may picture herself being overwhelmed by an aggressive stranger or being romanced by a sexy movie star. A man may conjure images of *Playboy* bunnies or a harem full of sex slaves. These fantasy images may be spontaneous, or one may consciously create them to try to improve his or her sexual experience. Whatever the case, the images and feelings are woven into the real lovemaking and can intensify the sensuality and feelings of closeness with one's partner.

Psychologist John Money feels that fantasy is at its best when it incorporates the real sex partner into the imagined scenario. According to Money, "When two lovers are really engrossed in each other, the fantasy eventually fades. After a while, the couple becomes totally absorbed in skin feelings, sex organ feelings, and motions of the body, and sex becomes a body trip" (Belson, 1980, p. 200).

The hazard of such fantasy is forgetting one's partner altogether. If the imagined scene is dwelled on compulsively, one's partner may become totally blocked out, creating feelings of detachment, distance, and alienation. Some people may become so dependent on certain fantasies that they are unable to become aroused without them. Others may use fantasies to cover up real problems. As psychiatrist Maj-Britt Rosenbaum has pointed out, "If a woman relies solely on her inner world to deal with problems, she defuses some anxiety that could be channeled into solving them" (Belson, 1980, p. 200).

How can one tell whether his or her fantasies are healthful or harmful? Apparently, content is not a good indication. According to Dr. Rosenbaum, "The very same visualization that helps one couple enjoy sex can constrict another. What matters is how and why we fantasize and how we react to it" (p. 153). Thus a better clue to a fantasy's value is how one feels about it. Does it cause anxiety? Is it an obsession? Does it create a feeling of distance from one's partner? If fantasies appear to interfere with a relationship rather than to enhance it, they may be a sign of psychological or interpersonal problems that need to be resolved.

For the most part, however, fantasy should be seen as a positive aspect of sexuality. Sex therapist Shirley Zussman encourages healthy fantasy involving one's partner: "Fantasy is one of the higher levels of human function. People can build bridges and write music because there is something in their heads that is not reality. For many men and women, life may be richer when they enjoy the same creativity during love" (Belson, p. 200).

Young adults are told little about the changes in sexual relationships that occur over time. In fact, most popular romance stories conclude with the couple living "happily ever after"—the assumption being that sexual attraction lasts forever. What is more typical, however, is that long-term sexual relationships have a tendency to become dull and boring. It is up to the couple to actively work against this tendency.

There are several approaches a couple can take to prevent boredom. First, they should be realistic and recognize that boredom is not only possible but, unless actively countered, highly likely. This knowledge will prepare the couple for any adjustments they will have to make.

Second, the couple should be inventive and imaginative. The use of new positions or new settings may greatly enhance excitement. Thus, variety should be built into the sexual relationship.

Third, the couple might examine their expectations. The quality of sexual experience usually varies from one time to the next; yet there is a tendency to expect every sexual encounter to be wonderful. In fact, some individuals may feel let down or may feel they have let their partner down if the sexual tensions are not quite as high as on a previous occasion. Such people would seem to have unrealistically high expectations for sexual behavior and to fail to take into account normal variation in sexual responsiveness.

Finally, boring sexual encounters may signify a more general problem of boredom with each other. In such cases, the relationship may need to be renewed either through increasing the amount of attention paid to each other or through doing more things together. This increase in togetherness may also improve the sexual relationship.

Maintaining sexual interest in long-term relationships also has much to do with communicating, listening, and learning about one's partner. Some people argue that it takes a lifetime to get to know another person. If so, then the dynamic ebb and flow of a long-term relationship must be based not only on sexual attraction but also on getting to know and understand another human being as intimately as one knows oneself.

In a long-term relationship each partner has the opportunity to explore the needs of the other person, to find out what stimulates and arouses the other person, and to develop a strong, intimate bond of sexual sharing and caring. The extent to which these goals are realized depends in part on how the partners communicate with each other about sex. In our society, however, people often find it difficult to engage in "sex talk." Even partners who readily express both complementary and contrasting opinions about a wide variety of controversial subjects may remain mute when it comes to their own sexual pleasure.

The uncomfortable aura that often surrounds the initiation of sex talk can be attributed to three main factors: (1) socialization experiences, (2) lack of a comfortable sex vocabulary, and (3) fear of revealing too much about oneself. Childhood social experiences in which talk of sex was discouraged or suppressed can profoundly affect the person's ability to converse freely about sex as an adult. Such persons may become acutely embarrassed and back away from intimate conversations. Other people may find it difficult to talk about sex because they lack a comfortable sex vocabulary. Many of our words for sex or sexual anatomy come from slang, derogatory expressions that cast sexual behavior in a negative, sinful, or dirty light. Finally, some people find it difficult to discuss sex because they feel vulnerable—they are afraid of exposing their inner self to scrutiny and evaluation by others. Knowledge and under-standing may help overcome these barriers to initiating effective communica-tion.

Communication alone does not necessarily mean effective communication. Consider, for example, the common question, "Was it good for you?" If the sexual encounter did not meet the partner's expectations, he or she may be in a dilemma. The person may fib and say, "Yes," thereby eliminating any oppor-tunity for improvement. But if the person says, "No," he or she risks offending the partner. Such yes-no questions are often judgmental and do not promote effective communication. It is better to use open-ended questions, such as "What parts of your body do you like to have stroked?" and free choice questions, such as "Do you prefer this or that?" Such questions focus on each individual's preferences rather than on judgments of performance. Another part of communication that should not be forgotten is body language, which can also convey or increase sexual excitement. Touches, caresses, provocative ges-tures, a knowing glance can vitalize and enhance sexual encounters.

SUMMARY

1   Masters and Johnson found that the *human sexual response* occurs in four main stages that gradually unfold from one to the next, along a a continu-um. These stages are characterized by dramatic changes in two main processes: *vasocongestion* (engorgement of tissues) and *myotonia* (muscle contractions).

2   The first stage of the human sexual response is the *excitement* phase. In males, the phase is characterized by erection of the penis and increased heart rate and blood pressure in response to sexual stimulation. In females, it is characterized by vaginal lubrication, enlargement of the clitoris, gradual ballooning of the vagina and tenting of the cervical area, color changes in the vaginal wall, vasocongestion in the breasts and erection of the nipples, and increased blood pressure and heart rate.

3   The second stage is called the *plateau* stage. During this phase vaso-congestive reactions reach a peak in the male, and a *sex flush* may appear. In the female, the tissues surrounding the outer third of the vagina swell to form the *orgasmic platform;* the clitoris retracts; the sex flush appears; and the inner lips change color.

4   During the *orgasmic* stage, the male experiences a series of rhythmic penile contractions resulting in the *ejaculation* of semen. Ejaculation occurs in two phases: *emission* and *expulsion*. The female also experiences a series of rhythmic contractions in the genital area, and some women expel a clear liquid at orgasm. Masters and Johnson have demonstrated that there is only one kind of female orgasm, not two as was previously thought.

5   During the *resolution* stage, the body returns to its previous, una-roused state. In males, erection is lost; any sex flush disappears; and heart rate,

blood pressure, and breathing rate return to normal. Men enter a *refractory period* after orgasm during which they are not responsive to sexual stimulation. In women, breasts decrease in size; the sex flush fades; the orgasmic platform relaxes; and the vagina and uterus return to their original size and shape. Body perspiration may occur in both men and women. Women do not experience a refractory period and may be rearoused quickly to additional orgasms.

6 During sexual arousal, or *foreplay,* men become excited more quickly than women, so partners need to adjust their actions accordingly. Foreplay typically consists of touching or licking of the partner's *erogenous zones*—areas that are particularly sensitive to sexual stimulation. The lips, breasts, and genitals are the most obvious erogenous zones. Different methods of touching, stroking, and kissing can be used to enhance arousal in particular partners. Factors that can affect sexual arousal include vocalizations, grooming, time spent in foreplay and *intromission* (penile thrusting), setting, and tempo.

7 Sex acts may be genital-genital, oral-genital, or anal-genital. The most common genital-genital positions are *man-on-top, woman-on-top, rear-entry,* and *side-to-side.* Oral-genital sex consists of *cunnilingus* (stimulation of the female genitals by the partner's mouth) and *fellatio* (stimulation of the male genitals by the partner's mouth). The occurrence of cunnilingus and fellatio together is called *sixty-nine.*

8 Autoeroticism, or *masturbation,* is self-stimulation for sexual pleasure. Women usually masturbate by stimulating their genitals with their hands or with a vibrator, but they may also rub their breasts or use thigh pressure. Men usually masturbate by grasping the penis and rhythmically pumping it up and down. The ideas that masturbation is harmful, that it leads to sexual frustration, and that it produces asocial tendencies are all untrue. Masturbation is a normal, healthy sexual outlet for both sexes at all ages.

9 Sexual fantasy plays an important role in masturbation and in other sexual activities. Women tend to be romantic in their fantasies, while men are more likely to fantasize about impersonal sex.

10 In order to maintain sexual excitement in a long-term relationship, couples must realize that boredom can occur, must be realistic in their expectations, and should be inventive and imaginative to keep variety in their sex life. Effective communication, both verbal and nonverbal, is of key importance in developing and maintaining a satisfying sexual relationship.

**ADDITIONAL
READING**

* **Brecher, Ruth, and Brecher, Edward.** *An Analysis of Human Sexual Response.* New York: Signet, 1966.
> *A simplified explanation of Masters and Johnson's* Human Sexual Response. *Less detailed and technical than the original, but easier to read.*

* **Comfort, Alex.** *The Joy of Sex.* New York: Crown, 1972.
> *A well-illustrated manual of sexual arousal and enhancement techniques.*

Heiman, Julia. The physiology of erotica: Woman's sexual arousal. *Psychology Today,* August 1975, pp. 90–94.
> *An interesting report on female and male differences and similarities in response to erotic materials.*

* **Vatsyayana.** *The Kama Sutra.* Translated by R. F. Burton and F. F. Arbuthnot. New York: Putnam, 1963.
> *The most famous of the ancient sex manuals.*

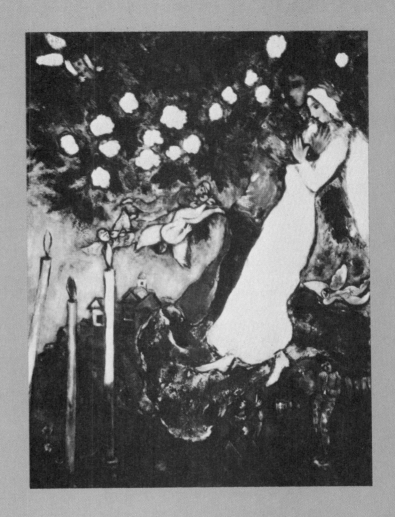

*Marital status and
sexual behavior*

12

chapter

12

Marriage is the most licentious of human institutions—that is the secret of its popularity.
GEORGE BERNARD SHAW

The central relationship in all human societies is marriage. Marriage as an institution seems to have been invented to provide a socially acceptable context for sexual behavior. Societies realize that sexual behavior must be permitted and encouraged if the group is to be perpetuated; yet they also realize that it must be regulated to maintain harmonious group living (Kenkel, 1980). So they have evolved rules to govern who can have what kind of sex, with whom, and when. And in all cases these rules are built around the marriage relationship.

Of course, not all sexual behavior occurs within marriage. There are important differences between the formal, recognized sexual unions of married couples and less formal sexual relationships. Ford and Beach (1951) divided these two types into **mateships**—formalized, sanctioned, and recognized unions—and **liaisons**—sexual relationships formed outside the formal mateship arrangements of a particular society. Mateships are the basis for many of the nonsexual aspects of social structure. They form the core relationship of the family and usually serve to legitimize offspring, establish lines of inheritance, and provide other formal dimensions of the social structure. Liaisons, on the other hand, are primarily sexual. They are not always violations of the rules of society; in fact, most societies permit various kinds of liaisons but place limits on who are considered permissible partners (blood relatives are usually prohibited, for example).

In American society, much attention has been focused on the fact that the traditional form of marriage seems not to be meeting people's needs. This fact is demonstrated by the ever increasing divorce rate, the high incidence of extramarital sex, the burgeoning number of young people living together without marriage, and the increased visibility of various alternatives to traditional marriage. The truth is, however, that we are still a rather conservative and traditional society with regard to marriage. The actual marriage rate has changed little in recent years, and 90 percent of the current adult population will be married for some portion of their adult lives.

It would appear that Americans are as inclined to marry as they have ever been, but they are more likely to change marital partners than at any other time in our history. Sequential marriages, also called **serial monogamy**, with each person eventually having two or more marital unions, may well be the marriage pattern of the future if current trends continue. So it is not really marriage itself that individuals become dissatisfied with—just specific marriages.

In this chapter we will look at how marriage fulfills its function of providing a context for sexual behavior. We will also look at sexual relationships that occur outside of marriage—relationships that are generally frowned on by society but that occur quite frequently anyway. These include premarital, extramarital, and postmarital relationships. We will also look at some alterna-

tives to traditional marital sexual arrangements to see whether they are por-
tents of things to come in this fundamental social institution.

Much of the information in this chapter is based on data from the Hunt
and *Redbook* surveys, which are described in Chap. 3. You will benefit from
reviewing the background information and issues related to this kind of research.

PREMARITAL SEX

Premarital sex has become a somewhat confusing label in our society. It
was a useful label in the not-too-distant past, when marriage in the early adult
years was nearly universal. At that time *premarital sex* was used to refer to
sexual behavior between young people just prior to their entry into marriage.
Most of this premarital sexual behavior was part of the mateship process, in
that it was engaged in with the prospective marital partner in preparation for,
and as a way to evaluate, marital compatibility.

In the 1980s, early marriage is much less common, even though most
people eventually marry. Now many young people live together without formal
marriage and without a requirement to marry their first sexual partner. However, even though the term *premarital sex* has come to be inaccurate, it does
have a formal status among researchers, for whom it means sexual behavior
among those members of the society who are below the expected age of
marriage.

*Attitudes toward
premarital sex*

Our society's attitudes toward premarital sex have become much more
accepting in the past few years. The moral-religious traditions of our society
have always disapproved of this kind of behavior. In fact, compared to other
societies ours has been unusually restrictive in this area. Murdock (1967) found
that 70 percent of the 849 societies he studied permitted premarital intercourse
for both sexes. Almost all of the other groups permitted premarital sex for
at least the males. Only 5 percent of the societies totally prohibited all premarital intercourse; ours was in that group. One common feature of the restrictive
societies was that they all placed a great value on virginity in the female. This
was certainly an important issue in the Judeo-Christian tradition of our society.

We can see how American attitudes toward premarital sex have moved
away from this tradition by looking at the results of surveys taken in the last
four decades. In 1939 the Roper survey asked a national sample of people about
their views of premarital sex. At that time only 22 percent felt that sex was all
right for both partners prior to their marriage; 8 percent felt it was all right for
men only; and 56 percent said it was right for neither. Twenty years later the
same question was asked again by the Roper pollsters and almost identical
results were found. However, several attitude surveys taken between 1958 and
1968 began to show increases in the percentage of people who felt premarital
sex was acceptable in those relationships that were likely to end in marriage.

In the early 1970s Morton Hunt (1974) found a significant rise in the
percentage of people who considered premarital sex to be an acceptable behavior. His findings are summarized in Table 12.1. If the 18–24 age group is taken
separately, the figures show an even more dramatic rise, as illustrated in Table

12.2. Does this mean that we are becoming radically liberated about premarital sexual relationships in general? Hunt doesn't think so. He notes that premarital sex without love or strong affection is still relatively unaccepted, especially among the older population. However, the response of the youngest age group may indicate a liberalizing trend, even in this underlying social rule that sex and love should go together.

	Males	Females
For a man:		
Where strong affection exists	75	55
Couple in love, but not engaged	82	68
Couple engaged	84	73
For a woman:		
Where strong affection exists	66	41
Couple in love, but not engaged	77	61
Couple engaged	81	68

TABLE 12.1

Percent of sample who think premarital coitus is acceptable

Source: Hunt (1974), p. 116.

	Males		Females	
	18–24	*55 and over*	*18–24*	*55 and over*
For a man:				
Where strong affection exists	86	57	73	32
For a woman:				
Where strong affection exists	80	48	59	11

TABLE 12.2

Percent of selected age groups who think premarital coitus is acceptable

Source: Hunt (1974), p. 117.

Premarital sexual behavior

The attitudes people hold toward premarital sex may not be directly reflected by their behavior. It is one thing to accept or reject the premarital sexual behaviors of others; it is another to engage in the behavior oneself.

Incidence   The actual incidence of premarital sex has been evaluated by several large-scale surveys. Kinsey was the first to pursue this question, and the data from his sample indicated that premarital sex occurred more often than expected. Kinsey found that 53 percent of males had engaged in premarital intercourse by age 20, while 20 percent of females had had premarital intercourse by that age. By age 25, 71 percent of the males and 33 percent of the females had engaged in premarital sex (Kinsey et al., 1948, 1953).

Perhaps the figure that most startled the general public in the 1950s was that 50 percent of the women in Kinsey's sample were not virgins at the time of their marriages. To make matters worse for the more conservative members of that society, nearly 70 percent of those nonvirgin women felt neither regret nor guilt (Duberman, 1977).

Between the time of Kinsey's surveys and the surveys conducted in the 1960s, there was relatively little change in the incidence of premarital sexual intercourse. By 1974, however, Hunt noted that changing attitudes, particularly among college students, were accompanied by an explosive rise in the incidence of premarital sex (see Table 12.3). Note the higher rate for younger age groups relative to the older age groups. These data support the idea that the liberalizing trend is continuing, and the incidence figures are expected to continue to climb as more young people reach the age where they can engage in premarital sexual behavior.

			Age		
	18–24	*25–34*	*35–44*	*45–54*	*55 and over*
Males	95	92	86	89	84
Females	81	65	41	36	31

Source: Hunt (1974), p. 150.

TABLE 12.3

Percentage of married sample who have ever had premarital coitus

The *Redbook* survey, which assessed women only, also showed the trend toward higher incidence of premarital sex. In the youngest age group (under 20), premarital sex had been engaged in by 96 percent of the respondents, and in the 20–24 group, 91 percent said they had engaged in this behavior. The percentages were progressively smaller for each age group, reaching 68 percent for the women 40 and older. Even considering that the *Redbook* respondents were probably more sexually liberal and active than the general population, these high figures indicate that the trend noted by Hunt at the beginning of the seventies had indeed continued and in fact had probably accelerated.

Number of partners People often cite the increase in the incidence of premarital sexual intercourse as evidence of a "new morality" in our society. A great deal has been written about this new morality, and for many of the more conservative members of the society, these figures have brought deep concern and much public hand-wringing about excessive sexual activity, promiscuity, and the casualness of sexual encounters among the young. However, such worries are often based on misunderstanding and misuse of the research data.

Promiscuity and a casual attitude toward sex are not in fact reflected in the incidence figures at all. Such figures report only the percentage of people who have engaged in premarital sex. They say nothing about the numbers of partners or the degree of emotional attachment to partners, both of which are better indications of promiscuity. When these data are examined, a different picture emerges—one of continued conformity to many of the more traditional moral values attached to sexual behavior. In fact, as a society we still show basically conservative attitudes toward sexual behavior.

If we consider just women, Hunt (1974) and *Redbook* (Tavris and Sadd, 1977), as well as many other surveys, found that most women have had only one premarital sex partner. Surprisingly, these more recent figures vary little from Kinsey's 1940s data. Table 12.4 presents the *Redbook* findings for women. When it comes to men, fewer data are available. Kinsey did not gather such data at all. Hunt (1974) did ask men about their number of partners and learned that the men in his sample had had a median of six premarital partners. However, because the men Hunt surveyed tended to be active members of the "singles scene," this figure is probably higher than would be true for most men.

TABLE 12.4

Number of lovers for women having premarital sex

Number of lovers	Kinsey (1953)	Total Redbook (1977)	Redbook by age			
			20–24	*25–30*	*35–39*	*40+*
1	53%	51%	53%	50%	56%	51%
2–5	34	34	33	33	31	36
6–10	7	9	9	9	7	7
10+	6	6	6	6	7	5

Source: Tavris and Sadd (1977), p. 77.

The nature and quality of premarital sex The survey questionnaires on which so much of our knowledge about sexual behavior is based usually asked only those questions that could be answered *quantitatively*, that is, how often, how many, at what age, and so on. Questions about the *qualitative* aspects of sexual behavior are much more difficult to ask and rate, so they were usually not included. Yet the qualitative aspects of premarital sexual interactions would seem to be of great importance. They represent the person's initial experiences with intercourse, and the quality of such experiences may well set the tone for future sexual interest and satisfaction. Individuals enter premarital sexual relationships with a variety of hopes and fears. It would be valuable to know what their initial experiences are like and how they affect later sexual adjustment. Many sexologists who have felt this need have conducted interviews and administered questionnaires designed to learn more about the quality of premarital sex.

As might be expected, the news about the quality of initial sexual experiences is not good. Our society tends to set up young people for early difficulty in their sex lives by not adequately preparing them for sexual experiences. Many of the studies have indicated that initial introductions to direct sexuality are often tense, awkward, unpleasant, anxiety provoking, and, in some cases, traumatizing. The perfect recipe for developing problems in sexual interaction would be to place two young people in a situation where they are forced to fumble unknowledgeably through the sex act and to provide pressure by putting high psychological importance on the act. The interview data suggest that this is exactly what happens. The result is a problematic beginning to sexual life.

Although the data vary with the particular survey, population sample, and phrasing of the questions, the overall picture that emerges is one of only moderate enjoyment of the initial sexual experience for men and far less enjoyment and satisfaction for women. Hunt listed the negative aspects of the initial experience as: nervousness, uncertainty, embarrassment, fear of failure, fear of discovery, lack of skill, and physical discomfort. He noted that 80 percent of the men but only 33 percent of the women in his survey reported feelings of pride after the initial experience. One-third of the men and two-thirds of the women felt regret. Half the women and a quarter of the men indicated that intercourse had not met their expectations.

Such negative beginnings to such a pleasurable part of life are truly unfortunate. But at least with such a dismal start sexual experiences can only improve. For many of Hunt's respondents this was exactly the course of events. They indicated that intercourse did get better with time. This was especially true when the relationship with one particular partner continued long enough for feelings of relative ease and comfort to develop.

With regard to the quality of premarital sexual experiences beyond the initial encounters, the research has indicated that people in the 1970s were engaging in more satisfying and varied sexual relationships than was true of previous generations. Hunt (1974) reported that there had been an increase in the incidence and frequency of sexual activity in premarital couples and a greater use of arousal techniques that had been avoided or used infrequently in the past. Total interaction time, duration of foreplay, and amount of time spent engaging in intercourse had all increased from previous studies.

Hunt found that single people under 25 spent approximately 15 minutes in foreplay. This increased to 20 minutes in the 25–35 age group. With regard to intercourse, the medium duration was 12 minutes in the 18–24 age group as estimated by the males and 15 minutes as estimated by the females. For the 25–34 age group, the estimates were 15 and 17 minutes, respectively.

The use of a greater variety of foreplay techniques was also noted by Hunt. He contrasted the variations described with those reported by Kinsey, as shown in Table 12.5. Variety was clearly higher among the 1970s sample than among the 1940s sample.

TABLE 12.5	Foreplay technique	Kinsey sample (adolescent to 25)	Hunt survey (18–24)
Percent of men who used selected techniques of foreplay in premarital sex	Male manual play with female genitals	91	90
	Female manual play with male genitals	75	89
	Fellatio	33	72
	Cunnilingus	14	69
	Source: Hunt (1974), p. 166.		

Frequency of premarital sex was also noticeably higher for the 1970s group. For females, the frequency of sexual intercourse was strikingly higher. Males engaged in sexual intercourse half again as often as those in Kinsey's sample, but females were having intercourse three times as often as those in the Kinsey study.

One oft-cited measure of the adequacy of the sexual experience, questionable as it might be, is the occurrence of orgasm in the female. Have the increases in the frequency, duration, foreplay, and variety of sex resulted in any changes in the female "big O," as Tavris and Sadd (1977) facetiously call it? These investigators asked the *Redbook* respondents this question and compared their results with Kinsey's data on women's orgasms in the first year of marriage. Kinsey found that 25 percent of the women never reached orgasm in the first year; 39 percent almost always did; and the remainder ranged between these two extremes. The comparable percentages from the *Redbook* study are shown in Table 12.6. In this case, the contemporary data do not indicate any increase in incidence of orgasm as compared to Kinsey's findings. Note, however, that the youngest women in the *Redbook* survey indicated more orgasmic responsiveness. If the trend continues, this particular area of sexual satisfaction may show further gains in the near future. For now, however, all of the change in premarital sexual behavior has not greatly increased the frequency of female orgasm. Given the tensions inherent in the sexual experience as it is arranged in our society, especially for women, this finding is not surprising.

	Age of respondent		
TABLE 12.6			
Female orgasm during premarital sex	**How often orgasm reached**	*Under 24*	*25–34*	*35+*
	Always	7%	6%	9%
	Most of the time	27	21	19
	Sometimes	38	38	31
	Never	29	35	41

Source: Tavris and Sadd (1977), p. 83.

Living together Premarital sexual behavior may occur in the context of a living-together arrangement. ***Cohabitation*** of a man and a woman without benefit of marriage is not new. "Shacking up," as it was once called, has been around for a long time. However, there has probably never been a time in which the activity has had such a high incidence, has been so openly practiced, and has had as much social acceptance.

Because studies of cohabitation have been conducted mostly with college students, how much of the research can be generalized to the noncollege community is questionable. College life more easily supports living-together arrangements. Both members of the couple are away from home and their respective families. Many are also away from the hometown community's disapproval that noncollege couples may face. Perhaps most important, the more liberal environment of the college community, especially with regard to sexual mores, is supportive of couples living together.

The publicity on cohabitation makes one feel that everyone is doing it. What are the actual percentages of couples living together? Among the college studies, the estimates of couples cohabiting range from 30 to 40 percent of the campus population. One study conducted on noncollege subjects pursued this question indirectly. Whitehurst (1974) asked, "What proportion of your friends are now involved in heterosexual living arrangements?" The responses ranged between 20 and 50 percent. Clayton and Voss (1977) found that 18 percent of

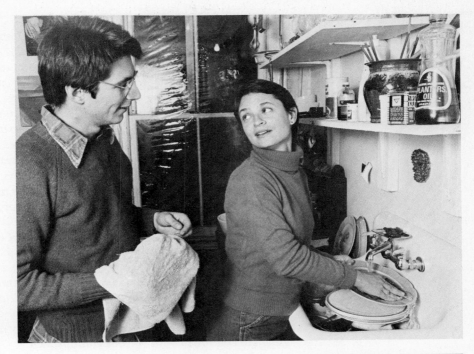

In our society there has been a dramatic rise in the number of unmarried couples living together.

the 2510 young noncollege men they contacted had lived with a woman for 6 months or more. All of the investigators have noted that the incidence figures appear to be increasing, indicating that a greater percentage of people are likely to be cohabiting in the future.

Why do people choose to live together? Cohabitants today are less likely to be "playing house" to see if the marriage will work than was true in the past. When asked why they live together, most current cohabitors focus on aspects and benefits of the arrangement itself rather than on its testing or practice features (see Box 12.1). When marriage is mentioned, it is more likely to be introduced by the woman. The men focus more on the ease and availability of sexual intercourse without the "hassles" of dating. Other reasons mentioned for living together are economic advantages, avoidance of living alone, and, especially, "establishing a meaningful relationship." Butler (1979) noted that few of the individuals in his study planned their cohabitation around a specific reason; they had just drifted together and found a variety of mutually beneficial reasons for staying together. Sociologists have found many similarities between the living-together couple of today and the "going-steady" couple of previous generations. The same level of commitment and exclusivity is involved, with the exception that marriage is not a part of the "contract" made between the cohabiting individuals.

BOX 12.1

The pros and cons of cohabitation

Steve and Janice met a year ago at the home of a mutual friend. They were immediately attracted to each other and began dating. They found they liked the same music, had similar upbringings, and worked in similar jobs related to photography. It didn't take long for sex to enter the relationship, and Steve ended up spending three or four nights a week at Janice's apartment. Now the rent has been raised on Steve's place, and the two are considering moving in together. Aside from moral considerations, what are some of the factors they should take into account when making their decision?

Their attitude toward marriage. Most couples who choose cohabitation say they are interested in marriage at some time in the future, but for the present they are more concerned with personal growth and achieving financial security. They also want to make sure they've chosen the "right" person before committing themselves to a legal relationship. Some feel that marriage can actually be destructive to an intimate relationship—that marriage makes couples take each other for granted. Nevertheless, research has found that cohabiting couples do not seem to differ from married couples in their amount of affection, their degree of satisfaction with the relationship, or their overall happiness.

Their attitude toward dating. Many couples feel that the "dating game" is a superficial means of courtship that places men and women in roles that severely constrict their ability to get to know each other as individuals. Cohabitation, on the other hand, allows for a more complex and realistic interaction on a day-to-day basis.

Their sexual needs and attitudes. Traditional dating places a heavy emphasis on sex, whereas cohabitation tends to put sex into perspective as just one part of an intimate relationship. Nevertheless, studies have found that men list ease of sexual gratification as a main reason for living together, whereas women are much more likely to list preparation for marriage as the main reason.

Their feelings of commitment. Many couples have a deep emotional involvement, yet are not ready to make a long-term commitment. Cohabitation can serve as a "trial marriage" for some such couples, but for others, it may provide a handy way of avoiding serious commitment.

Their sex-role attitudes. Many women entering living-together arrangements expect an egalitarian relationship in which both partners share household chores. Numerous studies have shown, however, that traditional sex-role patterns tend to be maintained by cohabiting couples; that is, women tend to do the cooking, cleaning, and laundry, whereas men handle the "handyman" jobs.

Parental attitudes. Many parents belong to the generation that considers cohabitation to be "living in sin." As a result, many couples are reluctant to let their parents know about their living arrangement. In one national survey of college students, more than half of those who had cohabited said their parents didn't know about it (Hassett, 1977). Although living together is becoming much more acceptable, couples often have to deal with the problem of telling their parents and risking conflict or not telling and thus having to deal with deceit and guilt.

Attitudes toward the relationship itself. Cohabitation can mean different things to different people. One person may see it as a convenient arrangement —friendly and casual. Another may see it as a trial marriage—a testing of the relationship before moving on to a more permanent commitment. And a third may see it as a long-term alternative to marriage. If a couple's attitudes differ, one person may end up feeling overpowered and trapped, while the other may feel jealous, anxious, and hurt. For example, Steve may feel that living together should not entail sexual exclusivity, whereas Janice may see it as tantamount to marriage. Thus, if Steve sees other women, Janice is likely to feel betrayed and threatened.

If Janice and Steve do move in together, what are they likely to derive from the experience? In general, college students who have cohabited report that they consider the experience to have been successful, pleasurable, and maturing (Knox, 1979). They say that living together is a good way of getting to know another person and that it fosters personal growth. A few report negative experiences, however. Cohabitation can be harmful if the individual comes out of the relationship with reduced self-esteem, inability to form new relationships, or hostility toward the opposite sex.

Will Janice and Steve find it easy to split up if the relationship doesn't work out? Studies have shown that co-habiting couples have the same rate of breaking up as do long-term dating couples. However, although terminating a living together arrangement is often as simple as packing one's bags and moving out—with no divorce proceedings, financial hassles, or custody battles—it can be just as emotionally devastating as a divorce.

Will successful cohabitation ensure a successful marriage? Studies comparing couples who lived together before marriage with couples who went through traditional engagement have found no significant differences in the happiness or success of the marriages (Macklin, 1978). It appears that although living together does provide close interaction, in many cases it is on a superficial level. It does not really prepare couples for making important life decisions regarding work, finances, and children—the kinds of decisions that can create the greatest conflict and unity in marriage.

In short, for many couples cohabitation has replaced dating as a means of assessing the compatibility of partners during courtship. But because of the lack of commitment involved, it is not really a substitute for marriage and cannot be equated to marriage.

Couples who choose cohabitation are usually well aware of its benefits and advantages but are less aware of its pitfalls. Certainly this life-style has great appeal for those who want intimate relationships but are wary of rushing into marriage in our divorce-prone society. But those who enter it must realize that it is not a panacea for all their problems and that, like marriage, it has its own set of drawbacks.

BOX 12.2

Sex and the single person

Howard is a 33-year-old businessman with his own small publishing company. He works 50–60 hours a week to put out the three magazines he publishes. A "bachelor," he lives in a one-bedroom apartment filled with an odd assortment of belongings he has collected over the years. Although he has been "in love" several times and has even lived with a couple of women, he doesn't picture himself ever getting married. He feels that he is already "set in his ways."

Audrey is a schoolteacher in her later thirties. She has a teenage son, the offspring of a marriage that ended tragically when her husband was killed in a car accident 10 years ago. Audrey has dated several men, but for the last year or so she has been spending most of her time with a zoologist she met at a party. They are happy with their "going-together" arrangement and have no plans for marriage.

Gene is a 55-year-old management consultant who has been married and divorced twice. He has led a single life for the last 15 years, dating from time to time but not finding anyone to get "serious" about. He remains close to his now-grown children and has a group of male friends.

Marcie is a 24-year-old student nurse planning a career in hospital administration. She has lived in the same house for the last 5 years and in that time has had a succession of roommates, male and female. She has an active sex life and enjoys dating but expects some day to meet "Mr. Right" and to get married.

These four people are all part of the burgeoning singles population in America today. This population consists of the never married, the separated, the divorced, and the widowed. In fact, at any given time, single people make up one-third of all individuals over 18. It is estimated that by 1990, the number of U.S. households composed of unmarried individuals will nearly equal the number of households of married people. As it is, 31 million households are already headed by singles (Wolfe, 1982).

If we look at the statistics for people living alone (no children, no roommates), we find that in 1980 there were almost 18 million such individuals—an increase of 64 percent over 1970. Although many more women live alone than men (11 million to 7 million), the number of men turning to the single life in the last decade increased at a much greater rate than that for women (92 percent to 64 percent). For men, the singles group is made up primarily of the never married (45 percent), while more of the single women are widowed (56 percent) (Wolfe, 1982).

What has led to the boom in the number of singles, particularly people living alone? Divorce is one contributor. The number of divorced single men increased 150 percent between 1970 and 1980; the comparable increase for divorced single women was 109 percent. The high percentage of widowed women among singles is accounted for by the fact that women tend to live longer than men. For example, 41 percent of all women in the 65–74 age group are widows. But we are still left with the fact that increasing numbers of individuals are choosing never to marry or are remaining unmarried until late in their twenties. Two main factors seem to be involved in this trend. First, greater occupational opportunities for women have made it less necessary for them to marry for purposes of financial security. Second, the relaxed social rules against sex outside of marriage has made it less necessary for men to marry for purposes of sexual access.

Another factor that has contributed to the singles population explosion is the increasing acceptance of singlehood as an alternative life-style. Not too long ago, anyone who didn't marry was considered to be a lonely reject ("old maid") or an irresponsible, self-indulgent hedonist. These stereotypes have to some extent fallen by the wayside as more and more people have purposely chosen the freedom and autonomy of the single life or have put off marriage a few years in order to accomplish personal and career goals.

However, today the image of the single person has acquired a new stereotype: the Cosmopolitan woman and the Playboy man, who drive fancy sports cars, wear designer clothes, live in singles' apartment complexes, vacation in luxury resorts, and pick each other up in singles' bars. This stereotype has some element of truth, in that single people tend to have more money to spend on themselves than married people do and thus are able to afford expensive cars, clothes, vacations, and so on. Nevertheless, like all stereotypes, this one applies to only a small, if conspicuous, group of singles. As the four people described in this box demonstrate, singles vary greatly in their backgrounds and lifestyles.

Like married people, singles have careers, family, friends, and hobbies. But they do not have "built in" companions or sex partners. Thus, they must find ways to fulfill their needs for attachment, for intimate relationships. Some, like Audrey, have a steady partner whom they may or may not live with. Others, like Howard, seem satisfied with an ever-changing series of partners. For people like Gene, the need for attachment is met primarily by family and friends. And for many singles, like Marcie, the hope is to someday find that perfect partner, fall in love, and get married, so social activities are geared to looking for that future partner.

In general, single people tend to gravitate toward large cities, where there are not only greater career opportunities and a variety of recreational and entertainment activities but also more places to meet potential partners. Singles' bars are indeed popular, but so are special groups and activities designed to bring singles together in a comfortable atmosphere. In New York City, for example, there are social, sports, and travel groups; counseling groups for the divorced and widowed; publications; courses and seminars; and special services all geared to singles.

Although few studies have been done on the sex lives of singles, Hunt (1974) did find that the wild and promiscuous sex life often attributed to today's singles is characteristic of only a few people. Although single men and women have intercourse rates comparable to those for married men and women, they apparently have sex with steady partners rather than with a parade of strangers. Single men between the ages of 25 and 34, for example, reported an average of four partners in the previous year, while women in this age group reported an average of three partners. Thus, as Keith Melville (1980) concludes, "Sexual standards for most singles are apparently still closely related to feelings of intimacy and affection" (p. 156).

Sexual activities among cohabiting couples have been found to be similar to those of recently married couples. With regard to sexual frequency, duration, arousal, and techniques, there are no differences between cohabiting couples and newlyweds. Cohabiting couples also experience many of the same sexual difficulties as newlyweds. However, with cohabitors these problems are more likely to lead to a breakup of the arrangement than to sex therapy or counseling.

One side effect of the increase in living-together arrangements is that marriages are tending to be delayed; that is, there has been a significant upward shift in the average age of first marriage. (See Box 12.2.) Other ripple effects of living together may show in society after a significant number of couples have been living together for a longer period of time.

MARITAL SEXUAL BEHAVIOR

Marriage is usually presented as the *end* of the romantic, sexually exciting part of life rather than as the beginning of a special love relationship. People often refer to their mates as "my old man," "my old lady," "the old ball and chain," and in other less than endearing terms. These are the same people they referred to, prior to marriage, as their "sweetie," "darling," or "sweetheart." Comedians have endless jokes about wives and husbands, from "Take my wife—please" to "My husband, Fang." It is difficult to think of any great love

While other ways of relating may be increasing, the traditional marriage is still the most common adult heterosexual relationship.

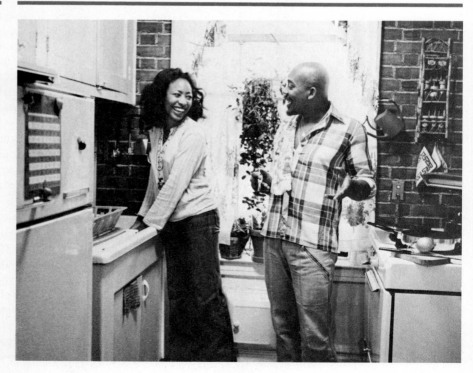

stories written about a married couple. It seems that marriage suffers from a very poor reputation. Yet it is the relationship that is at the very core of our social structure and that is the center of our sexual lives. What implications do these negative attitudes have for sexual adjustment to married life?

According to our moral imperatives and cultural traditions, marriage is the only acceptable context for sexual behavior. But like marriage itself, the sexual component is thought of as boring and possibly even unpleasant. There would seem to be some kind of divine injustice to a system in which the only sex that is allowed is described as not worth having. But is it really like that? And where it is, does it have to be? Do love and passionate sexual relationships have to end at marriage? Or is marital sex simply a victim of bad press and, in reality, not as awful as we are led to believe? These kinds of questions can only be answered by studying the sexual behavior of married couples.

Many of the same studies that we called upon in our discussion of premarital sex also form the basis for our knowledge of marital sexual behavior. Basically, they are questionnaire-type studies and as such suffer the problems inherent in all self-report studies. Thus, as we examine the contributions of these studies to our knowledge of marital sexuality, we should keep in mind the warnings about the limits to the generality of these studies that were noted in Chap. 3.

Frequency of
sexual intercourse

Every researcher interested in marital sexual behavior has studied the frequency of sexual intercourse in marriage. How many times a month, a week, a day do couples have intercourse? This focus reflects the common view that frequency indicates sexual interest, enjoyment, and so on. Yet most people would agree that quantity and quality cannot be so easily equated. Still, the search for an accurate report on the frequency of marital intercourse continues.

To complicate the issue further, the various survey studies have asked the question of frequency of sexual intercourse somewhat differently. With such variations we would expect large differences in the results. However, remarkably similar statistics have been obtained in the various studies. Even more interesting is the fact that the findings from studies conducted in the 1940s and 1950s are not very different from current figures. The studies also agree on the general decrease in frequency of marital intercourse with age.

Figure 12.1 summarizes the important studies on frequency and presents them in a single illustration for purposes of comparison. This figure clearly shows the similarity of the frequency rates and of the decline in frequency with age. Another look at the decrease in frequency with age is provided by Table 12.7, which combines the male and female data and gives the overall averages for five age groups (Hunt, 1974). It should be noted that all these figures represent group averages. Any particular married couple may have very different rates. In fact, the variability is very wide indeed, with couples engaging in intercourse anywhere from several times a day to only a few times a year, or even never.

It is not unusual for one or both members of a couple to be dissatisfied with the frequency of sexual intercourse. Some want more, some less. Studies

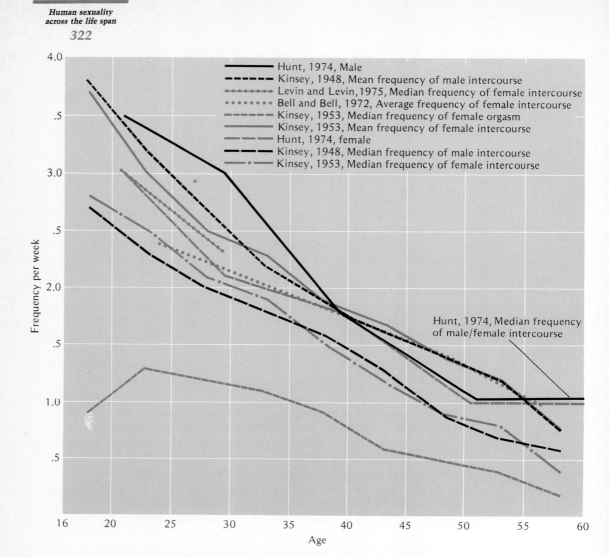

4.0

.5

3.0

.5

2.0

.5

1.0

.5

Frequency per week

——— Hunt, 1974, Male
- - - - Kinsey, 1948, Mean frequency of male intercourse
•-•-•-• Levin and Levin,1975, Median frequency of female intercourse
•••••• Bell and Bell, 1972, Average frequency of female intercourse
- - - Kinsey, 1953, Median frequency of female orgasm
——— Kinsey, 1953, Mean frequency of female intercourse
— — Hunt, 1974, female
— — Kinsey, 1948, Median frequency of male intercourse
—•—•— Kinsey, 1953, Median frequency of female intercourse

Hunt, 1974, Median frequency
of male/female intercourse

16   20   25   30   35   40   45   50   55   60

Age

FIGURE 12.1

As age increases, the weekly occurrence of sexual intercourse decreases. Several studies summarized here all show a similar slope to the decline in sexual frequency.

have typically found that men desire more sex, while women prefer less. (This difference has been cited as the reason for the constant, though small, discrepancy between the sexes in the estimates of frequency; that is, husbands tend to underestimate the frequency, and wives tend to overestimate.) Hunt has argued that this difference in ideal frequency is beginning to disappear with sexual liberation and, in fact, has been reversed for some of the younger women who find they desire intercourse more often than their husbands. Tavris and Sadd's (1977) data support Hunt's conclusions. In their *Redbook* study, 58 percent of the women said their sexual frequency was about right, and only 4 percent said it was too high. However, 38 percent felt it was not frequent enough.

TABLE 12.7	Age	Median frequency /week
Frequency of intercourse in marriage	18–24	3.25
	25–34	2.55
	35–44	2.00
	46–55	1.00
	55+	1.00

Source: Hunt (1974), p. 191.

Duration of sexual intercourse

Kinsey surprised everyone with his now famous finding that 75 percent of the married men in his study reached orgasm within 2 minutes or less of intromission. His subjects also indicated a median time of 12 minutes for sexual arousal prior to intromission. This amounts to a total of 14 minutes of sexual stimulation prior to orgasm. In contrast, most women in the *Redbook* study said they needed 6–15 minutes for arousal and another 6–15 minutes of coitus for orgasm (see Table 12.8). This is a total range of 12–30 minutes. The lack of overlap between women's needs and men's average times is striking. In light of this discrepancy, it is no wonder that large numbers of women have been unable to experience orgasm through intercourse.

TABLE 12.8	Average number of minutes needed	For arousal	For intercourse to orgasm
Time needed for arousal and orgasm (by percentage of women responding)	1–5	29%	28%
	6–10	43	37
	11–15	20	20
	16–20	5	9
	21–25	1	3
	25+	2	3

Source: Tavris and Sadd (1977), p. 115.

The duration figures have been changing, however. Hunt found a definite and dramatic increase in the duration of intercourse in his sample. His respondents averaged 10 minutes for the duration of coitus after intromission, as reported by both males and females. The average time spent in arousal activities was 15 minutes. This puts the total average time at 25 minutes. This more closely matches the woman's need for duration of stimulation to achieve satisfaction. Skill at maintaining the duration of sexual stimulation has become highly valued among males in our society since the publication of Kinsey's figures. If Hunt's data are accurate, it would appear that the problem of the "too rapidly ejaculating male" may be lessening. The drop in the percentage of nonorgasmic women and the increased satisfaction reported by many women may also reflect this increase in male duration.

Sexual techniques among married couples

In recent years the general liberalization of sexual attitudes has led to greater dissemination of information about sexual stimulation techniques. The moral restrictions against the use of certain sexual practices and positions in marriage have also relaxed. How have these changes affected marital sexual behavior? Unfortunately, not enough research has been done in this area to provide an adequate answer. Hunt, who has pursued some of these issues, presented his findings in his book, *Sex in the Seventies* (1974). Data from the *Redbook* survey (1977) and the *Hite Report* (1976) also touched on some of these issues but only for female subjects. All of these surveys were of subjects who were probably more sexually active and adventurous than the general public, so the results can only be taken as suggestive of possible current practices and future trends.

To summarize some of these findings in the area of sexual technique, there does seem to be a more liberal approach to sexual activities among married partners. The most noticeable changes are a greater variation in coital positions and a greater willingness to experiment in other aspects of the sexual encounter (setting, time, clothing, and so on). When Hunt compared his results to Kinsey's, he felt that the differences were dramatic. He found sharp rises in mouth-breast contact, manual stimulation of the partner, anal stimulation, and amount of time spent in fellatio and cunnilingus.

TABLE 12.9		Age group		
	Position	18–24	35–44	55+
Percentage of couples often using variant positions in coitus	Female above	37	29	17
	Side-by-side	21	15	15
	Rear-entry (vaginal)	20	8	1
	Sitting	4	2	2

Source: Hunt (1974), p. 203.

Table 12.9 presents Hunt's findings on variant coital positions by age group. Although the male-above position still dominates in our society, note that a large percentage of respondents indicated that they often use other positions. The differences among the age groups shown in Table 12.9 indicate that younger people engage in more variety. These data are thought to reflect the increased knowledge and more liberal attitudes of the youngest married couples compared to the older married couples.

*Orgasm in
marital sex*

Orgasm is often used as a measure of sexual adjustment for the married female, just as it was for the female who engaged in premarital sex. Kinsey found that although married women experienced orgasm, they did not experience it as often as they wanted to and that many did not experience it at all in their first year of marriage. Kinsey's findings focused attention on the fact that inorgasmic women were more than just a small minority of the married population. The *Redbook* researchers wanted to know just how important orgasm is to a woman. Had Kinsey created a pseudoissue? They found that the more often a woman reached orgasm, the more she liked her sex life. They noted that 85 percent of the women who thought their sex lives were terrific were orgasmic all or most of the time.

Males also consider the female orgasm a sign of success in their sex lives. Most men take a greal deal of (inappropriate) pride in their wives' orgasms and work mightily to produce the desired effect. This male need to achieve success through the female's orgasmic response has become as big a problem of contemporary sexual behavior as was the selfish lack of awareness among men in the Kinsey era. It has led to the woman sometimes feeling forced to fake orgasm when the sexual experience has not led to natural orgasm just to provide the man with a sense of accomplishment. Some women may also fake orgasm as a way of ending coitus in order to prevent further stimulation in an experience that may have moved beyond pleasure to irritation and pain.

While the overemphasis on female orgasm may have become a problem, orgasm is still a desirable outcome of sexual intercourse for the woman. Given an appropriate weighting, it can be a worthwhile measure for assessing the success of the relationship; therefore, it will be useful to review the findings in this area.

Almost all the major surveys have explored the question of female orgasmic response. In general, the picture that has emerged is one of improvement over the years in this aspect of marital sexual functioning. Unfortunately, the various studies have presented this question so differently from one another that direct comparisons are difficult. Hunt's findings are presented in Table 12.10. The *Redbook* results are summarized in Table 12.11. Both of these studies show substantial improvement in female orgasmic response over the Kinsey studies of the 1940s. More important, it appears that even between the Hunt sample of the early 1970s and the more recent *Redbook* surveys there has been a trend toward higher frequency of female orgasm. Overall, the data on female orgasm indicate that gains have already been made and that marital sexual experiences should continue to improve.

TABLE 12.10	Orgasm frequency	Percent of wives
Percent of wives in Hunt survey who reached coital orgasm	All or almost all of the time	53
	About $\frac{3}{4}$ of the time	21
	About $\frac{1}{2}$ of the time	11
	About $\frac{1}{4}$ of the time	8
	Almost none or none of the time	7
	Source: Hunt (1974), p. 221.	

TABLE 12.11	Orgasm frequency	Percent of wives
Percent of wives in Redbook *survey who reached coital orgasm*	All the time	15
	Most of the time	48
	Sometimes	19
	Once in a while	11
	Never	7
	Source: Tavris and Sadd (1977), p. 110.	

Orgasm for men has rarely been questioned. The assumption has always been that men reach orgasm at every sexual intercourse experience. Hunt was one of the few investigators to ask his male sample about their orgasmic frequency and surprisingly found that many men reported problems in the area of orgasm. Failure to experience orgasm, though it was reported by a small percentage of men, is every bit as important a problem for the men involved as it is for nonorgasmic women. Age turns out to be an important factor in the orgasmic problems of men. Hunt found that 8 percent of men aged 45 and older failed to have an orgasm "occasionally to often." When failure in 25 percent of intercourse experiences was used as the criterion for defining an orgasmic problem, Hunt found that 7 percent of men between ages 25 and 44 and 15 percent of those under 25 would be considered to have such a problem.

It is clear that the 100 percent orgasm rate for men, even young men, is a myth. This myth has probably caused more doubt and fear of impotence than is warranted when we consider that it may be perfectly natural to occasionally not carry the sexual act to orgasm. What do men do when they cannot complete the sex act? Clinicians know that some men engage in a practice everyone assumes to be a purely female behavior: They fake orgasm. Unfortunately, most men do not admit to such deception, and none of the surveys have asked about this practice. Thus, its extent is unknown. There are, of course, no cases of men faking erections!

*Communicating
about marital
sexual function*

If asked to indicate the most important aspect of a marital relationship that will increase sexual satisfaction, most counselors would say it is the ability of the couple to communicate with each other. Unfortunately, the increased openness in our society about sexual behavior has not necessarily been reflected in the way marital couples communicate about sex. The marital bedroom is a very silent room in most homes.

As we noted in Chap. 11, talking about sex is viewed as inappropriate and "dirty" in our society. The words for sexual organs and acts are more likely to be used as curse words than as part of normal conversation. As a result, marital partners find it embarrassing to discuss sexual problems, to make suggestions for change, to verbalize their fantasies and desires, and to indicate what is pleasant and unpleasant so that sexual feelings might be enhanced. This is particularly unfortunate when we realize that both partners in the relationship would really like to know what would give pleasure to the other as well as to be able to express their own desires.

Even indicating an interest in having sex becomes complicated when communication is poor. Such interest must often be signaled through subtle cues and symbolic language rather than through direct statements. The husband might say, "I feel so relaxed tonight," meaning, "Let's have sex." The wife might respond with, "I have a slight headache," meaning "No." For another couple, the wife might say, "Let's go to bed early tonight," as her signal of interest in sex, and her husband might reply, "Good idea, I have a busy day tomorrow," as his way of saying, "No." Note that the offers and refusals or acceptances are never delivered directly. This allows for misinterpretation, projection of one's own feelings, and an inability of the rejected partner to react to and deal with the rejection directly.

This brings up another issue about marital sexual behavior: Who initiates the sexual interaction? In our society the traditional initiator has been the male. The female is supposed to be passive and respond to the male's advances. A more contemporary view is that men and women having more equal sexual interest, and feminists have argued strongly against the power differences implied by women's submission to the more active male. Has there been any change in the traditional initiator-responder sexual roles as a result of the changing views of male-female dominance in other areas? Tavris and Sadd (1977) reported that a majority of women in their *Redbook* sample said their husbands were the most likely initiators of intercourse. However, there has been a rising trend toward female initiation. The data showed that 44 percent of the women initiated sex at least half of the time, 42 percent initiated sex sometimes, and only 4 percent never initiated sex. A surprisingly large group (11 percent) said they "always or usually" initiated sex. It is important to note, however, that these last two groups (always or never initiated sex) were the least satisfied with their sex lives.

In general, the various studies of marital sexuality show that it has its problems, but marriage is probably less of a negative experience than its bad press would indicate. The data demonstrate some important strengths and positive trends in marital sexual interactions as well as the problem areas and sources of dissatisfaction. If the data show ambivalence toward marriage, that is an accurate reflection of how most Americans feel. Our marriage, divorce, and remarriage rates seem to show that we desire to be married when we are single and to be single when we are married. And around and around we go. . . .

<table>
<tr><td>

EXTRAMARITAL
SEX

</td><td>

Extramarital sex, or **adultery**, is sexual intercourse by a married person with anyone other than his or her spouse. The term *affair* has become the most popular label for extramarital sexual involvement, perhaps because it makes this behavior sound less serious. Although we may lump them all together, extramarital affairs involve a rather wide range of sexual involvements. The actual encounters can be anything from a one-night stand to a lifelong relationship. Because affairs can be so varied, it seems questionable to categorize such diverse human relationships under one heading. Despite the fact that each extramarital affair may be very different, some of the general issues of such liaisons may help us to understand all of them better.

</td></tr>
</table>

Ford and Beach (1951) found that our society is one of a very few that have rules demanding total and lifelong monogamy. Most of the societies they studied not only permit sex partners other than the spouse but actually require them under certain conditions. No society, however, allows totally free reign to sexual impulses on the part of the married members of the group. In actual practice, on the other hand, our society does not differ markedly from most others. Our lifelong, single-pair monogamy exists primarily in our moral-legal rules about relationships and much less in our actual behavior. This difference means that people engaging in extramarital behavior must break the rules to do so, which has some far-reaching implications, as we shall see.

An important aspect of extramarital behavior is the strong influence of the sex-role double standard. The married woman who has an extramarital affair is viewed as having committed a much more serious violation and is treated much more harshly than the married man who has an affair. Such a double standard exists in many other societies as well. The double standard seems to be weakening in other areas of life as equality of women has increased. It will be interesting to see whether greater equality in the area of extramarital sexual behavior will come about as well.

*Incidence of
extramarital affairs*

Kinsey and others (1948, 1953) provided the first comprehensive view of the extent of extramarital sexual behavior in the United States. The results were a shock to the conservative American society of the time. He found that 50 percent of the men and 26 percent of the women had had an extramarital affair by age 40. There was much questioning of what seemed like an impossibly high figure, but these data were supported in several additional large-scale studies by subsequent investigators. These percentages may actually have been on the low side, since some people would never admit to an affair, even with full guarantees of anonymity.

Hunt (1974) performed an extensive analysis of comparable figures from his more recent survey. One important question that he sought to answer was whether there had been any change in the frequency of extramarital involvements since Kinsey's study. He was surprised to find relatively little change from the 1940s to the 1970s. The only exception came in one group: the under-25-year-old females. Three times as many women in this group had had an extramarital affair compared to that same age group in Kinsey's sample. None of Hunt's male groups had shown increases over their comparable Kinsey group. Despite this rise in the younger women, men were still ahead in the percentage who had had an affair, but the gap was closing. Hunt sees this as a move toward equality of the sexes and feels that it represents a reduction in the strength of the double standard in our society.

The *Redbook* survey indicates that the trend noted by Hunt has continued to rise, with the *Redbook* respondents showing near equality to men in the percentage having had an extramarital affair. While this may not be the activity for which we would want men and women to attain equality, the reduction of the double standard does seem appropriate.

*The nature of
extramarital affairs*

Extramarital affairs are usually presented as highly romantic encounters with intense emotional involvement and sensual sex far better than the marital sex the person has experienced. Once again the reality falls far short of the myth. The data show that extramarital affairs do not go on for very long periods of time and that the actual sexual interactions are comparatively few. Both the Kinsey and *Redbook* surveys found that the typical affair lasts for 1 year or less. Sexual interactions during the course of an affair average less than five occasions of actual sexual contact. Extramarital affairs, it seems, are rather short-lived experiences, especially in comparison to marriage, where the longevity of the relationship is several years, with average sexual contact of two or three times a week.

Another myth about the "adulterer" is that he or she has many affairs with many partners—that the person is promiscuous. The data indicate that this is far from the case. Kinsey found that people tended to engage in extramarital affairs with an average of only two partners. Tavris and Sadd (1977) make it even clearer that the adulterous women were neither promiscuous nor particularly sexually active. Table 12.12 shows the number of partners and the number of sexual interactions with each partner. From both the *Redbook* and Kinsey studies it is clear that most of those who had had an extramarital affair did not "sleep around" a lot of the time with a lot of people. In fact, they hardly got to sleep around at all. Considering the findings of the very limited nature of affairs, it is intriguing that they are given such great importance in marriage and can have such a dramatic impact on the lives and futures of everyone concerned. Once again, the emotional significance of the event has little to do with the "numbers" involved.

TABLE 12.12	Number of partners		Number of times with each partner	
Extramarital affairs among wives	1	50%	1	18%
	2–5	40	2–5	33
	6–10	5	6–10	10
	10+	5	10+	19
			Varied greatly from partner to partner	21

Source: Tavris and Sadd (1977), p. 166.

Sexual behavior in extramarital affairs

Literature has often portrayed the romance and excitement of the extramarital affair. Lady Chatterly, who found sexual excitement for the first time in her life in her affair with her husband's gamekeeper, comes to the minds of many who may fantasize about this romantic notion. The realities of this aspect of affairs are difficult to study. However, some of the surveys, interview studies, and clinical case records have shed a little light on the qualitative experiences in extramarital affairs. Again, romantic myth and reality are far apart. From much of the data, one gets the impression that many people come away from extramarital experiences wondering, "Is that all there is?" Two books that report extensively on the subjective experience of affairs, Wolfe's *Playing Around* (1975) and Hunt's *The Affair* (1969), are worth reading for their more personal views of extramarital sex. Both of these extensive, qualitative investigations revealed that many of the participants did have generally positive feelings about their affairs but, more interestingly, also felt that their marriages were as, or even more, interesting than the affairs. A frequent outcome of affairs was for the individuals to decide that their marriage was more important to them than they thought and that it could be salvaged.

The actual sexual behavior in the affairs also fell short of the stereotype of the extramarital partner as being a greater lover than the spouse. The *Redbook* survey found that women engaged in less experimentation and variation of sexual technique in their affairs than in their marriages. The researchers summed up their findings as suggesting that "sometimes the anticipation of an affair is much better than its execution." This may help to explain why affairs are as short-lived as they are and why there is so little sexual contact involved. The fact that affairs are so often disappointing to the participants has led several researchers to the hypothesis that affairs may actually be good for some marriages. Affairs demystify the "desirable stranger" fantasy; they make the marital partner look better than he or she seemed prior to the affair; and they lead the person to a reevaluation of and eventually a greater commitment to the marriage. With these experiences behind them, people return to their marriage and work harder to try to enhance the relationship rather than continually fantasizing about some unreal, magical salvation from outside.

POSTMARITAL SEXUAL BEHAVIOR

There are two life-change events that result in people becoming single people again after being married: divorce and the death of a spouse. Both of these situations create special problems, as the person must confront life in a totally new role. Individuals involved in these types of readjustments encounter important personal and social issues as they try to find a new place for themselves as sexual beings.

Divorce and separation

In 1975 there were 460 divorces per 1000 marriages. Since then this rate has been rising, and current estimates are that there are approximately 500 divorces per 1000 marriages, or one divorce for every two marriages. Separation, either through agreement to separate or desertion, is impossible to measure since there is no formal reporting except for the few couples who go through the formalities of legal separation. From both the available divorce statistics and from the estimates of the separations, however, it seems clear that there are a large number of people confronted with the task of adjusting to postmarital life.

There are many stereotypes of the divorced or separated person. On the one hand there is the "gay divorcee," the person who, released from the bonds and burdens of marriage, supposedly lives a life of gay abandon with constant entertainment, plentiful sex, and general irresponsibility in sexual and other areas of life. At the other extreme is the image of the sad, depressed, psychologically devastated victim struggling over the shock of this life change and experiencing numerous problems in his or her interpersonal and sexual relationships. Of course, neither stereotype is completely accurate, but both probably contain elements of truth applicable to many people's adjustment to divorce or separation.

Interview and clinical data indicate that divorced individuals must go through a period of adjustment that, at the very least, is difficult and quite often traumatic. After this period, however, the person's life settles down into its own pattern. It is this postadjustment period we are interested in: How do divorced and separated individuals adjust sexually to the new situations?

Not many of the major survey studies have focused on this aspect of sexual life. Hunt (1974) has done the most extensive work of the recent surveys and has also compared his findings to Kinsey's results. In general, Kinsey had found that divorced males and females were engaging in less sexual activity than were married men and women of comparable ages. These individuals also indicated that they were less happy with their sex lives than were married men and women. Hunt found a very different picture 25 years later. He found that 100 percent of the men and 90 percent of the women in his divorced sample had had sexual intercourse in the year prior to the survey. The frequency of intercourse for the divorced males averaged more than twice a week, which was slightly higher than that for the married men in the comparison group. The divorced females were having intercourse on the average of twice a week, which was equal to their married comparison group. However, this rate was four times the rate reported by divorced women in Kinsey's study.

Does this mean that the myth of the gay divorcee is now starting to come true? If we look at the number of partners, there has been a definite increase from the time of Kinsey's survey to the 1970s. The divorced men had a median of eight partners over the year prior to Hunt's survey. This was two to four times higher than the number of partners for premarital single males (who, it should be noted, were much younger as a group than the divorced men). For divorced women the median number of partners over the previous year was four. This was nearly twice the median number of partners of premarital single women. From Hunt's findings it appears that sexual activity was quite a bit higher among divorced people than might have been expected and much higher than previous measures had shown.

The divorced group in Hunt's study also indicated that some of the qualitative dimensions of their sexual lives were better than their marital sexual experiences. Divorced men and women both reported greater variety of sexual arousal techniques and sexual positions, and the women reported higher orgasm rates. Almost all of the divorced subjects rated their current sex lives as "very pleasurable" or "mostly pleasurable." Although they rated their current sexual pleasure as higher than their experiences in marriage, it should be remembered that they were evaluating disintegrating marriages in which they had probably experienced numerous sexual and related problems.

There is also a negative side to all this increased sexual activity. Many of the divorced subjects indicated that there was far less emotional attachment and commitment to their sexual relationships. The interviewees also complained about the difficulties of suddenly finding themselves required to date and engage in various types of courtship behaviors after years of "being out of circulation." They often didn't know the current rules of the game and frequently felt unsure, insecure, and in conflict about their actions. It was not unusual for men to experience occasions of erectile dysfunction as they tried to

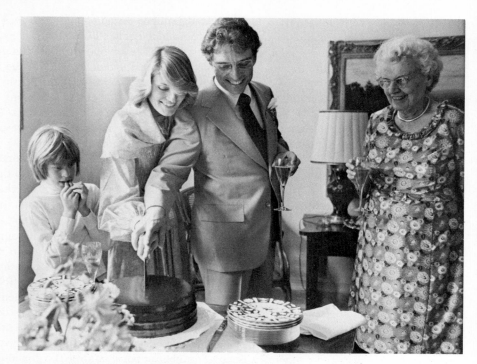

*While divorce
rates are rising, so
are remarriage
rates. Our society
thus remains
primarily one of
married adults
living together.*

have intercourse with new partners whom they perceived as being sexually
more demanding and forward than their wives. For some of the men, the
anxiety and insecurity led to postmarital sexual dysfunctions, which will be
discussed further in Chap. 15.

There is no possible simple summation of the positive and negative features of divorced life as compared to married life. How postmarital individuals
feel about marriage versus singlehood is perhaps best revealed by an interesting
statistic: five out of every six divorced males and three out of four divorced
females eventually remarry.

Widowhood

Widows and widowers are likely to be quite a bit older than divorcees.
Statistically, a person is more likely to lose a marital partner in the later years
than in the early or middle years of life. There is also an imbalance of widows
to widowers of five to one. This complicates the problems of the widowed
woman, since the pool of available men is small relative to the number of
women looking for partners.

There have been no direct studies of the postmarital sexual adjustment of
widows and widowers. This does not mean that they do not have sexual
problems. In fact, the problems for such people may be far more complex than
they are for younger people. It does reflect the fact that our society holds the
view that older people should be nonsexual and that any sexual interest among

the older population is abnormal or immoral (see Chap. 14). Researchers of sexuality appear to have accepted this view, at least as evidenced by their lack of attention to this group. With the increased awareness that sexual interest and activity can continue indefinitely, perhaps there will be greater concern about and interest in the special problems of widowed individuals as they face postmarital sexual adjustment.

VARIATIONS OF MARITAL SEXUAL RELATIONSHIPS

Some special types of sexual relationships related to marital status exist at the outer fringe of our moral structure and cultural traditions and often receive more publicity than more ordinary types of relationships. The publicity is far out of proportion to the rather limited numbers of people actually involved in these arrangements. Yet they deserve our attention in that they explore many of the issues of marriage we have discussed by pushing the marital sexual roles to, and occasionally beyond, their limits. The three types we will explore are open marriages, swinging, and group marriages.

Open marriage

The concept of the **open marriage** was popularized by Nena and George O'Neill and others who followed their ideas. The books *Open Marriage* by the O'Neills (1972) and *The Joys of Open Marriage* by Hecks (1974) are among those that have put forth the concepts and practices of this approach.

The most publicized aspect of open marriage is the option of each partner to have sexual partners other than the spouse. But open marriage is more than just broadened sexual contact. True open marriage includes having real attachments with others besides the marital partner. This takes open marriage beyond sleeping around or having affairs with the spouse's permission. The proponents of open marriage stress the growth of each individual and the value of nonownership of one's partner. They feel that marriage should not be expected to satisfy all of a person's emotional and social needs and that marriage partners should be free to form other deep relationships. According to the O'Neills, love and sex should never be seen as an obligation, which is true of traditional marriages with their guarantees of exclusive sexual privilege of one partner to the other.

Unfortunately, no research that objectively evaluates open marriages is available. The writers in this area are usually participants in such marriages and are intensely partisan and positive. The proponents argue that open marriages are the life-style of the future (Butler, 1979). At present, however, there has been no great movement of people toward this type of marriage.

Swinging

Swinging shares certain features with open marriage, but there are some fundamental differences as well. Basically, swinging is mate swapping for the purpose of recreational sexual intercourse. Typically, swingers attend or host parties of from two to several couples. People may pair off and go to separate rooms; there may be several partner changes in an evening; and sometimes group sex occurs. However, the individuals do not form lasting relationships with their swinging partners. In fact, continued contact is frowned upon and is as much a violation of the swinging subculture's rules as this type of casual sex is a violation of the ideals of open marriage. For swingers, sex is a recreational activity meant to be enjoyed for its own sake and not a vehicle for relationship building or personal growth.

Studies of swinging have yielded some interesting data. Although many different types of couples swing, the most typical are a married, middle-class couple who are quite conventional in other aspects of their lives. The researchers have generally found that swingers derive great satisfaction from their sexual life-style (Gilmartin, 1975). They have a strong belief in what they are doing and desire to have others do it as well (recruitment has some obvious secondary gains for the swinger). Swingers also report an increase in marital happiness as a result of their swinging behavior. Some claim it has saved their faltering marriages. The idea that engaging in sex with others could strengthen the marital bonds is ironic. Some of the features that maintain the marital bond include the fact (1) that the couple does it together (the couple that swings together, stays together), (2) that it provides a variety of partners, (3) that there is no emotional commitment to these outside partners, and (4) that there is no secrecy or lying and, presumably, no one's ego is punctured by being "cheated" on. Some of the proponents feel that swinging functions as a safety valve for the problems most marriages naturally experience from time to time.

The problems caused by swinging are not as visible as the benefits since the casualties of the swinging scene are not readily available for study. Jealousy is a major issue. Despite the fact that both people participate, one partner may feel that his or her possession of the other is slipping away. Another source of friction is for one partner to feel that he or she is being compared unfavorably to outside partners. Also, some of the couples with children indicate concern about what the children would think if they found out. Perhaps the least often stated but most important problem is that one partner may come to feel that this whole view of sexual involvement is distorted. The swingers come together for purely physical, mechanical sex. They often do not know each other as people, and the time constraints do not allow for extensive emotional involvement. For some participants, this nonromantic sexual experience does not meet the need for affectionate sex they may feel is absent from their marriage. Swinging then becomes more of the same kind of unsatisfactory sex that may have sent them into the swinging scene in the first place.

Group marriage

The idea of communal living caught the imagination of young people in the mid-1960s, and many communes were begun in that period. Many had a counterculture theme and were as much political statements of faith in group living as they were a chosen life-style. **Group marriages** differ from communes in many ways, but the most important is that in a group marriage the members make a marital-type commitment to one another. This includes sexual access of all the partners to each other. This differs from most communes, where couples tend to live together within the context of a larger group with whom they share resources and work. The group marriage also implies long-term commitment of all the participants to one another. Because there is no formal legal status to group marriages and there is no recognized status in our society for such marriages, the arrangement is totally dependent on the mutual agreement of the participants.

Research on group marriages is sparse. The only direct studies of group marriages have been done by Constantine and Constantine (1973). They observed group marriages involving young, middle-class individuals of varied educational backgrounds and careers. The groups had usually formed around several pair-bonded couples who came together, pooling their resources and their earnings and sharing all jobs in the household. The children were raised communally. The term **multilateral family** has been used to describe such arrangements.

As one can imagine, such marriages present many problems. Not the least complicated are the sexual arrangements. While it is possible that couples could remain pair-bonded in a multilateral family, the Constantines found that none of them did. All engaged in general sexual behavior with most other opposite-sex members of the group. Many of the groups used a fixed rotation for sexual relations (if this is Tuesday, you must be Fred). Other groups were less structured, and group decisions were made as to who would go where each night. Group sex and orgies were not found to be frequent events. The degree of sexual satisfaction was reported as high and better than participants felt was true of their previous, monogamous relationships.

Problems in the group marriages were less often concentrated on sexual aspects than might be expected. Jealousies and other sex-related issues did occur, but they were ranked third in the listing of problems gathered by the Constantines. The first two major problems were communicating and decision making.

Group marriages solve the problem among swingers of the lack of emotional attachment and meaningfulness in a multipartner sexual life-style. The ideal of the group marriage is for there to be multiple emotional love bonds between the participants. Living together, being concerned with one another, and sexual involvement are all intertwined in a complex matrix. Group marriage participants feel they have the sexual variety of swinging and the intimacies of open marriage. But how capable are people of maintaining intense emotional involvement with several others simultaneously? One factor that may keep some group marriages going is that breaking up implies all the difficulties of monogamous marriage breakup multiplied several times over. Can you imagine the complexities of a group divorce? The Constantines have promised follow-up research on the group marriages they have studied to see how they have survived. As with all these unusual marital arrangements, the future will tell us whether they are viable and valuable alternatives to traditional monogamous marriage.

SUMMARY

1   Marriage is a *mateship:* a formalized, sanctioned, recognized union in society. Sexual relationships outside of the formal mateship arrangements of

a society are called *liaisons*. Whereas mateships play an important role in a society's social structures, liaisons are strictly sexual in nature.

2   Although marriage in American society has seemed to be under attack, traditional marriage continues to be the choice of most men and women. They may be dissatisfied with specific marriages, as shown by high divorce rates, but they still feel marriage is an important institution, as shown by high marriage rates and high remarriage rates after divorce. In fact, *serial monogamy* has become a major trend.

3   *Premarital sex* is a term used by researchers to refer to sexual behavior among those members of society who are below the expected age of marriage. In recent years, premarital sex has become much more accepted in our society, although most people still think such sex should be engaged in only if strong affection exists between the couple.

4   Whereas Kinsey found that 53 percent of men and 20 percent of women had engaged in premarital sex by age 20, the Hunt and *Redbook* studies found that more than 90 percent of men and 80–95 percent of women in the 18–24 age group had engaged in premarital sex. However, this high incidence is not evidence of promiscuity or a casual attitude toward sex. A large majority of those involved in premarital sex have very few partners. Although initial experiences with sex are often negative, sexual experiences among premarital couples become more satisfying and varied with time.

5   *Cohabitation* of unmarried couples is on the increase. The sexual activities of cohabitors appear to be similar to those of newlyweds.

6   Various studies on the frequency of intercourse in marriage have found remarkably similar results. In general, young couples have intercourse 3.25 times a week; couples in the 25–34 age range have intercourse about 3 times a week; and the rate continues to decrease progressively with age.

7   The men in Kinsey's sample spent a median time of 12 minutes in foreplay and 2 minutes in intromission prior to orgasm. Since women need 6–15 minutes of foreplay and another 6–15 minutes of coitus to experience orgasm, the discrepancy in duration times explains Kinsey's findings of low orgasm rates for women during intercourse. However, more recent studies have shown that duration of foreplay and intercourse is increasing.

8   Today's couples appear to be using more varied sexual techniques and more variant coital positions than did the couples of Kinsey's day. Although female orgasm as a measure of the "success" of a couple's sex life has been overemphasized, studies do show that the incidence of female orgasm has increased over the years.

9   Many couples find it difficult to discuss sex and often resort to subtle cues and symbolic language in their efforts to communicate sexual desires. Such poor communication can lead to problems in the couple's sex life.

10   *Extramarital sex*, or *adultery*, is sexual intercourse by a married person with anyone other than his or her spouse. Kinsey's finding that 50 percent of husbands and 26 percent of wives had had extramarital affairs generally holds up today, although incidence figures for women appear to be on the rise.

11   Although extramarital affairs have been romanticized in our society, most affairs tend to be characterized by activities less adventurous than those found in marital sex, to be short-lived, and to consist of relatively few contacts. Furthermore, those who engage in such affairs tend to have few extramarital partners. Some researchers have suggested that affairs may even be

good for a marriage because they lead the person to a reevaluation of the marriage and perhaps greater commitment to it.

12 Divorced people are faced with many adjustment problems, including reassessing themselves as sexual beings. Kinsey found that divorced people engaged in less sexual activity and enjoyed it less than married couples, but Hunt found quite a bit more sexual activity in divorced men and women, who also said their postmarital sex lives were better than their married sex lives. However, many divorcees complained of a lack of attachment and commitment in their postmarital relationships and felt uncomfortable reentering the dating scene.

13 Widows and widowers also face postmarital sexual adjustment, but little research on their problems has been done. Widowed individuals tend to be older than other single people, and widows outnumber widowers five to one.

14 *Open marriage* is a variation on marriage relationships that stresses the growth of each individual and nonownership of one's partner. It therefore allows for extramarital relationships that help meet a partner's emotional needs.

15 *Swinging* is mate swapping for the purpose of recreational sexual intercourse. Unlike open marriage, emotional ties to casual partners are discouraged. Swingers believe that this behavior strengthens their marital bonds. However, swinging can also create problems, such as jealousy and a realization that neither marital sex nor swinging sex is providing the partners with the emotional satisfaction they need.

16 *Group marriages* are made up of men and women who make a long-term commitment to one another. Such marriages have also been called *multilateral families.* They provide both the sexual variety of swinging and the strong emotional attachments of open marriage, but they also are beset with problems of communication, decision making, jealousy, and other sex-related issues.

ADDITIONAL READING

* **Colgrove, Melba; Bloomfield, Harold; and McWilliams, Peter.** How to Survive the Loss of a Love. New York: Bantam, 1977.
   A warm and practical book about overcoming the emotional effects of the end of a love relationship.

Kaplan, Helen S. and Sage, Clifford J. Sexual patterns at different ages. *Medical Aspects of Human Sexuality,* June 1971, pp. 10–23.
   A well-written article on the course of male and female sexual patterns over the life span. Nontechnical, easy to ready.

* **Murstein, Bernard (Ed.).** Exploring Intimate Lifestyles. New York: Springer, 1978.
   A series of essays by different authors on different types of adult intimate and sexual relationships. Covers a wide range of alternatives.

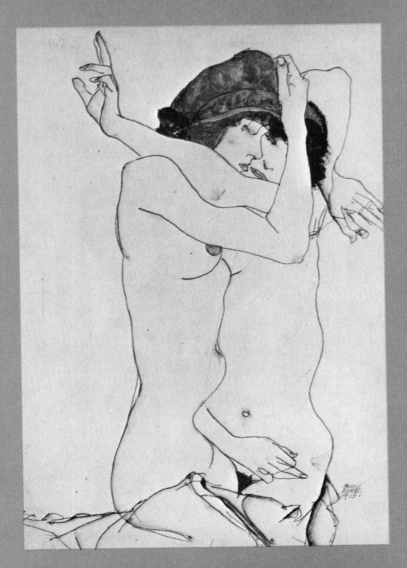

Homosexuality: An alternative sexual orientation

13

chapter
13

Aristotle. Alexander the Great. Leonardo da Vinci. King James I. Lord Byron. Queen Christina of Sweden. Hans Christian Andersen. Walt Whitman. Emily Dickinson. Marcel Proust. John Maynard Keynes. Gertrude Stein. Lawrence of Arabia. Dag Hammarskjold. Noel Coward. Virginia Woolf. These and many other famous men and women—monarchs, artists, politicians, writers, philosophers, composers—are known to have been homosexual or bisexual (Wallechinsky and Wallace, 1975). Some lived in societies where their homosexuality was accepted or ignored; others lived their homosexual lives in secret. But all made major contributions that live on today.

Obviously, homosexuality did not prevent these people from being productive members of their societies (although society may have prevented many of them from openly expressing their sexual preferences). In a few cases, societal repression may actually have contributed to their creative pursuits. But for the most part, it is difficult to distinguish the lives of these celebrated people from those of famous heterosexuals. Whatever their sexual preferences, socially approved or disapproved, they pursued their muses and careers, became leaders and innovators, and left lasting impressions on society.

In this chapter we will see that homosexuality in contemporary society is a complex issue. Homosexuals today are subject to both greater acceptance and greater rejection than in the past and continue to be misunderstood by the rest of society. We will be discussing this dichotomy in contemporary attitudes toward gays as well as the prevalence of homosexuality in American society. We will examine homosexual behavior and theories of homosexuality in order to try to dispel some of the myths about this sexual orientation. And throughout we will emphasize that, like heterosexuals, homosexuals are people who lead ordinary lives and for whom sexuality is just one aspect they must deal with and integrate into their way of functioning in the world.

ATTITUDES TOWARD HOMOSEXUALITY

Our society is struggling through a period of conflict and change in its view of homosexuality. In the United States, sexual attraction to members of one's own sex has been viewed as unnatural, as a sin, and as a mental disorder. Not only have people's feelings about homosexuality been generally negative, but they also have been very intense. In fact, few topics in the study of human sexual behavior arouse as much emotion as does homosexuality.

The upheaval in our views of homosexuality is the result of the interaction of numerous moral, legal, political, religious, psychological, economic, and social forces—probably too many to ever be totally disentangled. Civil rights and political power struggles have led to highly publicized confrontations, of which there are likely to be more. All this activity would seem to indicate that attitudes about homosexuality are in transition. The results cannot be easily predicted, but the changes will determine how we will eventually view homosexuality and the level of acceptance homosexuals are likely to experience in society.

Are people's attitudes toward homosexuality less negative than they were a decade or two ago? An initial impression of current attitudes might indicate a liberalization of views. As a society, we like to point to the negative attitudes and punitive laws of past decades as evidence that today we are more accepting of homosexual behavior. We note the exploration of homosexual themes in magazines, in films, on television, and in other media as evidence of our movement toward greater understanding. The increased visibility of homosexuals in our society—in gay demonstrations and parades, gay marriages, and gay bars—is similarly used as an indication that attitudes have become more accepting.

While there may indeed have been some softening of attitudes in a more positive direction, there have also been sharp negative reactions to this movement. Deeply held negative feelings about homosexuality exist in a sizable portion of the population. The popular appeal of antigay movements such as Anita Bryant's Save Our Children Foundation is surprisingly strong. In many communities hard-won gains in legislation of homosexual rights have all too quickly been reversed by public referendums. While gay demonstrations in cities like New York and San Francisco may be more visible in the media, the reaction of the rest of the country may be much more important in the long run. The attitudes of the "silent majority" appear to reflect a far less accepting stand toward homosexual behavior in general and homosexual life-styles in particular than popular media might lead us to believe. In fact, the highly publicized liberalization of attitudes and laws may be causing a quiet, but more pervasive, backlash that is just now being felt. What we may actually be experiencing is a *polarization* of attitudes rather than a liberalization. Thus, our society may be moving toward both positive and negative extremes on the issue of homosexuality.

The research on attitudes toward homosexuality does indicate some deeply held negative feelings. Levitt and Klassen (1974) used interview data from a nationwide representative sample of 3018 adults to arrive at some figures on the acceptability of homosexuality in the United States (see Table 13.1). Close

TABLE 13.1 *Moral attitudes (in percentages)*	*What is your opinion of sex acts between two people of the same sex when they:*	
	Have no special affection for each other?	Love each other?
Always wrong	77.7	70.2
Almost always wrong	8.4	8.4
Wrong only sometimes	6.3	7.2
Not wrong at all	5.6	11.4
Don't know	1.6	2.2
No answer	0.1	0.3
Total percent	99.7	99.7
Total sample	3018	3018

Source: Adapted from Levitt and Klassen (1974), p. 30.

to 80 percent of this sample thought it is always wrong for same-sex people to engage in sexual activities with each other, and 60 percent disapproved of actions by state legislators to decriminalize sex acts between people of the same sex. Most of those questioned would deny homosexuals jobs in teaching, law, the ministry, and other influential or sensitive positions. The majority felt that homosexuals are dangerous to children and that their acts are "vulgar and obscene," and over 80 percent indicated they would rather not associate with homosexual individuals. These findings differ little from similar surveys of the 1960s. An even more recent survey by Nyberg and Alston (1977) showed that 72 percent still believed that homosexual relationships are "always wrong."

These negative feelings have surfaced in the organized opposition to homosexuals demonstrated by the recent antigay rights crusades sponsored by various conservative and religious groups. They have reversed many of the changes that the gay rights groups have been able to effect in laws that discriminated against homosexuals. They have been able to get out the vote because antigay feelings seem to run deep in our society and are easily tapped by groups expressing these negative views. Such negative feelings are similar to the neurotic reactions psychologists call *phobias*. In fact, the term *homophobia* has been applied to this type of irrational reaction to homosexuals.

Our society shows many indications of **homophobia**—deeply felt fears and anxieties about homosexuality. It is not only on formal questionnaires that people indicate their disapproval of this sexual orientation. Homosexuals are discriminated against in a wide variety of ways, both obvious and subtle. Dishonorable discharges from the armed services, arrests for a variety of "victimless crimes," housing discrimination, loss of jobs and promotions, and dismissal from schools are just a few of the abuses heaped on homosexual individuals.

Our language regarding homosexuality is also highly derogatory: fruit, swish, dyke, fag, fairy, pansy, lesbo, homo, queer, and queen are just a few of the printable names applied to gays. The stereotypes of what homosexuals look and act like are equally negative and derogatory.

Such antagonistic attitudes and feelings have all too frequently resulted in violence toward homosexuals. It is considered great entertainment in many parts of the country for teenagers to spend an evening looking for homosexuals to beat up. Others prey off gays by luring them into sexual encounters only to rob and assault them. Gays do not fare much better with the legal authorities in many communities. If they complain about a crime, they are likely to find themselves in jail, with the criminal complaining that the victim solicited *him*. Police vice squads are active in arresting homosexuals through contacts in public places or in raids on gay bars and other meeting places. The arrested homosexual is then often subject to brutal handling by the police and by other prisoners.

What is the source of the deep feelings of fear, hate, and anger that support such actions toward homosexuals? The negative cultural view, as it has evolved from our Judeo-Christian heritage, is learned early. We are taught that

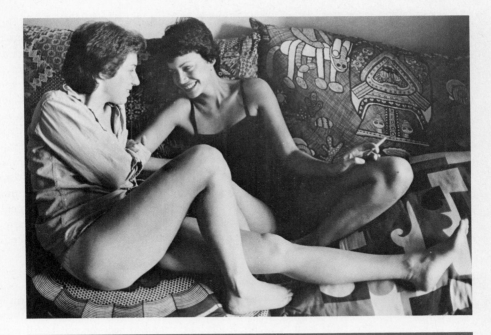

As we lift the cloud from homosexual relationships, we can see how closely they parallel those of heterosexual couples.

homosexual behavior is wrong and sinful. Added to this early conditioning is the fact that we receive very little actual information about homosexuality while growing up. This allows the myths to become stronger, with no disconfirming information. Since homosexuals themselves tend to stay hidden from public view, they are not known to us as actual people. What we know and believe are the stereotypes about homosexuals and their behavior. Among the stereotypes are the notions that homosexuals engage in bizarre sexual acts, that they seduce young children at every opportunity, that they are sadomasochists, that many are insane mass murderers, that they exist in a gay world of drugs and constant sex, and that they are at the very least neurotic but more likely seriously emotionally disturbed. Other stereotypes, while less fearsome, are equally distorted. These include the ideas that homosexual men are effeminate and work as hairdressers and interior decorators, while homosexual women are masculine in appearance and manner, work in men's jobs, are angry toward "real" men, and are "women's lib types."

Other sources of homophobia have been ascribed to subtle psychological factors within the heterosexual person. It has been suggested that for some, the homophobia is a projected fear of their own homosexual impulses. Similarly, it has been proposed that some people are reacting to repressed envy of the imagined sexual freedom of the gay life-style.

All of these issues are involved in individual and collective distrust of homosexuals, even for those of us who consider ourselves quite liberal on this issue. These attitudes and the intense feelings that accompany them are similar to racism or sexism in how deeply ingrained and unconscious they are. When gay groups take organized action, these strong feelings are all too easily aroused. However, unlike the situation of racial hatreds, there are few moral voices in the community saying that the hatred itself is wrong and unacceptable. In a discussion of public attitudes toward homosexuality, Tripp (1974) noted, "The truth is that almost nobody is very liberated." The various homosexual action groups have been very naive in not realizing the depth of the general public's negative feelings toward homosexuality. In attempting to counter such homophobia, it is important to help the public toward real knowledge about homosexuality. Hatred toward any group thrives on lack of knowledge. Debunking the myths and showing the essential human condition of people struggling with their adaptation to the world brings a greater acceptance of the supposedly deviant group when it is shown to be more similar than different. This chapter is devoted to the goal of making the reader aware of the realities of the homosexual orientation.

THE HOMOSEXUAL LABEL

The names and labels we apply to people become the basis of how we respond to them. In effect, the categories we place people in form our stereotype of how we expect them to behave. The labels we place on ourselves also affect our own behavior. Such labels tend to become self-fulfilling prophecies.

The label *homosexual* has a strong impact on how one is viewed and on one's self-perception. The word *homosexual*, by itself and devoid of any extra meanings, refers only to men and women who are sexually aroused by and prefer to achieve sexual gratification with a person of their own sex. The label *homosexual*, however, goes far beyond just the sexual preferences of the person. It carries implications for every aspect of the person's character, behavior, and life-style. The label evokes all the stereotyped images the listener has learned about homosexuals. It takes us beyond the simple statement of sexual preferences to a description of the person and everything about him or her. The sociologist would note that at this point we have moved from labeling the *act* or behavior to labeling the *actor*.

While labels can create many problems, they also help us organize the world so that we can communicate effectively. Because of the problem of labels in the study of homosexuality, it is important that the terminology we use be clearly defined. In this book, the term **homosexuals** refers to those *adults* of *either* sex who are sexually attracted to and prefer to achieve sexual gratification with members of their own sex. **Heterosexuals** are adults who are sexually attracted to and prefer to achieve sexual gratification with members of the opposite sex. We are applying the term *homosexual* to both males and females, using the Greek meaning for the root word *homo*, which means "same," in contrast to *hetero*, which means "different." (Some apply the term *homosexual* to males only, using the Latin root meaning "man"; they would then use the word **lesbian** for female homosexuality. We will use both *homosexual* and *lesbian* in reference to females.)

In our definition of homosexuality we refer to both psychological orientation and overt sexual behavior. Both components should be present. We also add the qualifier "adult" to exclude the same-sex attachments and sexual experimentation that commonly occur among adolescents.

Transsexualism and *transvestism* are two labels that are sometimes confused with homosexuality. **Transsexuals** are individuals who feel they are really of the opposite gender from their biological sex. They feel they have been put in the wrong body and seek to change to the opposite sex. They may seek out sex-change surgery to realize their goal. Thus, a biological male will feel that he is really a woman and wants to be and to function as a biological female. He is attracted to men sexually but does not consider himself homosexual since he is "really" a heterosexual woman. **Transvestites** derive sexual pleasure from dressing in the clothing of the opposite sex but do not necessarily prefer same-sex partners for sexual experiences. Both of these variations are discussed in further detail in later chapters.

THE PREVALENCE OF HOMOSEXUALITY

Does homosexuality occur in all cultures throughout the world? Does it occur in other animals? These questions are of more than just passing interest. For a behavior sometimes described as unnatural, or even more forcefully as an "abomination against nature," the answers become useful in trying to understand more about the "naturalness" of homosexuality.

Ford and Beach (1951) directly explored the question of whether homosexuality occurs in a large number of human social groups. Of the 76 societies for which they could obtain data, 49 (64 percent) showed evidence of homosexual activity of various types and degrees. These were societies in which there was a socially acceptable role for homosexual behavior for certain people or specific time periods. The remaining 27 societies did not show any type of homosexuality. Because homosexuality was viewed negatively in these cultures, it was not possible for Ford and Beach to learn whether homosexuality was totally absent or whether it was simply being practiced "underground."

In those societies in which homosexual behavior was reported, there was often a social role for the homosexual. In some groups, the homosexual individual lived totally as a member of the opposite sex. In others, there were special religious or magical powers attached to the role, and being a homosexual often elevated the individual to high status. In most of these societies, homosexuals were primarily men. The dominant behavioral expression was anal intercourse for the males and mutual clitoral stimulation for the females.

Among subhuman species, the primates show the clearest examples of homosexual behavior. Monkeys and apes have been observed engaging in a variety of homosexual behaviors (Chevalier-Skolnikoff, 1974; Gordon and Bernstein, 1973). These behaviors are relatively infrequent, however. No individual animals have been found to be exclusively homosexual, and almost all show heterosexual preferences when presented with the appropriate stimuli. Some of the male sexual displays seem to be more related to establishing dominance within the group rather than to purely sexual relations.

The question of just how many people in the United States are homosexual is difficult to answer. Kinsey's (1948) findings are the most frequently cited. That study indicated that 37 percent of males had at least one experience of a homosexual nature leading to orgasm at some time after puberty or in their adult lives. But is this evidence for homosexuality? By our definition, one or only a few homosexual experiences (especially prior to adulthood) should not be considered a homosexual orientation. Occasional homosexual experiences may be examples of **transient homosexuality** if the person's predominant orientation is heterosexual.

Gagnon and Simon (1967) reexamined Kinsey's data and found that only 6 percent of the males reported having several homosexual experiences after age 20, and only 3 percent considered themselves to be exclusively homosexual. These figures are consistent with the data for women: 6–8 percent of the female respondents in Kinsey's (1953) study had several homosexual experiences, and 2–3 percent considered themselves exclusively homosexual. Some contemporary studies indicate that there has been little change in these incidence figures from the 1940s to the 1980s despite large changes in most other types of sexual behavior.

An overall summary of current incidence figures shows that approximately 80 percent of men and women consider themselves to be exclusively heterosexual (though many of them have had a few homosexual experiences at some time). Approximately 2–3 percent of all men and 1–2 percent of women consider themselves exclusively homosexual. The remaining 17–19 percent of the population have engaged in varying amounts of homosexual behavior or have considered themselves homosexual for short periods of time.

Between the extremes of those who are exclusively heterosexual and those who are exclusively homosexual fall a large number of people who have varying degrees of interest in homosexual behavior. In observing this fact, Kinsey (1948) suggested that there is a *continuum* of sexual interest. He proposed using a 7-point scale, with 0 representing those who are exclusively heterosexual and 6 representing those who are exclusively homosexual. Between these extremes are several gradations of involvement with members of the same sex. The Kinsey scale is particularly valuable in supporting the view that sexual orientation is not a dichotomy; that is, homosexuality is not something one is or is not but a sexual orientation that can be felt or expressed in degrees.

On the Kinsey **sexual orientation continuum,** the middle range designates those individuals who are attracted in varying degrees to members of their own and of the opposite sex. A score of 3, for example, should be given to a person who finds both sexes equally attractive. Such people are termed **bisexuals.**

In some ways the identity problems of bisexuals are even more complex than those of homosexuals. Since our society tends to think in terms of sexual orientation dichotomously, bisexuals often feel that they should commit themselves to one orientation or the other. They are criticized by both homosexual and heterosexual cultures and find themselves unwelcome in both. Support groups are much more difficult for the bisexual person to find. Bisexual groups exist in only a few large urban areas; thus, most bisexuals remain closeted from both the heterosexual and homosexual communities.

Comfort for the bisexual is dependent on society's awareness of the plasticity and flexibility of sexual orientation. This enlightened view, if held more generally, would lead to greater social acceptance of bisexuality and, more important, to greater self-acceptance of this orientation.

The development of a homosexual orientation starts with a process of self-awareness of homosexual feelings and a labeling of oneself as homosexual. Those who enter the homosexual community begin with this self-labeling. Actual entrance into the gay community is called the *"coming-out" process.*

When and how does a person make this kind of identity statement? Dank (1971) gathered data on this subject from a large number of homosexual men. Gagnon and Simon (1967, 1973) interviewed a smaller group of female homosexuals. Jay and Young's *The Gay Report* (1980) and the *Spada Report* (1979), both large-scale surveys of homosexuals, included questions about the coming-out process.

Most of the data reported in these studies suffer from a subject selection bias that we must keep in mind as we review the findings. Most subjects were contacted through sources such as gay rights groups, homosexual organizations and clubs, and homosexual magazines and radio programs in large cities. In the Jay and Young study, the questionnaires were even handed out at a homosexual meeting place at a rest stop on a major interstate highway in the Northeast. Thus, most of the respondents were people who were active and involved in the homosexual subculture. It seems reasonable to assume that most of the respondents in the studies were more active in their homosexual roles than those who did not get contacted or who did not choose to be subjects. However, with these sampling drawbacks in mind, we can still derive some insights from the results of these studies.

With regard to the process of coming out, all of the studies found that awareness of one's homosexual orientation came slowly and with much doubt and conflict. Subjects reported early, vague feelings of being "different." There were frequent reports of unfocused attraction to same-sex peers or adults that was experienced as confusing or embarrassing. There may even have been one or two homosexual encounters that were not labeled as such by the participants. Since almost all of the subjects had acquired the usual negative attitudes toward homosexuality, their last thought was that they themselves might be homosexual. The point where this thought did enter consciousness was almost always a time of psychological crisis.

The patterns of homosexual self-awareness for males were found to be different from those for females. For most males, the average age of awareness was in early adolescence, with the majority indicating the ages of 13–15 as the pivotal time. For females, the average age of awareness was more likely to be early adulthood. Jay and Young (1980) found a mean age for women of 29.6;

however, this seems somewhat distorted by the fact that their study included several women who didn't become aware of their homosexual interest until their middle and later years—one woman was 60 when she made this discovery.

The respondents reported that their initial homosexual experience was extremely stressful. However, they indicated that the physical pleasure they experienced in that first encounter was quite high. Many reported stumbling into their first encounter with little planning but with quite a bit of prior fantasy. This gave it a "dream-come-true" quality. For most of the men and women, their initial reaction at being involved in a homosexual encounter was embarrassment, quickly followed by a feeling of the essential correctness of what was happening. This was reported to be an important feeling in providing support for their emergence as a homosexual.

One stereotype that proved not to be true is the general belief that older homosexuals initiate young people into a homosexual orientation. Neither the male nor female accounts of initial experiences contained frequent involvement with older homosexuals. Most of the early contacts were reported to be with peers. The Spada study (1979) found that 62 percent of men had their first experience with a same-sex friend before the age of 14. The relative lack of the adult homosexual seducer in these reports invalidates the arguments of the antigay groups that homosexuality should be outlawed to protect children from the clutches of the adult homosexual. Anita Bryant's Save Our Children Foundation and similar antigay groups appear to be built on this mythical fear.

Coming out in one's own eyes was not automatically followed by coming-out publicly. In fact, most of the homosexuals never did go completely public but instead lived as homosexuals in part of their lives and simply allowed others to assume they were heterosexual in the remainder. About half of the respondents indicated they had never told their families about their homosexuality. Colleagues and co-workers were similarly uninformed. Some had never told anyone except their immediate partners. Dank (1971) refers to this group as the **closet queens** and feels that they are the ones experiencing the greatest difficulty with their homosexual orientation. Basically, they view their homosexuality as unacceptable but are driven to it by their sexual needs. The result is a self-loathing because of their sexual activities. These individuals experienced the most conflict of the homosexual sample and were the most likely to present themselves for treatment to change their orientation.

The subjects in these studies consisted of individuals who were actively homosexual. There are few data on those who go through a crisis of questioning their sexual orientation but eventually reject homosexuality. We know from other sources (Kinsey, 1954, for example) that many people go through transient homosexuality. How these individuals resolve their conflicts remains unknown. Do they remain concerned about their orientation? Does the existence of the label **latent homosexual** forever plague them with doubts? Coming out seems to force a dichotomous decision; that is, one must choose either homosexuality or heterosexuality. With increasing knowledge may come a more realistic appraisal of these early experiences and less concern about being of one orientation or the other. By most current definitions, a person who experiments with same-sex relations once or twice is not considered homosexual and such a person should not feel that these experiences have determined his or her future sexual orientation.

Most people know very little about the actual sexual behavior of homosexuals. While much has been written about the gay life-style, little has been mentioned of gay sexual practices. Without knowledge, we tend to fill in the gaps with visions of fantastic and strange sexual behaviors. We also lack knowledge of how homosexuals relate to each other and thus have developed myths and stereotypes about gay relationships.

Because our misconceptions and ignorance tend to create an even wider gap between nonhomosexual society and the homosexual subculture, it is important to demystify these areas. And the best way to do so is to learn the facts about homosexual practices and relationships. In this section we will describe what is known about the sexual practices, sex roles, levels of sexual activity, number of partners, long-term relationships, and special problems of homosexuals. Because male and female patterns differ somewhat, we will describe them separately.

Male patterns of homosexuality

Despite the myths that indicate vast differences in the sexual practices of homosexuals and heterosexuals, the practices of homosexual men are not really unusual. In most cases their sexual practices are exactly the same as those used by heterosexuals, with the obvious exception of vaginal-penile contact. However, the lack of that sexual act means only that orgasm must be achieved with other kinds of stimulation.

Sexual practices All of the major surveys have gathered information on sexual practices. There is general agreement on the nature of the sexual activities and the relative popularity of each. Ranked in order of frequency, the most popular practices are: fellatio (mouth-genital contact), mutual masturbation through manual stimulation, anal intercourse, body rubbing, and interfemoral stimulation (inserting the penis between the thighs of the partner).

These techniques are performed exactly as they would be in heterosexual lovemaking. And, just as with heterosexual couples, there are individual and couple preferences, so that particular activities are included or excluded in any particular encounter. One of the myths about homosexual men is that they engage in various sexual techniques for arousal but always achieve orgasm through anal intercourse. This is not supported by the descriptions given by homosexual men. In one study only 11 percent said they achieved orgasm through anal intercourse. This mistaken idea arises quite naturally as an extension of the heterosexual lovemaking script, in which other sources of stimulation always serve as preliminaries to penile insertion in the vagina for the final climax. The lack of that possibility in homosexual men does not mean they substitute anal intercourse for vaginal intercourse. In fact, homosexual men do not seem to have any set sequence in their sexual script, and they achieve orgasm in any of a variety of ways.

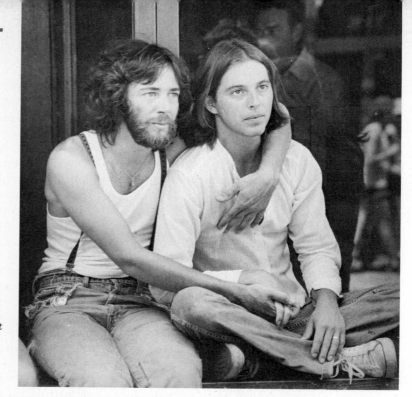

Care, concern, support, and love are as much a part of homosexual relationships as they are of heterosexual relationships.

Another distortion of homosexual behavior in our society is caused by focusing attention on orgasm and forgetting that lovemaking occurs in as elaborate a fashion as it does for heterosexuals. Undressing each other, kissing, pillow talk, fondling, hugging, and mutual stimulation alternating with periods of relaxation are all part of the sexual behavior of gay men. It is this part of homosexual behavior that the general public has the greatest difficulty imagining and accepting. But as Masters and Johnson (1979) have reported, homosexual couples may have more satisfying sexual foreplay with greater arousal than do heterosexual couples.

Accurate description of homosexual behaviors was one of the goals of a study by Bell and Weinberg (1978). Their questionnaire asked homosexual men whether they had engaged in any of a long list of sexual activities over the previous 12 months. On the average, the men indicated that they had engaged in 5 or more activities from the list. In order of decreasing incidence, these activities were: fellatio of their partner, fellatio by their partner, masturbation by their partner, masturbation of their partner, performing anal intercourse, having anal intercourse performed on them, and body rubbing.

Which activities do homosexuals enjoy most? According to the *Spada Report* (1979), 88 percent enjoyed giving fellatio; 90 percent enjoyed receiving fellatio; and 77 percent enjoyed anal intercourse (no distinction was made between giving and receiving). When asked, "Do you enjoy affection during sex?" 90 percent replied positively. In response to the question, "How do you most often reach orgasm?" 53 percent indicated masturbation, 11 percent anal intercourse, and 10 percent fellatio. However, 24 percent simply said, "It varies," which supports the observation that much of homosexual behavior is unstructured.

The lack of a single way of experiencing orgasm is logical if one remembers that there is no prior socially determined script for the "right way" to participate in homosexual behavior. In addition, no particular sexual practice has an anatomical advantage over any other, and, of course, reproductive advantage is not an issue. Thus, choice is more likely to be determined by the personal preferences of the individuals.

Sex roles What sex roles do male partners play? Is one man submissive and the other dominant? Is one more masculine in behavior and the other more feminine? Is one the initiator and the other the responder? These questions are valid to the extent that the heterosexual script for sex-role behavior can be applied to homosexual lovemaking. The question of sex roles also relates to other aspects of the relationship. Does one man wear the pants and the other wear the apron?

Psychoanalytic theory suggests that the personality development problems that produce a homosexual orientation would lead to a predominantly masculine or predominantly feminine type of homosexual, depending on the timing and nature of the developmental conflict. Bieber and others (1962), for example, proposed that there are two types of homosexual men: the **inserter** and the **insertee.** The inserter represents the active partner, while the insertee is the receiver. The perfect homosexual couple would consist of both types. Once again we see the attempt to find a parallel to heterosexual relationships.

Harry and DeVall (1978) studied this proposed division of roles in homosexual couples and could find no support for such differences. Most of the men varied their roles, sometimes being more active, sometimes more passive. Furthermore, these researchers found that interpersonal dominance-submission patterns were unrelated to the sex roles during sex. Research conducted by Peplau (1981) arrived at similar conclusions.

Levels of sexual activity The sexual activity of homosexual men has alternately been described as being far more frequent than that of heterosexual men and far less frequent. Several of the recent studies have addressed this issue. Bell and Weinberg (1978) asked their subjects how often they had had sex each week during the previous year. Approximately half the men indicated a frequency of two to three times per week. The rest of the subjects ranged about equally above and below this figure. This frequency is approximately the same as that reported for heterosexual men in the same age groups. Bell and Weinberg concluded that the homosexual men could not be characterized as either sexually hyperactive or underactive.

Number of partners, impersonal sex, and cruising A common stereotype of male homosexuals is that their lives consist of an unending series of fleeting relationships. All of the various studies found this stereotype to be true to some extent. While figures vary slightly from study to study, most researchers have found that homosexual males experience sex with a large number of partners and that their lifetime average number of partners is much higher than that of heterosexual men.

Homosexual men indicate that they seek out and are sought out by others for sexual encounters several times a month. Most of these encounters are one-night stands. The men contact each other at parties, social gatherings, gay bars, Turkish baths, public parks, men's rooms, and other such locations. The places of likely contact are widely known in the homosexual community.

The searching for partners is called **cruising.** This term refers to the finding of a partner, mutual evaluation, and communication of the desire for sex. Cruising is an important feature of male homosexual life that differs greatly from both heterosexual and lesbian practices. It is often viewed by nonhomosexuals, and even by many homosexuals themselves, as being promiscuous and devoid of warm human contact. Although gay men are divided on whether such sexual encounters are debasing, all agree that they are a fact of gay life.

The *Spada Report* (1979) and the Bell and Weinberg (1978) study further suggest that cruising is increasing with today's increased sexual freedom, the more open display of homosexuality, and decreased concern about police entrapment.

As an indication of just how extensive cruising is, Bell and Weinberg found that 80 percent of the men reported more than half of their partners to be complete strangers, mostly one-night stands. When Spada asked gays whether they enjoyed one-night stands, 53 percent said yes; 30 percent said no; and 12 percent said sometimes. In the majority of cases, then, the impersonal sexual experience was evaluated positively.

There is no one explanation for the predominance of impersonal sex in homosexual males. It has been argued that all men prefer quick and immediate biological sexual gratification, so when two men get together to satisfy their needs, the sex tends to be impersonal. A similar argument is that men in our society are socialized to try to get sex whenever they can. Without the constraints of heterosexual scripts, men simply engage in free and easy sexual encounters. There is no virginity issue, no dating requirements prior to intimacy, no pregnancy scare, no worry over ruining someone's "reputation." In fact, there is no script, and the impersonal sex seems to have evolved to fill the role of a homosexual script. Some of this behavior may have arisen from the problems of being homosexual in an unaccepting society. In addition, the need to hide one's identity, which many homosexuals still do, would support impersonal encounters with no continuing relationship.

It has also been proposed that this is the type of sex that heterosexual men and women would actually prefer but avoid because of social sanctions. *Fear of Flying*, the best-seller by Erica Jong, owes much of its popularity to its introduction of the "zipless fuck"—basically impersonal sex that could occur instantaneously and with no emotional commitment. According to this approach, homosexuals, freed as they are of the usual social constraints, are actually living the life all would choose if they were free to do so. The current heterosexual singles scene, in fact, shows many parallels to the homosexual cruising scene.

The behavior of male homosexuals does show a high frequency of impersonal sex with a large number of partners. However, several of the investigators have pointed out that this does not mean the sexual interactions are without affection and feeling. Some of the qualitative descriptions given in the various interviews indicate warm, tender, and deeply felt interrelationships. Some, in fact, do become long-lasting relationships. On the other side of the coin, many of the men describe cruising as the source of some of the more unpleasant and difficult aspects of gay life. Robberies, extortion, blackmail, beatings, and epidemic venereal disease are part of the price of this style of sexual interaction.

Long-term relationships   Not all homosexuals engage in a cruising life-style. Some never do, and most others stop at various times to engage in longer-lasting intense relationships with another man—an "affair." Some partnerships can be likened to heterosexual marriage, with a sense of total commitment of the two men to each other.

Among the various survey respondents, it was found that long-time relationships were highly desired but less frequently achieved than an unattached life. The *Spada Report* found that to the question "Do you have a lover?" 52 percent of respondents answered no; 41 percent said yes; and the remainder did not answer. Of the group that had lovers, 60 percent lived with their partners. Most interesting, however, is the fact that 88 percent said yes when asked "Would you like to have a lover?" It seems clear that while only a minority achieve long-lasting relationships, many more would like to be in this situation.

Given the desire for such relationships, why is there not more frequent pair bonding among homosexual men? Recall from Chap. 10 that complementarity (the matching of differences) is an important component in maintaining long-term relationships. Since two men are likely to have many of the same needs, skills, interests, and so on, Tripp (1974) has argued that it is the high degree of similarity between men that makes gay relationships unstable.

The cruising life-style is also a poor training ground for learning how to live in a long-term relationship. The social values of this life-style give little importance to commitment and to maintaining relationships. The social standing of the man in the gay community is based on his number of partners and his attractiveness as a pickup, not on the longevity of his interactions.

Finally, a more subtle factor working against long-term gay relationships is that two men living together are immediately suspected of being homosexual by the nonhomosexual community. To avoid the social sanctions that come with the label of *homosexual*, many men choose not to live together. In effect, the negative public attitudes toward gay relationships inadvertently help maintain the less socially acceptable cruising life-style.

Despite the many factors that hamper long-term relationships, many exist. Bell and Weinberg (1978) found several long-term pairs within their sample.

They referred to these pairs as **close-coupled homosexuals.** They described these relationships as being very similar to heterosexual marriages. Most of the couple's life gratifications were found in each other, and their lives revolved around the home. They were the best-adjusted group in the larger study. They had fewer sexual problems, less regret about their homosexuality, and more happiness with their lives in general.

Bell and Weinberg also identified gay pairs that they called **open-coupled homosexuals.** This group contained men who lived together but who had not made the same degree of commitment to their partners as close-coupled homo- sexuals. They sought sexual and emotional gratification both in and outside the relationship and thus were still doing considerable cruising. In general adjustment, they were slightly better off than the nonconnected homosexuals but had more problems than the close-coupled ones. Thus, it appears that the stability of long-term relationships is associated with better psychological ad- justment.

Special problems of male homosexuals Homosexual men have many of the same sexual problems as heterosexual men as well as a few that are special to their situation. Sexual dysfunctions (erectile problems, premature ejacula- tion, and so on) occur frequently. However, sex therapists who are willing or able to work with homosexuals are few and far between. Many therapists consider homosexuality to be an illness and want to change their clients into heterosexuals.

Aging is an important issue for some men. After all, the life-style of the homosexual man requires a high level of sexual responsiveness, and the slow- ing down that results from aging takes its toll on the gay male. Aging can also erode the attractiveness and energy that are highly valued commodities in a cruising life-style. In some of the early studies, aging homosexual males de- scribed themselves negatively, and the researchers generalized that looking old was one of the greatest fears of the male homosexual. However, Weinberg and Williams (1974) found that this was not true in their sample: "Contrary to popular beliefs, our older homosexuals are no worse off than our younger homosexuals on various psychological dimensions and are, on some dimen- sions, better off." Aging in homosexuals is discussed in further detail in Chap. 14.

We have mentioned that venereal disease is rampant among homosexual males. It is, in fact, of epidemic proportions in this group. Several factors combine to make this problem difficult to control. The variety of partners is certainly a major factor, but if the infections did not exist in the group, numbers would not matter. VD is high because it is not adequately controlled. The embarrassment and realistic fear of admitting to homosexuality keeps some men from getting treatment when they should. Furthermore, the cruising life of impersonal sex makes it almost impossible to trace the source or the further contacts of someone who does come for treatment. In some states, admitting to homosexual practices amounts to confessing to a crime, which further reduces the likelihood that the infected man will want to present himself to public health authorities. If control over VD in the gay community is to be gained, legal protections and privacy must be guaranteed.

Although researchers have found many similarities between homosexual men and women, there are some distinct differences.

Sexual practices   As is the case with gay men, homosexual activities between female partners are more ordinary in reality than in the straight world's fantasies. One respondent in the Hite (1976) survey answered the question of how women relate physically with the statement, "Basically, the same things a man and woman can do without a penis and *usually don't!*"

Lesbians point out that sexual technique is far less important than the quality of the experience together. The actual sexual practices are only important in the context of lovemaking. Hugging, kissing, caressing, and touching are the main forms of physical expression. The three techniques used most frequently to produce orgasm are mutual masturbation, cunnilingus, and tribadism. Mutual masturbation between women involves light manual stimulation of the clitoris and labia, and penetration of the vagina. Cunnilingus involves stimulation of the same structures and the surrounding areas by the tongue of the partner. *Tribadism* is body rubbing in which one woman lies on top of the other and they move against each other, mutually stimulating each other's clitoris. The surveys show that lesbians rank the *frequency* of the methods used as masturbation first, cunnilingus second, and tribadism third. The *preference* of the women, however, is cunnilingus first, then masturbation and tribadism.

These methods do not exhaust all the possibilities, of course. As we noted for male homosexuals, there is no set sexual script to follow, and the absence of penile insertion for orgasm leaves the partners freer to improvise. (Interestingly, the use of a *dildo*—a penis substitute—is rare among lesbians.) Lesbians indicate that a female partner is much more aware of what would feel good than were the male partners they have had and is therefore better able to produce sexual excitement. Once again, the couples form their own scripts and tend to individualize their procedures with practice.

One aspect of lesbian interaction that differs from that of heterosexuals and male homosexuals is the amount of time spent in sexual stimulation. Lesbians report long time periods of mutual pleasuring, with far less attention paid to orgasm. There is more emphasis on the excitement phase of sex, and several orgasms may occur at different times during a single lovemaking session. Lesbian women also report that they prefer sequential—your turn, my turn—stimulation to simultaneous mutual stimulation.

Sex roles   The commonly held image of the lesbian couple is that one partner is a pseudomale figure, sometimes called a *butch* or a *dyke,* and that other is a more female type, called a *femme.* These two are presumed to play out the stereotypical heterosexual relationship, with the butch dominating, initiating, and directing behavior and the femme being passive and feminine and the receiver of stimulation. If the couple live together, these roles are presumed to spread to other aspects of their lives. The butch would be the one who works and makes important decisions, and the femme would cook, clean, and play the "wifely" role in the relationship.

Interestingly, this caricature of married life as put forth by nonhomosexuals used to be accepted by many lesbians, and many couples tried to live in this manner. However, present trends in the lesbian community are very much against these heterosexual role stereotypes. Most women claim they want a relationship with another woman on an equal and totally shared basis. In fact, many women originally rejected the heterosexual world because of the inequities they felt would be required if they lived with a man. Sex roles among homosexual women, both in lovemaking and in other aspects of their relationships, do not currently show any particular type of dominance-submission pattern (see Box 13.1).

Levels of sexual activity The lesbians sampled were somewhat lower in frequency of sex than the male homosexuals. Bell and Weinberg (1978) found that half of the females in their sample had sex less than once a week. However, variability was high: 20 percent indicated two to three times a week, another 20 percent indicated once a week, and a large 35 percent indicated only two to three times a month or less. Generally, in this and other surveys, an average of one to two times a week emerges, which is approximately the same frequency as that for heterosexual women.

Number of partners, impersonal sex, and cruising It is in this area that there are the most striking differences between female and male homosexuals. Bell and Weinberg (1978) found that 31 percent had had a total of 5–9 partners to date. The rest were just above or just below this number. Jay and Young (1980) found that 62 percent had had from 1–10 partners. These figures are much lower than those for gay males.

Similar differences appeared in other areas of impersonal sex. Most of the partners were not strangers, and a majority were people for whom the women had a strong emotional attachment. The majority of encounters were not one-night stands. Cruising was found to be relatively uncommon among lesbians. Less than 20 percent had cruised in the previous year. The little cruising that was done was limited to parties and lesbian bars; it was never done in public places. All these findings seem to support the conclusion that homosexual women are less involved in impersonal sex than are their male counterparts.

Long-term relationships The surveys all indicate that continuing relationships are more common among lesbians than among gay men. Women considered their first affair to have been especially important; it was often their initiation into a lesbian life-style. For more than 50 percent of the women, that first affair lasted from 1 to 3 years, and 25 percent lasted 4 years or more. More than 75 percent of the lesbian respondents to the various surveys were currently in a relationship, felt they were "in love" with their partners, and saw the relationship as lasting for some time to come. These women fit Bell and Weinberg's close-coupled description and were feeling quite positive about their current relationship and its future.

Special problems of homosexual females   Sex appeal and continued attractiveness are less of an issue for homosexual women than men—a striking reversal of the heterosexual world. However, given the central role of cruising for the males and its unimportance to the females, the difference is understandable.

Venereal diseases are almost totally absent among gay women. Sexual problems do occur, and getting counseling help is also a problem for the lesbian. As with male homosexuals, mental health centers and sex clinics are typically oriented toward changing a woman's sexual orientation, not toward helping her adjust to her lesbian sexual life.

HOMOSEXUAL SOCIAL STRUCTURE

The thought that you are gay is always with you and you know it's there even when other people don't. . . . That means there is always a certain amount of strain. . . . You know, the only time I really forget I'm gay is when I'm in a gay crowd. (Quoted in Gagnon and Simon, 1973, p. 186)

Homosexuals have tended to segregate themselves into separate social structures. This quote highlights the desire for a sense of social ease, which is only one of numerous factors that have fostered the development of **homosexual communities**—subcultures existing parallel to, but separate from, the nonhomosexual world.

The male and female homosexual worlds are also separate from each other. There is some contact, especially in the political sphere, but not as much as might be expected, given their common problems with the heterosexual world. As we have seen, male and female homosexuals have different needs, and the social structures useful in fulfilling the needs of one group have little value to the other.

Gay males have a more structured subculture than do gay females. Female homosexuals are less numerous and less public, and their modes of interacting do not require a wide variety of public gathering places. However, lesbian social support groups and businesses that represent and cater to the lesbian community are emerging. The future will certainly show a more visible lesbian subculture if present trends continue.

Gay bars, baths, and other meeting places

Cruising requires ways of meeting potential partners. The **gay bar** provides such a milieu. It is a bar-restaurant that serves a primarily homosexual clientele. The gay bar permits the people who use it to feel relaxed, to engage in their special type of interaction, and to cruise in relative safety from public embarrassment and police harassment. Lesbian bars and restaurants are more for socializing and meeting friends than for cruising. They are valued for excluding heterosexual males, who would assume that any female in a bar was "fair game."

While much about the activities of individuals in gay bars is imagined, these establishments are quite similar to neighborhood bars in urban areas or to singles' bars. Both types provide the time and place for meeting and interacting with other potential partners.

BOX 13.1

Gay relationships

How do homosexual relationships differ from heterosexual ones? Social psychologist Letitia Anne Peplau (1981) and her associates became intrigued with this question. So they devised a questionnaire designed to probe love relationships, both straight and gay. Among the questions they addressed through this survey were: Do homosexuals take heterosexual marriage as an ideal model for love relationships? Is there a "homosexual ethos"—a distinctive set of values about relationships unique to the gay world? Do lesbians and gay men want long-term relationships with a single partner, or do they prefer to live pretty much in the present? Do they feel emotionally close to their partners? Is their view of love cynical or romantic? The survey included questions that covered not only the respondents' attitudes toward intimate relationships but also their living arrangements, balance of power, sexual activity, and degree of commitment in ongoing relationships.

Peplau and her associates administered the survey to 127 lesbians, 128 gay men, 65 heterosexual women, and 65 heterosexual men. An effort was made to recruit a diverse sample of participants from the Los Angeles area. The homosexuals in the sample varied widely in age, education, career, and religion. For cross-group comparisons, 4 subgroups were selected: 50 each of lesbians, gay men, and heterosexual men and women. These subsamples, all white students, were carefully matched for age, educational level, and length of their romantic relationships.

What did the researchers find? In general, they learned that homosexual relationships are very similar to heterosexual relationships. In fact, they found only one major difference: "Heterosexual couples—whether they are dating casually, living together, or married—are powerfully influenced by the model of traditional marriage, a social institution that prescribes very different roles for men and women. In contrast, most homosexual couples reject husband-wife roles as a basis for love relationships. Instead, gay relationships resemble 'best friendships,' with the added component of romantic and erotic attraction" (Peplau, 1981, p. 29). The researchers discovered, for example, that it was unusual in gay relationships for one partner to financially support the other and that both partners shared household chores more or less equally.

Other researchers have also found that gay couples tend to reject traditional roles. Contrary to the popular notion that homosexual partners take on dominant and submissive roles, most homosexuals say they look for egalitarianism in their relationships. When Karla Jay and Allen Young (1980) interviewed homosexuals for The Gay Report, they learned that the absence of rigid sex roles was one of the major attractions of the homosexual life-style. As one lesbian told them, "If ever I felt we were getting locked into any roles, especially those of butch-femme, I would run to escape this relationship" (Peplau, 1981, p. 30).

Without dominant-submissive role playing, homosexual relationships are more like best friendships. As Peplau points out, "Same-sex friends often have similar interests, skills, and resources—in part because they are exposed to the same gender-role socialization in growing up. It is easier to share responsibilities in a relationship when both partners are equally skilled—or inept—at cooking, making money, disclosing feelings, or whatever" (p. 32).

As Peplau and her co-researchers examined heterosexual and homosexual attitudes toward intimate relationships, they found that the majority of respondents placed emphasis on both having a close, secure relationship and maintaining independence, regardless of sexual orientation. In general, the researchers found that in the matched subsamples all four groups were "remarkably similar in the priorities they set for relationships." The only notable difference between gays and straights seemed to be that sexual exclusivity was more important to the heterosexuals than to the homosexuals.

Analysis of gay and straight participants' reports on their current relationships revealed an almost identical degree of closeness and of satisfaction in the relationships. Furthermore, no differences were found between lesbians, gay men, and heterosexuals in the depth of love or liking felt for one's partner, and few differences were found in the frequency and enjoyment of sex among all groups.

One way in which gay men tend to differ from lesbians and straights was in their ability to separate love from sex. Gay men were much more likely to have had sex with people other than their steady partner. Peplau conjectures that the difference may in part be a result of sex-role socialization that emphasizes the double standard for men

and that, in addition, sexual openness, including "cruising," is supported in the male gay community.

Peplau concludes from this study that "homosexual relationships are often emotionally close and personally gratifying" and that they provide the same sort of satisfactions—and conflicts—as heterosexual relationships. She is quick to emphasize, however, that this one study is not definitive. The questionnaires explored only certain topics, so there may indeed be other differences between straights and gays that were not touched upon. Furthermore, as with any kind of survey, there is the possibility that respondents did not answer all questions truthfully. Finally, the sample was probably not representative, since the participants tended to be white, middle-class, well-educated, and open about their sexual preference. And, as Peplau mentions, people dissatisfied with their relationships were not likely to volunteer for this type of research.

Nevertheless, other researchers have been reaching similar conclusions in their examination of homosexual relationships. In fact, the main differences they are finding are not between straights and gays but between men and women, whatever their sexual orientation. Women tend to have certain goals in an intimate relationship, and men tend to have different, although related, goals. Thus, as Peplau says, "the character of a particular relationship may depend less on whether the partners are homosexual or heterosexual than on whether they are men or women."

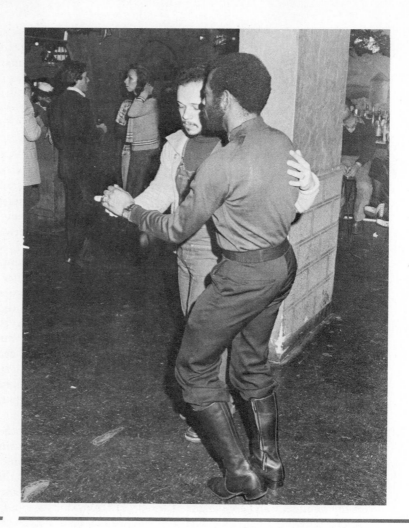

*A male
homosexual
couple in a bar.*

The **gay Turkish baths** are a male homosexual phenomenon. They have a much more direct sexual function. Here the physical setting is meant to promote and support direct sexual behavior right on the premises. Private rooms, baths, and facilities for dressing and undressing are all conducive to sexual encounters. Some baths are very elaborate, offering bars, food, and even entertainment. Contacts made in the baths may move on to sex immediately.

In addition to the structured settings, homosexuals often have designated areas in parks, public bathrooms, bookstores, film parlors, and so on, where anonymous contacts can be made.

The social subculture of the homosexual community is structured in other ways as well. There are gay "ghettos" in most of the larger cities. These are geographical areas that have a reputation of being favored by homosexuals. Once such areas become identified as homosexual hangouts, gay bars, restaurants, nightclubs, and other businesses will locate there. The result is an area that is highly visible to the nonhomosexual community and that gives the impression that all homosexuals form isolated communities.

The members of the male gay world sometimes seem to be desperately trying to live up to the "gay" name. The life-style favors partying, entertainment, drinking, and, of course, cruising. However, this gay sociability is really serious business. It serves the purpose of providing the context for meeting and relating to one another as homosexuals. However, this may be a distortion of the subculture based on the high visibility of the activities of its younger members. Older homosexuals may stay closeted, so we see only these younger and more active representatives.

In contrast to this version of gay life, Warren (1974) has described the social structure of a group of older and more settled male homosexuals in a western city. These men are primarily in more stable relationships, live in their own homes, and move in a social circle of similarly settled and sedate homosexuals *and* heterosexuals. While they are a small group, they provide evidence that there is a "silent minority" of homosexuals who do not live the stereotyped gay life and who are underrepresented in much of the research on homosexuality.

Legal issues

Both civil and criminal laws make homosexual life very difficult. Our laws contain a wide variety of statutes against homosexual behavior and individuals, many of which violate their basic human rights. The laws make it illegal to live as a homosexual, and various statutes make it legal to discriminate against homosexuals; that is, homosexuals can be barred from certain jobs or from the military, they can be refused housing, and so on. The law also works against the homosexual in more subtle ways. Because most laws are written with the basic heterosexual married couple in mind, the homosexual is frequently penalized by tax laws, community property rights, child custody laws, and other such legislation.

Although the laws themselves are a problem, it is the way they are applied that often creates the most unpleasant situation for the homosexual. Police vice squads often use entrapment to catch homosexuals for soliciting. Raids on gay bars, baths, and parties have created a deep resentment and distrust between gays and law enforcement officers. Activism against these practices is a new feature of the homosexual community. The Stonewall Rebellion in Greenwich Village in 1962 was a group reaction to a brutal raid on a gay bar and is considered to have been the beginning of the modern gay rights movement. Some of the laws are now being changed to decriminalize sexual practices between consenting adults and to protect the civil rights of homosexuals. Gould (1979) has noted, however, that many of the legal gains of the 1970s are

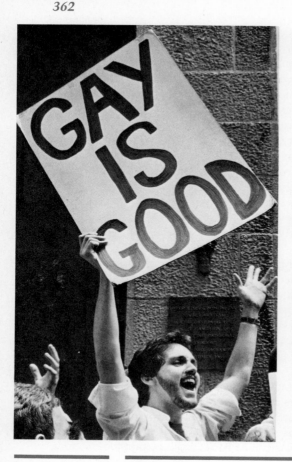

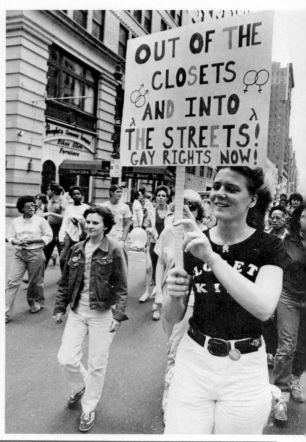

being reversed by well-financed campaigns against homosexuals in many communities. The loss of these protections can only support the spread of suppression and brutality and drive further wedges between the homosexual community and heterosexual society.

THEORIES OF THE DEVELOPMENT OF HOMOSEXUALITY

When asked, "Why do you think you are gay?" one male homosexual responded, "God made me gay, bless her," (Spada, 1979). This is one way of looking at causality. Unfortunately, science has little of greater substance to offer about the causes of homosexuality.

The question of why some people are homosexual is usually asked from an *etiologic* perspective; that is, the "why" question seeks the *cause* of the difference from heterosexuals. This type of thinking tends to imply that the homosexual orientation is an abnormal deviation from the norm of heterosexuality. The question might better be posed as "*How* does a person develop *any* particular sexual orientation, heterosexual, homosexual, or something between the two?" Numerous theories have been proposed to explain homosexuality; we will review only a few here.

Genetic theories of homosexuality were very popular in the 1950s. One study of twins showed higher concordance rates for homosexuality in identical twins than in fraternal twins and nontwin control subjects (Kallman, 1952). These data were used to support the hypothesis that homosexuality is an inherited trait. However, this finding has not been verified by other researchers. In fact, one study (Kolb, 1963) found just the opposite—no concordance at all in several homosexual men with identical twins.

Another set of biological theories starts with the premise that hormonal imbalances create the potential for homosexual behavior. After all, hormones do play a central role in sexual behavior and thus are likely to be involved in the development of homosexuality. So far, however, the data have shown that hormones affect the *level* of sexual interest, but not the specific *direction* of that interest. Although some studies have shown hormonal and other biochemical differences between heterosexuals and gays, no persuasive evidence has yet appeared. Another hormonal hypothesis, the idea that prenatal hormonal abnormalities affect postnatal sexual orientation, was discussed in Chap. 5.

Freud proposed that we are all **pansexual** (arousable by both sexes) and that during normal development we all go through both homoerotic and heteroerotic stages. If conflict develops at a key stage, particularly with regard to resolution of the Oedipal complex, the result is a homosexual orientation.

According to other psychodynamic approaches, fixations in particular psychosexual stages—such as the oral or the anal—result in the individual continuing to seek his or her gratification in these erogenous zones and becoming unable to move on to the genital orientation necessary for heterosexuality.

One psychodynamic view with a large following is the one put forth by Bieber (Bieber et al., 1962). He proposed that everyone is heterosexual (that is, that this is the *normal* state) and can only be diverted from this course by psychological events. The male homosexuals he studied in the course of psychoanalytic treatment showed an overattachment to their mothers, who had become too close and psychologically intimate with their sons. The fathers tended to be passive and detached, thus further forcing the boys to identify with their mothers. Bieber has been criticized for generalizing from dissatisfied, neurotic patients to all homosexuals.

Behavioral theories start with the observation that human sexual behavior can easily become associated with a wide variety of environmental cues; that is, it is learned behavior. According to this approach, homosexuality is basically normal sexual behavior attached to the stimulus of a same-sex partner. Such behavior can be learned by direct rewards or by being inhibited or punished in relationships with opposite-sex partners. However the original learning may have occurred, once sexual satisfaction is experienced in the presence of homosexual stimuli, it will be strongly reinforced and is likely to be repeated. According to social-learning theory, once the behavior moves in a particular direction, the positive outcomes will maintain and strengthen that sexual orientation.

The debate about the cause or etiology of homosexuality tends to reinforce the view of homosexuality as an illness. This idea was considered a radical move when it was first proposed, since prior to that time homosexuality had been considered a sin. Having a psychiatric illness supposedly took the onus off the person and lessened the sense of blame and guilt. Being "ill" also implied that the person could get "well"—that he or she could be changed back to "normal." If homosexuality were a symptom of an emotional illness, therapies could be used to change the behavior. But while therapists did report that their homosexual clients showed much emotional disturbance, their success rates for changing them to heterosexuals were dismally low. In recent years everything from hormone treatments to psychoanalysis to aversion therapy with electric shock have been tried with little success.

Some have suggested that while homosexuality may not be caused by psychiatric illness, being homosexual may *produce* psychiatric illness. Do the stresses and strains of trying to live as a homosexual in a rejecting society create psychological casualties? The answer to this question is yes and no. The general finding of various studies is that homosexuals do *not* show more maladjustment than heterosexuals on the average, but there is an increase in the variability of adjustment in the homosexual groups (Hooker, 1957; Bell and Weinberg, 1978; Saghir and Robinson, 1973). This means that some are doing better than heterosexuals, but some are doing worse.

The contemporary mental health profession's response to such findings has been to suggest a movement away from the illness model as an approach to homosexual behavior. Both the National Institute of Mental Health and the American Psychiatric Association have removed the label of *homosexuality* from their formal listings of psychiatric disorders. The APA has indicated that homosexuality "by itself does not necessarily constitute a psychiatric disorder." Those homosexuals who are unhappy about their orientation are now given the designation of *sexual orientation disturbance* and can receive therapy either to help them adjust to homosexuality or, where appropriate, to help them change their orientation. Individuals who experience sexual orientation disturbance are further discussed in Chap. 17.

How should we now view homosexuality? It certainly is a sexual orientation different from the majority's. It is characteristic of only a small percentage of the population. Isn't that an abnormality? Our view is that homosexuality should be treated as an alternative sexual orientation rather than as a moral or psychiatric deviation. Certainly homosexuality is different, and as such it presents important issues to the study of human sexual functioning. But different is not abnormal, and different does not have to be treated or "cured" just because it is different. In fact, with greater knowledge and understanding, homosexual behavior may not look all that different after all.

SUMMARY

1   Attitudes toward homosexuality in American society are in a state of transition. On the one hand, homosexuality is being portrayed more positively in the media, and homosexuals have become more visible through their participation in gay groups and activities. On the other hand, antigay groups have managed to negate some of the gains of homosexuals, and the highly publicized liberalization of attitudes toward and laws affecting homosexuality has created a backlash in the more conservative parts of the country. A large percentage of Americans continue to believe that homosexuality is "always wrong," and many suffer from *homophobia*—deeply felt fears and anxieties about homosexuality.

2   *Homosexuals* are adults of either sex who are sexually attracted to and prefer to achieve sexual gratification with members of their own sex. Although the term *homosexual* refers only to sexual orientation, it is also a label that evokes stereotyped images of the person's character, behavior, and life-style. Homosexuals are not the same as *transsexuals*—people who feel they are really the gender opposite from their biological sex—and *transvestites*—people who derive sexual pleasure from dressing in clothing of the opposite sex.

3   The prevalence and acceptability of homosexuality varies from society to society. In the United States, most studies indicate that approximately 80 percent of men and women are exclusively heterosexual, while 2–3 percent of men and 1–2 percent of women are exclusively homosexual. The remaining 17–19 percent have engaged in varying amounts of homosexuality or have gone through periods of *transient homosexuality* but are predominantly heterosexual. Kinsey proposed that there is a *continuum* of sexual interest, with heterosexuality at one end and homosexuality at the other.

4   *Bisexuals* are individuals who fall midway on Kinsey's sexual orientation continuum. They are equally attracted to men and women as sexual partners. Bisexuals are often pressured to choose one orientation or the other because they are unwelcome in both the homosexual and heterosexual cultures.

5   The realization of one's own homosexuality is called *coming out*. For most males, the average age of awareness is early adolescence, while for females it tends to be in the twenties. Most homosexuals have their first same-sex experience with someone of similar age, putting lie to the myth that older homosexuals are the main initiators of young people into the gay world. Most homosexuals do not tell their families, co-workers, or anyone other than their closest friends and partners about their homosexuality. Those who take the greatest pains to conceal their orientation, the so-called *closet queens*, are likely to have the most psychological problems regarding their homosexuality.

6   Among gay men, the most frequent sexual practices are fellatio, mutual masturbation, anal intercourse, body rubbing, and interfemoral stimulation. Despite the stereotype to the contrary, most gay men do not use anal intercourse as their main technique for achieving orgasm. In fact, many techniques are used to reach orgasm, with mutual masturbation the most common. As with heterosexual lovemaking, foreplay is an important part of the sexual encounter.

7   Although it is commonly believed that there is a division of roles in homosexual male couples, with one man becoming dominant and the other submissive, no evidence has been found to support this belief.

8 An important feature of homosexual life for many males is *cruising*, the searching for partners with whom to have casual sex. One study found that 80 percent of gay men reported more than half their partners to be complete strangers. More than half said they enjoyed such impersonal sexual experiences. However, many homosexuals consider cruising to be demeaning and devoid of warm human contact, and even those who do cruise find many aspects of this behavior to be unpleasant.

9 Most homosexual men would prefer to have long-lasting relationships, but such relationships are less common than the single life among gay men. Of those long-term relationships that do exist, some are *close-coupled* exclusive pairings, similar to heterosexual marriage, and some are *open-coupled*, in which one or both partners continue to cruise. Close-coupled homosexuals tend to be the most well adjusted psychologically of all gays.

10 The problems of homosexual men include sexual dysfunctions, difficulties related to aging, and venereal disease.

11 Sexual practices among *lesbians*—female homosexuals—are centered around mutual pleasuring, with less concern for orgasm. The three techniques used most often to produce orgasm are mutual masturbation, cunnilingus, and *tribadism* (body rubbing in which one woman lies on top of the other).

12 Although the social stereotype of lesbian couples is a masculine *butch* or *dyke* coupled with a "wifely" *femme*, the relationships of gay women tend to more closely resemble best friendships, without any role stereotyping.

13 Unlike gay males, gay females do not tend to engage in cruising and impersonal sex. They prefer long-term relationships involving strong emotional commitment.

14 In many cities *homosexual communities* or subcultures have developed to provide a separate social structure for gay individuals. Gay males have a more structured subculture than gay females; it consists of *gay bars*, *gay Turkish baths*, and other such meeting places. Gay women tend to get together more for social purposes than for cruising.

15 Homosexual behavior is illegal in most states, and homosexuals themselves are discriminated against on the job, in the military, in housing, in tax laws, and in other areas. Furthermore, law enforcement officers often use entrapment and raids to catch homosexuals. Gay rights activists are currently working to decriminalize homosexual behavior and to win civil rights for gays.

16 There are many theories as to what "causes" homosexuality. According to biological theories, homosexuality may be genetic or brought about by hormonal imbalances. According to psychodynamic theories, homosexuality is the result of fixation in an early psychosexual state or of identification with the opposite-sex parent. According to learning theories, homosexuality is a type of incorrect learning. Depending on the theory, different "treatments" have been proposed for "curing" homosexuality.

17 Current studies of homosexuals do not find them to be any more or less psychologically maladjusted than heterosexuals, on the average. Mental health professionals no longer consider homosexuality to be a psychiatric disorder. The main thing that is abnormal about homosexuality is that it is characteristic of only a small percentage of the population. The authors believe that homosexuality should be seen as an alternative sexual orientation rather than as a moral or psychiatric deviation.

ADDITIONAL
READING

* **Bell, Alan, and Weinberg, Martin.** *Homosexualities: A Study of Diversity Among Men and Women.* New York: Simon & Schuster, 1978.

> *The results of a large survey of gay men and women. The book is surprisingly extensive and quite readable, even though technical material is included in the text.*

* **Bullough, Vern.** *Homosexuality: A History.* New York: New American Library, 1979.

> *A short but excellent history of homosexuality.*

* **Loovis, David.** *Straight Answers About Homosexuality for Straight Readers.* Englewood Cliffs, NJ: Prentice-Hall, 1977.

> *A well-written book of questions and answers by a gay author aimed at straight readers unfamiliar with the gay world.*

* **Wolf, Deborah.** *The Lesbian Community.* Berkeley, CA: University of California Press, 1979.

> *An anthropological investigation of a lesbian community in California. Intensive, detailed, and interesting.*

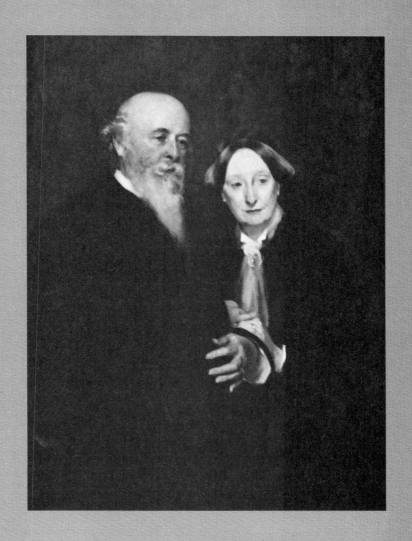

*Sexuality in
the later years*

14

chapter 14

DEAR ABBY: I'm 81 and when my husband was alive, I thought sex was the most fun in the world. Now that I am a widow, it is hard to find someone to play with.

—HAVING FUN AT 81

DEAR ABBY: I am pushing 85 and hope that the last healthy breath God gives me will be spent in an intimate embrace with my man.

—M. IN SAN DIEGO

What is your reaction to these letters? If you think they are funny, or unseemly, or disgusting, you've got a lot of company. Our society has typically viewed the elderly as incapable of sexual behavior and as uninterested in sexual matters. Furthermore, we feel that they shouldn't be capable or interested. Pfeiffer (1969) had difficulty obtaining subjects for his study of sexuality in the aged because younger family members felt that it was inappropriate for their elderly parents to participate. Sons and daughters often demanded that their parents withdraw from "such foolishness." Thus, the elderly person is stamped by both society and family as asexual—as being sexless by virtue of being old.

This transition to sexlessness is marked in the public eye by certain events that are normal concomitants to the aging process. In women, menopause heralds the end of the childbearing years and is often erroneously equated with the end of sexuality. In men, retirement is an event that signifies a loss of usefulness, productivity, and eventually virility as well. It is as if some switch is suddenly turned off, causing sexuality to disappear. But just as sexuality does not suddenly emerge at puberty, neither is it suddenly lost by virtue of menopause, retirement, or other events associated with aging.

THE BIOLOGY OF AGING

As we grow older, many of our bodily systems deteriorate or at least become altered in function. This is a gradual process, with some alterations occurring early in life (range of hearing begins to diminish by age 15) and others occurring later in life. The reproductive system is no exception. Major changes in reproductive functioning occur during late middle age and on into old age. In women, such changes tend to be more clearly marked, as the capacity for reproduction typically ceases around age 50. In men, reproductive capacity declines more gradually.

Changes in women

As women grow older, various internal processes decline or slow down. The **climacteric** is the reproductive aging process that extends over a 15-year period from about age 45 to 60. **Menopause** is a highly distinguishable event in this gradual process: the cessation of menstruation. Over 50 percent of all women experience menopause between the ages of 45 and 50, while 25 percent become menopausal before age 45 and 25 percent after 50 (Ganong, 1967).

Menopause is usually a significant event in a woman's life, both physiologically and psychologically. It marks the end of her reproductive years and is not without bodily and emotional stress. How a woman reacts to menopause has a major effect on her and on those around her. Understanding and support

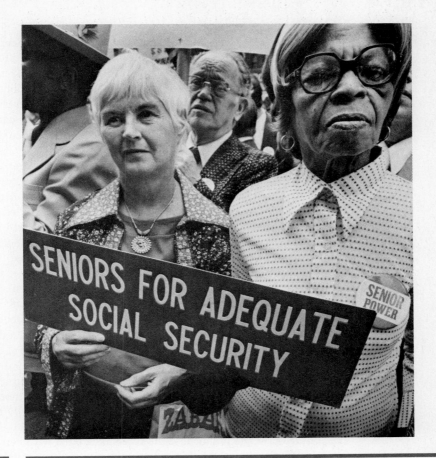

*The elderly have
been given a
negative social
position in our
society. Today,
more and more
older people are
speaking out
against age
discrimination.*

from family members and from friends can help her to make the appropriate adjustments.

The onset of menopause is seldom abrupt. Rather, menstrual cycles become increasingly irregular, with decreased blood flow and increased time between successive menstrual periods. The time between menstrual periods keeps increasing until the cycles stop altogether. Although menopause is said to have occurred after a 1-year absence of menstrual flow, it is still possible for a woman to ovulate after this period of time. Thus, women are advised to practice some form of birth control for at least 2 years after menopause has been confirmed.

Physiological effects of menopause   Nearly 85 percent of all women exhibit some kind of physical reaction to the reproductive aging process. However, less than half seek treatment, and fewer than 10 percent are severely affected (Huff, 1979). Most of these reactions or "symptoms" disappear within 5 years.

Other than amenorrhea, the most common symptom of menopause is the **hot flash**, which occurs in 4 out of 5 menopausal women. Typically, hot flashes appear in the upper part of the body and consist of a red flush, profuse sweating, and a feeling of suffocation. The hot flash lasts from 1 to 3 minutes, and the woman may feel chilled afterward. Hot flashes occur about 4 or 5 times a day. They commonly appear at night when the woman is quiet, and they frequently disrupt sleep. Hot flashes are severe enough to constitute a significant problem for approximately 25 percent of all menopausal women (McKinlay and Jeffreys, 1974).

The second predominant symptom of menopause is a decrease in the moisture and elasticity of the vagina. This condition is referred to as **vaginal atrophy** or **senile vagina**. The vaginal walls lose their rough, corrugated appearance and become thin and smooth. Such vaginal changes may lead to painful intercourse. A lubricant such as K-Y jelly is often effective in reducing the unpleasant sensations associated with the increased friction. Vaginal dryness may also make a woman more susceptible to vaginal infections.

A number of other symptoms have been reported in conjunction with menopause. These include dizziness, heart palpitations, swollen ankles, and dry and wrinkled skin. Some of these symptoms may be side effects of the hot flashes or vaginal atrophy rather than direct consequences of menopause. However, a frequent occurrence in older postmenopausal women of a disease called **osteoporosis**, in which the bones become brittle, can be traced to the drop in estrogen levels that occurs with menopause.

Emotional effects of menopause Menopause may also trigger a wide range of emotional problems, including apathy, anxiety, depression, morning fatigue, insomnia, and even severe depression. These effects are generally temporary and may or may not require treatment.

The climacteric and menopause are often associated with certain types of life stresses. This is not to say that menopause causes these stresses, or vice versa. Rather, menopause may act as a reminder that brings these events to the forefront of the woman's thoughts. The four most common life stresses associated with menopause are:

1   Changes in the family unit and loss of the maternal role. *This crisis occurs for women who have spent the majority of their adult lives occupied with child rearing. As their children grow up and move away, they develop feelings of uselessness. This is sometimes called the* empty nest syndrome. *For other women, however, the leaving of their children may bring a sense of freedom from child rearing with the possibility of entering a second career of their choosing (Deutscher, 1964).*
2   Success or failure in reaching goals. *For women who are strongly career oriented, failure to achieve desired goals by the time of menopause can lead to feelings of frustration and hopelessness. These women may feel that they do not have enough time left to succeed. Conversely, a woman who has been very successful may believe that there is nothing left for her to pursue or enjoy.*

3   Decrease in self-esteem. *This is a direct function of the aging process.
Aging causes changes in appearance and a decline in ability to perform.
Both can lead to a negative self-image.*

4   Loss of sexuality. *Menopause heralds the end of reproductive life for
women. For women who think that femininity and sexuality are synonymous with menstruation, the loss of these cycles may lead to feelings of
sexual inferiority. Furthermore, some women believe that sexual intercourse ends with menstruation, a view that is simply not true. Women can
continue to receive sexual fulfillment after menopause with little or no
adjustments.*

It is generally the case, then, that menopause coincides with some major
life stresses. It serves to remind women that their lives are two-thirds over and
that their childbearing years are gone. In a culture that emphasizes youth and
youthfulness, this can be a devastating time. Fortunately, sexuality does not
have to end—nor should it—when menopause occurs. Women can expect
to have sexual fulfillment for as long as they desire it. The aging process is a
real one, however. Youth cannot be regained, and the changes are inevitable.
Thus, women must learn to cope with the onset of middle and old age—a
process that may be achieved easily or with some difficulty, depending on the
individual.

The causes of menopause   The actual causes of menopause are not known
with any certainty, although a complex set of biological events must clearly be
involved. One aspect of this process that has been identified is a disruption of
part of the negative feedback loop involving the hypothalamus, pituitary, and
ovaries. Disruption is not primarily at the pituitary level but at the ovarian
level. The ovaries become progressively less responsive to stimulation by the
pituitary gonadotropins, resulting in a decline in estrogen levels. For example,
in the 50- to 60-year-old woman, ovarian synthesis of estrogen is reduced to 40
percent of premenopausal rates. This figure drops to 20 percent for women over
the age of 65. On the other hand, LH and particularly FSH levels actually
increase (see Fig. 14.1) because of the loss of negative feedback from estrogen
(Yen, 1977). (One diagnostic test for menopause looks for higher levels of FSH
in the bloodstream.) These changes, in turn, cause a decline in follicular
development and ovulation.

The ultimate stimulus for this chain of events is still a mystery. According
to one theory, the depletion of eggs that begins before birth is almost complete
by the time of menopause (Block, 1952). The reduction in estrogen is therefore
attributed to the loss of functioning ova. Other researchers discount this notion and suggest that the ovary has an inherent life expectancy that differs
from woman to woman and that is unrelated to the age at which menstruation
first occurs or to the use of birth control pills (Huff, 1979).

As estrogen levels decline, menopausal symptoms begin to appear. It is not
surprising, then, that the majority of menopausal symptoms are presumed to
be linked to a reduction in estrogen levels. This explanation for menopausal
symptoms is called the ***estrogen deficiency hypothesis***. The best support for

FIGURE 14.1
Changes in the circulating levels of hormones in postmenopausal women. Following menopause, FSH and LH levels increase, while estrogen levels (E_1 and E_2) decline. The label A represents androgen levels. (Yen, 1977)

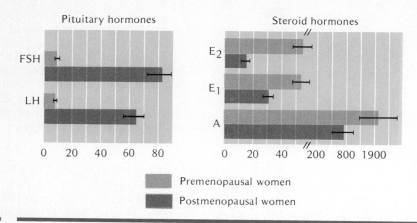

this hypothesis comes from the success of **estrogen replacement therapy** (ERT). Women who are given Premarin, Stilbestrol, Progynon, or Meprane (trade names for various estrogen preparations) report a significant reduction in hot flashes, osteoporosis, and other physical complaints (see Box 14.1). Thus, raising estrogen levels in the blood causes most of the physical symptoms of menopause to disappear. There is some question, however, as to whether estrogen provides any relief from the emotional distress that may also be present (Bardwick, 1971; Huff, 1979). Furthermore, ERT has been found to pose some major risks when used in significant dosages over long periods, as discussed in the box.

Although there is considerable evidence to support a hormonal interpretation of many of the physical symptoms of menopause, some researchers have suggested that part of the menopausal syndrome may be due to or at least exacerbated by cultural factors. They suggest that the emotional responses could be triggered by cultural expectations, thereby leading to the types of life stresses we have mentioned. In support of this argument, Bart (1971) found that depression, a fairly common menopausal symptom in our society, occurs much less frequently in cultures where a woman's status increases with age. It is likely that the changes that take place during menopause will eventually be attributed to a combination of hormonal and cultural factors. The exact interplay between the two is currently unknown and probably varies from woman to woman.

Treatment of menopause often depends on the orientation of the woman's physician. Physicians who view menopause as a part of the natural aging process may prescribe little in the way of treatment unless symptoms such as osteoporosis are present. On the other hand, doctors who believe that menopause is an estrogen deficiency disorder typically recommend estrogen replacement therapy for as long as the woman seems to need it.

BOX 14.1

Estrogen replacement therapy

When women reach menopause and their ovaries reduce hormone production, they may experience a number of uncomfortable symptoms, including the well-known "hot flashes." For more than 35 years physicians have dealt with these symptoms by prescribing estrogen replacement therapy (ERT). The woman takes a daily pill containing synthetic or natural estrogens to help reduce the effects of menopause. This method of therapy became particularly popular in the 1960s and early 1970s—prescriptions nearly tripled between 1965 and 1975 (Consumers Union, 1980). In 1975 alone, 27 million such prescriptions were written for postmenopausal women (Klinck, 1979). But then the popularity of ERT began to fall, because physicians and women began to hear of research reports suggesting that ERT may cause endometrial cancer, breast cancer, and a number of other problems. Many women who had taken their estrogen therapy for granted suddenly became worried. Were the risks involved in ERT worth the benefits? Reports since then have often been confusing. What are the facts about estrogen replacement therapy?

Let us look first at the benefits of ERT. Estrogen is primarily prescribed to deal with three problems that often accompany menopause: hot flashes, vaginal atrophy, and osteoporosis. A hot flash is a sudden change in body temperature that may last a few seconds or a few minutes. It is often experienced as a wave of heat spreading over the face, head, and upper body. The woman may turn red, and she may become drenched in perspiration. Such hot flashes may occur several times a day and can be quite stressful. Some women experience them for a few months following cessation of menstruation; others may have them for a year or more. Although the precise cause of these episodes is unknown, they seem to be linked to reduced hormone production, and estrogen therapy definitely helps to alleviate them. However, hot flashes generally subside and disappear on their own whether or not the woman is given estrogen supplements.

Vaginal atrophy, a thinning and hardening of the vaginal lining, is a well-documented consequence of reduced estrogen in the body. With menopause, vaginal lubrication decreases, and the women may experience itching, burning, urinary discomfort, and pain during sexual intercourse. This condition is slow to develop and may not appear until 10 years after menstruation has ceased.

Estrogen replacement therapy has been shown to be effective in dealing with the problem of vaginal atrophy. As Isaac Schiff and Kenneth Ryan of the Boston Hospital for Women, Harvard University, have pointed out, "Vaginal atrophy progressively worsens. If the patient is sexually active she may complain of both vaginal dryness and pain in intercourse. Unfortunately, some women are reluctant to discuss this with their physicians; and at the same time some physicians feel ill at ease in bringing up sexual matters with older patients. The silence that may enshroud this problem is all the sadder in that sexual intercourse may remain an important part of the life of the aging women. The symptoms of [painful intercourse] may respond very dra-

matically to estrogen therapy" (Consumers Union, 1980, p. 268).

But what about the other benefits of ERT? Many women say they take estrogen because it helps them to stay young, it alleviates such psychological problems as postmenopausal depression, or it protects against heart attack. At a recent conference sponsored by the National Institute of Aging of the National Institutes of Health (NIH), participants concluded that "there is no evidence at present to justify the use of estrogens in treatment of primary psychological problems." In fact, there is no evidence that such psychological difficulties as depression, irritability, and nervousness often associated with menopause have anything to do with hormones. Marvin Fogel, of the Mount Sinai Medical Center in New York, has noted that although menopause does not induce depression, in a person who already has a tendency toward depression, menopause may trigger a depressive episode. But such depression cannot be treated with hormone therapy.

Participants at the NIH conference also failed to find any connection between hormone replacement and youthful appearance. ERT does not prevent skin wrinkling, nor does it halt the natural aging process. Furthermore, ERT is not a preventive measure against heart attack in women, as was once believed.

A final possible benefit of ERT is prevention and treatment of osteoporosis. Osteoporosis is a condition in which the bones become brittle and fracture easily. This problem occurs in some form in 25 percent of all postmenopausal women, and it can be quite serious—16 percent of women who suffer hip fractures die of related

complications within 3 months of the accident (Science News, 1979). Estrogen deficiency has been shown to be a causative factor in osteoporosis—young women who have had their ovaries removed and have not taken estrogen tend to develop osteoporosis sooner and more severely than do other women. Estrogen treatment for osteoporosis has been proven to delay bone loss, although it cannot cure the problem. But can ERT prevent this bone condition? Apparently it can be quite helpful for the 25 percent of women who are at high risk for developing the problem. Unfortunately, there is no way at present to identify those women who are at risk, and the remaining 75 percent may actually be harmed by taking estrogen if recent reports of the dangers of ERT are accurate.

What, then, are the dangers of ERT? The primary danger seems to be the risk of developing cancer of the endometrium (uterine lining). Several studies have now shown that postmenopausal women with intact uteruses who are on ERT are at much greater risk for developing endometrial cancer than are postmenopausal women who are not on estrogen. And the longer a woman remains on estrogen, the greater her risk. One study found that users of estrogen in general run a 6 times greater risk of this cancer than do nonusers, but those who have been taking estrogen for more than 5 years run a 15 times greater risk (Consumers Union, 1980). So far all of these studies have been epidemiological—they have compared cancer rates for women who have and haven't used ERT. No study has proved that estrogen does indeed cause endometrial cancer. It is interesting to note, however, that since 1976 both the incidence of endometrial cancer and the use of ERT have declined significantly (Schildkraut, 1979). Furthermore, women who go off ERT reduce their risk of endometrial cancer to normal within about 2 years.

ERT has also been linked to breast cancer in recent years, although the evidence is not conclusive. One study found that women on high doses of estrogen for at least 3 years run a 2.5-fold higher than normal risk of developing breast cancer (Science News, 1980). However, this study has been criticized on the basis of the high dosages involved.

In addition to the major risk of cancer and possible hazards of high blood pressure and gall bladder disease, the normal regimen of estrogen replacement therapy carries with it some annoying side effects. Among those that have been reported are nausea, vomiting, abdominal cramps, bloating, headache, dizziness, and breast tenderness. Some of these side effects are eliminated or reduced by a regimen in which the woman takes the estrogen for 21 days and then forgoes it for 7 days.

In balancing the benefits against the dangers of ERT, the participants in

the NIH conference advocated an overall policy of "lowest dose for the shortest time" for women whose menopausal symptoms are severe enough to warrant estrogen therapy (Science News, 1979). They warned that women who have a previous history of cancer, heart attack, or stroke or who have other contraindicated conditions should not use ERT and that those who do use it should be aware of the risks involved.

The general conclusion is that although much research is still required, there is enough evidence to suggest that for some women the risks of long-term use of estrogen replacement therapy outweigh the possible benefits. One must carefully assess the risk of cancer against the benefit of controlling osteoporosis, for example. However, the decision on whether to use ERT ultimately rests on the individual case. If a woman finds that her menopausal symptoms interfere with her life and if she doesn't have a contraindicated condition, she may choose estrogens at the lowest effective dose for a short period of time to help alleviate those symptoms while running the fewest risks of suffering from the potential harmful effects of the therapy.

Attitudes toward menopause Menopause is a major life event, and we might expect women to have strong feelings about it. This may not be the case, however. In Bernice Neugarten's (1963) survey of 100 women aged 43–53, only 4 viewed menopause as a major source of worry. "Losing one's husband," "just getting older," and "fear of cancer" were much more frequent concerns. In a more recent survey conducted by the Boston Women's Health Book Collective (1976), younger women were more fearful and felt more negative about menopause than women who had already experienced it. The anticipation of menopause appears to be far worse than the actual event. In general, about two-thirds of menopausal and postmenopausal women felt neutral or even positive about the changes they had experienced. Sexuality remained relatively unchanged in half the respondents, while the remainder reported either an increase or decrease in sexual desire. Despite the fact that menopause is a major life event producing some unpleasant side effects in many cases, the women who have made it through this period find that they have survived it quite well.

Changes in men

There is no male counterpart to menopause, that is, no clear sign indicating the loss of reproductive capacity. Nonetheless, men do exhibit biological and physical changes with aging that may contribute to a reduction in sexual functioning. Male hormonal changes tend to be more gradual, to be less pronounced, and to occur at older ages than do those in women. Paradoxically, however, men tend to display a decline in sexual functioning more severe than that of women, either because of psychological reasons or because they may be more dependent on hormones for their sexual potency (Silny, 1980).

Physiological changes include a decrease in the production of testosterone and a decline in the sensitivity of the penis, both of which may contribute to a decrease in sexual activity. In addition, spermatogenesis declines and sometimes stops altogether. Associated with falling sperm counts are changes in the concentration of sperm and in the volume and quality of semen. The testicles appear smaller and less firm with age (Rubin, 1965).

The most common physical complaint in elderly men is an enlargement of the prostate gland that may result from changing hormone levels. Although prostate enlargement is found in only 10 percent of men in their forties, it is characteristic of 50 percent of all men age 80 and older. As the prostate enlarges, it begins to press against the urethra, producing painful and/or frequent urination. Successful treatment depends on surgical removal of the part of the gland at fault. Often a partial **prostatectomy** can be performed. If a total prostatectomy is performed, however, sexual activities may be impaired because of possible damage to the nerves involved in penile erection. Loss of the ability to have an erection occurs in only a small percentage of these cases (Zimring, 1979). Despite current folklore, neither masturbation nor high levels of sexual activity cause prostate enlargement.

Men also experience some emotional changes during aging, but these changes often occur more gradually than with women. Again, such emotional changes are probably related to specific life stresses. The four most common life stresses in aging men are:

1   Changes in the family unit. *Although this is generally a more serious problem for women, men must also adjust to the absence of children in the household.*
2   Success or failure in reaching goals. *During the period of middle to old age, men often judge themselves in terms of success or failure in achieving some set of goals. Self-evaluation of present accomplishments and future development may not lead to satisfying answers. In this situation, the older man is likely to feel that time is running out for him.*

3   Retirement. *Regardless of health and general well-being, most older men are forced to retire between the ages of 65 and 70. For those who strongly identify with their work, this can be a difficult time of transition—a time that brings feelings of insecurity and uselessness. This is especially true if the man has made little preparation for retirement (Comfort, 1976). Pleasure in his new-found leisure may be short-lived, and boredom may set in quickly. Those who have realistic plans for their retirement, however, tend to view the event in a different light. Such individuals approach it as an opportunity to explore hobbies or new careers, not as a marker for the conclusion of their reproductive life. For them, retirement is a new beginning, not an ending.*

4   Loss of sexuality. *Two factors may contribute to a loss of sexuality in older men. First, the inevitable changes in physical appearance can have a deleterious effect on the man's self-esteem. Second, the sexual responses slow down in the later years, and more time and stimulation are needed to produce erection and orgasm. Because of these two factors, men may fear failure or may regard the required changes as unpleasant and may thus show a decreased interest in sex. Partners who adapt to the inevitable slowing down of sexual response by altering their patterns, positions, and so on, continue to maintain their sexual activity well into their advanced years.*

THE SEXUAL
RESPONSE CYCLE
IN THE ADVANCED
YEARS

The changes in the reproductive system that occur with age are accompanied by changes in sexual responsivity. In 1966 Masters and Johnson published their landmark work on human sexual response (see Chap. 11). Although most of their subjects were in their twenties and thirties, Masters and Johnson did study the sexual responsiveness of older men and women. The 61 older women in their sample ranged in age from 40 to 78, while the 39 older men were 50–90 years old.

Despite the significant hormonal and anatomical changes that occur with aging, Masters and Johnson found that older people tended to show a pattern of sexual response similar to that of younger people. During sexual encounters, older people progressed through the same stages of excitement, plateau, orgasm, and resolution. The primary differences in the sexual response of older versus younger people were in timing and sensation. In general, older people took longer to become aroused, seemed less sensitive to stimulation, and experienced orgasms of weaker intensity than their younger counterparts. Interestingly, the extent of the differences between the old and the young was related to sexual activity in youth and mid-life. Those who showed a consistent and frequent pattern of sexual activity up to and into their advanced years had little decrease in sexual response as a function of aging. The effects of aging were much more pronounced if sexual activity had ceased or declined to low levels by mid-life. Most of the changes in timing and sensation can best be explained by alterations in the physiology and anatomy of the male and female sex organs.

*Changes
in women*

There are a number of significant bodily changes in women that may contribute to some alteration in sexual responsivity. As women age, the labia or lips become progressively flattened and lose their capacity to undergo extensive color changes during arousal and orgasm. Of even greater significance for sexual activity are the changes that occur in the vagina. The vaginal barrel becomes increasingly less able to expand in length and width. The walls become thin and inelastic, and vaginal lubrication occurs more slowly and in reduced amounts. Taken together, these changes may make penile insertion difficult and unpleasant. Some of these labial and vaginal alterations can be reversed with estrogen replacement therapy or with topically applied jelly or cream. Masters and Johnson also noted that lubrication declined little in elderly women who continued to have sexual relations once or twice a week. Furthermore, not all sex acts require insertion of the penis into the vagina, and variation may be a desired element of sex in the later years. Older women continue to have a capacity for orgasm despite these changes. However, the number and intensity of orgasmic contractions tend to decline with age.

*Changes
in men*

Sexual activity in men may extend well into the eighties or nineties, although the percentage of individuals experiencing erectile failure increases with age (Kinsey, et al., 1948). The proportions at 50, 70, and 75 years of age were 8 percent, 27 percent, and 55 percent, respectively. No one has fully evaluated the extent to which poor health and other physical factors contribute to erectile failure. Advanced age is synonymous with slower arousal and a delay in sexual response. The speed of penile erections, for example, increases from 3–5 seconds in the adolescent years to 30 seconds or longer after age 50. The amount of precoital mucus also generally decreases.

As with females, the orgasmic response is altered over time. In the young adult male, orgasm is experienced in two stages: emission and expulsion (see Chap. 11). As men age, however, the first stage is typically foreshortened so that the feeling of ejaculatory inevitability is reduced or lost. In a few cases, the first stage may actually be lengthened, creating a continued feeling of ejaculatory inevitability without the expulsion of seminal fluid. According to Masters and Johnson, this latter condition is usually transitory.

Other aspects of the orgasmic response also change. There is a decline in both the number and intensity of orgasmic contractions, a lessening of the force with which the semen is expelled, and a reduction in the total volume of semen. The refractory period between ejaculations, which is relatively short in adolescence (30 minutes), increases to 24 hours or more in the forties and fifties. The incidence of morning erections and nocturnal emissions also declines.

One of the advantages of male aging, however, is an increased ability to delay ejaculation. Thus, sexual encounters may be more prolonged and enjoyable for the man's partner. Whether this prolongation of arousal is due to experiental factors (older men have had more opportunities in which to learn to delay orgasm) or to decreased sensitivity has not yet been determined. In general, though, male sexual functioning decreases with age. Men may find it more difficult to attain an erection and to reach orgasmic levels of sexual arousal. Despite this decrease in sexual functioning, there may not be corresponding decrease in fertility. Older men continue to produce viable sperm (although at reduced levels) that can impregnate a fertile woman.

As we have already indicated, sexual functioning declines more dramatically in men than in women. This may be a cause of concern or anxiety for a sexually active partnership. Women, however, can play a positive role in alleviating such anxiety by being as supportive as possible. They must remember that failure to achieve or to maintain an erection is much more obvious and more difficult to correct than insufficient vaginal lubrication (Silny, 1980).

SEXUALITY IN THE
ADVANCED YEARS

Although biological studies can tell us much about the sexual functioning of the elderly, other factors, such as attitudes and beliefs, also play an important role in shaping sexuality in the later years. In addition, although physiological studies of the human sexual response reveal much about sexual *capacity* in older men and women, they tell us little about the typical sexual *activities* of the elderly. It is to these attitudes and activities among older individuals that we now turn.

The influence
of attitudes

Our attitudes indicate what behaviors we consider acceptable or unacceptable, comfortable or uncomfortable. Our own attitudes are often shaped by the attitudes of others around us and more generally by the predominant attitudes of the society in which we live. Societal pressures can also be a more direct force in our behavior by explicitly sanctioning certain kinds of actions while prohibiting others. The sexual activities of older people therefore reflect not only their own attitudes but societal expectations and admonitions as well.

Societal attitudes and expectations The views of our society toward sexuality in the elderly, as we have noted, are generally negative, even harsh. At the very least, sex is thought to be inapplicable to older people. They are, in fact, expected to be sexless. In the extreme, some consider sexual interest and activity in the elderly to be an indication of psychopathology or of moral degeneration. This attitude is expressed in such statements as "He's a dirty and disgusting old man," and "That's indecent for a person of your age."

A number of studies have now verified the pervasiveness in our society of this negative view of elderly sexuality. In 1959, Golde and Kogan found that college students considered sex to be inappropriate for the elderly. They gave one group of students the opportunity to complete a sentence beginning "Sex for most old people . . ." and another group the task of completing the sentence "Sex for most people . . ." Whereas 92 percent of the subjects in the first group finished the sentence with "negligible" or "unimportant," only 4.9 percent of the subjects in the second group used such terms. In a more recent survey of sexual attitudes, Harris (1976) found that 46 percent of the general public viewed people over the age of 65 as being quite physically active, but only 5 percent saw them as being sexually active. In yet another study, sex in the aged was viewed as less believable than sex in young and middle-aged adults (LaTorre and Kear, 1977).

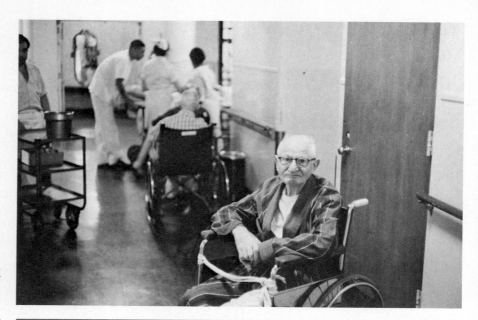

*Some elderly
people feel
isolated and lonely
in nursing home
environments.*

One of the most damaging aspects of these negative attitudes is the fact that they seem to be held most strongly by those who have professional and clinical contact with the elderly, such as nursing staff personnel (Rosencrane, 1969). Nursing homes in general are not supportive of sexual interactions. Facilities for having sexual relations are not available to married or unmarried couples (Burnside, 1975; Schlessinger and Miller, 1973); the physical settings are not well suited to fostering expressions of tenderness; and the nursing staff actively discourages sexual expression of all kinds, including masturbation (Butler and Lewis, 1976). More recently, however, LaTorre and Kear (1977) have argued that nursing personnel are generally more negative about sexuality in all groups of people than are students or people in other professions. Their restrictive view may therefore not be limited to the elderly patients they serve.

The asexual quality that society attributes to older people may stem from a number of sources. First, because Western society is generally youth-oriented, sexuality and youthfulness are usually linked with each other. This point of view is widely reinforced in literature, the arts, and the media. The "Pepsi generation," for example, is not over 30. Older people are seldom presented in television commercials unless they are selling coffee or endorsing various medications for arthritis or "irregularity." Thus, we are exposed to few cultural examples that connect sexuality with the elderly. Second, some people erroneously equate sexuality with reproduction. As a woman's reproductive years come to an end at menopause, it is sometimes assumed that all her sexual activities will automatically cease. Finally, many individuals believe that sex is meant primarily for procreative purposes. Accordingly, once people are past their fertile period, they should not engage in sex even if they retain the ability to do so (Pfeiffer, 1975). Whatever the reasons for society's negative view of sex in the elderly, this attitude probably contributes greatly to the decline in sexual functioning and activities with age. Older people are not supposed to be sexually motivated, and so, through self-fulfilling prophecy, they aren't.

Attitudes in the elderly The attitudes of elderly people themselves obviously play a major role in their sexual expression. Yet few attempts have been made to investigate the sexual attitudes of this segment of the population. As we consider what is known about this topic, keep in mind that the views of older people are likely to have been influenced by the culture in which they grew up.

It is clear that health concerns are often uppermost in the minds of older people when they think about sex. For example, some women who are adversely affected by menopause may erroneously assume that sexual activity will intensify their menopausal symptoms. Some men believe that sex will trigger a heart attack, despite the fact that most doctors consider the benefits of sexual activity to outweigh the risks (Hellerstein and Friedman, 1969). In fact, only 1 percent of all coronary deaths occur during sexual intercourse. Interestingly, these instances often involve an extramarital affair, where anxiety might just as reasonably be the prime factor in the attack (Zimring, 1979). In general, both men and women sometimes believe that sex weakens them and makes them more vulnerable to numerous diseases. There is little evidence to support this belief; in fact, the reverse may actually be true.

More detailed information on the sexual attitudes held by the elderly is difficult to obtain. Individuals are often reticent to participate in surveys on this topic, and nursing home personnel may put up strong resistance to studies of their residents. In one recent study, however, Wasow and Loeb (1979) did succeed in assessing the sexual attitudes of a group of nursing home residents. Despite great initial resistance, 63 individuals (27 men and 36 women) finally agreed to be interviewed.

Wasow and Loeb first asked their subjects two questions about sexual activity: "Should a person your age have sex?" and "Should older people be allowed to have sex?" Surprisingly, the subjects responded much more positively to the second question (81 percent of the women and 75 percent of the women said yes) than to the first. The investigators reasoned that the respondents were interpreting the first question in a personal manner but not the second. The subjects appeared to be saying that sex should be available to older people, but as individuals it was not for them. This attitude was further reflected by a predominantly negative view toward masturbation. Over 60 percent of the women and 42 percent of the men felt that masturbation was abnormal. The majority of the residents were embarrassed by this subject and denied that they masturbated. Most of them had also given up sexual intercourse, either because of the lack of a partner or because of poor health. One woman flatly commented, "My husband died and that was the end of it."

When asked about sexual thoughts and fantasies, 75 percent of the women and 31 percent of the men indicated that they did not currently experience such fantasies. In responding to subsequent open-ended questions, however, these same subjects commonly spoke of a "person down the hall" who was preoccupied with sexual thoughts. The investigators concluded that "either every nursing home keeps their big fantasizer down the hall or a lot of projecting is going on!"

The final part of this interesting study examined the relationship between sexual knowledge and attitudes among the nursing home residents. In general, the subjects were quite ignorant about sexual matters. This was particularly true of women. Furthermore, the extent to which they were knowledgeable was strongly related to the degree of permissiveness of their sexual attitudes. Accurate knowledge seemed to foster more permissive opinions about sexuality. This finding reinforces the more general notion that knowledge and understanding are beneficial in promoting positive and healthy views toward sex.

Sexual behavior

Most of what is known about sexual practices (rather than attitudes) in the elderly comes from Kinsey's survey data collected in the 1940s (Kinsey et al., 1948, 1953). These findings are still considered to provide the most comprehensive picture of sexuality from the teenage years to old age (Silny, 1980). As is the case of most studies conducted with elderly people, Kinsey had relatively few subjects (126 men and 56 women) in his "old" age group.

If there is one basic trend common to all aspects of sexual behavior across the life span, it is one of decline. Kinsey found that all forms of sexual expression tended to decrease with age. However, he also noted that males reported a higher incidence of sexual activity than did females at all ages. If we consider all the forms of sexual behavior leading to orgasm, men reported a frequency of 3.3 sexual acts per week at age 20, 2 such acts per week at age 45, 0.8 at age 60, and 0.2 at age 75. Married men were more active sexually than single men overall, although this difference tended to disappear by age 50. More recently, Martin (1977) demonstrated a steady decrease in orgasmic frequency beginning at about age 35 for a group of well-educated, middle-class white subjects (Fig. 14.2).

Kinsey used orgasm as an index of sexual activity in women as well. Although there was not much decline in the number of orgasms per week in single women across time (it averaged about 0.3 per week), there was a decline for married women from 2 orgasms per week at age 20 to 0.6 per week by age 55.

Although masturbation is most common in young unmarried men, Kinsey did find some evidence for masturbation in both sexes at various ages. For the single, sexually active male, masturbation decreased from 1.7 times per week in the teen years to less than once per week in the forties. These frequencies were 4–5 times lower in married men in each age bracket. Although single females showed little reduction in the frequency of masturbation (about once per week) across time, married women had the same pattern of decline as married men.

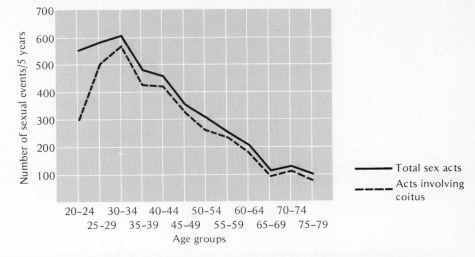

FIGURE 14.2
*Declining sexual
activity in men as
a function of age.
The solid line
refers to all sexual
events, the dotted
line to those
involving coitus.
(Martin, 1977)*

A number of researchers besides Kinsey have examined the frequency of marital intercourse as it varies across time (Bell and Bell, 1972; Pearlman, 1972). They all agree that marital intercourse declines with advancing age. Intercourse in married women decreases from a frequency of 4 times a week at age 20 to twice per week at age 40 and finally to once per week by age 60 (Kinsey et al., 1953; Bell and Bell, 1972). Similar declines have been noted for married men. Pearlman (1972) also found that by ages 60–70, 25 percent of the men he surveyed engaged in sexual intercourse less than once per month, and 33 percent were not having intercourse at all.

Extramarital intercourse is the only form of sexual activity surveyed by Kinsey that did not show the typical decline from youth to old age. In Kinsey's overall sample, about 35 percent of all married men reported having had at least 1 extramarital affair. More important, the frequency of such affairs was about the same for all age groups. In the case of married women, 26 percent reported having engaged in at least 1 extramarital relationship. However, the frequency was lowest in the woman's twenties, rose sharply in her thirties, and declined thereafter.

The results of a more recent, extensive longitudinal study of sexuality in the elderly complement much of Kinsey's prior work (Pfeiffer, Verwoerdt, and Wang, 1968; Pfeiffer, 1969; Pfeiffer and Davis, 1972). This study employed interviews of individuals ranging in age from 60 to 94. Each subject was interviewed 3 times: in 1957, in 1961, and in 1964. Pfeiffer and Davis (1972) noted, as had Kinsey, that females generally showed levels of sexual activity lower than that of males. This difference is particularly compelling if we look at those subjects who reported total sexual inactivity. In the fifties, the proportion of men who were completely inactive was 7 percent, and in the sixties, it was 24 percent. For women, the comparable figures were 42 percent and 73 percent.

Verwoerdt, Pfeiffer, and Wang (1969) looked at changing patterns of sexual activity across Pfeiffer's first 2 interview periods and classified behavior patterns into 4 types. They used *C* to denote activity that continued from the first to the second interview period, *A* to denote an *absence* of sexual activity in both the first and second interviews, *D* to indicate a *decline* in sexuality activity between the 2 periods, and *R* to signify a *rise* in activity between the periods. The most typical pattern for women respondents was *A* (74 percent), while the most common pattern for males was *D* (31 percent). The same classification was also used to study sexual interest. As one might expect from the other results, the most common pattern of sexual interest for females was *A* (always absent), while the most common patterns for males were *C* (continuing) and *D* (declining).

What all these studies tell us, in summary, is that as people grow older, their interest in sex and their frequency of sexual activity both decline. This trend is more rapid in women than it is in men. However, we do not know to what extent this sex difference might be attributable to lack of an available partner. Women tend to live, on the average, 7–8 years longer than men. Because women usually marry men who are slightly older than themselves, it is highly likely that their husbands will die before they do. Given the fact that there are 4 times as many women as men over age 70, widows are likely to have difficulty finding another husband if they desire one. More generally, there may indeed be no available partner for older women who are interested in a sexual relationship either within or outside the confines of marriage. This factor may help explain why the surveys consistently report that elderly men are more sexually active than elderly women, despite the fact that men tend to be more adversely affected physically by aging.

In addition to the problems posed by physiological changes, negative attitudes, and difficulties in finding a suitable partner, other problems can also affect sexuality in older men and women. These factors include: (1) boredom with one's partner, (2) preoccupation with one's job, (3) mental or physical fatigue, (4) obesity, (5) poor physical health, (6) alcoholism or drug addiction, and (7) fear of failure in sexual encounters, especially on the part of men.

Diseases of the elderly and the drugs they take to control these diseases may also alter sexual functioning. Diabetes mellitus, for example, is a major cause of sexual dysfunction in both men and women. The painful symptoms of arthritis are a possible source of interference with certain forms of sexual expression. A wide variety of drugs used to treat various chronic ailments can diminish or curtail sexual functioning. Antihistamines, antihypertensives (drugs used to control high blood pressure), antipsychotics, antidepressants, cardiac drugs, and certain diuretics are only a few of the medications that fall into this category. In addition, the popular tranquilizer Valium can produce enough muscle relaxation to retard or inhibit orgasm in both sexes (Zimring, 1979). As people age, they become more susceptible to various diseases; fortunately, a number of these ailments can be treated. However, patients should be aware of the fact that many of the drugs that provide symptomatic relief may also produce the unwanted side effects of reduced sexual interest, activity, and satisfaction.

The new morality—living together at 70?

Within recent years, the phenomenon of living together, which has become common among people in their twenties, has also been occurring more frequently in the elderly (Wax, 1977). Elderly widows and widowers are moving in with each other in increasing numbers. Does this represent a new morality for the aged? Is this a version of "sexual liberation" among the elderly? Probably not. The basic impetus for such arrangements appears to be economic, not romantic, although romance is certainly not excluded. The simple fact of life is that many of the elderly must subsist on social security benefits, which are often quite meager. Pooling 2 monthly checks while paying only 1 monthly bill for housing, utilities, and so on, can be quite advantageous. If 2 people who have agreed to live together for economic reasons later decide to get married, they each stand to lose half of their social security benefits. It is little wonder, then, that cohabitation is becoming increasingly more popular among the elderly. Recent estimates indicate that there may be as many as 16,000 elderly couples living together in the United States.

Will this living arrangement create a new standard of increased sexuality for the aged? As we have already indicated, this phenomenon is unlikely to occur on a large scale. Many older people resort to this arrangement in desperation and are fearful that their relatives will find out. Some of them assuage their discomfort by going through a marriage ceremony that recognizes the

The need for sexual intimacy is not restricted to the young.

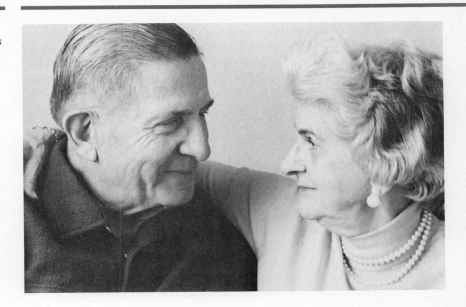

union in the eyes of God although not in the eyes of the State. For others, however, such a ceremony is an affirmation of love rather than a reflection of guilt. It is gratifying to see that people can, in fact, reaffirm their sexuality and "have fun" in their old age (Wax, 1977). Even if the present elderly generation did grow up under circumstances that shaped a more restrictive attitude toward sex, their present actions may have an impact on younger people in fostering a greater recognition of sexuality in the older members of society.

AGING IN THE
HOMOSEXUAL

There is no evidence to suggest that the biological effects of aging are any different for homosexuals than for heterosexuals. No consistent hormonal differences have been detected, nor do these groups reliably differ in any other biological dimension. However, homosexuals and heterosexuals may experience different psychological reactions to aging. The common assumption has been that homosexuals have particular difficulty in adjusting to the changes brought on by aging. As we noted in Chap. 13, gay men may worry about becoming less attractive and therefore less successful in the cruising aspect of homosexual life. The typical picture of aging in the homosexual has been one of increasing social isolation, especially in the case of men. Recent studies, however, are challenging these views of the older homosexual.

Weinberg and Williams (1974) found only a part of this stereotype to be accurate. Using a questionnaire to obtain information on homosexual life experiences, they found that older homosexuals did tend to be less involved in the social aspects of gay life than younger homosexuals. The older gays associated less frequently with other homosexuals and spent less time in gay bars. However, older homosexuals were no different from their younger counterparts in self-acceptance, degree of anxiety, depression, or loneliness, and were more stable.

Some of the research findings suggest that homosexuals undergo role changes qualitatively different from those of heterosexuals. These differences may actually make adjustment to aging easier for the homosexual than for the hesterosexual. Francher and Henkin (1973) indicated that the major life crisis for the homosexual is acceptance of his or her orientation. Once this crisis has been faced, usually early in life, the homosexual avoids some of the later-life crises of the heterosexual, such as the empty nest syndrome.

A more recent report of in-depth life-history interviews of 14 aging homosexual men also contradicts the stereotype (Kimmel, 1980). The average age of the subjects in the sample was 64.9 years, with a range of 55–81. When asked about aging, the typical attitude was expressed by one man who said, "Preparation for old age is much better among gays than it is among heterosexuals. Because you've always been that way, you haven't expected anyone to take care of you, except yourself." Others spoke of a freedom from role playing and the importance of friendship networks in maintaining the continuity of life. Still others mentioned the adjustment to living alone that heterosexuals sometimes encounter with the death of a spouse. Homosexuals, they argue, have lived alone for substantial periods and are used to it.

These studies do not deny that homosexual men and women may become more isolated as they grow older (which may also be more generally true of all elderly). There is no evidence to suggest, however, that such individuals have more difficulty adjusting to the aging process than do heterosexuals. In fact, the opposite may be true at certain times and under certain conditions.

*PROBLEMS OF
RESEARCH ON
AGING AND
SEXUALITY*

We have been discussing various research findings as if they represent an accurate picture of sexuality in the aged. And, indeed, we would like to think that this is so. However, there are two very important issues that may limit in important ways the validity of the work by Kinsey, Masters and Johnson, and others as applied to the elderly. First, most of the studies of sexuality in older people have involved small numbers of subjects. Both Kinsey and Masters and Johnson had many fewer subjects in their elderly samples than in other age groups. Wasow and Loeb's (1979) conclusions were based on 63 subjects, and Kimmel's (1980) observations were based on a mere 14 homosexual subjects. Clearly, it is important to survey and interview greater numbers of the elderly if a broader perspective is to be achieved.

Second, there is probably a particularly strong selection bias in terms of those individuals who have been willing (or have been allowed) to serve as subjects in these studies. A selection bias always exists in sex research, but the bias may be even more severe in the case of the elderly. This is true at least partially because the likelihood of an older person participating in such research is often determined not only by his or her own views but also by the pressures that may be applied by children, relatives, and perhaps nursing home staffs. As a result, the subjects who have been studied are likely to have been more sexually liberated and to have come from families that, as a general rule, were more supportive of sexuality in the elderly. Thus, our present views on sexual practices in older people may not accurately reflect the attitudes and practices of this population as a whole. For these reasons, the current findings about sexual activity in the aged should be treated as tentative until further studies have been performed.

In this chapter we have discovered that sexuality can and does extend well into old age. However, this discovery should not be taken as a directive for what older people *should* do. Knowledge should be used to free people from the repression of old ideas without imprisoning them in a set of equally dogmatic new ones. Knowledge should not be used to create a set of immutable expectations. That we are prone to this way of thinking can be demonstrated by our attitudes toward female orgasm. Once researchers uncovered new information about the ability of women to experience orgasm, there developed the general expectation that women should have orgasms every time they engage in sex. We must be careful not to develop similar expectations concerning sexuality in the elderly. Sexual activity can continue for a longer period of time than was originally thought, but all individuals should feel free to make their own choices in this as in any other area of life. All people, elderly or otherwise, must be able to select whatever life-style is comfortable for them.

SUMMARY

1   The aging process in women is marked by the *climacteric*, which extends from about age 45 to 60. The most significant aspect of this period is *menopause*, the cessation of menstruation. Menopause is said to have occurred after a 1-year absence of menstrual flow. The physicial changes that occur with menopause include *hot flashes*, *vaginal atrophy*, and symptoms such as heart palpitations and swollen ankles. Some women also develop *osteoporosis*, a condition in which the bones become brittle.

2   Menopause is associated with certain life stresses, including changes in the family unit and loss of the maternal role (the *empty nest syndrome*), success or failure in reaching goals, and loss of sexuality.

3   Although the exact causes of menopause are not known, many of the physical symptoms are known to be related to lowered levels of estrogen in the body. Evidence for this *estrogen deficiency hypothesis* of menopause comes from the success of *estrogen replacement therapy* in treating the physical symptoms. It has also been suggested that many symptoms of menopause are actually culturally induced. This may be particularly true in the case of psychological symptoms such as depression.

4   Although menopause is a major event in every woman's life, a majority of menopausal and postmenopausal women do not view it as a source of worry. In fact, younger women are much more fearful and negative about menopause than those who have already experienced it.

5   Although there is no male counterpart to menopause, men do experience biological and psychological changes with age that affect their sexual functioning. Physical changes include decline in sensitivity of the penis, falling sperm counts, and possible enlargement of the prostate gland. Psychological changes are related to such life events as changes in the family unit, success or failure in reaching goals, retirement, and loss of sexuality.

6   Changes in the sexual response cycle occur with age. In general, older people take longer to become aroused, seem less sensitive to stimulation, and experience orgasms of weaker intensity than do younger people. It seems that the more sexually active a person is throughout his or her life, the less effect aging has on sexual responsiveness.

7   The woman's sexual response is altered with age because the vagina becomes less flexible and produces less lubrication, in some cases making intercourse painful. Older women continue to have a capacity for orgasm despite such changes.

8   Aging also affects the male response. Older men are slower to develop erections, produce less precoital mucus, and may lose the emission aspect of ejaculation. However, they have an increased ability to delay ejaculation, which can be an advantage for their partners.

9   Our society has a strong negative attitude toward sexuality in the elderly, and this attitude probably contributes strongly to the decline in sexual functioning and activities with age. Few studies of sexual attitudes and behaviors among the elderly have been done because researchers are discouraged from questioning older people about their sex lives.

10   Studies such as Kinsey's have shown a general decline in all forms of sexual behavior with age. The only form of sexual activity that has not shown this pattern of decline is extramarital affairs, which show a similar frequency for all age groups. In general, men stay more sexually active than women into

the later years. This difference may be explained in part by the fact that women live longer than men and that there are more older women than older men, reducing women's access to sex partners.

11   Sexuality in the elderly can be adversely affected by a number of factors, including poor health, chronic diseases, and the side effects of medications.

12   Many older men and women are choosing to live together without marrying for economic reasons. Such couples who are romantically and sexually involved may be presenting a positive example of sexuality in the aged from which the rest of society can learn.

13   There is some evidence that homosexuals adapt better to the sexual aspects of the aging process, despite stereotypes to the contrary.

14   Because our knowledge of sexual behavior in the elderly is based on highly limited samples, it may not accurately reflect the elderly population as a whole. However, we do know that sexuality is not something that suddenly ends in mid-life but rather is an important part of life that can continue indefinitely.

**ADDITIONAL
READING**

* *Masters, William, and Johnson, Virginia. Human Sexual Response.* Boston: Little, Brown, 1966.
    This book contains a special section on geriatric sexual responding.
Rubin, Isadore. Sexual Life After Sixty. New York: Basic Books, 1965.
    A well-written discussion of sex and the elderly. Less technical than Masters and Johnson.
Starr, Bernard, and Weiner, Marcella. Sex and Sexuality in the Mature Years. New York: Stein & Day, 1981.
    A methodologically sound survey of older adults regarding their sexual experiences, attitudes, and values. A comprehensive and readable book.

four

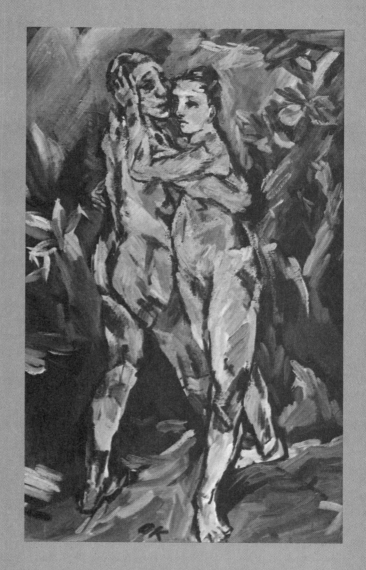

Sexual dysfunctions
and sex therapy

15

chapter

15

Fred, a 23-year-old teacher, has been having trouble sustaining an erection with his new girlfriend. He has been dating her only a short time, but she has been eager to establish a sexual relationship. The first time they had sex, he experienced premature ejaculation, and on three occasions since then, the inability to sustain an erection has plagued him. His girlfriend says she has never encountered this problem with other men and she's sure there is something wrong with him.

Marilyn, a 35-year-old sales manager, does not like the way her partner makes love to her. If he touches her gently, she feels ticklish rather than aroused. If he touches her too roughly, it irritates her. She is also annoyed by all his attempts to caress her breasts. She has too many other things on her mind to have to pay attention to his seemingly constant desires.

Sam is a 28-year-old musician who has been married for 6 months. He is troubled by the fact that he ejaculates too soon after entering his wife's vagina. Before they were married, their primary method of birth control was withdrawal; now Sam wonders whether that has affected his ability to have normal intercourse.

Doris, a 42-year-old housewife, has been reading a lot about orgasms in books and magazines, but she doubts that she's ever had one. She has always done her "duty" by being available for sexual intercourse with her husband, but she's never seen the attraction of it. "Ten minutes and it's over," she has often commented. Now she wonders what all the hubbub is about.

What do these four people have in common? They are all experiencing some form of **sexual dysfunction**, or an inability to engage in or enjoy sexual encounters. In this chapter we will be describing the most common sorts of sexual dysfunction among men and women and the treatments that have been developed to deal with these problems. But the question first arises, what causes sexual dysfunctions?

In a few cases, physical problems, such as certain medical conditions, can affect the normal sexual response cycle. (Some of these medical problems are discussed in Chap. 18.) Because of this possibility, it is standard practice for people experiencing sexual problems to be medically evaluated to make sure such conditions are not operating and that they are in good physical health.

In most cases, however, failure to function under normal circumstances and given appropriate sexual stimuli is the result of psychological factors that interfere with the person's natural reactions. Such factors can include anxiety about pleasing the partner, anxiety about failing to perform adequately, ignorance of sexual techniques, inability to communicate well, and a myriad of other feelings, attitudes, and behaviors. The specific elements at work in a particular person's situation may be difficult to pin down. Even factors like job stress, financial difficulties, or general fatigue can alter sexual functioning, so any one problem may be the result of the interaction of a number of aspects of the person's life. As a further complication, the other person—the sexual partner—brings all his or her potential areas of difficulty into the picture. Given all the possible factors that can contribute to sexual dysfunction, it begins to seem incredible that anyone has a normal sex life. As a matter of fact, sexual dysfunctions are so common that they should really be considered an unavoidable part of sexual behavior (see Box 15.1). Almost everyone experiences occasional problems of this kind. It is only when they come to seriously affect the person's general and sexual adjustment that they require special attention and possibly sex therapy.

Sexual dysfunction is a broad label that encompasses a number of specific problem areas. The American Psychiatric Association, in its *Diagnostic and Statistical Manual*, 3rd edition (DSM-III), has developed formal names for the most common dysfunctions that are treated by mental health professionals, and we will be using this terminology throughout the chapter. For convenience, we have separated the dysfunctions into those that affect men and those that affect women.

**SEXUAL
DYSFUNCTIONS
IN MEN**
*Inhibited male
sexual excitement*

Male sexual dysfunctions can involve problems of getting or maintaining an erection and problems with ejaculation.

Inhibited sexual excitement (ISE) is the inability to achieve or maintain an erection of sufficient quality to engage in sexual intercourse. This problem used to be called **impotence.** That term is no longer used, because it connotes a loss of strength or power. There are two types of ISE. **Primary inhibited sexual excitement** is used to refer to those cases in which the man has never experienced an erection that has been maintained during sexual intercourse. **Secondary inhibited sexual excitement** is used to refer to cases in which the man has functioned adequately at some time in his life but has since developed inhibited sexual excitement.

Primary inhibited sexual excitement   The actual physical reaction in ISE is a failure of the reflexes involved in penile erection. From our earlier discussion of the functioning of the sexual organs (Chaps. 4 and 11), recall that part of the male sexual arousal response is a flow of blood into the penile cavernous bodies, making the penis firm enough for sexual intercourse. In ISE, this vasocongestive response fails or reverses itself prematurely, and the erection is not sufficient for intercourse. There are some rare physical conditions that can cause such a problem, but by far the most usual causes are psychological. The man with psychologically based primary ISE may have little problem achieving erection under the conditions of masturbation or oral sex, but is unable to maintain an erection for intercourse.

The causes of primary ISE vary greatly from individual to individual. Because the man has never experienced the usual erectile response for intercourse, early experiences in development are thought to be involved in creating this problem. Masters and Johnson (1970) noted in several cases that overinvolvement of the mother in the child's early sexual reactions had produced sexual confusion and guilt in the child. (Freud would explain this type of situation as lack of resolution of the Oedipal conflict.) Masters and Johnson also found that several of the primary ISE individuals they treated had been raised in homes where religious training stressed the idea that sexuality was sinful. This training created great conflicts in the person about the acceptabili-

BOX 15.1

Sexual dysfunction in "normal" couples

What is "normal" when it comes to sexual problems in marriage? Should a couple expect their sex life to be relatively free of dysfunctions or difficulties? If not, how can they tell whether their sexual problems are in the "acceptable" range?

Researchers at the University of Pittsburgh's Western Psychiatric Institute were concerned with this question —with establishing some baseline data for dysfunctions in "normal" couples (most studies of sexual dysfunction are based on data from individuals who have sought professional help for sexual or marital difficulties). They wanted to determine the prevalence of sexual problems in couples who believed their marriages were working well and who had not felt the need for marital counseling or sex therapy.

The researchers gathered their data by administering a 15-page marriage questionnaire to 100 couples who were predominantly white, middle class, and well educated (Frank, Anderson, and Rubinstein, 1978). The questionnaire dealt with many aspects of marriage; sexual relations constituted only a portion of the questions.

The results? Although more than 80 percent of the couples reported that their marital and sexual relations were happy and satisfying, they also reported high frequencies of various sexual problems. Among the men, 40 percent reported erectile or ejaculatory dysfunction, and a striking 63 percent of the women reported arousal or orgasmic difficulties. The researchers noted that the discrepancy in frequencies of reported dysfunctions in men and women "may represent a real difference or may be an artifact of the wives' greater willingness to admit to having problems. In fact, the difference is probably explained by a combination of the two: the women were probably experiencing greater dysfunction and were more willing to admit it" (p. 114).

Although there were no major differences between how wives saw their husbands' dysfunctions and the husbands' self-reports, the husbands tended to underestimate dysfunctions in their wives. For example, 15 percent of the men said their wives had trouble maintaining excitement, yet 33 percent of the women reported having this problem. The researchers pointed out that this underestimation "seems consistent with the typical American pattern of sexual interaction in which as long as the wife neither complains nor refuses to have intercourse, the husband assumes that all is well" (p. 115).

In addition to sexual dysfunctions, the couples were asked to report on the prevalence of various "difficulties" in their sex life, including such things as "inability to relax," "partner chooses inconvenient time," "too little foreplay," and "turned off." Women reported more of these difficulties than did men (77 percent to 50 percent), which the researchers said "may support the notion that women require more emotional sensitivity accompanying the sexual act, or are at least more aware of the absence of such amenities" (p. 115). The researchers found that, in general, the number of sexual difficulties in a marriage made a greater contribution to sexual dissatisfaction than the number of dysfunctions.

In summarizing their findings, the

researchers concluded, "It should be reassuring to many that these couples were apparently able to tolerate a relatively high frequency of specific sexual dysfunctions and difficulties and still feel very positive about their sexual relations and their marriages" (p. 115).

As a result of this study and others like it, we are learning that sexual dysfunctions and difficulties are a normal part of marriage. Apparently, it is how these problems are dealt with and how they relate to the couple's overall interaction that counts in a couple's marital satisfaction, not their existence or frequency.

ty of sexual feelings and behavior. Other factors also noted by Masters and Johnson included early homosexual experiences and experiences with prostitutes that led to confusion and guilt.

In the psychological literature there are numerous cases suggesting that a single, traumatic sexual intercourse experience can result in a life of erectile problems. While such single-incident learning is indeed possible, especially in a high-anxiety situation such as an early sexual encounter, traumatic experiences may be overemphasized. Those who have problems with erection may find comfort in blaming all of their difficulty on a single negative experience, but it is more likely that such a long-standing problem as primary ISE has much more complex origins.

Masters and Johnson discovered that many of the men whom they treated for primary ISE seemed to experience high levels of anxiety in many aspects of their lives besides sex. Such anxiety levels, when added to any of the other causal factors, could create a difficult situation for men to overcome. Perhaps their maladaptive response to sexual interactions was a natural end product of a highly anxious general nature, negative early training experiences, and stressful initial sexual encounters. Thus, the recipe for primary ISE is more than likely to contain several important ingredients.

Secondary inhibited sexual excitement It is quite normal for most men to experience occasional erectile failure. How then, do we determine whether a man is experiencing "normal" problems or has secondary ISE? Masters and Johnson have used an arbitrary cutoff point to indicate secondary ISE. They say that the point at which there is an ISE problem worthy of concern is when a man is unable to function sexually in 25 percent or more of the opportunities for sexual intercourse.

It is difficult to get reliable figures for the incidence of this problem. Although secondary ISE is reported much more frequently than primary ISE, embarrassment still keeps many men from seeking professional help for their problem. Kinsey's (1948) studies found a consistent relationship between the existence of secondary ISE and age. It was infrequently reported below age 35 and rose rapidly after age 55. Of men over age 70, 27 percent were experiencing erectile problems, and the figure was 75 percent for those over age 80. As we saw in Chap. 14, many men accept such problems as a normal part of aging when, in reality, they need not occur.

As with primary ISE, secondary ISE can be caused by a number of factors. However, it is more likely for there to be an identifiable **precipitating event** that initiates the ISE pattern. Some typical situational events noted by Masters and Johnson include fatigue, overindulgence in alcohol, guilt over an affair, work pressure, financial insecurity, depression, and arguments.

One frequently reported precipitating event is a change in sexual partners. The recently divorced or separated man may experience difficulty in his first sexual encounters with a new partner. Similarly, a man having an extramarital affair may experience ISE with his new partner or with his wife. In such situations, guilt, anxiety, and the change in sexual patterns that occur with a new partner can all contribute to the problem. Once a difficulty occurs, the man may begin to question his adequacy, making the next sexual opportunity a highly anxiety-provoking occasion, thereby increasing the chances of a second failure.

How is it possible that infrequent erectile failure (or, even more puzzling, a single failure) can create a condition of continuing ISE? To see how this can happen, let's consider a possible sequence of events. We have noted that anxiety is incompatible with sexual performance. It makes biological sense for an animal in an anxious state, which is basically a reflex preparation for fighting or fleeing, to not be aroused by sexual stimuli at such a time. Now, in our society, the sexual situation itself has come to be a source of anxiety. Many men view sexual behavior as a *performance* in which they can either succeed or fail. The man is responsible for making coitus possible, and his erection is a necessary precondition for sexual intercourse. Thus, his "manhood" is on the line every time he engages in sex, and any failure is a reflection on his masculine identity. This prevailing attitude is reflected by the fact that the older terms **potent** and **impotent** were really references to the success-failure aspects of erection and sexual functioning.

Thus, the man in a sexual situation is in a highly vulnerable position. He feels that his sexual prowess is being evaluated by his partner as well as by himself. The **performance anxiety** this belief creates ironically interferes with the very response he is trying to achieve. The resulting failure creates an even greater tension during the next sexual encounter. It is not unlikely, then, that the next occasion for sex will be too highly charged with anxiety and that another erectile problem is not only possible but probable. This vicious cycle of initial erectile failure leading to anxiety, which in turn heightens the probability of further difficulty, and so on, is a common sequence in the development of serious secondary ISE.

Premature ejaculation

Premature ejaculation is a sexual dysfunction in which the male reaches orgasm too quickly. In its most basic form, the male climaxes just before entering his partner or immediately after entering. There is little or no opportunity for movement, so stimulation of his partner does not occur. The result is dissatisfaction for both sexual partners. Although this description makes the problem sound easy to identify, there is actually a great deal of debate among the experts as to what constitutes prematurity. Just how quickly is too quickly? Because two people are involved, "long enough" has to be defined by the satisfaction of both.

Among the definitions that have been proposed for prematurity have been those based on time after entry (within 1½ minutes), number of thrusts (12 or fewer), and even minutes since the initiation of foreplay. In an attempt to avoid the problems of measuring everyone against some yardstick, Masters and Johnson (1970) proposed that the partner's sexual satisfaction be considered an important part of the definition. They suggested that premature ejaculation exists if the man cannot control his ejaculation for a length of time sufficient to satisfy his partner on at least 50 percent of the occasions they engage in sexual intercourse.

When all is said and done, the arguments among the professionals are unimportant to the people involved. Most sufferers define the problem for themselves. The man feels he has climaxed too quickly for himself and his partner, and he is embarrassed, frustrated, and fearful of further sexual encounters. Such self-diagnosis is quite common—premature ejaculation is one of the most frequently reported problems dealt with by sexologists and therapists (Sadock, Kaplan, and Freedman, 1976).

What causes premature ejaculation? The primary characteristic of the problem is that once arousal begins, the man seems to move to orgasm rapidly and uncontrollably. Anxiety is an important component in the process, as it is in erectile problems, but here it serves to heighten arousal rather than to interfere with it. Instead of inhibiting the central nervous system, the anxiety actively excites it. In this vicious cycle, the anxiety over premature ejaculation raises arousal levels to the extremes, ensuring that prematurity will occur.

As with primary ISE, early learning may play an important role in the development of this problem. Because young males who masturbate learn to reach orgasm quickly, they may transfer this experience to intercourse. In addition, the early intercourse experiences in our society are likely to occur under circumstances of haste, worry about being caught, and physical discomfort (such as in the ubiquitous backseat of a car). Young men are also led to believe that orgasm is the all-important end result of sex, so they tend to accomplish it as quickly as possible. This emphasis on speed must certainly leave its mark on later sexual functioning.

Masters and Johnson found that the individual's first few sexual experiences are often instrumental in the development of premature ejaculation. Among the factors they noted were initial experiences with prostitutes, who routinely rush their clients, use of withdrawal before ejaculation as a birth control method so that ejaculation outside the vagina is trained, and intensive sexual stimulation to ejaculation without intercourse.

A different explanation of premature ejaculation comes from the psychoanalytic viewpoint. Freud proposed that early in their psychological development men with this problem experienced conflicts that left them feeling rejected or angry. As adults, they transfer this unconscious anger to their partners and express it by having their orgasm but not allowing the woman to experience her sexual pleasure and release.

Because it is likely that each man with this problem has developed it through a unique combination of causes, it is important to examine each case individually rather than assume any standard development of the problem for everyone.

*Inhibited male
orgasm*

Inhibited male orgasm, which has also been called **ejaculatory incompetence, inhibited ejaculation,** and **retarded ejaculation,** refers to the man's inability to ejaculate during sexual intercourse. There is no sense of orgasm or of completion and satisfaction that the climax usually brings. Fluid containing sperm may leave the penis and enter the vagina, so pregnancy is still possible, but the muscle contractions of orgasm do not occur. If the man has never experienced ejaculation during coitus, the problem is called **primary inhibited orgasm.** If he has had orgasm and ejaculation in the past but now experiences difficulty, the condition is called **secondary inhibited orgasm.** In all cases the ability to have an erection is not impaired.

Sometimes the inhibition is quite specific. Some men can have orgasm in other ways, either by themselves or with their partner, but cannot achieve orgasm with the penis in the vagina. In other cases, the man cannot experience orgasm under any conditions. Despite the fact that sexual intercourse can take place, the partner is no less disturbed about the problem than the sufferer himself. The partner may see the problem as a personal rejection, may interpret it as a failure of her sexual performance, or may just be saddened at the plight of her partner. It is also not unusual for the attempts to achieve orgasm to go on for so long that discomfort and pain for the partner become likely side effects of the man's problem.

Incidence figures from various sources indicate that the secondary type of inhibited orgasm occurs quite frequently, whereas the primary type is relatively rare.

What causes inhibited male orgasm? In this problem, the orgasmic-ejaculatory response at the height of the excitement phase is somehow prevented from occurring. In most cases, the cause is anxiety. Worrying about not climaxing as the feeling approaches is likely to create the kind of anxiety that can inhibit the orgasm. Masters and Johnson (1970) used the term **spectator role** to describe the self-absorption and overawareness characteristic of the man experiencing this type of problem.

Several kinds of early experience have been implicated in creating an environment for the development of this problem. Traumatic episodes, such as being discovered by parents while masturbating, being interrupted during early sexual encounters, and even having sex in a situation where interruption is simply a possibility, can lead to the effects of fear, embarrassment, and punishment coming to be associated with impending orgasm. The feeling of impending ejaculation could thus become conditioned to produce the response of fear or anxiety, which in turn effectively inhibits orgasm.

The approach taken by psychoanalytic theorists is that during childhood the man developed an unconscious fear of being castrated should he ejaculate. This unconscious fear effectively turns off the individual at the height of arousal.

Some cases of inhibited orgasm can be explained in terms of severe religious training. If the man has been taught to view ejaculation as being sinful, he may be unable to feel comfortable and unself-conscious during the sex act, even if he has intellectually rejected this religious idea. The internalized training may still be strong enough to interfere with the lack of inhibitions necessary for orgasm.

SEXUAL DYSFUNCTIONS IN WOMEN

In the past, the term *frigidity* has been used as a blanket label for a wide variety of female sexual dysfunctions. One of the problems with this label is that it has the negative connotation of a cold, unfeeling woman who withholds her natural sexual responsiveness in order to spite men. Despite its value-laden connotations and the fact that it confuses several distinct and different problems, frigidity is still included as a formal category in most current medical texts. However, those working in the field of human sexual behavior have generally abandoned this term in favor of more specific categories referring to the individual problems involved.

Masters and Johnson (1970) were prime movers in questioning both the term *frigidity* and the general view it represented. They successfully argued that new labels more appropriate to the actual problems women experience were needed. Kaplan (1974) further elaborated on their work by adding and discussing specific problems with arousal. The result has been a revised terminology, which is now reflected in DSM-III. The important sexual dysfunctions in women have been identified as inhibited female sexual excitement, inhibited female orgasm, functional vaginismus, and functional dyspareunia.

Inhibited female sexual excitement

Inhibited sexual excitement (ISE) refers to a lack of responsiveness to sexual stimuli during sexual encounters. The woman reports little or no erotic feeling and does not show the physiological manifestations of arousal, such as vaginal lubrication, nipple erection, expansion of the vagina, and so on. The woman reports little pleasure from sexual intercourse and may even experience it as uncomfortable or painful. As with male ISE, the problem may be primary, in which case the woman has never experienced arousal, or secondary, in which case arousal has occurred previously but is not being experienced currently. Inhibited sexual excitement must be distinguished from **inhibited sexual desire**, another category included in the DSM-III. Inhibited sexual desire is a general lack of interest in all sexual aspects of life in either men or women, although it is much more frequently reported in women. Unlike other dysfunctions, which involve specific responses that are not functioning adequately, this problem is a generalized lack of desire that frequently results in the avoidance of sexual contact. Inhibited sexual excitement, on the other hand, is specific to certain occasions of sexual contact. The woman experiencing ISE may be desirous of sex and may be aroused under other conditions, but at the time of sexual intercourse she does not show the normal physiological excitatory responses.

Incidence figures are not a useful gauge of the extent of this problem. Many women feel it is inappropriate for them to complain about a lack of sexual feelings. Our Victorian heritage still has many women questioning whether a "normal" woman should have such feelings. Even if there are no moral rules against feelings of arousal, many women have had no training, instruction, or experience to help them know what they should be feeling. Because self-exploration and self-stimulation have been discouraged for women, many have never experienced the sensual-erotic sensations they are capable of. Thus, women such as Doris, described at the beginning of this chapter, are unaware that they may be missing an important part of their sexual lives.

Inhibited sexual desire is a common problem in women. The famous female "headache" was not made famous by its rarity. The many couples in the process of separation, divorce, marital counseling, and sexual enhancement therapies often indicate that female ISE is one of the most significant problems in their relationship. The feminist movement has made women more aware of, and more concerned about, enhancing their own sexuality. Now that women are more aware of the missing eroticism in their lives, more and more are reporting problems with ISE to their gynecologists and physicians. One result has been a rise in the number of couples taking the positive step of seeking help for this problem.

The causes of female ISE are many. As with the male sexual response, the female excitement state is highly sensitive to interference. The emotional reactions, the feelings of arousal, and the physiological events of vasocongestion and lubrication are all part of the autonomic arousal system of the body. Any stimulus, current or remote, that creates tension or distracts from the sexual situation can reverse the excitement response. Unlike inhibited excitement in the male, with its resulting erectile problems, ISE in the female does not prevent sexual intercourse. However, it may be experienced as mechanical, lacking in eroticism, and perhaps uncomfortable.

An important causal factor in this problem is the partner's sexual behavior. Since the woman's buildup of excitement is more gradual and more fragile than the man's, a certain amount of patience and skill is required from the partner for successful arousal. An insensitive partner whose sexual arousal techniques are too rough or too fast is a commonly reported cause of ISE in women. The woman is not, however, just an innocent bystander. Her ability, and responsibility, to effectively communicate her desires and dislikes plays a significant role in her partner's arousal techniques. Without guidance, the partner may develop behaviors that are actually antierotic, despite the best of intentions to the contrary. Later in this chapter we will see how recent approaches to sex therapy have focused on improved communication between partners as an important part of the treatment for women experiencing ISE.

The psychoanalytic approach to ISE explains the development of this problem in terms of the ***Electra*** complex. According to this explanation, the girl's incestuous desire for the father figure is so frightening that residual feelings in adulthood cause intense anxiety that effectively shuts down sexual responsiveness to male partners.

*Inhibited female
orgasm*

Although ***orgasmic dysfunction***, ***orgastic dysfunction***, and *frigidity* are all terms that have been applied to lack of orgasm in women, the formal label used in DSM-III is ***inhibited female orgasm***. In this type of dysfunction, the woman does not experience the orgasmic phase of the sexual response cycle. The woman may feel sexually aroused, may experience vaginal lubrication, and may show other signs of sexual responsiveness, yet she does not experience orgasm.

Inhibited female orgasm is usually divided into two types. In the primary type, the woman has never experienced orgasm, regardless of the type of stimulation tried (intercourse, masturbation, oral genital contact, and so on). In the secondary type, the woman has experienced orgasm in the past but is not currently orgasmic. Masters and Johnson have added a third type, a category they call ***situational orgasmic dysfunction***. They use this term in describing women who experience orgasm under certain specific conditions but not others. For example, a woman might have orgasms during masturbation but not during intercourse, or she might experience it in motel rooms but not in her own bedroom.

Women have been asked about their orgasmic responsiveness since the 1930s, and it is interesting to note the changes in the statistics for dysfunction since then. In a 1931 study, Dickman and Beam reported that only 40 percent of the 1000 women they sampled had experienced orgasm during intercourse. Kinsey's (1953) study, which included 6000 women, found that 28 percent had never experienced orgasm from any type of sexual encounter. Half of the women who were married did not experience it in their first year of marriage, but eventually 95 percent of the married group did experience orgasm at least once. However, only 45 percent of that group indicated that they expected orgasm on every or almost every occasion of sexual contact. More recent surveys, such as Hunt's (1974), have found that 53 percent of married women expect orgasm on every or almost every occasion of intercourse. In Hunt's survey only 15 percent of the women reported experiencing orgasm "sometimes or never." Both Hunt and Kaplan (1974) determined the figure for inhibited female orgasm to be approximately 10 percent of women in the United States.

There may be a problem with such incidence figures because of the difficulty women may have in defining orgasm or lack of it. Orgasm is a highly subjective event and varies greatly from one woman to another. There is no ejaculation as in the male to give a distinct signal of orgasm's occurrence. It can be experienced in any of a variety of ways, from dramatic to subtle. For many women it is actually felt as a series of experiences rather than as a single event. Furthermore, expectancy as to what the feelings should be plays an important role in the self-labeling of orgasm. If a woman is expecting an earthquake and experiences only mild tremors, she may not think she has actually experienced orgasm.

The woman who does not experience orgasm may feel disappointed and frustrated. For her there is a sense of something missing in the excitement phase, and resolution is slow and unsatisfying. Because of this dissatisfaction, the woman may avoid sexual encounters altogether.

What causes inhibited female orgasm? The immediate cause is an involuntary inhibition of the natural orgasmic reflex, but there are many factors that can contribute to this inhibition. One such factor is the double standard regarding the acceptability of sexual feelings in men and women. The view that women should not enjoy sex is still part of some family-trained moral codes and some religious upbringing. Such training could be expected to affect excitement and arousal, or it could interfere with the woman's ability to relax and enjoy her sexual sensations.

Masters and Johnson have noted that anything that puts the woman into the spectator role at the point of orgasmic release is incompatible with the freedom to experience orgasm. A wide range of stimuli, feelings, thoughts, and conditioned reactions can provide such self-consciousness and thus interfere with the natural course of the sexual response cycle. These interfering factors are highly specific to the individual; counseling is usually required to determine what factors are involved and to provide procedures for neutralizing them.

Vaginismus

Vaginismus is a condition in which the muscles of the vagina contract involuntarily, thereby making penile entry extremely difficult or impossible. It does not appear to be a common disorder, but as with other disorders involving sexual dysfunction, statistics are not highly reliable.

In the fully developed type of vaginismus, the muscles of the lower third of the vaginal barrel and those controlling the entrance to the vagina go into **spasm**, closing the vagina almost totally. The spasm is initially brought on by the man's attempts to penetrate the vaginal tract during intercourse. While failure to be able to introduce the penis into the vagina is the usual complaint, the woman may also have the same involuntary muscle response to any attempt to enter the vagina. Thus, sexual foreplay by manual stimulation and even gynecological examination of the vagina may produce the involuntary closure.

The problem can be highly specific to vaginal entry and not affect any other aspect of sexual responsiveness. For example, the woman may be totally arousable and orgasmic in response to other stimulation but cannot experience penile insertion.

What causes vaginismus? The spasm is much like the protective reactions of other muscle groups in response to pain. Traumatic attempts at vaginal entry from any source during the woman's formative years would be a likely basis for the flinchlike reaction of the vaginal muscles. However, in most cases no specific previous event is reported. More often, the problem appears to be a result of psychological fear rather than a repercussion from some actual physical event. A variety of such psychological prior conditions were found by Masters and Johnson (1970) in a group of women experiencing vaginismus. Among the events found to contribute to the problem were strict religious upbringing, mothers training their daughters that sex is unpleasant and painful, and psychological reactions to rape even when no physical trauma has occurred.

Dyspareunia

Basically, **dyspareunia** is painful intercourse. Most of the physical conditions that are likely to cause discomfort can be successfully treated by appropriate medical procedures. For some women, however, there is no structural or physical problem to explain the discomfort. They are referred for psychological study and treatment.

The extent of this problem among American women is difficult to determine. Dyspareunia is a subjective state, and if no physical pathology is found, the complaint may be dismissed by the physician or gynecologist as imaginary or hysterical. Whether or not the doctor thinks the problem is real, the woman may refuse to engage in further sexual encounters.

In some cases, dyspareunia may be secondary to nonlubrication of the vaginal tract during the excitement stage of sexual response. The resulting irritation leads to a sense of discomfort, and eventually the woman avoids further stimulation because of the pain. In such cases the dyspareunia is really secondary to ISE and should be approached with treatment appropriate for that problem.

In those cases where dyspareunia is indeed a separate psychological problem, it may be the result of a low threshold for pain or of a high threshold for pleasure sensations, so that the movement of the penis is sensed as nonpleasurable stimulation. Everyone has experienced occasions when a previously pleasurable type of stimulation was found to be unpleasant. For the sufferer from dyspareunia, this situation may have become the rule rather than the exception. The complications in dealing with such a subjective state are obvious; thus, each case must be approached individually and with a great deal of empathy for the woman's concerns. After all, she experiences pain where everyone else tells her she should feel pleasure. Not only does she miss out on the pleasures of sex, but she is made to feel guilty for somehow not reacting appropriately.

**APPROACHES TO
SEX THERAPY**

Once a problem is identified and labeled as a sexual dysfunction, the individual may seek sexual therapy. There are a number of different therapeutic approaches available to choose from, but two main theoretical models have come to dominate thinking about the causes and treatment of sexual dysfunction: the psychodynamic approach and the behavioral approach.

According to the ***psychodynamic (psychoanalytic)*** perspective in its simplest form, sexual dysfunctions are ***symptoms*** of ***intrapsychic conflicts*** that remain unresolved from earlier stages of psychosexual development (see Chap. 9). The goal of therapy is to make the individual aware of these conflicts and to enable him or her to ***work through*** them so that they no longer create sexual dysfunctions, thereby allowing the person to have a normal sex life. (It is important to note that the psychoanalytic perspective generally equates "normal" sexuality with heterosexual behavior. For Freud, the final positive result of psychosexual development was adequate psychosexual adjustment to the opposite sex.)

According to the ***behavioral*** perspective, on the other hand, sexual dysfunction is a ***learned maladaptive behavior*** or a failure to learn appropriate sexual behavior. The goal of treatment is ***relearning.*** Therapy is designed to increase the frequency of adaptive responses and to decrease the frequency of maladaptive responses.

Despite the major differences between these theoretical approaches, there has been a growing consensus on the treatment of sexual dysfunctions. This consensus has followed from the successes of Masters and Johnson (1970, 1974) in their use of specially designed procedures based on their research. The newer approaches based on the Masters and Johnson model are basically behavioral. They directly confront the dysfunctional behavior rather than approach it as a symptom of some more fundamental problem. However, they also recognize developmental events in the person's earlier life as important contributors to current problems.

Masters and Johnson's research (1966) on the nature of the normal sexual response demonstrated how sexual dysfunctions result from distortions of the natural sexual response cycle. Therefore, they devised ways for clients to "relearn" more adaptive behaviors and to eliminate interfering behaviors. The result was a set of treatment procedures designed to reestablish the natural sexual response.

The growing popularity of what has come to be called the ***new sex therapy*** (Kaplan, 1974) does not mean that no other therapeutic approaches are available. Psychoanalysis and other insight-type approaches still have a place in the treatment of certain kinds of problems. There are also more specific behavioral procedures that do not employ the complete Masters and Johnson approach, such as LoPiccolo and Lobitz's (1972) treatment for inhibited female orgasm. In addition, there is a wide array of other treatment procedures based on a variety of theoretical models of the development of psychological problems. Client-centered therapy, gestalt therapy, existential therapy, transactional analysis, and rational emotive therapy are just a few of the psychotherapeutic approaches used for helping people who are experiencing sexual dysfunctions. And while psychotherapists have had to learn to double as sex therapists, many sex therapists are learning that clients must be treated for more than just sexual problems, as is discussed in Box 15.2.

BOX 15.2

The increasing complexity of sex therapy

During the last few years, the field of sex therapy has gone through some gradual yet major changes. Originally, the focus of sex therapy, as initiated by Masters and Johnson, had been on individual problems, such as premature ejaculation and inhibited female orgasm. Specific therapeutic procedures were developed and used to deal with such problems and were found to be quite successful. As a result, these procedures came to be well publicized, and people experiencing such problems could learn how to deal with them from reading books, from talking to their family doctors, or from seeing a psychologist, as well as from visiting a sex therapist.

Because people have become better able to deal with their sexual dysfunctions on their own, they are less likely to go to a sex therapist with such problems. Instead, sex therapists have begun to see a greater percentage of individuals with complex sexual problems. As Avodah K. Offit, coordinator of sex therapy at Lenox Hill Hospital in New York City has put it, "What seems to be happening more and more is that people who are unable to put their other conflicts into words often find they have a sexual symptom—and this is very easy to verbalize. Most couples now coming for sex therapy really need marital counseling for the major part of their difficulties" (Kosner, 1979, p. 85).

Furthermore, more and more couples are seeing therapists about sexual dissatisfaction rather than dysfunction. For example, Leon and Shirley Zussman, sex therapists in New York City, say that about 50 percent of their clients complain of lack of sexual desire. And it's not that lack of desire has become more prevalent; rather, more people are just wanting to do something about it. The more they hear and read about sexual behavior in the popular media, the more they begin to suspect that they're abnormal. Thus, whereas in the past sex therapy has relied heavily on correcting behavioral problems, today it must deal with each person's psychological problems and with the interpersonal dynamics of each couple.

In response to the need for changes in sex therapy, many practitioners have developed more eclectic approaches to treatment. One such therapist is Helen Singer Kaplan of Cornell University Medical College, who believes that brief behavioral therapy works best for couples whose relationship is basically sound and who are psychologically healthy. But if the relationship is bad, one person may try to sabotage the therapy, and if one of the persons has neurotic fears and anxieties, behavioral treatment may be difficult to implement. So Kaplan emphasizes an approach that deals at first with surface problems, such as dysfunctions, and then probes deeper if emotional conflicts are uncovered. Using a psychoanalytic approach, she may go into interpretation, trying to give the client insights into the deeper sources of his or her problems (Adams, 1980b).

The Zussmans also favor an eclectic therapy. They use the basic Masters and Johnson techniques to start with. But even if this short-term behavioral treatment is successful in curing the problem, they often refer the couple to *another therapist or provide counseling themselves to help the couple work through nonsexual problems that have emerged in the relationship.*

What is the outcome of the new sex therapy? In a large percentage of cases, the "simple" dysfunctional problems are cured. And the psychological counseling at least helps couples to learn more about their sexual selves and their sexual relationship. But therapy cannot guarantee a happy outcome for the couple. They may learn, for example, that their sexual problems are a sign of overall dissatisfaction with the relationship. As James Maddock of the University of Minnesota Medical School has pointed out, "People can reverse their symptoms and still find themselves very unhappy. You cure impotence and then you find that the

marriage is a mess—that the impotence was an adaptive coping mechanism for keeping distance from each other. Now it becomes obvious how much conflict there really is" (Kosner, 1979, p. 141).

On the other hand, sex therapy can also breathe life into marriages that seem dead. Even though it may not succeed in improving the couple's sexual performance, they may feel happier as a result of the therapy. As with other kinds of psychotherapy, the new sex therapy is subject to so many variables that it is difficult to judge its success or failure. The main thing is for couples who seek therapy to have realistic expectations. According to psychiatrist Stephen Levine, "Therapists should not promise quick cures, and people should not expect them" (Adams, 1980b, p. 36).

Although there are variations in how the new sex therapy procedures are applied, most sex therapy clinics and sex therapists follow the same basic format and use the same basic techniques.

The format of the therapy is the way the treatment is conducted—the formal aspects of the therapy. It is in these formal aspects that the impact of the behavioral approach is most noticeable. Prior to the work of Masters and Johnson, individual psychotherapy was the usual approach. A client was seen by a therapist, who tried to help the person achieve a more satisfactory sexual adjustment. The problem was considered to be in the patient's psyche, and the procedures were designed to change the person.

By not looking for the "cause" of the problem within the individual client, Masters and Johnson (1970) began to see the problem as existing within the sexual relationship. Thus, they saw the nonorgasmic woman not as a "frigid" female with a problem in her psyche, but as a person with an interactional difficulty in the sexual part of her relationship with a partner. This led to one of the most important changes in the treatment format: the treatment of sexual partners together as a unit. In fact, except in cases with unusual circumstances, Masters and Johnson refused to treat individuals alone. Today this has generally become accepted as standard practice in the various sexual dysfunction treatment centers. A related development has been the use of mixed-gender co-therapists. Since most couples are male-female pairs, Masters

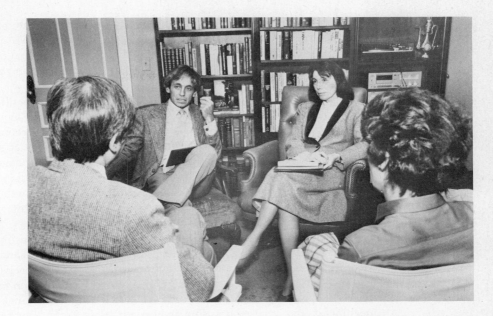

*Male and female
co-therapists are
considered the
ideal therapist
combination in
treating mixed
gender dysfunc-
tional couples.*

and Johnson have found that the greatest gains are made when there is a male
and a female therapist working with the couple. This eases some of the natural
discomfort involved in discussing intimate sexual details with a therapist.

*Treatment
techniques*

Several of the techniques first employed by Masters and Johnson have been
incorporated into modern treatment programs. These techniques include coital
abstinence, sensate focusing, and use of sexual surrogates.

Coital abstinence The most frequent first "homework" assignment for
couples experiencing dysfunction is to stop having sexual intercourse. This
coital abstinence is imposed to eliminate all sexual demands on the individuals
and to reduce the tension created by their efforts to achieve a goal. It also
serves to stop the ineffective behaviors and helps build up sexual desire in the
couple. Although they are not to engage in intercourse, the couple are told to
engage in closeness, touching, and other forms of mutual arousal without
moving on to intercourse.

Sensate focusing The couple are given instruction in **sensate focusing**—
mutual sensual pleasuring in which each partner takes turns actively producing erotic sensations in the other, who remains passive. Coitus is still not
allowed, so there is no pressure to reach any specific level of performance.
Genital stimulation may be left out at first, but eventually it is included,
although orgasm is still avoided. The couple are encouraged to communicate
their feelings about what is pleasant and unpleasant during the sensate focusing process. They thus learn to give and receive pleasure and to communicate
about sexual feelings. The verbal instruction is provided by the therapists

during the office visit, and the couple use the procedure at home when the therapists indicate it is appropriate. This process is meant to *densensitize* the anxious feelings that may arise during sexual encounter and to allow arousal to occur without the performance anxiety that is typically a part of the couple's dysfunction problem.

Sexual surrogates We have noted that the treatment of couples is the preferred treatment format. Because so many of the procedures require two people practicing various techniques together, this really has become a necessity. Yet many victims of sexual dysfunction are not in sexual relationships, often because of the problems that have driven them to seek therapy. The problems may have destroyed prior relationships or have kept them from forming adequate relationships in the first place. How, then, are therapists to deal with such unattached clients? One solution has been the interesting and rather controversial use of **sexual surrogates**.

Sexual surrogates are people who have had no prior relationship with the client but who are willing to go through the sexual experiences and treatment with the client. They are sometimes found by the clients themselves, or they may be supplied by the therapist and clinic. Masters and Johnson have argued against the use of surrogates for women clients, saying that women require a meaningful emotional relationship and cannot relate to the "mechanical" nature of the use of a surrogate. Some view this argument as chauvinistic and say the female client should be allowed to decide for herself whether a surrogate should be tried. Nevertheless, many clinics follow Masters and Johnson's rule and do not use surrogates with female clients.

Finding individuals willing to act as surrogates for males experiencing dysfunctions has not been as difficult as might be expected. Most therapists prefer not to use prostitutes. The general feeling is that a prostitute's approach to sexual relationships is distorted by her attitudes and experiences. Paid and unpaid respondents to advertisements are the most common types of surrogates. Many of the people who respond to such ads are altruistic in their desire to help dysfunctional individuals. The use of surrogates raises many ethical and moral issues. But at present this is the only method available for treating the unconnected client in the new sex therapy and is therefore seen as a complex but necessary part of the therapeutic approach.

Other techniques A variety of other innovations have come from the behavioral approach to treatment. Erotic films may be shown to a couple to heighten arousal. Or a couple may be moved to a motel or cabin for a few nights, thus providing a new environment that serves to reduce the tensions of the home situation (children, pets, noises, and so on) and to remove the stimuli associated with prior failures and frustrations.

In rare instances, direct observation of the couple's lovemaking has been used in order to analyze and correct problems in lovemaking skills. Because the obvious increase in tension and self-consciousness that occurs with such observation is likely to be counterproductive, most therapists feel the gains do not justify the potential problems.

THERAPEUTIC
PROCEDURES FOR
SPECIFIC
DYSFUNCTIONS
Inhibited male
sexual excitement

Now that we have introduced the basic sex therapy techniques, let us see how they are applied to the specific types of dysfunctions.

Primary and secondary ISE are primarily fear-based reactions. Thus, therapy is directed at *removing* the anxiety response that prevents the natural erection from occurring. Masters and Johnson (1970) stated the specific goals of therapy for ISE as (1) removing the male's fears about sexual performance, (2) making him an active participant in the sexual experience rather than allowing him to maintain the spectator role he has probably adopted, and (3) relieving the partner's fears about the man's performance.

The steps to be used in treatment were outlined by Kaplan (1974) as follows:

1   **Nondemand pleasuring.** *Coitus is not permitted during this phase, and sensate focusing is employed, with no demand for intercourse. By alternating active and passive erotic activities, the man usually experiences erection. Although this is encouraging, it does not dispel the man's fear about how he will perform when it comes to intercourse.*

2   Dispelling fear of failure. *Here the **squeeze technique** (originally designed to prevent premature ejaculation) is used. At the height of the erection, the partner squeezes the penis just below the glans until the erection subsides. Then stimulation is resumed until the erection returns. The reestablishment of the erection forms the basis of a new learned confidence that the erection will return if lost during stimulation.*

3   Removing distracting thoughts. *Any thoughts about losing the erection or other self-conscious thoughts need to be dispelled. Many mental techniques can be used, including thinking about sexually stimulating ideas or fantasies, visualizing nude women, or even thinking of nonsexual but pleasant non-anxiety-producing images or events.*

4   Coitus. *The first reestablished coital experience is extremely important and is approached slowly, with no pressure. Every possible support is arranged. The woman-on-top position is used, the woman guides the initial entry, and no orgasm is sought on the first few occasions.*

These procedures and variations on them are the current therapeutic techniques for curing ISE. As we will see in our discussion of outcome, they have proved to be remarkably successful.

Premature
ejaculation

The goal of treatment for premature ejaculation is to help the man experience nonanxious, nondemand erotic stimulation. In this way he can learn to withhold ejaculation. The main technique used is nondemand pleasuring, which leads to an increase in the excitement phase without proceeding to ejaculation.

The therapists instruct the couple in coital abstinence and teach them sensate focusing. The man is told to focus on his own sensations and to note when ejaculation seems imminent. At his signal, the woman is to use the squeeze technique or to cease stimulation until the feeling of imminent ejaculation passes. Then stimulation is resumed. This method, called the **start-stop technique**, also opens lines of communication between the partners that were probably not available before.

After several sessions of the start-stop technique, nondemand intromission is begun. The female superior position is used; once the penis is in place, no thrusting is tried at first. After several sessions, light movements are allowed, but only until the preejaculatory sensations occur. Then the penis is withdrawn and the squeeze technique is used, or the couple just relaxes until the sensations have passed and then start again.

The lack of orgasm is seen as a learned inhibition imposed on the natural process of stimulation leading to orgasm. The relearning here takes the form of reconditioning the ejaculatory response in the presence of the sexual partner.

The initial steps of treatment are the same as for ISE. Sexual intercourse is forbidden for a time, and sensate focusing is initiated. Next, the partner is instructed to use noncoital stimulation techniques on the man. These masturbatory activities can be of any kind, presumably those most comfortable for the couple. They are performed slowly, with no pressure and with the prime focus on enjoyment and pleasure. When ejaculation seems imminent, the man fixes his attention on his partner, to connect her to the orgasm.

When orgasm is occurring fairly regularly with these procedures, the next step is reestablishing coitus. Using the woman superior position, the stimulation activities are used until ejaculation seems near. At this point the penis is inserted. Intercourse may not work the first time or two, but the couple are told to expect this and to not feel angry or frustrated. Eventually the man will experience orgasm with intercourse; once this happens, there is usually a rapid return to natural responsiveness.

Masters and Johnson strongly recommend that the sexual needs of the partner be attended to during the masturbatory phase of the treatment. Because she is experiencing arousal, if no orgasm occurs, she may eventually develop a negative reaction to the treatment or perhaps sexual problems of her own. The woman should therefore also achieve orgasm using masturbation. Masters and Johnson refer to this as the *"give-to-get" principle.* It maintains good relationships during the noncoital phase of the treatment and guarantees that the treatment will not create other problems that replace those it was designed to help.

As we noted earlier, female ISE is a complex problem. Before treatment is begun, it is important to determine the point in the sexual arousal sequence at which natural positive erotic feelings stop. If no sexual feelings are aroused at any point in the sexual encounter process, the problem may be more accurately described as inhibited sexual desire, in which case treatment should be oriented more toward general issues of the psychological meaning of sexual encounters for the woman.

ISE can start quite early in the sexual sequence. *Phobic reactions* (irrational fears) may be so severe that the slightest hint of sex may stimulate them. Even thinking about sex or a slight indication of sexual desire from the partner may begin the inhibitory response. The starting point for treatment must be just prior to where the inhibition occurs.

If the client's negative reactions are so strong that the partner cannot be included, the first phase of treatment may be designed for the woman alone until she can become comfortable in experiencing sexual feelings by herself. The initial arousal stimulus could be erotic literature or fantasies. Once the woman experiences arousal, she is instructed to move on to exploring her own body and to experiencing arousal and pleasure from self-stimulation (LoPicolo and Lobitz, 1974). Being comfortable with and knowledgeable about one's own body is often a new experience for the woman. The prohibitions against such self-exploration and eroticism in our society are so strong that many women are totally ignorant and ashamed of such experiences.

When the woman can achieve arousal alone and feels reasonably secure doing so, the partner is reintroduced into the picture. Kaplan (1974) provides a detailed step-by-step procedure, based on the Masters and Johnson approach, for the couple to follow:

1 Sensate focus I. *The partners take turns pleasuring and caressing each other, but they avoid genital stimulation.*
2 Sensate focus II. *They take turns pleasuring in a nondemanding way, but they do not try to produce orgasm.*
3 Genital stimulation. *This is done in a slow, teasing manner, stopping just prior to orgasm. The couple continues after the woman is in a less-aroused state.*
4 Heightening. *Arousal continues, but intercourse is still avoided to assure heightened desire and lubrication.*
5 Intercourse. *When intercourse is intiated, the woman-on-top position is used so that the woman can control the degree of sensation, speed, pene-tration, angle, and so on. She is instructed to maximize the sensation and still withold orgasm as long as possible.*

A variety of cognitive procedures are also used by many of the behavioral approaches. Erotic fantasies can be shared by the partners, and erotic materials (films, books, magazines) may be used. The goal is arousal in the presence of the partner, and any help in achieving this in a nonthreatening manner is welcomed.

Finally, the importance of communication is critical. Sensitivity to mood and pace are highly important, and since the woman can easily be turned off, it is necessary that the partners be able to communicate openly about their needs, desires, and so on. After all, sexual intercourse is basically a social interaction, and communication is a central component in any successful social interaction.

Inhibited female orgasm

The techniques for treating inhibited female orgasm are similar to those for treating ISE. However, they must be tailored to whether the dysfunction is evidenced in all situations or just during intercourse. If the woman has never achieved orgasm through masturbation, the therapist will start here, with the first level of learning orgasmic responsiveness. It is important to establish the feeling of arousal and orgasm and to know they are achieved under psychologically safe conditions. Vibrators have been used as one method for treating inorgasmic women. They are, however, simply a means of heightening sensation and do not "cure" inhibited orgasm.

Once self-knowledge, eroticism, and orgasm are well established in the woman, the partner is introduced into the situation. The program is much the same as for ISE, with the various stages of sensate focusing and slow arousal. Now, however, the emphasis is on increasing sexual tension to high levels and avoiding inhibitory responses at the point of orgasm.

For some women, the standard procedures are all that is necessary, and orgasm soon follows. Others are able to masturbate to orgasm but do not achieve orgasm with their partner. One way to bring the orgasm and the partner together is to have the partner use the woman's recently learned masturbatory techniques, with her help. In this way the association of the partner with orgasmic experiences is accomplished, and the increase in the partner's knowledge about what is exciting to the woman will be an important aid in their continued growth as a sexual couple.

Vaginismus and dyspareunia

Treatment of vaginismus follows the **systematic desensitization** model for overcoming conditioned reactions. It is important that the woman and her partner understand the nature of the problem and realize that there is nothing physically wrong with her. A typical desensitization sequence begins with the woman stimulating herself alone, very gradually introducing her fingers into the opening of the vagina and then gradually inserting them inside. This is always done under arousal conditions and is stopped if the arousal subsides. The woman gradually tries deeper and wider penetration. Then the partner is instructed to use his fingers in following this same gradual sequence. Once the woman is comfortable with finger insertion, the couple may move on to intercourse. The female superior position is used at the beginning, so that the woman has total control over the amount of stimulation. Generally, this procedure works rapidly and is quite effective.

Dyspareunia, as we noted earlier, can be a reaction to a variety of conditions. Most are local physical conditions and can be treated medically. The psychological type is difficult to recognize or treat. The few cases that have been treated have been helped by gentleness and graded exposure to sexual activity.

THE OUTCOME OF SEX THERAPY

Sexual problems have traditionally been among the most difficult to treat psychotherapeutically. Low success rates, even after years of treatment, were the norm. Even more disappointing were high rates of recurrence of problems that were thought to be cured. Furthermore, traditional psychodynamic procedures usually entailed a great deal of time and exposure.

The results of the new sex therapy stand in sharp contrast to previous success rates. Masters and Johnson (1970) reported high success rates with their clients and, even more important, low levels of recurrence. The new therapy also takes less time and less money than have previous treatment

TABLE 15.1	Dysfunction	Percent not cured
Failure rates for sexual therapy	Primary impotence	40
	Secondary impotence	26
	Retarded ejaculation	2
	Orgasmic dysfunction	20
	Vaginismus	0

Source: Masters and Johnson (1970), p. 359.

approaches. Some of the figures cited by Masters and Johnson in their outcome studies are given in Table 15.1. (Note that labels are older, DSM-II-type labels.)

Since Masters and Johnson's initial reports, similar results have been obtained by several other sex therapists. The results have even been improved on as the techniques have been refined. There are failures; there are relapses; and there are individual therapists and sex clinics that provide inadequate treatment. The problems of sexual dysfunction have not been eradicated from our society, and treatment is not always readily available—nor are cures easy. Not all reports have been positive. Zilbergeld and Evans (1980) have criticized the Masters and Johnson outcome statistics. This questioning has stimulated lively debate about how such statistics should be gathered. Despite the debate, a person experiencing a sexual dysfunction today should be able to receive adequate and reasonably rapid treatment with a high probability of return to a fulfilling sex life. Thus, sexual problems, which seemed to be so resistent to treatment just a few years ago, can now in large part be overcome with contemporary treatment approaches.

SUMMARY

1 *Sexual dysfunction* is an inability to engage in or to enjoy sexual encounters. Although some dysfunctions are the result of physical problems, most are attributable to psychological factors that interfere with the person's natural reactions.

2 *Inhibited sexual excitement* (ISE) in men (formerly called *impotence*), is the inability to achieve or maintain an erection of sufficient quality to engage in sexual intercourse. It may be primary or secondary. Primary ISE is usually the result of early experiences, such as repressive religious training and stressful initial sexual encounters. Secondary ISE is more likely to be caused by a specific *precipitating event* (such as fatigue or work pressure) that creates difficulty in achieving or maintaining erection. This first occasion creates anxiety over future ISE, which in turn increases the likelihood of future ISE. *Performance anxiety* plays a major role in the problem.

3 *Premature ejaculation* is difficult to define precisely, but in general it refers to the man's coming to orgasm too quickly. The main causes of the problem appear to be anxiety as well as early sexual experiences.

4 *Inhibited male orgasm* is the inability to ejaculate during sexual intercourse. This problem may be primary or secondary. The usual cause is anxiety, with the man often taking a *spectator role* in his efforts to achieve orgasm.

Traumatic sexual experiences in which orgasm has been interrupted may contribute to this problem.

5   In women, *inhibited sexual excitement* refers to a lack of responsiveness to sexual stimuli during sexual encounters. It must be distinguished from *inhibited sexual desire*, which is a general lack of interest in sex. ISE in women may be primary or secondary. This problem is very common, given the repressive Victorian heritage governing female sexual responsiveness. One major factor in the development of ISE is the partner's inappropriate sexual arousal techniques.

6   *Inhibited female orgasm* is the lack of orgasm in women. The woman may experience arousal and excitement but does not experience orgasm. There are three types: primary, secondary, and *situational orgasmic dysfunction*, in which the woman is orgasmic in some situations but not in others. Research has shown that the percentage of women with this problem has been declining in recent years. The main causes of this problem seem to be residual childhood training against female sexuality and interfering factors that distract the woman during intercourse, putting her into the spectator role.

7   *Vaginismus* is an involuntarily conditioned response in which the muscles of the vagina *spasm*, thereby preventing penile entry.

8   *Dyspareunia* is painful intercourse. It may be caused by a physical condition or may be psychological in origin.

9   The two major approaches to sexual therapy are the *psychodynamic* (psychoanalytic) and the *behavioral*. According to the psychodynamic approach, dysfunction is the result of unresolved *intrapsychic conflicts* in psychosexual development and requires long-term psychoanalysis as treatment. According to the behavioral approach, dysfunction is *learned maladaptive behavior*; the goal of therapy is therefore *relearning*.

10   The *new sex therapy* is basically a behavioral approach based on the research and methods of Masters and Johnson. The treatment of both partners, using mixed-gender co-therapists, is the basic format of the new therapy. The main treatment techniques used are *coital abstinence* and *sensate focusing*. If the dysfunctional person does not have a partner, a *sexual surrogate* may be used.

11   The specific treatment methods used depend on the particular dysfunction. In male ISE, for example, the sequence involves nondemand pleasuring, dispelling fear of failure, removing distracting thoughts, and gradual movement toward coitus. Other techniques used with male problems include the *squeeze technique* for halting ejaculation, the *stop-start technique* for prolonging arousal, and the *"give-to-get" principle*, in which the man ensures the woman's sexual pleasure during his own treatment so that she will not develop problems of her own.

12   Treatment techniques for women often focus on teaching them to explore their own bodies and to become comfortable with self-arousal before involving the partner. A method used for treating vaginismus is *systematic desensitization*, in which entering of the vagina is done very gradually, beginning with the woman's fingers, then the man's fingers, and eventually the penis.

13   The new sex therapy appears to be highly successful in treating the various sexual dysfunctions, although the statistics that have been used are controversial.

ADDITIONAL READING

* **Barbach, Lonnie Garfield.** *For Yourself: The Fulfillment of Female Sexuality.* Garden City, NY: Doubleday, 1976.

> *A sensitively written book aimed at helping each woman fulfill her sexual potential. Presents a clear set of steps to help the preorgasmic woman explore and accept the sensations of her body.*

* **Kaplan, Helen Singer.** *The New Sex Therapy.* New York: Brunner-Mazel, 1974.

> *The most comprehensive book on the treatment of sexual dysfunctions in both men and women to date. A clear and concise discussion of treatment issues and techniques. Somewhat more clinical than Barbach or Zilbergeld.*

* **Masters, William H., and Johnson, Virginia E.** *Human Sexual Inadequacy.* Boston: Little, Brown, 1970.

> *The classic volume that revolutionized the treatment of sexual dysfunctions. Includes a complete description of their treatment program and their research findings.*

* **Zilbergeld, Bernie.** *Male Sexuality.* New York: Bantam Books, 1978.

> *A book that addresses male sexual myths and problems. A clear discussion of what men can do to aid their own sexual functioning. Witty and easy to read.*

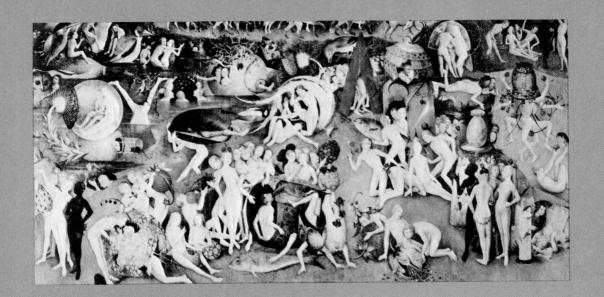

Sexual variance

16

chapter

16

On August 28, 1889, P. was arrested at the Trocadero, in Paris, in the act, as he forcibly cut off a young girl's hair. He was arrested with the hair in his hand and a pair of scissors in his pocket. He excused himself on the ground of momentary mental confusion and an unfortunate, irresistible passion; he confessed that he had ten times cut off hair, which he took great delight in keeping at home. On searching his home, sixty-five switches and tresses of hair were found, assorted in packets. P. had already been once arrested on December 15, 1886, under similar circumstances, but was released for lack of evidence.

P. stated that, for the last three years, when he was alone in his room at night he fell ill, anxious, excited and dizzy, and then was troubled by the impulse to touch female hair. When it happened that he could actually take a young girl's hair in his hand he felt intensely excited sexually, and had erection and ejaculation without touching the girl in any other way. (Krafft-Ebing, 1965, p. 267)

The case of P. is an example of a sexually related problem that is quite different from sexual dysfunction. Problems such as P.'s involve sexual behavior that differs markedly enough from a society's usual patterns for it to be considered "abnormal." Such problems are called **sexual variances**.

The term *variance* implies a difference from other, presumably more "normal," patterns of behavior. But how do we decide what constitutes normal behavior? Normality is typically defined according to one or more of three basic standards: psychological standards, societal standards, and legal-moral standards. Each of these sets of standards provides a different perspective on normality and thus a different interpretation of what should be considered variant from the normal.

According to *psychological standards* of normality, sexual behavior that varies sufficiently from the usual is considered psychopathological. Such behavior is seen as a deviation from expected psychological functioning in an otherwise psychologically intact person. Thus, the behavior is thought to entail some developmental distortion, personality defect, or learned maladaptive response that is now part of the person. According to this approach, change in the variant behavior is brought about by changing the psychological factors that produced the behavior.

When a sexual behavior is viewed as varying from *social standards*, the criterion is a normative-statistical one; that is, the majority of people engage in sexual behavior *X*, while the variant minority engage in sexual behavior *Y*. In this context, Gagnon (1977) prefers the term **sexual minorities** to *sexual variants*. According to the sociological viewpoint, either the individual must adapt to society (either by changing to fit the norms or by learning to live with the existing difference), or society must adapt to the variant minority (such as by being more tolerant of the variant behavior).

Finally, variant behavior can be defined in terms of the *legal-moral standards* of a society. The legal statutes are the source of such definition and demonstrate the "cost" of engaging in a specific behavior by indicating the legal penalties involved. Similar rules and penalties are invoked by religious standards. Legal and religious laws are, of course, socially determined, but they tend to label behavior as being "right" or "wrong" rather than just different. According to the legal approach, change is brought about through punishment, removal from society, and reeducation or retraining. According to the religious-moral approach, change is brought about through guilt and shame, as the variant individuals see the "error of their ways."

Because each of these three systems of standards sees variant behavior differently, the approach that is taken to deal with such behaviors depends on which system (psychological, social, or legal-moral) is invoked. As we examine the various types of sexual variance in this chapter, we will be noting how each is predominantly treated in our society. Toward the end of the chapter, we will assume the psychological perspective in order to discuss therapy and treatment for individuals who engage in variant sexual behavior.

In discussing specific variant behaviors, it is useful to be able to put them into some distinct categories. Thus, in this chapter we have chosen to use three main categories for classifying variant sexual behaviors: (1) variations in the mode of the sexual expression, (2) variations in the choice of sexual object or outlet, and (3) variations in the strength of the sexual response.

VARIANCES IN SEXUAL EXPRESSION

This category emphasizes variations in the *nature* of the sexual behavior the person prefers. The way the sexual behavior is performed and the way sexual satisfaction is achieved differ for individuals in this category when compared with those of most of the other people in society. However, the variant behaviors are also frequently part of "normal" sexual behavior. It is often the amount or degree of the behavior that is problematic rather than the type of behavior. It is when the problem behavior comes to dominate the person's sexual life that it comes to be considered variant. Included in this category are voyeurism, exhibitionism, sadism, masochism, and transvestism.

Voyeurism

We are all voyeurs to some extent. In our society there are many socially acceptable ways to view nudity or erotic activities, from nightclub acts to "nudie" magazines, X-rated films, and coin-operated peep shows. The act of looking at any of these is not considered a deviation. Presumably these "normal" visual activities only serve to heighten sexual interest, which is then directed to more usual sexual outlets. But in the case of true **voyeurism**, watching other people in various stages of undress or engaging in sexual acts is the *primary* or *exclusive* source of sexual satisfaction. There is usually a clandestine aspect to voyeurism. The person becomes a *Peeping Tom* or *peeper*, seeking unsuspecting targets by peering in windows, through keyholes, over fences, and so on.

The original name *Peeping Tom* comes from the legend of Lady Godiva's famous nude horseback ride in 1057. Her husband, the Lord of Coventry, had decreed that everyone was to stay inside with the shutters closed during his wife's ride. Tom, the tailor, "peeped" through his shutter and, depending on which account you read, was either blinded or put to death for his transgression. It is interesting that the penalty was so severe relative to the crime. It is also interesting that the first recorded peeper was looking *out* his window and not *in* someone else's.

The need for an unsuspecting victim and the invasion of someone's privacy seem to be important parts of voyeurism. The secret, even illegal viewing of the innocent victim adds to the voyeur's excitement. Viewing is the ultimate sexual pleasure, and the true voyeur does not seek out more usual sexual outlets. Viewing itself can lead directly to orgasm or can do so with masturbation. This activity replaces sexual intercourse as the mode of sexual satisfaction. Voyeurs generally do not seek or want contact with the object of their peeping behavior.

It is unusual for voyeurs to present themselves for treatment of their problem. They are most often identified as the result of the complaints of others or as a result of arrest while engaging in the behavior. Arrested voyeurs are almost always men; thus, voyeurism has been considered to be a problem of males only.

Voyeurs are often emotionally and sexually immature men who do not have ordinary sexual outlets available. Only one-fourth of men arrested for this behavior are married, far below the average for the society. Voyeurism is also commonly a repeat offense: 50 percent of first arrests are typically followed by a second offense. Obviously, many more repeat the act but are not caught.

Exhibitionism

The man in the rumpled raincoat with nothing underneath who suddenly opens his coat to reveal all to unsuspecting passers-by has become a comic figure in our society. The "flasher" has been depicted in cartoons, television shows, movies, and comedy routines as a humorous subject, played for laughs. But for the person who engages in the behavior and his victims, it is not quite as entertaining an experience.

Exhibitionism generally refers to exposing one's sexual organs to someone else who is not seeking or expecting such exposure. The exhibitionist is usually a man and the victims are usually women or children. Sexual excitement is experienced by the exhibitionist, and orgasm may occur at the time of exposure or shortly thereafter, with or without masturbation. Exhibitionism is usually a repetitive pattern that is performed compulsively. Some exhibitionists report trying to withstand the compulsion but failing, find themselves "yielding to the urge."

While the actual exposure behavior may follow a similar pattern from case to case, the reasons for the behavior may differ greatly from one exhibitionist to the next. The most frequently reported type of exhibitionism is designed to shock the victim. In such cases the man tends to choose younger women as his victims and becomes greatly disturbed if the victim makes any derisive comments or does not show surprise. A second type of exhibitionist exposes himself primarily to children. Although this type seems more oriented toward interesting or attracting the child to sexual activity, he rarely actually approaches the child.

Exhibitionism accounts for one-third of all arrests for sex offenses in the United States. After a first arrest, about 20 percent are arrested again. But these statistics do not really indicate the extent of this behavior, since most reports of exhibitionism do not result in an arrest and many incidents are never reported to the police in the first place.

An arrest often precipitates a crisis in the exhibitionist's life and is the impetus for seeking help from mental health professionals. Because arrest leads to shame, guilt, and embarrassment and to negative reactions from wives, friends, and employers, the exhibitionist acknowledges the need for professional help. Nevertheless, his compulsion to repeat the act is often as strong or even stronger than ever.

In addition to being a cause of stress in a man's life, exhibitionism may be a result of it. It seems that some men respond to stressful periods in their lives by committing exhibitionist acts. In these cases, stresses such as impending marriage, the birth of a child, or loss of a job tend to precede the exposure incident. Such men may perform subsequent exhibitionist actions but only after additional life stresses.

Some investigators note that the angry, hostile nature of exhibitionism and the desire to shock and scare are important parts of the act (Lester, 1975). Since it does not require physical contact, exposing oneself is seen as a "safe" way of expressing angry feelings. Getting caught and punished for these unacceptable feelings may also be part of the script for some exhibitionists. Once they have been caught, the guilt for having these angry feelings has been responded to, so they feel better. This explanation also accounts for the fact that many exhibitionists seem to deliberately get themselves caught and then offer little defense for their actions.

Sadism

This married man in his twenties requested psychiatric help because he feared he would soon commit murder. Since adolescence, he has been excited by fantasies and pornography depicting women bound and tortured. During courtship of his wife, he introduced mild versions of his fantasy into their sex play, and in this manner only was able to proceed on to intercourse. Now, after eight years of marriage, they invariably have intercourse by his first binding her tightly with ropes and then, with her still bound, having intercourse. She has noticed that gradually the binding has been less and less symbolic and more and more painful. On two occasions in the last year, binding around her neck choked her into unconsciousness. (Stoller, 1976, pp. 204–205)

One would think that the pleasurable sensations we associate with sexual activity should preclude hurting one's partner—that hurtful behavior toward another person would be antithetical to sexual encounter. Physical sensations are, of course, difficult to define and highly subjective. Biting and scratching, which can be painful under other circumstances, may become pleasurable in a sexual context, and the giving and receiving of such stimulation is, for many, a

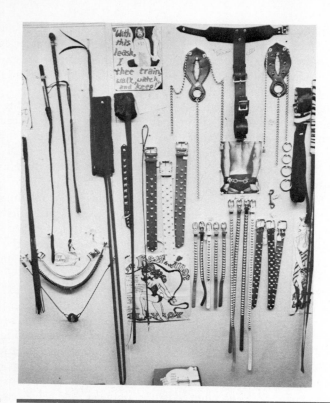

*Some of the
equipment sold in
shops catering to
sadomasochistic
customers.*

normal part of sexual behavior. The same could be said for psychological dominance and submission: Under certain circumstances, they may serve to enhance sexual encounters for a particular couple.

Sadism, however, involves an extreme use of pain and dominance. The sadist is a person who derives heightened sexual stimulation from administering physical or psychological pain to others. Sadism at a deviant level goes far beyond the typical biting and scratching of vigorous lovemaking and is meant to be hurtful and cruel; the sexual excitement and orgasm of the sadist are dependent on the discomfort of the victim.

The term *sadism* comes from the Marquis de Sade (1740–1814), who wrote vividly about his own imagined and actual sadistic practices of torture, cruelty, and debasement of others for his own sexual pleasure. That he was widely read in Europe suggests that he may have struck a responsive chord in many of his readers. The sexual deviation derived from his name is reserved today for those who engage in sadistic activities as their primary means of achieving sexual excitement and orgasm.

The American Psychiatric Association's DSM-III (1980) indicates that the diagnosis of sexual sadism is appropriate in any of the following three situations:

1   *The individual has repeatedly intentionally inflicted psychological or physical suffering on a nonconsenting partner in order to produce sexual excitement.*

2   *The preferred or exclusive mode of sexual excitement combines humiliation of a consenting partner with simulated or mildly injurious bodily suffering.*

3   *As in (2), the partner consents, but bodily injury is extensive, permanent, and possibly mortal.*

Sadistic activity may thus vary from mild levels, involving a need to fantasize sadistic activities in order to have adequate intercourse, all the way to the rare but horrifying extreme in which acts of mutilation and even murder are performed.

The description of sadistic activities in case studies, novels, and biographies of famous sadists constitutes a large body of literature demonstrating the ingenuity of humans in hurting and degrading others. There does not seem to be any particular pattern or specific acts that sadists prefer. Various paraphernalia (whips, bonds, masks, chains) are also used and today are sold in **sex shops** or **"leather" shops**. Use of such devices to enhance more usual types of sexual intercourse would probably not be labeled formally as sexual sadism. It is only when the criteria specified by the DSM-III are met that the person can be said to be a true sadist.

Masochism   As with sadism, **masochism** involves the pairing of erotic pleasure with physical or psychological pain. But instead of inflicting pain, the masochist wants to experience it. The term *masochism* comes from another author who wrote about his personal experiences with this form of sexual desire: Leopold von Sacher-Masoch (1836–1905).

The types of masochistic behaviors reported in the psychological literature are amazingly varied. Some of the more frequently reported activities include humiliation, beatings, whippings, spankings, and being tied up or bound in such a way as to feel helpless.

It is important to the masochist that the humiliation or pain be of a specific type administered in a specific manner. The case of Frank B. described in Chap. 1 illustrates this important aspect. Unexpected pain or pain administered in a way different from the one prescribed may be as antierotic to a masochist as it is to a nonmasochist. This scripted quality of the masochistic experience would seem to indicate that the experience is related to specific fantasies rather than to a desire for generalized pain.

The desire to experience pain seems an even greater violation of the natural rules of sexual behavior than sadism. Not only is pain antithetical to sexual pleasure, but it would seem to invalidate most of our theories of how behavior is learned and maintained. Living organisms are thought to seek out pleasure and to avoid pain, not the other way around. But pain, we must remember, is a highly subjective experience. Observing someone else receiving stimulation that we think should be painful leads us to believe that this person is experiencing the stimulation in the same way we would expect to experience it. But we may be mistaken. To any nonsmoker who has deeply inhaled cigarette smoke, the experience is extremely painful. But experienced smokers obviously derive a great deal of pleasure from this behavior. So we are on shaky ground when we try to describe what is or is not painful from other than our own perspective.

One factor that may contribute to our understanding of masochistic behavior is the role of physical punishment in child rearing. Masochists often report that such punishment played a central role in their childhood and remains a vivid memory of their relationship with their parents. They also note that the beatings and scoldings sometimes had sexual overtones. For some of these individuals, the occasions of being punished were among the few times they had close physical contact or direct attention of any kind from the important adult figures in their lives.

Punishment as a release of guilt is another childhood pattern that could be generalized to a confused adult reaction to punishment. In such cases the child may have felt terribly guilty about some thought or deed and only experienced relief from such feelings by being physically punished. In both of these examples we can see how being punished, either physically or psychologically, can become a desired experience quite early in a child's development.

It is often thought that sadists and masochists make the ideal sexual match, with each supplying what the other needs. In actuality, however, they make poor bedfellows! The sadist desires someone who experiences pain or degradation as just what it is—a highly unpleasant experience. The sadist does not want the partner to be enjoying himself or herself. For the masochist, the ideal is to have the scripted masochistic acts administered in the proper manner. The masochist does not want a partner who will punish or degrade in unexpected ways for his or her own pleasure. The point of both of these patterns is not just to hurt someone or to be hurt oneself in random ways but rather to enhance sexual arousal and responsiveness. Masochists actually tend to choose other masochists for sexual partners and to alternate dominance-submission roles so that each achieves satisfaction. A study of such **sadomasochists** in West Germany is described in Box 16.1.

Transvestism

In **transvestism**, the person experiences sexual arousal by dressing in the clothing of the opposite sex. The main focus of the person's sexual behavior is the cross-dressing, and transvestism, as such, is not an indication that the person wishes to become a member of the opposite sex or that the person wants to have homosexual experiences while dressed as a member of the opposite sex.

Transvestism has been reported primarily in men. Such men dress in one or more articles of women's clothing as a central part of their sexual behavior. In Prince and Butler's (1972) survey of readers of a transvestism magazine, they found that over 64 percent were married and another 14 percent had been married. Furthermore, 89 percent considered themselves to be heterosexual, 10 percent bisexual, and 1 percent homosexual. This percentage of homosexuality is lower than that found in the population as a whole.

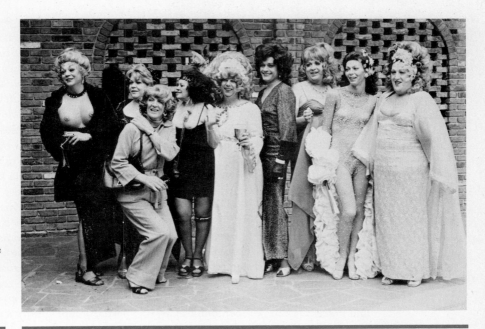

These transvestite males take great pride in their ability to look as feminine as possible.

The initial cross-dressing experience usually occurred in childhood or adolescence. In the Prince and Butler sample, 54 percent had their first transvestite experience before the age of 10. These early forays into cross-dressing became more sexually oriented as the person entered adolescence.

Transvestism is rarely a public problem. Most often it is not considered to be a problem by the transvestite, although it may create adjustment problems for mates, children, and other close people. It is often the concern of others that causes the transvestite to seek therapy.

Lester (1975) noted that there are few studies of the development of transvestism. He did find that the available data indicate that identification with the opposite-sex parent is highly important—if not central—to the development of transvestism.

VARIANCES IN SEXUAL OBJECT

For individuals in this category, it is the object of sexual desire that varies from the usual sex objects of most members of society. It is toward whom or what the individual directs his or her sexual interest that is at issue here rather than the actual sexual behavior. Variations included in this category are fetishism, zoophilia, pedophilia, incest, and necrophilia.

Fetishism

In **fetishism**, sexual arousal occurs in response to inanimate objects rather than to human partners. The most typical fetish objects are articles of clothing, particularly underwear, nightclothes, shoes, stockings, and other items worn close to the body. Besides physical objects, sounds, smells, tastes, and tactile sensations may become the chief focus of sexual arousal. Individuals can also

BOX 16.1

A study
of sado–
masochism

Sadomasochism is a sexual preference for inflicting and receiving pain or for acting out roles of submission and dominance. How do sadomasochists fit into the rest of society? How do they feel about their behavior? How do they deal with the social conflicts involved? Few studies that address such questions have been done. However, research conducted by Andreas Spengler (1977) in West Germany has shed some light on the sociocultural aspects of sadomasochism.

Spengler and his associates at the University of Hamburg devised a questionnaire to be filled out anonymously by sadomasochists. It covered such topics as sadomasochistic (S/M) activities and practices, the number and availability of partners, attitudes toward one's sexual preferences, and "coming out." One of the main problems, however, was finding subjects to complete the questionnaires, since people with this sexual orientation make a point of keeping it a secret. However, such people do try to contact each other through ads in special publications and may belong to sadomasochism clubs. So the researchers distributed over 800 questionnaires to addresses listed in contact ads and to cooperating clubs. Responses were received from 245 men. (Women were not included in the study.)

Of the respondents, 30 percent said they were exclusively heterosexual, 38 percent homosexual, and 31 percent bisexual. The men tended to be older (75 percent were over 31), well educated, of high social status, and financially well off. According to the researchers, the strong representation of such people might be explained by the way in which the sample was obtained. Participation in the subculture (through ads and clubs) might be easier for people with more disposable time and money, and the better educated might be more motivated to complete a questionnaire.

What did the researchers learn? A major discovery was that many sadomasochists are part of a subculture that provides them with a special set of behavioral norms. These norms, used as a point of reference, "make possible the deviant behavior," according to Spengler. "Where the sadomasochism practice is affirmed . . . and made possible, a social arena is created in which the usual social stigmatization of sadomasochistic behavior is suspended and is partially replaced by a positive counter norm" (p. 442).

The degree to which the participants in the study were integrated into this subculture varied. About 60 percent said they had friends who had S/M interests, and one-third reported attending sadomasochist parties. However, heterosexuals were less likely than homosexuals and bisexuals to have such direct contact with others in the subculture. Indirect contact, through S/M correspondence, had been used by about 80 percent of the men. All the respondents reported having purchased at least some S/M books and magazines, and most said they read such publications regularly.

Most of the men said they found their partners through contact ads in the various specialized publications. These S/M liaisons tended to be brief, since the men reported an average of 4.5 partners a year and 5 S/M experiences a year. The researchers therefore concluded that the sexual forms of behavior of sadomasochists "are characterized by low frequency and relatively great number of partners." Many of the men had wives or steady partners with whom they rarely engaged in S/M activities, so they went to outside partners to indulge in their special preference. Homosexual men in particular were 3 times as likely to engage in S/M activities with casual partners than with their steady partner.

Few of the men (16 percent) were devoted exclusively to sadomasochistic practices for their sexual pleasure. More than 60 percent indicated they had a medium or strong preference for S/M practices, while 16 percent said they only occasionally desired sadomasochistic sex. Very few of the men said they used extreme or dangerous S/M methods. Most preferred spanking or beating with a cane or whip, and about a third had fixations on fetishes, such as leather and boots.

A large percentage of the men (43 percent) said they hadn't become aware of their S/M desires until after age 19, although the heterosexual men were more likely to have "come out" in their younger years (63 percent before age 20). When asked how they had reacted when they first realized their preference for S/M, the majority (69 percent) said, "I wanted to do it again," and many reported feelings of pride and

happiness. Only 11 percent said they felt guilty, although 40 percent said, "I was troubled." Those who were active in the subculture tended to give the more positive responses.

All the men made a point of keeping their sexual orientation secret from the outside world. Their families rarely knew about it, and of those who were married, only 35 percent of the wives knew of or suspected their husband's S/M preference. Nevertheless, the majority of the men felt positive about their orientation. They felt it was "different from the ordinary but all right" (78 percent) and that "many more people ought to be like this" (49 percent). Only 1 percent considered the behavior to be immoral. Most considered S/M sex to be "fun" (84 percent) and "sexually satisfying" (79 percent). Only 4 percent reported feeling depressed or regretful. When asked whether they would accept or reject sadomasochism if they could decide freely on their sexual disposition, 70 percent chose acceptance.

Spengler found that positive self-judgments and positive emotional reactions were highest among men who were active in the S/M subculture. Thus, he felt that this study confirmed his hypothesis: that social roots in the S/M subculture contribute to a man's self-acceptance of his deviant behavior.

develop fetishes for parts of the body that are not the primary sexual organs, such as feet, nails, and hair. This type of fetish is called **partialism** Unlike the "breast man" or "leg man" who is aroused by particular body parts but then proceeds to more usual types of intercourse, the partialist is interested solely in the body part and has little if any interest in sexual intercourse with the person possessing the part. The following case is an example of a fetish involving partialism:

*An unmarried man in his twenties begins to be sexually excited whenever
he looks at women's feet with shoes on. He becomes more so if he sees
the feet naked, and is brought to orgasm if a woman steps on his penis
with her naked feet, or if in masturbation he fantasies this action. He can
only be aroused by feet. (Stoller, 1976, p. 196)*

Discussions of fetishism sometimes make people feel uncomfortable, since
most of us are aroused to some extent by various nonsexual objects, such as
the feel of silk underwear. But for sexual arousal to be considered a fetish, the
person must be primarily interested in the fetish object to the exclusion of
other sexual stimuli. In fact, given a choice, the fetishist would choose the
fetish object over an available sexual partner.

As with the other variant sexual behaviors we have discussed, men are
more likely to be fetishists than women. However, this imbalance may simply
reflect the fact that male fetishists are more likely to be visible than female
ones, since they tend to engage in the kind of fetishes that result in arrests.
The actual relative incidence of males to females is unknown.

Where violations of the law are involved, it is usually because the fetishist
is caught stealing the fetish object. Occasionally a more bizarre crime is
involved such as the cutting of hair described in the case of P. at the beginning
of this chapter. While such events are dramatic, they are also rather rare.

Zoophilia

Throughout history people seem to have had a fascination with the idea of
sexual contact between animals and humans. Myths of various cultures describe such activities, often in romantic terms: Beauty and the Beast, Leda and
the swan, and so on. *Zoophilia,* or **bestiality,** is the name for the desire for
animals as the preferred object of sexual arousal and orgasm. To be a true
variant, an individual must prefer the animal contact despite the availability of
other, more usual, sexual partners. Thus, the sexual contact with animals
occasionally found among adolescents growing up on farms or that of people
isolated for long periods of time would not be included in this category.

The incidence of those having had even a passing experience with an
animal is not high. Kinsey et al. (1953) found that 8 percent of the men and 3
percent of the women he had interviewed had had an erotic experience with an
animal, usually a farm animal or household pet. Actual zoophilia, in which
there is continued contact with the preferred animal, is much more rare.

Despite the romantic myths of love between human and animal, the
actual cases are much less than ideal experiences. In the few cases available for
study, the initial encounter was a result of close living arrangements with the
animals. When more usual sexual objects were not available or were lost
through death or divorce, the person maintained or reestablished the animal
contact. In most of the cases the person was not well equipped to deal with
society in general and with interpersonal relationships in particular.

Pedophilia

Pedophilia is direction of sexual desires toward children. The types of
sexual behavior may vary greatly in nature and intensity from pedophile to
pedophile. However, because children are involved, social and legal reactions
tend to be strong, even toward benign advances. There is concern not only for

the current safety of the child but for the child's future life adjustment. Criminal arrests for pedophilia involve men almost exclusively. Women may experience attraction to children and some may even act on their impulses, but if they do, they are usually not found out.

Pedophilia is usually divided into heterosexual pedophilia and homosexual pedophilia. The heterosexual pedophile often knows the child, and incidents often occur in the child's home. The children in such cases tend to be young (8–10 years old), and the pedophile is more likely to experience arousal simply by touching the child and viewing him or her undressed than to attempt direct sexual contact.

The homosexual pedophile seems to prefer older children who are complete strangers. The behavior is more oriented toward sexual contact and orgasm by any of several types of homosexual encounter. The events typically occur outside the child's home. A common pattern of the pedophile is "cruising" in his car and propositioning youngsters on the street. The homosexual pedophile is more likely to be a repeat offender than the heterosexual type. Furthermore, homosexual pedophiles are less likely to be married than heterosexual pedophiles (Stoller, 1976).

Arrest statistics and records of police complaints indicate that pedophilia constitutes a significant portion of sexually related crimes. Problems in the reporting of this behavior make the true incidence difficult to determine, however. On the one hand, families may refuse to report such acts when they occur for fear of the effect of publicity on the child, the stress of the police-legal system, and further harassment from the pedophile. On the other hand, some parents or guardians may tend to overreact to totally innocent approaches to children by elderly, retarded, or alcoholic men, who are then unable to defend themselves adequately against the charges. Both of these extremes hamper efforts to determine the extent of the problem of pedophilia.

The displacement of the sexual drive from adult objects to children seems predictable from the general pattern of poor life adjustment shown by most pedophiles. They have been consistently found to be immature, to be inadequate in social situations, to be lacking in heterosocial behaviors, and to have a higher than average rate of other problems in sexual functioning. They are, in fact, poorly equipped to compete for sexual favors in the adult world. In this light, their turning to children does not seem so unusual. The severe social penalties and negative social reactions to pedophilia do not seem to control their behavior, which fits with another characteristic ascribed to this group—a lack of control over impulses.

Incest

A problem related to pedophilia is ***incest***, or sexual desire for a blood relative. Although there are many types of incest (brother-sister, cousin-cousin, and so on), the type that creates the greatest concern is parent-child, especially father-daughter.

Interestingly enough, incest is not considered a formal sexual variance. There is no category for it in the DSM-III. Yet our society, and almost all others, specifically prohibit incest. The problem of incest has received greater attention in recent years because it is becoming evident that it is more widespread than was previously thought. With the support of feminist groups, many women have revealed childhood incest experiences that have had a significant effect on their later adjustment. The reporting of such events has always been a problem, and despite the increased openness, many women are still reluctant to discuss such matters. Incest is, so to speak, "all in the family," and everyone is hurt by its disclosure. Underreporting is therefore likely to continue. The actual effect on the family and the adult sexual adjustment problems of the women who have experienced incest would certainly argue for increased attention to this problem.

Because of the shroud of secrecy over incest, there have been few formal investigations of the problem. What research has been done seems to indicate that the fathers in incest relationships are similar to pedophiles. Their wives may have emotionally, and perhaps physically, rejected them, yet they have stayed in the home. Lacking control over their impulses, they turn to the accessible children of the family for emotional and sexual support (Lester, 1972).

It is interesting how often **blaming the victim** occurs in psychological discussions of incest; that is, the child may be seen as seducing the parent. It has been suggested that the girl is playing out the Freudian pattern of competing with the mother for the attention of the father. This explanation fits psychoanalytic theory better than it fits reality. If we consider the relative levels of knowledge and sexual sophistication between father and child, it becomes obvious who must bear responsibility for the behavior.

Incest has more recently been viewed as an example of child abuse as well as sexual variance. This seems like a constructive development. With the educational and community resources already available for help with child abuse, incest may receive more appropriate attention.

Necrophilia

Perhaps the strangest variance in choice of sexual object is **necrophilia**—desire to have sexual intercourse with a dead body. Although this deviation is rare, it occurs often enough to have earned a place in the psychological literature.

In most of the reported cases, the individuals were people who were quite disturbed in other ways as well. Their necrophiliac behavior was only one element in a disorganized personality and was often accompanied by other disturbed behaviors, such as mutilating the body, self-mutilation, and bizarre rituals. It is probably best to view this problem as part of a more severe state of psychopathology such as schizophrenia rather than as simply a sexually variant behavior.

VARIANCES IN THE STRENGTH OF THE SEXUAL DRIVE

This category includes variations in the amount of sexual interest and activity. Interestingly, only excessive sexual interest is considered variant. Diminished interest in sex, or even total absence of sexual interest, is considered a sexual dysfunction (see Chap. 15). Excessive sex drive or *insatiable* sexual desire, as it is sometimes more forcefully labeled, has two subcategories: nymphomania and satyriasis. Occasionally the term **hypersexuality** is used to describe these problems. In addition, **promiscuity**, in which the variance is an unusually large number of partners, is sometimes viewed as an aspect of hypersexuality.

Nymphomania

The **nymphomaniac** is an important figure in myth, literature, and the fantasies of most young men. In actuality, however, if there is such a sexual variance, it is exceedingly rare. Presumably, the nymphomaniac is insatiable in her sexual needs. She is immediately arousable, requires endless sexual intercourse, never feels sexually fulfilled, and eventually may become promiscuous in her attempt to find this elusive fulfillment.

Kinsey argued that the label *nymphomaniac* has been applied too widely. He felt that a strong sex drive does not represent an extreme pathological overinterest in sex but rather is a statistical fact of the normal curve of sexual interest; in other words, someone has to be higher than the rest.

In many of the cases presented for clinical treatment, it turns out that there is not actually an unusually strong sexual interest on the woman's part but rather a difference in relative sexual interest between her and her partner. In such cases the partner is less interested in sex and responds to the woman's requests for more sexual interaction with the explanation that she must be a nymphomaniac. We can see the self-protective nature of this response for the less active partner. The woman, having no standard to compare herself against, might accept her partner's diagnosis of deviation and think of herself as abnormal.

In those cases where there does appear to be more sexual activity compared to that of most other women, the issue is primarily one of promiscuity, or a large number and variety of partners. As Box 16.2 explains, such promiscuity may in fact be an attempt to try to resolve basic psychological problems in the woman's life and thus is not based on an excessive sex drive as such.

Is there, then, any such thing as true nymphomania? There are a few extremely rare physical conditions in which a woman affected by hormonal factors experiences hypersexuality, but such cases are so rare that they have little to do with the existence of the idea of nymphomania in our society. It is much more likely that the excessive interest in this idea is a sociopsychological phenomenon related to our culturally ingrained idea that women should have little interest in sex. Nymphomania does not appear in DSM-III.

Satyriasis

Satyriasis, or insatiable sexual desire in men, is named for the half-men, half-beasts of Greek mythology who were always interested in sexual encounters—the satyrs. In our society, men are supposed to be sexually insatiable; thus, few men seek therapy to have their sex drives toned down. However, they may, as in nymphomania, be convinced by their partner that their higher relative interest in sex is some kind of sexual deviation. Questions of excessive sexual drive are also raised in the case of sex offenders. Castration and drug suppression of sexual interest are still practiced as treatment for sexual offenses in some states. (We will discuss some of these legal issues in Chap. 20.)

Whether satyriasis actually exists is questionable, but as with women,

BOX 16.2

The "promiscuous" woman

"When is an active sex life with a large number of partners to be viewed as high spirits, and when is it sexual acting out? When is a person's sexuality an affirmation of life, and when is it to be seen as self-defeating, masochistic, hurtful of the self and others?" These complex questions are among many raised by science writer Maggie Scarf (1980) in her research on "promiscuous" women.

Although the real focus of Scarf's research has been on the problem of depression in women, in the course of interviewing hundreds of subjects she has regularly encountered a type of woman who is not only depressed but who has been promiscuous and is distressed about it. A far cry from the stereotypical "nymphomaniac," this type of promiscuous woman is not driven by an insatiable need for physical satisfaction; rather, she appears to be driven by feelings of despair, grief, and anger into a series of superficial sexual affairs with a variety of men.

What is such a woman like? What causes her to pick up and discard sexual partners as if they were Kleenex? According to Scarf, many such women become promiscuous following the breakup of a love affair or marriage. The promiscuous behavior serves not only to reaffirm the woman's attractiveness after suffering rejection, but it can be a way of expressing anger at men. As Scarf puts it, "To offer one's body and at the same time withhold the self is a wonderful way of expressing a good deal of underlying fury—and wonderfully confusing for the other person."

Also, promiscuity can help combat feelings of abandonment, emptiness, and aloneness by serving as an antidepressant; that is, the sexual behavior increases the woman's overall level of excitement, thus temporarily masking her depressed state. Says Scarf, "Promiscuity, like amphetamines, promotes a short-term high. It surely won't cure feelings of despair, grief, and depression (neither will amphetamines), but it may keep them at bay, keep them contained for a while" (p. 84).

Scarf also points out that sleeping around has an element of risk or danger to it that helps the woman divert her attention away from inner anxieties and fears, such as feelings of unattractiveness, undesirability, and desertion. By focusing on the risk of being discovered by someone's wife or partner or of contracting a sexually transmitted disease, the woman avoids attending to the painful feelings within her. The risk element also helps counter feelings of emptiness by providing a "sense of aliveness."

Another function of casual sexual encounters is simply to provide contact with another human being. Scarf suggests that it may actually be the body contact rather than sexual interaction that many women seek in such affairs. Such contact is a form of reassurance; it can, if only fleetingly, make one feel loved, protected, and comforted.

Many women use promiscuous behavior as a means of avoiding the grief and mourning necessary to getting over the breakup of an important love relationship. Yet, as Scarf notes, such avoidance of the mourning process actually makes it impossible for the woman to develop new relationships: "The promiscuous woman is thus, in some extraordinarily curious way, remaining faithful to the old love tie, the one that has been severed. Her real emotional connection, her true bond, is with the person whom she 'hates' and has lost" (p. 87).

Scarf sees the promiscuous woman's behavior as a continuation of a desperate, lifelong quest for someone who will nurture and care for her. Yet the woman is so angry at those who have failed her in the past—especially parents who were uncaring—that the inner rage is expressed by diminishing others—by treating them as mere sexual objects. Thus, for her "sex is robbed of its most rewarding and human elements, which have to do with loving communication and intimacy and the mutual reinforcement of self-esteem— and with the shelter and security of an emotional bond" (p. 87).

So the promiscuous woman, in effect, sabotages all her relationships not only by subconsciously venting her anger and resentment but by unrealistically expecting each new man to be the ideal nurturing, accepting partner she has been searching for. As a result of her indiscriminate sexual behavior, the woman feels shame and self-hatred in addition to her unacknowledged feelings of loneliness, loss, and rage. As one woman told Scarf, she felt "low down, rotten, and cheap . . . just not worth that much to anyone."

Obviously, not all women who have promiscuous sex lives follow the pattern that Scarf describes. There are indeed many psychological routes to an active sex life with many partners, and certainly not all of them are as negative as this one. It does seem, however, that in many cases promiscuity serves as a coping mechanism for dealing with problems in a woman's life that are otherwise nonsexual.

---

promiscuity is the basis of many men being labeled "oversexed." Clinical cases of promiscuity in men are referred to as the *Don Juan syndrome.* Men in this category have a large number of partners, change partners frequently, and seem to lack any deep emotional feeling for their partners. Promiscuous men seem to be motivated by many of the same psychological factors as promiscuous women (see Box 16.2). Sexuality is less the issue than are some other basic psychological needs and conflicts. As with promiscuous women, the man is using sexual behavior to accomplish other goals that are not related to sexual appetite at all.

CAUSAL THEORIES OF SEXUAL VARIANCE

Two theoretical perspectives dominate current thinking about sexual variance: the psychodynamic approach and the behavioral-learning approach. While there are other theoretical views, none has received the widespread support that these two have. They also dominate current psychotherapeutic practice, as we will see in the next section of the chapter.

Psychodynamic theory

The **psychodynamic view** of sexually variant behavior is based on Freud's theory of psychosexual development described in Chap. 9. According to this theory, each stage of psychosexual development can give rise to conflicts that, if left unresolved, may lead to variant sexual behavior in adulthood. The phallic stage of development is particularly critical. It is during this period that the Oedipal conflict occurs, and unresolved issues from this conflict are considered to be central factors in the development of sexual variance. In the male, the Oedipal conflict leads to sexual desire for the mother and fear of retribution (in the form of castration) from the father. "Normal" development requires that this conflict be resolved with the boy identifying with his father and rejecting his mother as a sexual object. Freud was less clear about the female conflict at this stage. Freud and his followers have all suggested that for females this stage is more complex. Basically, it takes the form of desiring the father as the sexual object and competing with the mother. While there is no castration anxiety, there is fear of losing the mother's love and care. Satisfactory resolution is achieved when the girl rejects her desire for her father and begins to identify with her mother.

Lack of resolution of these conflicts in the phallic stage leaves the person vulnerable to the development of variant sexual patterns. In the male, adult heterosexual relations become overshadowed by fear of castration. In the female, heterosexual relationships suggest a loss of the mother's love and guilt over any sexual encounters, since the lover is a symbolic father figure. In both cases attempts at "normal" adult sexual relationships are hampered by the unresolved conflicts. Because heterosexual encounters threaten to bring the unconscious conflicts into full consciousness, they are avoided. Instead, the person turns to sexually variant behavior both as a defense against becoming aware of the conflicts and as a replacement sexual outlet.

Behavioral-learning approaches

Behavioral-learning theories see sexual variance as **learned maladaptive behavior.** Just as most of us learn "normal" heterosexual behavior, some people are subjected to unusual situations in which they learn atypical connections between sexuality and their environment. These connections are then maintained and strengthened by the sexual pleasure obtained each time the behavior is performed. According to this approach, the type of variance demonstrated by a particular person is a function of his or her specific learning experiences and is therefore unique. Thus, unlike psychodynamic theory, which focuses on personality, learning theory focuses on behavior.

In order to understand how variant behaviors might develop, behavioral analysts discuss various learning sequences that have the potential for leading to maladaptive sexual behavior. For example, the initial experiences associated with masturbation or intercourse might rapidly condition any response to a sexual situation by relating it to the intense arousal and sexual release of orgasm. Sexual experiences in early adolescence are particularly important in developing learned connections to both usual and unusual stimuli. It is at this time that the emerging sexual behavior can be sent in a direction that may result in maladaptive behavior.

When Albert Bandura (1969) reviewed the literature on types of maladaptive learning, he noted some common routes along which variant behavior might develop. First, parents may model variant behavior, which the child comes to imitate. He cited the work of Stoller (1976), who documented the direct and subtle ways in which transvestite behavior was taught to children who later became transvestites. Second, Bandura noted that positive reinforcement may follow initial instances of variant behavior, leading to its repetition. Parents or peers may, for example, directly or indirectly approve of a deviant pattern. Take the situation of certain teenage gangs in New York, whose members consider physical abuse an appropriate part of sexual behavior. Girls proudly wear bruises, bite marks, and knife-carved names on their arms as if they were medals. It may be difficult for such females to abandon masochistic behaviors as they grow older. In addition, fantasizing about a variant sexual behavior during masturbation may also serve to condition this behavior.

An important learning factor we noted in several of our examples of sexual variance is inadequate interpersonal and sociosexual skills, which make it difficult for the person to function adequately in sexual situations. To learning theorists, this *lack* of adaptive learning, called a **behavioral deficit** is an important part of the development of sexual variance. Thus, it is not only what individuals learn directly but also what they fail to learn that helps create many of the problems of sexual variance. The maladaptive response comes to fill the void left by the failure to learn socially appropriate sexual behavior.

Let us use the example of fetishism to further amplify the differences between the psychodynamic and behavioral-learning approaches. According to psychodynamic theory, the fetishist was made fearful of normal sexual intercourse by the lack of resolution of the Oedipal conflict. Because any heterosexual behavior would symbolize sexual intercourse with the parent, it raises fears of castration and guilt. The person is thus forced to seek other, safer sexual stimuli. According to psychodynamic thinking, the chosen stimulus is symbolic of the forbidden parent figure. The sexual energy directed toward the parent is thus *displaced* to the fetish object, and the person, in effect, "loves" the object. In this view, the fetish serves as a defense against the anxiety about sexual behavior by allowing the person to experience sexual arousal and gratification from a nonthreatening representation of the denied love object.

According to learning theory, a fetish is a learned connection of the sexual arousal response to unusual stimuli. Remember how Pavlov's dog responded to the ring of a bell with salivation after the bell had been repeatedly paired with food? Sexual responses can similarly come to be paired with neutral (nonsexual) stimuli. The long period of time during adolescence when the sexually mature person is not given access to direct sexual behavior creates a strong drive or need with no appropriate outlet. The possibility that the sexual response can become attached to nonsexual stimuli is therefore not surprising. How strong this connection becomes and how much it dominates later behavior depends on when and how much more usual sexual stimuli become available. As we noted earlier, everyone finds some nonsexual stimuli to be sexually arousing. The difference between most people and the fetishist is thus not one of kind but of degree. Thus, we can see that the development of fetishlike responses can be part of the natural learning process. It is where the fetish becomes overlearned that it is maladaptive.

The psychodynamic and behavioral-learning theories have led to quite different approaches to the treatment of variant behavior. Perhaps the relative effectiveness of these two approaches will give us some insights into which theory is the most useful in explaining sexually variant behavior.

THERAPY FOR VARIANT BEHAVIORS

Now that we have identified the variety of variant behaviors in our society and two different theories of causality, the question arises as to what should be done for people who exhibit such behaviors. In this section we will examine some specific therapeutic techniques that are used for changing variant behavior. First, however, we should point out that many issues must be resolved before treatment is considered in a particular case. Is the behavior doing anyone harm? Who is uncomfortable about the behavior? Is there **informed consent** to the treatment? Because many of the sexual variances are also considered legal offenses and the offenders are under legal constraint, important questions of social values and individual freedom are also raised. Thus, it must be realized that issues of ethics, morality, and individual rights are frequently involved in both the decision to treat and the type of treatment chosen.

The type of treatment an individual will receive depends in part on whether the variant behavior is seen as a symptom of some more basic pathological process or as a learned behavior maintained by the environment. As we have noted, psychodynamic theorists have taken the first view, and behavioral theorists have taken the second. Specific treatment methods based on both theories have been developed.

Psychodynamic approaches

The object of psychodynamic (psychoanalytic) therapy is to make unconscious conflicts available to the conscious mind so that they can be resolved. Whatever the type of variance involved, the therapy method is basically the same. The patient is asked to **free associate**—to say whatever comes to mind—while the analyst patiently listens. The analyst uses **interpretation** to guide the patient toward dealing with the problems of early psychosexual development that are uncovered. As the patient works through the previously unconscious conflicts, he or she becomes freed of these irrational childhood feelings and can begin to develop more adult-like relationships.

This may sound like a simple procedure, but it is actually highly complex and may require years of regular sessions. The unconscious feelings at the heart of the person's problem are old, deep, and highly **repressed**, that is, actively kept out of the person's conscious awareness. A great deal of **psychic energy** is expended in keeping this material repressed, and removing the repression is a long, tedious process.

How does "normal" sexual behavior result from psychoanalytic treatment? The procedures of psychodynamic therapy are aimed at removing the conflicts that cause variant behavior, and it is presumed that once they are gone, sexual behavior will be able to occur in a nonvariant, normal way. The analyst does not tell the patient how to function at any time and, in fact, says very little about the patient's day-to-day life.

Psychoanalysts consider sexual variance to be among the problems that are most resistant to treatment. For other types of problems, a consistent figure of 65 percent improvement or cure has been reported with use of psychoanalysis. O'Conner and Stein (1972) have shown similar results for the application of psychoanalytic techniques to sexual variances. However, because approximately 65 percent of people improve without treatment, the effectiveness of psychoanalysis has been difficult to establish.

Behavior therapies

In behavioral approaches to therapy, it is not really necessary to know what originally created the sexual variance. Rather, it is more important to know what keeps it going and what can be done to change it.

A wide variety of **behavior therapy techniques** have been developed for the treatment of sexual variance. The choice of technique depends on the type of learning considered to be most helpful to the particular person for a particular problem. If the problem involves an unwanted behavior, the treatment may involve methods for inhibiting a response or removing it from the person's behavioral repertoire. If the problem involves lack of appropriate sexual behavior, the treatment may involve the conditioning or learning of new behaviors.

Extinction is one method of reducing a behavior. In extinction, the arousing stimulus (such as a fetish object) is presented over and over, but arousal or approach is prevented. However, because arousal is difficult to control, it is sometimes necessary to provide more active interference with the person's response. In such cases **aversive therapies** are used. In these procedures the arousing but unwanted stimulus is paired with an unpleasant stimulus. For example, the person might be instructed to think of something unpleasant while being shown a picture of a fetish object. This is called **cognitive aversion** or **covert sensitization**. Or a safe but painful shock may be administered whenever the person is in the presence of the fetish object. This is called **physical aversion**.

In another technique, called **fading**, the arousal response is allowed to occur but is transferred to a more appropriate object. For example, a pedophile may be shown pictures of children and asked to indicate when he begins to feel aroused. At that point a picture of an adult female is faded in (that is, superimposed on the child's picture, which then disappears), so that the arousal response can come to be paired with the more appropriate stimulus.

Modeling techniques using films can be valuable in demonstrating acceptable sexual practices that the person may never have had the opportunity to learn. Sex education procedures are also helpful in conjunction with other procedures, since lack of knowledge is often an important part of the problem.

Many clients suffer from anxiety—they may have avoided the more usual channels of sexual interaction for fear of failure or rejection. Thus anxiety-reducing procedures are often useful in helping people with variances. A technique commonly used in such cases is **systematic desensitization** (described in Chap. 15).

Numerous other behavioral procedures are also available. Behavioral rehearsal, cognitive restructuring, assertiveness training, and self-modification are just a few of the many techniques that have proved valuable in treating sexual variances. In actual clinical work, the usual approach is to select the most effective methods for the particular person and to design a program that seems most appropriate to both the person and the problem. Development of such individualized programs avoids some of the mechanistic qualities for which behavioral treatment has sometimes been criticized.

Success rates vary with the problem. "Cure" rates range from 70 to 98 percent. Behavioral procedures are thus one of the most successful approaches to sexual variance. In addition, the duration of treatment is much shorter than that of other procedures. This type of treatment also seems to be better suited to the type of clients who most need the help. Because a large number of people with sexual variances are less verbal and are from lower educational levels, they are less likely to benefit from insight therapies such as psychoanalysis. They are also less able to afford long-term psychotherapy. Behavior therapy may be more suitable not only because it is relatively fast but because it can be administered by nonprofessional counselors, can be self-administered, or can be administered by family members.

The possibility of helping more people, more quickly, more effectively, and at less expense has made behavior therapy techniques quite popular in the treatment of sexual variance in recent years. The rapidly growing demand has also led to some misuses of the procedures. Concern for the psychological well-being of clients, awareness of the limitations in terms of applications, and ethical consideration must be taken into account in evaluating the success of this approach.

SUMMARY

1 *Sexual variances* are sexual behaviors that differ markedly enough from a society's usual patterns for them to be considered abnormal. Normality may be defined in terms of psychological standards, social standards, or legal-moral standards. Variances can be classified into three main types: variations in the mode of sexual expression, variations in the choice of sexual outlet, and variations in the strength of the sexual response.

2 In variances of sexual expression, the way the sexual behavior is performed and the way sexual satisfaction is achieved differ from those of most other people in the society. Such variances include voyeurism, exhibitionism, sadism, masochism, and transvestism.

3 *Voyeurism* is the derivation of sexual satisfaction from secretly observing others in various stages of undress or engaging in sexual acts. Voyeurs are often emotionally and sexually immature men who do not have ordinary sexual outlets available.

4 *Exhibitionism* is the exposure of one's sexual organs to someone who is not seeking or expecting the exposure. Some exhibitionists are out to shock their victims; others are trying to entice children into sexual activity, although they rarely actually touch the children. Exhibitionism may be a "safe" way for a man to express hostile feelings, and getting caught may be experienced as punishment for these unacceptable feelings.

5   *Sadism* is the derivation of sexual pleasure from administering physical or psychological pain to others. The partner may be nonconsenting or may be consenting but experiences real suffering and pain (as opposed to masochists, who may experience painful stimuli as pleasurable).

6   *Masochism* involves the pairing of erotic pleasure with physical or psychological pain. However, the pain must be of a specific type administered in a specific manner for it to be experienced as sexually pleasurable. Punishment in childhood may be one source of adult masochism.

7   In *transvestism*, the person experiences sexual arousal by dressing in the clothing of the opposite sex. Most transvestites are not homosexual, nor do they desire to become the opposite sex.

8   In variances of sexual object, the object of sexual desire varies from the usual sex objects of most members of a society. Variances included in this category are fetishism, zoophilia, pedophilia, incest, and necrophilia.

9   In *fetishism* sexual arousal occurs in response to inanimate objects rather than to human partners. Fetishes for specific parts of the body may also develop; this is termed *partialism*.

10   *Zoophilia*, or *bestiality*, is desire for animals as the preferred objects of sexual arousal. *Pedophilia* is sexual desire for children, which may be either heterosexual or homosexual. *Incest* is sexual desire for a blood relative, usually that of a father for his daughter. *Necrophilia* is the desire for sexual intercourse with a dead body.

11   In variances of the strength of the sexual drive, the man or woman has an excessive interest in sex. In women, the variance is called *nymphomania*, and although it is an extremely rare condition, the notion is highly popular. What is often referred to as nymphomania is really *promiscuity*, or an unusually large number of partners. Promiscuity is more often a woman's means of dealing with psychological problems in her life than it is an excessive interest in sex. In men, this variance is referred to as *satyriasis*.

12   According to the *psychodynamic view* of sexual variance, problems are the result of unresolved conflicts of psychosexual development, particularly in relation to the Oedipal complex. According to the *behavioral view* of sexual variance, problems are *learned maladaptive behaviors*. Thus, a variant behavior may be classically conditioned through unusual associations; it may be modeled on adult behavior; or it may even be a result of a *behavioral deficit*, or the lack of adaptive learning.

13   Psychodynamic treatment for variant behavior involves psychotherapy to help the person bring unconscious conflicts into consciousness and resolve them. This therapy may be time-consuming, because conflicts are often strongly *repressed*, and a number of techniques, such as *free association*, must be used to overcome the repression. The effectiveness of this therapy has been difficult to assess.

14   Behavioral treatment for variant behavior involves a wide variety of *behavior therapy techniques*. Some techniques, such as *extinction* and *aversive therapies*, are designed to reduce or remove unwanted behaviors. Other techniques, such as *fading* and *modeling*, are used to help the person develop appropriate responses to appropriate stimuli. Behavior therapy is relatively fast, is less expensive than psychoanalysis, and can be administered by nonprofessional counselors.

ADDITIONAL READING

Gebhard, Paul; Gagnon, John; Pomeroy, Wardell; and Christenson, Cornelia. *Sex Offenders: An Analysis of Types.* New York: Harper & Row, 1965.
  The largest study of convicted sex offenders to date.
Krafft-Ebing, R. V. *Psychopathia Sexualis.* New York: Pioneer Publications, 1950.
  The classic work on sexual variations. Full of interesting case examples and discussions.
Lester, David. *Unusual Sexual Behavior.* Springfield, IL: Charles C. Thomas, 1975.
  A readable and nontechnical overview of the sexual variations. Research is cited where applicable.

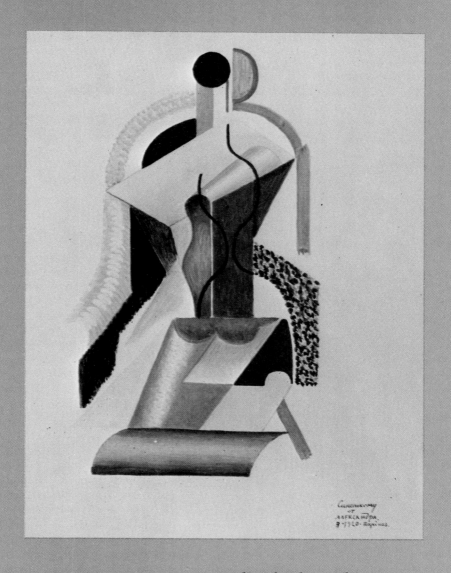

Individuals seeking change: Dissatisfied homosexuals and transsexuals

17

chapter

17

In the course of a May 1979 interview in *Playboy* magazine, musician Walter/Wendy Carlos described his/her problem of being biologically male and feeling psychologically female:

Carlos: . . . My awareness of it happens to be one of my first memories—when I was about five or six and didn't even know there was a real difference between boys and girls. . . . And I remember being convinced I was a little girl, much preferring long hair and girls' clothes . . . so I began hiding my feelings at a very early age. . . .

Playboy: Was there a period when you tried to deny your feelings?

Carlos: Yes. At some point during my teenage years, I tried to pretend they didn't exist. I told myself I didn't have all those inclinations, that I was straight, normal, that I was going to date and get married. I put up a great battle. But by the time I got through high school, the feelings were there, stronger than ever.

Playboy: What was college like?

Carlos: . . . I felt set apart. I felt that nature had made a cruel mistake. That's a cliché, but that's how I felt. Extreme confusion. From time to time, I was able to repress it—I don't know, maybe I thought I'd close my eyes one day and then suddenly wake up and find I was a woman.

Playboy: So by the time you were in college, you were definitely—

Carlos: Here's what I was: After puberty, my condition became more and more hellish, and by late adolescence, as I started to become more masculine, I began to hate my body, my corpus . . . It sounds mad, doesn't it? I feel myself to be a somewhat bright, fairly introspective person, normal in many ways, yet as I say these words, I sound like a madwoman to myself! . . .

Playboy: Were you conscious of your appearance?

Carlos: I hated the way I looked. I tried never to look in a mirror. I wouldn't look at my body when I bathed. Oh, I'd check in a mirror occasionally to make sure my tie was on straight or that the haircut I'd gotten wouldn't give away my aberration. I was always having slightly paranoid fears that I could be too easily spotted as some kind of sexual subdeviate. . . .

Playboy: Can you pinpoint a time when you decided to do something about your feelings?

Carlos: It was in the fall of 1962, when I came to New York as a graduate student at Columbia. I had become extremely despondent, and the idea of suicide was becoming stronger and stronger in me. There was a period, perhaps a little later than that, when I was daily taking a razor to my wrists and wondering . . . Anyway, that first year at Columbia, I made a list of things I needed to do with my life if I were going to survive. And at the top of the list was to find some doctor, someplace, who would help me change my sex. Whatever that meant. At the time, I was just putting pieces together, only dimly becoming aware that I might not be the only person in the world who felt the way I did. (pp. 75–106)

Being a male or female biologically, feeling masculine or feminine psychologically, acting with masculine or feminine overt behavior, and desiring a male or female sexual partner—all are separate but related aspects of gender identity and gender role. In our society each of these aspects is expected to conform to the others, and any failure to match along these dimensions almost certainly results in psychological difficulties for the individual, as it did for Walter/Wendy Carlos. We noted in Chap. 13 that both the individual and society can adapt to some differences, as in the case of adjusted homosexuals. However, some people, like Carlos, become so uncomfortable with their discrepancies in sexual identity that they are unable to function adequately and therefore seek change.

COMPONENTS OF
SEXUAL IDENTITY

The various components necessary to understand sexual identity and its potential disruptions are listed in Table 17.1. *Biological sex* refers to our genetic, hormonal, and anatomical designation as male or female. Our *gender identity* is how we are perceived and how we perceive ourselves as masculine or feminine. Our *gender role behavior* relates to whether we show masculine or feminine traits in situations where the sexes are expected to behave differently. Finally, *choice of sexual partners* refers to whether we prefer men or women as sexual partners or which sex most arouses us.

TABLE 17.1

Components of sexual identity

Sexual life-style	Biological sex	Gender identity	Gender role behavior	Sex of preferred partner
Heterosexual	Male	Masculine	Masculinity	Female
	Female	Feminine	Femininity	Male
Homosexual	Male	Masculine	Masculinity*	Male
	Female	Feminine	Femininity*	Female
Transsexual	Male	Feminine	Femininity	Male
	Female	Masculine	Masculinity	Female

Source: Adapted by Altrocchi (1980), p. 487, from Townes, Ferguson, and Gillam (1976).
*Some homosexually oriented individuals adopt the role behavior of the opposite sex.

In our society the dominant pattern is shown by the heterosexual person who is consistently oriented within one sex across all the categories and prefers members of the opposite sex as sexual partners. Homosexually oriented people are also consistent across all categories for their sex, but they prefer a same-sex sexual partner. As we noted in Chap. 13, homosexuality is now considered a normal variation of sexual life. Finally, there are **transsexuals**, like Carlos, who feel that their biological sex assignment is a bizarre mistake of nature and that they are actually members of the opposite sex. In every other way they are like heterosexuals; that is, their behavior, identity, and partner preference is consistently opposite their biological sex. Thus, they do not consider themselves to be homosexual even though they are attracted to individuals who are of the same biological sex as themselves.

The major problems that can arise because of discrepancies between the components of sexual identity are problems of sexual preference and problems of gender identity. **Sexual preference disturbance** refers primarily to those homosexuals who would prefer to be heterosexual. **Gender identity disturbance** refers to transsexuality. Table 17.1 would seem to indicate the potential for other types of sexual identity disturbances. For example, there could be **dissatisifed heterosexuals** who want to change to homosexuality. While many people who currently identify themselves as homosexual may have gone through such a process, they have rarely sought professional help in making the change. Thus there have been few recorded cases. There could also be males or females who feel, or are made to feel, that they show too much gender role behavior appropriate to the opposite sex ("effeminate" males and "butch" females). Such individuals are occasionally seen for treatment. Recently, children showing such discrepancies ("sissy" boys and "tomboy" girls) have been given more attention. Early treatment of gender identity conflicts in children is now thought to be important in preventing later identity problems in adulthood (Green, 1974).

Bisexuality (discussed in Chap. 13) is yet another form of gender identity that has important implications for understanding the conformity of the components of sexual identity. In this case individuals are attracted to sexual partners of both sexes. Except for the bisexual attraction, the person's sexual identity is completely consistent with the heterosexual model. As a variation of sexual life, it is rarely presented clinically as a sexual problem. Bisexuals typically see themselves as having greater opportunities for sexual experience—as Woody Allen has remarked, it definitely doubles their chances for dates on Saturday nights. Bisexuals who become dissatisfied with their dual preference can easily solve their problem by becoming exclusively homosexual or heterosexual—a choice that would not ordinarily require therapeutic help. In light of these factors, it is probably best to consider bisexuality a "normal" variation of sexual adjustment.

The two groups whose sexual identity problems are most likely to require therapeutic intervention—dissatisfied homosexuals and transsexuals—have both been recognized by the formal diagnostic system of the American Psychiatric Association. The DSM-III (1980) lists the following two categories for these problems:

1   **Ego-dystonic homosexuality** *refers to those homosexuals who are not comfortable as homosexuals and who may be seeking conversion or reversion to heterosexuality.*
2   **Gender identity disorders** *refers to transsexual individuals and to gender identity disturbances in children.*

THE NATURE OF SEXUAL PREFERENCE DISTURBANCE

As a society we are in the midst of a dramatic change in our views of homosexuality. In Chap. 13 we noted that the American Psychiatric Association (APA) no longer lists homosexuality as a disorder, and a homosexual orientation is no longer an automatic signal to mental health professionals that the person must be treated to change that orientation. The arguments favoring removal of homosexuality from the list were based on the fact that homosexuality does not *necessarily* cause distress or disability, nor does it entail any inherent disadvantage (the basic criteria used by the APA for including behaviors as disorders in the DSM-III). This does not mean that homosexuality never causes psychological distress. Given the current social, legal, and moral climate in the United States, the potential for problematic adjustment is certainly present. Because of this *potential* for psychological problems, the decision to drop homosexuality from the DSM listings was highly controversial among mental health professionals. Although the initial vote in favor of removing it was taken in December 1973, implementation was slow, and many attempts were made to reverse the decision.

As we have noted, the vote did not wipe out all the negative aspects of being a homosexual. The special problems of homosexual life in our society may lead many homosexuals to question their orientation. Some eventually decide that they would rather "switch than fight" and may request professional help in making the transition to heterosexual life. It is this subgroup of **dissatisfied homosexuals** that are the topic of this section.

In Chap. 13 we discussed the fact that homosexuals and heterosexuals do not differ greatly on a wide variety of psychological and adjustment measures. However, there are some homosexual individuals who indicate that they do have problems in dealing with their orientation. The best single study on the subject (Bell and Weinberg, 1978), which we described in detail in Chap. 13, helps shed some light on these individuals. In their sample of nearly 1000 homosexuals in the San Francisco Bay Area in 1969–1970, Bell and Weinberg found a small percentage of individuals who had difficulty accepting their homosexual orientation. In response to questions about whether they had any regrets about their homosexuality or had seriously considered stopping their homosexual behavior, 25 percent of the males said yes. For the females, a smaller percentage had regrets, but a larger percentage had considered stopping their activity and becoming heterosexual. Two clever questions that Bell and Weinberg used to reveal the person's feelings about being homosexual were: If there was a magic pill to make you heterosexual, would you take it now? Would you have wanted to be given it at birth? Only 14 percent of the men and 5 percent of the women indicated they would want to take such a pill if it were currently available. A slightly higher percentage (25 percent of the men and 15 percent of the women) said they would have wanted to take such a pill at birth. Bell and Weinberg concluded from these and other data that the great majority of homosexuals have accepted and have adjusted to their homosexual orientation and do not desire to change.

In pursuing information on the less well-adjusted homosexuals, Bell and Weinberg found two groups who were not experiencing fulfilling sexual lives through their homosexual orientation. They labeled these groups **dysfunctional homosexuals** and **asexual homosexuals**. *Dysfunctional* homosexuals were sexually active and had many partners. However, they reported a great deal of sexually related problems, had trouble finding partners that they could relate to, and had trouble maintaining relationships. *Asexual* homosexuals did not engage in much sexual activity, often had problems when they did, and reported low sexual interest. Both of these groups indicated regret about being homosexuals. Individuals from both these groups were the most likely to seek treatment with the desire to change their sexual orientation.

Dissatisfied homosexuals who try to deal with their problem on their own by pursuing heterosexual encounters may experience difficulties in achieving arousal or in maintaining a heterosexual relationship. At this point they may request help. But what leads to such dissatisfaction? There are a number of factors involved, and the particular reasons vary from individual to individual. Masters and Johnson (1979) noted several common patterns. In one pattern, the person had developed an attraction to a heterosexual partner. The relationship may have been nonsexual at first, but as it developed the homosexual partner may have decided to change his or her sexual preference to facilitate a heterosexual relationship. In another pattern, an already ongoing heterosexual relationship was threatened by the homosexual orientation and activities of one of the partners. Sometimes change was sought because of an ultimatum from the heterosexual partner. Masters and Johnson point out, however, that therapy has little chance for success when the homosexual is seeking change solely on the basis of threats from others.

The motivation to change a homosexual orientation often is the result of the social threats that are still a part of homosexual life in our society. The person's social, professional, or economic standing in the community may be affected if he or she maintains a homosexual orientation. Thus, the person may request conversion to heterosexuality as a means of living more comfortably in society.

Age is another factor that may come into play in creating dissatisfaction. While younger men and women may adapt to the gay life and all that it implies, they may find parts of that life-style too difficult as they grow older. The heterosexual life-style may become more attractive at that point, and the person may request help with assuming that sexual orientation. Finally, some homosexuals go to therapists seeking change with no clear motivating factors. They simply experience strong discomfort with their homosexuality and feel they would be happier as heterosexuals.

*Bisexuality as an
alternative*

Is heterosexuality the only response to homosexual dissatisfaction? One aspect of sexual reorientation that needs further exploration is the possibility that the best response to the request for change might be to help the person achieve heterosexual arousal and behavior *without* removing the existing arousal and response to homosexual stimuli. One of the major myths in our society is that people must be exclusively heterosexual or exclusively homosexual. In Chap. 13 we noted that Kinsey and his co-workers (1953) found a continuum of heterosexual to homosexual orientations and that in reality many people fall somewhere along the continuum and not exclusively at one end or the other. It thus seems odd that when changes for homosexuals are discussed the only outcome considered is exclusive heterosexuality. With additional investigation it may be found that many of the problems of homosexual dissatisfaction can be solved by promoting positive change to heterosexual responsiveness without negating homosexual responsiveness.

More than most other psychological problems presented for therapy, a request to change from homosexuality to heterosexuality requires serious discussion of the reasons for the change, the effects the change will have on the client, and the clarity of the client's decision to change. Many therapists have argued that even offering such treatment is unethical, since it implies that there is something wrong with maintaining a homosexual orientation (Davidson, 1976). In a similar vein, others have argued that, because such a change is always a response to an unaccepting society rather than a freely formed decision to become heterosexual, the only treatment that should be offered is to help the person adapt to homosexual life. The ethical and moral aspects of these therapeutic issues are beyond the scope of our discussion here, but you should be aware that there is great concern and discussion among both professional and gay groups about how to respond to requests for conversion to heterosexuality by dissatisfied homosexuals.

In moving toward heterosexuality, it is more than the sex of the desired partner that is at issue. We have already reviewed the many components that are part of a person's sexual identity and orientation. Any or all of these aspects may be in need of modification if heterosexuality is to be a viable life-style option. Barlow (1973) has indicated that special emphasis must be placed on four aspects of homosexuality in any attempt to change sexual orientation: inappropriate sexual arousal, lack of heterosexual responsiveness, inappropriate gender role behaviors, and lack of heterosexual skills.

In addition, another aspect of homosexuality that is not directly related to sexual behavior must be attended to: social supports. Most active homosexuals exist in a homosexual subculture that provides numerous supports for their homosexual identification. Friends, meeting places, jobs, clothing, vacation spots, and shopping places are just some of the many social aspects of the homosexual subculture. Thus, many elements of day-to-day life activity promote and support the homosexual's life-style. If therapeutic change is to be achieved, these influences must be replaced. Yet taking people out of their support groups and away from their only sources of attention, attachment, and reinforcement can be quite harmful psychologically. Thus, if such a change is made too abruptly, not only is the therapy doomed to failure, but, as could be expected of anyone who loses all social supports, the person may suffer other serious psychological effects. Therefore, the therapist must help the client to gradually embrace heterosexual supports, timing major steps to opportune points in the treatment process. Despite the importance of such timing, surprisingly few treatment programs take this factor into account when designing procedures for helping people move from a homosexual to a heterosexual life-style.

Once the decision for movement toward heterosexual functioning has been made and both the client and therapist are comfortable with the decision, the techniques for producing such movement become the central focus of treatment. The therapist's theoretical orientation toward the causes of homosexuality and its maintaining factors will strongly influence the selection of treatment methods. In Chap. 13 we described the major schools of thought and their explanations of homosexuality. These approaches give rise to three main types of therapy: biological approaches, psychodynamic approaches, and behavioral-learning approaches.

Biological therapies

The biological approach is based on the idea that homosexuality is caused by genetic, constitutional, physiological, or endocrinological factors. As a result, an extensive effort has been made to treat dissatisfied homosexuals by altering hormone levels. Lesbians are given estrogens to increase their female hormone level, and homosexual males are given testosterone to increase their male hormone levels. Such hormone therapy is designed to increase deficient levels or to combat high levels of opposite-sex hormone in the bloodstream.

How valid is this approach? Recent studies of hormone levels in both homosexuals and heterosexuals provide conflicting evidence for hormone effects. In some cases initial hormone deficiencies have been reported, while in others no hormone differences between homosexuals and heterosexuals have been found. A recent carefully controlled study suggests that homosexual men may have levels of FSH lower than that of heterosexual men (Newmark et al., 1979), but the ramifications of this finding have not yet been fully explored. When hormone therapy has been used, there has been little or no effect on sexual functioning. In some cases, raising the levels of hormones has increased the sex drive but has had absolutely no effect on sexual preference. As a result, hormone therapy has lost much of its popularity.

Psychodynamic therapy

Psychodynamic explanations of homosexuality revolve around conflicts developed early in childhood. Such conflicts may lead to homosexuality as the result of faulty or inadequate sexual identification, unusual infantile fixations, or defenses against Oedipal wishes and the fear of castration. As we saw in Chap. 16, the primary therapeutic approach of psychodynamic treatment is to analyze such conflicts, make them available to the conscious mind, and work them through so that they are no longer distressing. Once the conflict is neutralized, the natural process of heterosexuality should emerge. What produces this awareness is the insight achieved through the interpretive work of the analyst.

There have been few controlled studies of the effectiveness of psychodynamic treatment for the dissatisfied homosexual. When Bieber (1962) evaluated 106 cases, he found that only 27 percent were exclusively heterosexual and another 12 percent were bisexual after psychodynamic treatment. These meager results came after an investment of a great deal of therapeutic time and effort. Thus, psychodynamic treatment appears to have been a less than optimal approach to increasing heterosexual behavior.

Behavioral therapy

Behavior therapy starts with a ***functional analysis*** of the particular individual's behavior. The therapy procedures chosen are those anticipated to be the most effective for the particular complex of factors contributing to the maintenance of the individual's homosexual behavior. In such an approach, many aspects of the person's functioning become the focus of treatment, and the specific program of procedures is highly individualized to the client.

Most behavioral approaches to homosexuality address four basic areas: increasing heterosexual arousal responses, decreasing any responses that interfere with heterosexual behavior, building heterosocial skills in social and sexual areas so that the client can begin to function in a heterosexual context, and reducing homosexual responsiveness and behavior if it interferes with the developing heterosexual responsiveness.

Reducing homosexual responsiveness   Unfortunately, the last goal, that of decreasing or eliminating homosexual responses, has received the most attention. Many of the earliest applications of behavioral procedures to modification of homosexuality used aversive conditioning procedures as the total treatment. While they are still employed occasionally, they are rarely used alone. When aversive techniques were first used in behavioral treatments of homosexuality, there were understandably negative reactions from many sources, particularly from the homosexual community. These procedures were seen as being both manipulative and unpleasant. It also turns out that they are not the best procedures for producing change either. In fact, there is really little need for such aggressive suppression of the homosexual response. Instead, behavior therapy is more successful when it focuses on building positive heterosexual responses. Thus, techniques for removing the arousal value of homosexual stimuli should only be used when absolutely necessary, and when they *are* used, they should involve the more benign methods such as extinction before consideration of any painful or unpleasant methods.

Increasing heterosexual responsiveness   Increasing heterosexual arousal is the basic goal of individuals requesting change to heterosexual functioning. The therapeutic techniques used to accomplish this goal are designed to establish and strengthen a positive connection between the person's sexual arousal and heterosexual stimuli. **Classical conditioning** is one method used for this purpose. In this procedure, stimuli that already elicit a sexual arousal response, such as homosexual pictures, are connected to the currently neutral heterosexual stimuli by presenting them close together. A variation on this approach is **fading,** which we described in Chap. 16. In fading, the homosexual stimulus slowly fades and is gradually replaced by a heterosexual stimulus while the individual is still feeling aroused. Masturbation is another positive sexual event that can be paired with heterosexual stimuli. A secondary advantage of masturbation is that it results in sexual climax and release in addition to arousal. The procedure is the same as for **orgasmic reconditioning,** which was described in Chap. 15.

Reducing heterosexual anxiety   Some homosexual clients experience a well-developed anxiety-fear response in heterosexual situations. This response could have been learned in any of a large number of ways, many of which were mentioned in Chap. 13. The individual's fear interferes with any sexual arousal he or she might experience in heterosexual contact. This anxiety response is quite similar to the performance anxiety that is so much a part of the sexual dysfunctions. For this problem, the procedure of **systematic desensitization** is most useful. With this technique, the person learns to pair relaxation with

BOX 17.1

A behavioral approach to modifying homosexual behavior

We cite the following case study reported by R. W. Hanson and V. J. Adesso (1972).

History

The client was a 23-year-old, single, male hospital employee with a history of homosexual involvements beginning in early adolescence and continuing through 4 years in the military service. His only sexual experiences with females were two abortive attempts at intercourse with prostitutes.

Treatment

Phase 1: Assessment. During this phase, an attempt was made to determine the exact nature and history of his problem, to obtain a general sex history, and to estimate his motivation to change and his intellectual ability. He was given several questionnaires to assess his heterosexual anxiety, the extent of his sexual experience and the degree of arousal associated with a variety of sexual activities, his general heterosexual and homosexual orientation, the extent of his fears, and his level of assertiveness. The results indicated extensive heterosexual anxiety, an inability to relate to females on an intimate level, very little sexual attraction to females, and considerable sexual attraction to males. In contrast, the questionnaires did not suggest any significant lack of assertiveness or fears outside the problem area. A score of 119 on the Shipley Hartford Institute of Living Scale placed him in the bright-normal range of intelligence.

Phase 2: Preparation for treatment. After he was accepted as a suitable candidate for therapy, he was given a thorough explanation of the treatment procedures and their rationale. He was also asked to obtain medical clearance for electrical aversion. The client was then instructed to begin making a daily record of his hetero- and homoerotic thoughts and given training in deep muscle relaxation.

Phase 3: Application of systematic desensitization, aversive counterconditioning, and masturbation training.

. . . [T]he first priorities in treatment were to reduce the attraction value of homosexual stimuli and to abate his heterosexual anxiety. He was seen twice a week to allow an alternation between desensitization and aversion sessions. The desensitization dealt with a hierarchy of 22 items, developed from his responses to the Fear Survey Schedule and a heterosexual behavior anxiety scale. The items ranged from holding a girl's hand to engaging in complete sexual intercourse. Desensitization of the hierarchy was completed in five sessions.

In the aversion sessions he was shown pictures of nude males and asked to fantasize one of four scenes which depicted homosexual behaviors that were problematic for him, including masturbation or performing fellatio on the subject in the picture or having the subject masturbate or perform fellatio on him. When he had a clear image of the prescribed scene, he signaled to the therapist and received a painful 5-second shock to one of his forearms. After only four aversion sessions he reported an inability to imagine the prescribed homosexual activities despite earnest endeavors.

. . . [H]e was given masturbation instructions in order to increase the valence of heteroerotic stimuli. . . . [H]e was told to obtain an erection by any means, even if it required a temporary reversion to homosexual fantasies. Just before ejaculation, he was to switch to a heterosexual fantasy. He was then gradually to switch earlier to heterosexual fantasies.

Phase 4: In vivo training. Most homosexual clients possess a limited repertoire of heterosexual social skills. The client was given training in conversing with girls and asking them for dates by verbal instruction, modeling, and behavior rehearsal with two female assistants. He was then given graded behavioral assignments. The first assignment was to find a suitable dating partner, which he managed within a week. He was instructed to go no further sexually than he could with comfort. Therapy sessions were then devot-

ed to discussing his dates, the extent of his sexual activity, how he felt about it, and what to do next. His girlfriend knew nothing about his problem and fortunately was quite receptive to his amorous advances.

After 4 weeks of in vivo training, he was able to engage comfortably in heavy necking with his girlfriend. After 2 more weeks, he was able to engage in complete sexual intercourse for the first time in his life. At this point he considered himself "cured" and therapy was terminated. Altogether, his treatment took 14 weeks. . . .

The client, contacted 6 months after terminating treatment, reported that he was continuing to enjoy heterosexual activity and that his homosexual inclination was negligible. (pp. 325–326)

heterosexual situations of various types. Masters and Johnson's techniques for the treatment of interference anxiety (described in Chap. 15) also work well with heterosexual fear in homosexual conversion treatment.

Increasing heterosocial skills   Only recently has it been realized that an important part of changing sexual orientation is changing the person's **heterosocial skills**. The therapist first evaluates a variety of the individual's behaviors to see whether they have a positive or negative effect on the person's ability to function in the heterosexual social world. The therapist may then need to help the person modify his or her way of walking, using the hands, asking for a date, handling social anxiety, and so on. In particular, any previously learned inappropriate cross-sex behaviors must be modified or replaced if the individual is to function more adequately in those social situations that will be important in developing his or her budding heterosexuality. The various behavioral procedures are illustrated in a broad-spectrum approach to treatment like the one described in Box 17.1.

These behavioral procedures are a definite move away from the illness model of homosexuality described in Chap. 13. They focus on homosexuality as a complex of learned attractions to homosexual stimuli, of deficits in heterosexual arousal, and of social supports and deficits that maintain the homosexual status. As a response to requests for change, new learning is initiated to replace old patterns. The behavioral therapies have not been in use long enough to have established a record of success or failure, but initial data indicate positive results.

THE NATURE OF GENDER IDENTITY DISTURBANCE

Imagine that you woke up one morning and found yourself in the body of a person of the opposite sex. After the initial shock, you had to go on living in this body while every moment you felt that you were actually of the opposite sex. This may sound like the script of a horror movie, but for some people, like Walter Carlos, it has been their daily experience. They are transsexuals, or individuals with a gender identity disturbance. Essentially transsexuals feel that they are locked in the body of the opposite sex by some cruel mistake of nature. The interview with Carlos at the beginning of this chapter demonstrates many of the important features of gender identity disturbance. As a man, Carlos clearly felt he was a female despite his obvious male anatomical features. He was uncomfortable in male clothing, preferred female activities, and wanted to be a female anatomically. Eventually Carlos had surgery to become the woman she had always felt herself to be.

Transsexuality and other sex identity problems

Transsexuals do not consider themselves to be homosexual, as demonstrated in the following interview between a doctor and a woman requesting a sex-change operation to become a man:

Doctor: *Have you ever had a sexual relationship with a woman?*
Patient: *no.*
Doctor: *Have you thought about it?*
Patient: *Yes, I've thought about it. I've thought about it very much, but somehow or other I've never done it. Not as a girl I don't want to. It just bothers me, having sex. That's not what I want.*
Doctor: *Do you feel that if you could conduct a homosexual life, as many women do, and not feel guilty, this might make your life easier?*
Patient: *I don't really think so. Like even with my girlfriend I have to be careful, like opening doors or things like this. Maybe the way you look at somebody. You can't be free, and besides I don't think sexually that it would be satisfying. It's not meant to be.*
Doctor: *It's very common.*
Patient: *I know it's very common, but I don't see how they can be satisfied with it. I don't know. I don't think I would be. I definitely believe in God, and I have my own religious beliefs. (Green, R. 1974, p. 105)*

Note that this person cannot think of herself as a homosexual. She knows that she is sexually attracted to women but states that this is only because she is really a man herself. Transsexuals will often stress this point.

Another important distinction that must be made is between transvestites (see Chap. 16) and transsexuals. Transvestites dress in the clothing of the opposite sex for the sexual pleasure it brings them. Generally, transvestites retain their biological-anatomical sexual orientation and would be horrified at the thought of surgical change to the opposite sex.

Transsexualism has been well publicized in recent years because of several dramatic surgical transformations that have caught the public's attention. Walter/Wendy Carlos, professional tennis player Renée Richards, and writer James/Jan Morris are a few of the better known cases. But despite the high visibility of these people, transsexuality is still a relatively rare problem.

Transsexuality is not unique to our society or to our historical period. Before the availability of the surgical procedures for sex change, there was little reason for anyone to "go public" with the problem, but historians have noted many periods and cultures where transsexualism has been found. In some North American Indian tribes, for example, male members wore women's clothing and in every other way functioned as women in the tribe. Many lived out their lives in these reversed roles. In some cases such men were highly revered and were thought to be blessed with great magical powers.

Our own society has been less accepting and accommodating. Transsexuals generally remain well concealed, and if they do come out of the closet it is often to face a good deal of scorn and rejection. Their special problems frequently force them to live on the fringes of society. Driscoll (1971) described the situation of one group of male transsexuals who all lived in a San Francisco hotel that catered to them. Because of their cross-sex behavior, they could only work in rather undesirable jobs where their unusual life-style was accepted. Many also worked as prostitutes, trying to earn enough to live on, and more importantly, to save up for the expensive sex-change surgery that most felt would be their magic entry into a fulfilling life. As prostitutes, they would frequently try to pass as women and, while this worked surprisingly often, it sometimes resulted in severe beatings when they were discovered to be men. Driscoll's description of the lives these men led makes it clear that transsexuality may be one of the most difficult problems to live with in our society. It also clarifies why the drastic move of sex-reassignment surgery is pursued so relentlessly by many transsexuals.

Characteristics of transsexuals Transsexuality, being as atypical as it is, has not been studied extensively. The people involved are understandably reluctant to become guinea pigs for study. As a result, investigators have been forced to study only those individuals who have presented themselves for treatment, especially sex-reassignment surgery. Thus, our knowledge of transsexualism comes primarily from individuals experiencing the greatest difficulty in adjustment, since they are willing to experience the pain, expense, and trauma of complete physical change.

Given this caveat, we can make a few basic generalizations about transsexuals. For one thing, they have a strong identification with the opposite sex. They show interests, attitudes, behavior, and sexual arousal that are clearly opposite those of their own biological sex. As Carlos reported, these patterns appear quite early in life. Almost all transsexuals report having felt this way before puberty, and some say they felt they were the opposite sex as early as they could remember anything at all. In a group of male transsexuals studied by Pauly (1965), two-thirds claimed to have felt they were really of the opposite sex before age 5. Pauly noted that these memories may have been distorted by the transsexuals' current situation. He found in general that they were poor historians and even poorer reporters. Many of them had important psychological reasons for convincing themselves they had always been this way—much of their self-blame could be absolved if they could feel they had been born in the wrong body.

The idea of being born into the wrong-sex body is basically an appeal to an illness or biological accident explanation of transsexuality. However, the data do not support any chromosomal, hormonal, or physiological source for transsexual feelings. With regard to hormonal differences between transsexuals and normal heterosexuals, one study did show that testosterone levels were twice as high in transsexual women compared to normal women, but this study was the exception rather than the rule (Sipova and Starka, 1977).

One factor that may contribute to the early memories of opposite-sex identification is early parental influence. The studies of feminine boys and masculine girls discussed in Chaps. 5 and 9 (Green, 1974) indicated the great power that parents have in shaping sexual identification from a very early age. Nevertheless, there is no direct evidence that children whose parents treat them as if they belong to the opposite sex grow up to become transsexuals.

In some male and female transsexuals, homosexual impulses appeared in adolescence. These feelings were usually a serious problem for the individuals, most of whom had been raised to believe that such feelings are totally unacceptable. This fact raises the possibility that the transsexuals' view of the cause as being a biological accident may be an elaborate rationale for unacceptable homosexual feelings once they can no longer be denied.

TREATMENT OF GENDER IDENTITY DISTURBANCE

There are two directions in which treatment can proceed for a person experiencing gender identity disturbance: change the physical sex of the person or change the psychological gender of the person. In the first case, hormonal and surgical procedures have been developed for **sex reassignment**, thereby changing the anatomical sex of the person to conform to the strongly held identification with the opposite sex. In the second case, psychotherapy is used to help the person become more comfortable with, and adjusted to, his or her biological sex. The decision as to which of these two directions to follow is obviously important, and a great deal of thought and counseling should go into the decision-making process. Both of these methods have positive and negative aspects, but the sex-reassignment surgery has the additional problem of being irreversible.

Transsexuals are more likely to request physiological sexual reassignment than psychological adjustment. As we have noted, psychological forces that make the physiological change the more acceptable choice are at work. The result, however, has been that transsexuality has come to be viewed as a *medical* problem, and emphasis has been placed on that approach as a solution to the problem. The rationalization of the transsexual has thus been injected into society—perhaps inappropriately.

Physiological sex reassignment

The surgical changes of the sexual anatomy are the most publicized part of sex-reassignment procedures. However, they are actually only the last in a

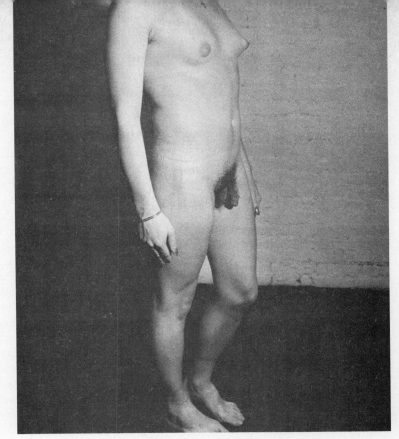

FIGURE 17.1

This is a male-to-female transsexual during the sexual reassignment process. He/she has had female hormones but has not yet had surgery to remove the penis and create a vagina.

series of physical interventions to change the biological-anatomical sex of the person. The few medical centers willing to do this type of work have typically established sex-reassignment clinics in which a team of medical and psychological specialists work with prospective clients.

The typical program begins with a discussion of the nature and totality of the changes and the kinds of physical and psychological problems that may occur. If the individual wants to proceed, a thorough assessment of the person's motivation, current adjustment, and likelihood of later adverse psychological effects is then made. Should the assessment prove favorable, the next step is **hormone therapy**. Hormones are injected to shift the hormonal balance toward that of the opposite anatomical sex. With the change in hormones, secondary sexual characteristics begin to change to conform to the new sexual orientation. Men lose their body hair, show breast enlargement, have increased fat deposits that result in a rounding of body contours, and undergo other similar changes (see Fig. 17.1). Women experience increased muscular development, appearance of facial hair, a lowered voice, cessation of menstruation, and so on. Most of the centers then require the person to live for at least a year in the sex role to which he or she has been changed. This is the crucial test for the final decision. If the person feels better in this new role and psychological assessment shows improvement during this test period, the decision will probably be made to proceed to actual surgical change.

Surgical modifications to produce further secondary sex characteristics is usually performed first. For anatomical males, breast implants, Adam's apple reduction, hair electrolysis, and other cosmetic changes are made. For females, breasts may be removed and hysterectomies performed. After recovery from these procedures, the individual is ready for actual change of the sex organs.

In the male-to-female transformation, the surgery consists of removing the testes and creating a functional vagina. The erectile tissue is removed from the penis but the external sheath, with all its nerve endings intact, is inverted and inserted into the body to form a vagina-like structure. For the female-to-male transformation, a penis and scrotum are fashioned from the clitoris and surrounding tissue. The penis is not totally functional, since it is small and not capable of spontaneous erection. Some penises are made permanently semierect so they can be used for sexual intercourse. Some experimentation has been done with implants that are pumped up manually to form an erect penis, but they have not gone into wide use. Many of the female-to-male transsexuals use an artificial penis if they want to include penile insertion as part of their sexual activities with a female partner.

Postsurgical adjustment has been highly variable. Many transsexuals who have gone through the procedure report they are functioning well in their new social roles and in their sexual activities. Such individuals also report being much happier after surgery than before. But for many others, the results are mixed. The life change does not reduce all problems. As of 1976, some 2500 people had undergone sex-change surgery in this country (Gagnon, 1977). Unfortunately, there are no overall figures on adjustment, since many of the clinics and surgeons do not do follow-up research on their clients. An early figure of 85 percent client satisfaction with this procedure was reported in 1968 by Pauly. However, a recent study at Johns Hopkins Medical Center, a pioneer in the area of sex reassignment, convinced that institution that the surgical procedures had not greatly improved the lives of the transsexuals who had been treated, and the sex-reassignment clinic had been closed (see Box 17.2). There is an obvious need for better evaluations of outcome so that a clearer picture of the overall value of sex reassignment surgery can emerge.

Although research is necessary to evaluate the surgical approach, the sense of desperation among transsexuals will probably keep sex-change surgery going. When the *Playboy* interviewer asked Wendy Carlos, "Do you have any idea what would have happened to you if you hadn't had the operation?" she responded, "Yes, I'd be dead." While this reply is rather dramatic, it does represent the kind of intense emotion that many transsexuals bring to discussions of potential surgical intervention.

*Psychological
treatment*

The less desperate measure of changing the psychological identification of the transsexual has received far less interest or emphasis as a method of treatment. Because transsexuals seem so definite in their desire for surgical change, they usually actively reject any possibility of psychotherapeutic resolu-

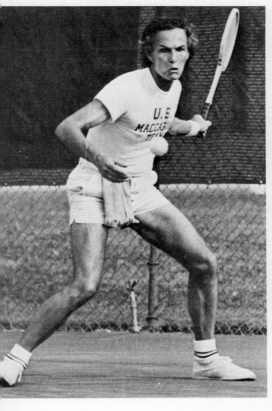
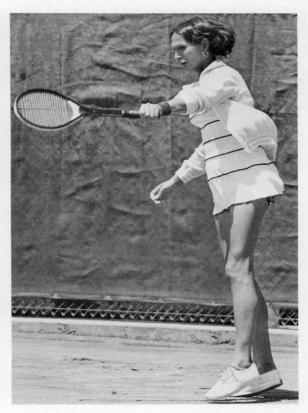

Renée Richards, a well-known transsexual, before and after his/her sex-change procedures.

tion of the problem. In addition, the mental health professions have done little to encourage them in this direction.

One demonstration of a carefully planned and executed program of psychological intervention with a gender identity disturbance was presented by Barlow, Agras, and Reynolds (1972). They worked with a 17-year-old male who desired to be a female. The particular methods used have been described previously; what is unique to this case is the great care that was taken to work with all the components of sexuality, so that a total identity of masculinity would have a chance to emerge in the client.

The young man was depressed, withdrawn, and isolated and was obviously mixed in his gender role, gender identity, and behavior. He felt his only hope for happiness was through sex-change surgery. The sex-reassignment clinics had turned him down because of his age. As a result, he agreed to try psychological treatment. An assessment indicated effeminate behavior, feminine life goals (he was the only male in a secretarial school), totally inadequate heterosocial skills, no sexual arousal response to women, and strong arousal to transsexual fantasies. The therapeutic work included changing gender role

BOX 17.2

The sex-change controversy

In 1979 Johns Hopkins Hospital, renowned as a pioneer in sex-change surgery, elected to phase out this surgical program. Why?

The hospital made its decision after reviewing research indicating that sex-change surgery provides no more benefits to a transsexual than does conventional psychotherapy. The key study was done by psychiatrist John K. Meyer, head of Johns Hopkins' Sexual Behaviors Consultation Unit. Starting in 1971, Meyer followed the progress of 50 transsexuals who had been treated at the Johns Hopkins gender identity clinic. Fewer than half of the patients (most of whom were men wishing to be women) underwent the sex-change surgery; the rest received counseling or therapy. Meyer assessed the life adjustment of these patients in four areas: job or work, legal difficulties, marriage and family, and psychiatric consultation.

After following the adjustment of these 50 individuals for several years, Meyer concluded that "surgery serves as a palliative measure, relieving some of the patients' symptoms of discomfort, but not necessarily improving the individual's adjustment in life" (Meyer and Reter, 1979, p. 1014). He suggested that positive adjustment was, if anything, greater among those who received therapy than among those who had the operation.

Critics of sex-reassignment surgery point out that the procedure is subject to hazardous complications, such as dangerous infections and failure of the new sex organs to "work" properly. These people say that the surgical procedure is "a mutilating, irreversible, and drastic approach to an essentially subjective complaint" (Restak, 1979, p. 20).

Psychiatrist Theodore Van Putten and others have pointed out that many studies of the "success" of transsexual surgery have relied on the patients' own reports of being happier or better adjusted. But self-reports are notoriously unreliable. Van Putten cites, for example, a case in which the patient's postoperative adjustment was rated between good and satisfactory even though he was a drug addict and homosexual prostitute.

Another critic, Richard Restak (1979), has compared sex-change surgery to the "crude 'ice-pick' psychosurgical operations of the 1940s and 1950s," which also provided an irreversible surgical solution to behavioral problems. He sees the surgery as "a drastic nonsolution to the problem" that should be sharply restricted. Restak suggests that medical authorities redefine transsexual operations as "experimental surgery" to be used in small, carefully selected trial populations. In this way he says, the proponents "will be forced to demonstrate the value of the operation through rigorous selection of patients, long-term follow-ups, and . . . full disclosure" of results. Otherwise, it is yet to be demonstrated, say Restak and the other critics, that the drastic changes produced by sex-change surgery can "cure" or rehabilitate the transsexual patient.

behavior through direct instruction, modeling, and videotape feedback. Similar methods were also used to increase heterosocial skills. An important component was instruction in how to interact with males and females from a masculine perspective. Behaviors such as eye contact, lowering of the voice, and talking about male topics all had to be trained.

Increasing heterosexual arousal involved several procedures. Fading was found to be particularly helpful. Slides of nude males were faded to nude females as soon as arousal began. The therapists measured penile response to assess the arousal and to maximize the transfer effect. Finally, decreasing homoerotic responsiveness was accomplished using both electrical aversion and covert sensitization.

The client was followed with visits for evaluation and support for several months after treatment. At a 2-year follow-up, the client was found to be attending college and dating regularly. Although this successful outcome is gratifying, it is, after all, only one case. However, it does suggest that such procedures deserve continued exploration, especially in light of the recent questioning of the value of physical sex-reassignment procedures.

We are currently reevaluating the actual nature of gender identity disturbances and sexual preference disturbances as well as the best approaches to their treatment. Through understanding of these problems, we are becoming more knowledgeable about the important components of sexual identity in all people, and such advances in our knowledge should prove valuable in understanding many aspects of human sexual behavior.

SUMMARY

1   The various components that make up a person's sexual identity include biological sex, gender identity, gender role behavior, and choice of sexual partners. The major problems that can arise because of discrepancies between the components of sexual identity are problems of sexual preference and gender identity disturbance.

2   *Sexual preference disturbance*, or *dissatisfied homosexuals*, refers to homosexuals who wish to change their sexual preference to heterosexuality. Only a small percentage of homosexuals are in this category. Their dissatisfaction may be a result of an attraction to a heterosexual partner, interference of their homosexuality with an ongoing heterosexual relationship, external social pressure, or a number of other factors.

3   It is usually assumed in our society that people must be exclusively heterosexual or exclusively homosexual. Kinsey found, however, that sexual orientation actually falls along a continuum. Thus, dissatisifed homosexuals may find a solution to their problem in some degree of bisexuality.

4   Treatment of sexual preference disturbance focuses on four main areas: inappropriate sexual arousal, lack of heterosexual responsiveness, inappropriate gender role behaviors, and lack of heterosocial skills. Homosexual social supports must also be replaced with heterosexual ones.

5   The biological approach to treatment of homosexuality relies on hormone therapy. The psychodynamic approach to homosexuality is to bring underlying conflicts into consciousness and to analyze them so that they are

no longer distressing. The behavioral approach to treatment begins with a *functional analysis* of the particular individual's behavior. Therapy techniques, such as classical conditioning, fading, and systematic desensitization, may be used to reduce homosexual responsiveness and heterosexual anxiety and to increase heterosexual responsiveness and social skills.

6   *Gender identity disturbances* refers to *transsexuality,* or the belief that one is locked inside the body of the opposite sex by some mistake of nature. Transsexuals do not consider themselves to be homosexual. Most transsexuals say they have felt they were really the opposite sex since early childhood. The causes of this type of disturbance are unknown, although physiological problems are unlikely to be involved.

7   Treatment of transsexuality consists of either physiological *sex reassignment,* in which the person is physically transformed into the opposite sex, or psychotherapy to help the person adapt to his or her biological sex. Sex-change procedures are highly controversial, and there is doubt whether they actually help the person. Behavior therapy procedures have been shown to be successful in specific cases.

**ADDITIONAL
READING**

Masters, William, and Johnson, Virginia. *Homosexuality in Perspective.* Boston: Little, Brown, 1979.

> *Contains chapters on male and female homosexual dissatisfaction and attempts at therapeutic interventions to change sexual orientation. The book presents the research findings on these groups.*

* **Morris, Jan.** *Conundrum.* New York: Harcourt Brace Jovanovich, 1974.

> *The fascinating autobiography of Jan/James Morris, a successful journalist, mountain climber, and World War II veteran who underwent sex reassignment surgery. A rare inside glimpse, sensitively written.*

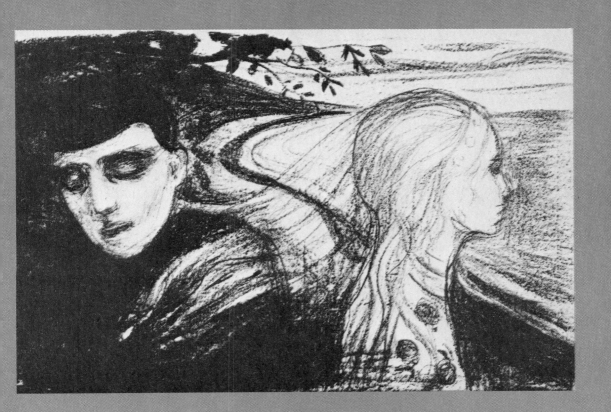

Sex-related diseases
and disorders

18

chapter

18

Sexual intercourse, that most intimate of human interactions, has the potential for passing along more than the beauty and pleasure of the sexual experience. It is perhaps one of the great ironies of nature that sexual interaction is the means by which a number of diseases, some of them quite serious, can be communicated from one person to another. These diseases are the **sexually transmitted diseases** (STDs). You may know them by their former name, **venereal diseases** (VD). In this chapter we will use these terms interchangeably as we describe the major types of diseases—their causes, clinical effects, diagnosis, and treatment. Toward the end of the chapter we will also describe some of the nonvenereal diseases of the sex organs as well as various disorders that can affect sexual functioning.

THE RISE OF THE SEXUALLY TRANSMITTED DISEASES

The venereal diseases (named after Venus) have been around since the beginning of recorded history. An Egyptian papyrus described a genital infection called *ucheda*, and the Old Testament has numerous references to sexually transmitted diseases, hygienic measures to avoid the diseases of sexual intercourse, and the dangers of the diseases of prostitutes. The Greeks and Romans also wrote about venereal disease (Brasch, 1973).

Although STDs have been present during all of human history, they need not be part of humanity's future. Many of the major venereal diseases are preventable with proper care and are curable with modern drugs when they are contracted. Thus, theoretically their spread could be managed with appropriate and coordinated efforts by public agencies and individuals. The most active effort to eradicate venereal diseases occurred in the 1950s. An all-out campaign by the U.S. Public Health Service with adequate funding produced dramatic results. However, a number of events, including lack of continued financial support, led to an easing of the effort, and the subsequent rise in the incidence of the diseases has been even more dramatic than the 1950s decline.

Figures 18.1 and 18.2 show the number of cases of gonorrhea and syphilis for the years 1950–1974. The real tragedy of these graphs is that victory over these two major STDs seemed within reach, only to have slipped away. Note that the rise since the 1950s, especially for gonorrhea, has been remarkably steep. Many public health officials consider the incidence of this disease to be at near epidemic proportions. The figures for other countries show similar rising trends, although not quite as dramatic.

What has caused this sharp rise in STD rates in the past few decades? This question is especially puzzling given our increased knowledge about the diseases and the availability of adequate treatment. Nevertheless, several factors have obviously contributed to this situation. One is increased sexual activity. The freedom to enjoy sex more often and with more partners has contributed greatly to the rise of STDs, particularly among young people. There has been a sharp decline worldwide in the age at which sexual activity begins. Younger people are more likely to get and spread STDs, and they are less likely to be aware of the problems of STDs, to know the signs and symptoms, and to know about techniques for preventing infection of themselves and others.

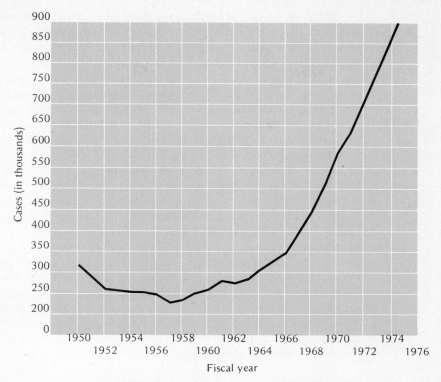

FIGURE 18.1
*Cases of gonorrhea
reported in the
United States for
1950–1974.
(Wiesner, Jones,
and Blount, 1976)*

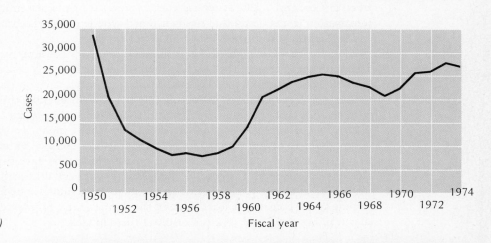

FIGURE 18.2
*Cases of syphilis
(primary and
secondary)
reported in the
United States for
1950–1974.
(Wiesner, Jones,
and Blount, 1976)*

A second important factor is the greatly increased use of oral contraceptives since the early 1960s. Use of the Pill has reduced the use of condoms, which, besides their birth control function, also help to control the spread of some organisms responsible for STDs. By reducing concerns about pregnancy, the Pill has also contributed to the higher rate of sexual activity and the younger age levels at which individuals are engaging in sexual behavior.

A third factor is that newer, stronger strains of the STD organisms that are more resistant to the various drugs used for treatment have developed. These new strains may be part of the natural evolution of the infectious agents, but they are also a result of inappropriate treatment of STDs. In some countries (Brazil, for example) penicillin is sold without prescription or medical control of dosage. People who medicate themselves often take only enough of the drug to reduce the external symptoms or to make them feel a little better. Not only are they unaware of the need for taking a full course of the antibiotic, but they tend to take the drug sparingly because of its high cost. Other people take antibiotics in a morning-after, preventive fashion. When people do not take a full course of these medications, they kill the weak organisms but leave the stronger ones alive, with greater potency than before. In addition, by reducing the external signs, they leave themselves and their potential partners without the obvious symptoms that could warn them that they are carriers of this even stronger strain of the disease. Such inadequate drug treatment is worse than no treatment at all if we consider that it is contributing to the creation of a worldwide epidemic of more highly resistant venereal disease organisms.

The lack of systematic programs of public education is still another factor in the rising incidence of STDs. Most of the peoples of the world, including the United States, do not get adequate information on how to recognize, prevent, treat, and control STDs. Schools are often prevented from disseminating such information to the group that needs it most—young people. So, many of them end up learning about the STDs from direct experience.

Finally, the public health effort in many countries has simply not kept pace with the problem. The diseases themselves are so costly to a society that it would seem to make good economic sense to control their spread rather than to just treat the victims. A socioeconomic factor counteracting this obvious good sense is that the usual victims of the diseases tend to be from the least politically powerful groups. Legislators are not usually inclined toward voting for programs to help the poor, and they are even less inclined to help those who are perceived as the *immoral* poor, that is, those who have the highest rates of VD. Funds for the control of STDs were cut back drastically in the United States in the 1950s, just when the major infections seemed to be coming under control. At least some of the dramatic rise in infection rates shown in Figs. 18.1 and 18.2 is a result of that cutback.

**CONTROL OF THE
SEXUALLY
TRANSMITTED
DISEASES**

Because many factors are involved in the spread of STDs, their eventual control will require a coordinated attack directed toward all the factors. The three main components of an effective control effort are (1) clinical care of the infected individuals, (2) epidemiological methods to control the spread of the disease, and (3) education of people about prevention.

Clinical treatment of diseases depends on the availability of medical services through clinics and hospitals. To serve this purpose adequately, such treatment must be readily available to the target population. The effectiveness of clinics depends on their number, the fees that are charged, and public knowledge of their existence. They must adequately diagnose the disease, provide the appropriate treatment, and do follow-up work to make sure the treatment was effective and to control relapse. Prompt treatment is necessary both for the health of the individual and for controlling the spread of the disease by reducing the person's ability to infect others. Currently, many European countries as well as England have a more extensive program of clinics than the United States.

Epidemiological methods focus on controlling the spread of diseases in the community. Two methods are most important in such control efforts: contact tracing and mass screening. ***Contact tracing*** involves finding all of the infected person's sexual contacts from the time of probable infection to the time of treatment. An effort is made to find the source of the infection as well as to control further spread of the disease. Contact tracing is often difficult and delicate, since the infected person will need to discuss sexual activities and reveal the names of sexual partners. Notifying the contacts is an even more sensitive problem, since both casual partners and long-term partners such as wives and husbands have to be informed that they might have the infection and need to be tested and possibly treated. It is no easier for the person who has an STD to discover that a loved one is the source of the infection. Contact tracing is best carried out by trained investigators rather than by physicians or untrained health clinic personnel. Time is of the essence, since the contacts may be spreading the infection further.

Mass screening involves checking members of the general populace for possible VD. People usually encounter such screening when they apply for a marriage license, as most states require a blood test before the license is granted. Routine blood screening is also done on all people who donate or sell blood to blood banks or who take certain jobs requiring the handling of food or drugs. One of the most important uses of screening is that of testing pregnant women for potential STDs. Several types of venereal infections can be transmitted to the newborn, causing serious disease in the child. A final type of screening is establishment of short-term walk-in clinics in various communities, where anyone who wants to can be tested. People can withhold their names if they wish to, and treatment is given to those whose tests prove positive. Contact tracing is initiated if the infected persons cooperate.

Public education is an important component of any comprehensive STD control program. An individual's personal vulnerability can be dramatically reduced with knowledge of how the diseases are transmitted from person to person and of what measures can be taken to protect oneself. Any educational programs must be available to the younger age groups to be really successful, since it is younger people who are most vulnerable, who have more partners, and who are least likely to have other sources of information.

The most common sexually transmitted diseases are gonorrhea, syphilis, genital herpes, trichomoniasis, moniliasis, granuloma inguinale, chanchroid, lymphogranuloma venereum, scabies, and crabs.

The causative agent of **gonorrhea** is a bacterium called **Neisseria gonorrhoeae**, named after Albert Neisser, who discovered it in 1879. Although he identified the disease organism, the disease itself has been around for centuries and is probably the disease described in the Old Testament as "an abnormal discharge from the genitals which was highly contagious" (Brasch, 1973).

The gonorrhea bacterium produces an acute, highly infectious disease. It has a strong affinity for the tissues of the genitals, the urinary tract, the fallopian tubes, and the anus. It is currently the most frequently found STD and is, in fact, one of the most common of all the infectious diseases of human beings.

Transmission is almost totally through sexual intercourse, since this organism cannot live outside the body. Gonorrhea can be transmitted by vaginal intercourse, anal intercourse, oral-genital contact, and oral-anal contact. It can also be transmitted to newborn infants during the birth process as they move through the vaginal canal.

Clinical effects   The **incubation period**—the amount of time it takes for symptoms to appear—is from 2 to 7 days after contact with an infected person. In men, the first signs are a milky-looking discharge from the penis (Fig. 18.3)

FIGURE 18.3 Symptom of gonorrhea as it appears on the male penis.

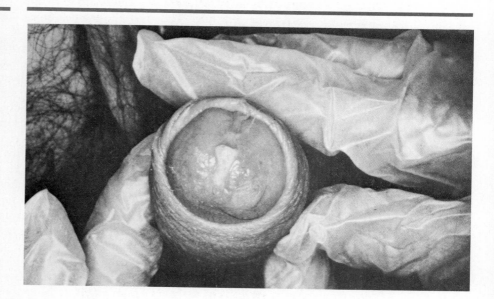

and a burning sensation when urinating. There is often general discomfort in the urethra and the sensation of needing to urinate but being unable to. If there has been anal contact, there may be discomfort in the anus. The severity of the symptoms varies widely, and approximately 5 percent of men who are infected show no symptoms at all, even though the infection is quite active within the body.

From 50 to 60 percent of infected women show no external clinical signs, and even when signs are present, they may be so mild as to be ignored. Thus, many women become carriers of the disease without knowing it. This is one of the reasons that gonorrhea has been so difficult to eradicate. When symptoms do appear in women, they usually consist of a discharge from the vagina and a burning sensation upon urinating. Sexual intercourse may be quite uncomfortable.

Gonorrhea that goes untreated sometimes gets better by itself, but all too often it gets worse. The effects of the full-blown infection can be quite damaging, including the possibility of sterility, especially in women.

In the male, the infection can extend into all of the sexual organs, including the epididymides, the prostate, the seminal vesicles, and the urinary tract. Like any infection that is out of control, gonorrhea can threaten the man's total health and may even be fatal.

In the female, the infection also extends into any or all of the sexual organs and the urinary tract. Since the infection is more likely to go undetected in the female than in the male, the damage to women is often more severe. For example, infection of the fallopian tubes can cause a buildup of scar tissue that blocks the tubes, resulting in sterility. If the infected woman is pregnant, the infection can be passed on to the infant as it is being born. Gonorrhea can have multiple damaging effects on the child, including mental retardation, heart defects, and blindness. Infant blindness from gonorrhea is so great a concern that all 50 states require that silver nitrate drops or penicillin ointment be placed in the eyes of all newborn infants as a protective measure.

Gonorrhea can occur in other areas of the body besides the sex organs. Common sites are the mouth, throat, and eyes. If the infection enters the bloodstream, it can affect other body systems. One type of arthritis that attacks all of the body's joints is thought to be a result of chronic gonorrhea infection.

Diagnosis Formal diagnosis of gonorrhea is made through finding the bacterium in cultures taken from the vagina, anus, or penis. It is important to find evidence of the actual organism, since there are many other disorders, including other types of STDs, that have similar symptoms and that require different treatment. If the disease is misdiagnosed and different treatment is given, the gonorrhea is likely to go on uncured.

Treatment In adequate doses, penicillin cures gonorrhea rapidly and completely. After a single injection, the discharge may disappear within a matter of hours, and the person may be totally symptom free in 2 to 3 days. In those few cases that do not respond immediately, higher doses usually prove successful.

If the person is allergic to penicillin, other antibiotics are available that work almost as effectively and quickly.

The problem with the availability of such an easy cure is that it has made people less concerned about becoming infected and about infecting others. Thus, in some cases, the effectiveness of the cure actually works against people taking precautions—one can always get a shot to take care of a "dose of the clap." As we have noted, people who self-medicate with penicillin often do not take enough of it, thereby creating "super strains" of the infectious gonococcus. While no strain has proven to be totally antibiotic resistant, it is still feared that such a strain could evolve if current trends continue.

Follow-up tests are important in the treatment of gonorrhea, since the stronger organisms may survive the initial treatment. Follow-up cultures are recommended for 3 months after the initial treatment to guard against relapse.

Of all the sexually transmitted diseases, **syphilis** is perhaps the most frightening. If allowed to run its full course, this disease can produce paralysis, madness, and finally a painful death. However, nowadays syphilis is usually halted in its early stages, and it is rare for these later damages to occur.

Syphilis is caused by the bacterium **Treponema pallidum** This type of bacterium, called a **spirochete**, has a long life once it has entered the body. It is capable of moving through the bloodstream to different locations, thereby producing the wide range of symptoms that mark the final phase of the disease. Although it has existed in Europe since the time of Columbus, the actual disease organism was not identified until 1905, and it was not until 1943 that penicillin was found to be the best treatment.

The transmission of syphilis is basically through sexual intercourse. The infectious organism is passed from one person to another through the skin or mucus membranes during sexual activity. Usually a small abrasion or sore is the site of entry for the infectious organisms. Once in the body, the spirochetes multiply and spread rapidly through the bloodstream. People can also be infected through kissing or living in close proximity with an infected person, although such cases are rare.

Pregnant women can pass the disease on to their unborn children through the placental barrier. The child is then born with **congenital syphilis** If it survives, the child is severely handicapped with a number of defects, including mental retardation, deafness, and abnormalities of the heart, bones, teeth, and facial features. Such a child will show the distinctive signs of syphilis for the rest of his or her life. Infected women can pass the disease on to their children for 5 years after becoming infected. Fortunately, an infected mother can be treated during pregnancy and the fetus can be treated while still in the uterus. The earlier the treatment, the less the potential damage. For this reason, routine blood screening of all pregnant women is required in most states.

Clinical effects The incubation period for syphilis is 10–90 days. The first sign of the infection is a small sore that appears at the site of the entry of the spirochetes, usually on the genitals (Fig. 18.4). This sore, called a **chancre** (shank-er), can look fairly innocent. It is round, approximately 10 millimeters

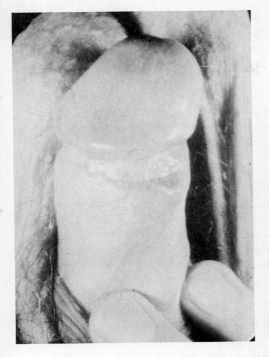

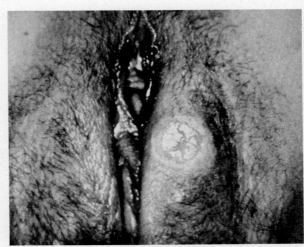

FIGURE 18.4
*The primary-stage
syphilitic chancre
as it appears on
the male penis
(left) and female
labia (right).*

(0.4 inch) across, and has a smooth edge. Because it is painless and heals with no scar, it may not be given any special significance. And should it occur inside the rectum or in the vagina, it may not be noticed at all. The sore goes away by itself in a few weeks, but the infection is only beginning. Up to this point, the person is in the **primary stage** of syphilis.

The **secondary stage** occurs anywhere from 4 to 8 weeks after the appearance of the primary signs. The dominant feature is a rash of rather ugly-looking sores over the entire body and in the mouth. The person also feels sick and feverish, has head and body aches, and has a sore throat. Some infected people dismiss even these symptoms as an allergic reaction, a cold, or the flu. This stage lasts 2–6 weeks.

If the disease is not treated, the visible signs and the general body reactions disappear by themselves, and the person believes he or she has shaken off the disease. But, in fact, the infection has once again gone "underground" into what is called the **latent stage**. For the next 5–20 years, the person is clear of external symptoms, but the spirochetes are actually doing their most destructive work. Infected individuals are actively contagious during the first 2 years of the latent stage. After this period, they are unlikely to pass on the disease. Although there are no external signs of syphilis during this stage, a blood test will show the presence of the spirochetes.

Third-stage or **tertiary** syphilis does not invariably follow the latent stage. Some people do fight off the infection and arrest any further damage. But many do not, and they will show the ultimate effects of syphilis. The relative degree of the original infection, the general health of the person, and the body sites affected all contribute to the extent of damage that occurs in the last stage. The systems of the body most likely to be affected are the heart, the blood vessels, the bones, the spinal cord, and the brain. If the brain is involved, the person may show the degenerative disease called **parenchymatous neurosyphilis** or **syphilitic psychosis**. At the turn of the century, this syndrome was called **general paresis** before its cause was traced to syphilis. The symptoms include intellectual deficits, memory loss, and eventual madness. There is also loss of muscle function, loss of speech, convulsions, and paralysis. Although death eventually results from the internal destruction, the process is long and slow. The connection of general paresis to syphilis helped establish syphilis as the most dreaded of the venereal diseases.

Diagnosis   There are several types of tests for syphilis. Where skin lesions are present, serum from the lesion can be examined under the microscope for presence of the spirochetes. Blood tests that make use of various staining methods will also show the infection. In any of the latent periods, blood tests must be relied on to show the presence of the infectious organisms. The **Wasserman test** is perhaps the best known of these tests, but several others that are considered more reliable are in greater use today. It is important to do follow-up blood tests for several years after treatment, because the infection can reappear.

Treatment   The best treatment for syphilis is penicillin. It is given in two large injections, a week apart, in order to kill all of the infectious spirochetes. If the person is allergic to penicillin, other antibiotics can be used. Treatment is effective at all stages of the disease. There is, however, no reversal of the damage the disease has already done, although additional damage can be prevented. Even in advanced, tertiary-stage syphilis, aggressive treatment with antibiotics is recommended, since the active bacteria will produce further damage if not stopped.

Genital herpes

It's just ruining my entire life! . . . I've been to three different doctors—a gynecologist, a dermatologist, and now another gynecologist who specializes in VD—and none of them has been able to cure me.

First I get this terrible itching. I feel tired and lousy all over. Then the sores come; usually four or five all bunched together. They are like fever blisters, but they hurt so much I can hardly stand it. Of course, I can't have sexual relations when I'm all broken out, so it is ruining my personal life, too. (Subak-Sharpe, 1975, p. 92)

This description, given by a 29-year-old woman, fits the typical pattern of the early stages of **genital herpes, herpes simplex type 2**, a viral disease of the genitals that is related to the herpes virus we generally associate with cold sores of the mouth. Genital herpes is a widespread problem; the number of cases has surpassed that for syphilis, and if present trends continue, herpes will soon challenge gonorrhea as the number one sexually transmitted disease.

Beyond the discomfort and inconvenience this disease produces in its victim, it has two serious implications. First, a pregnant woman can transmit the virus to her infant during the birth process. Of the infants so exposed, 50 percent get the infection, which causes severe damage and can even prove fatal. The second potential danger is cervical cancer. A strong statistical relationship has been found between herpes and incidence of this type of cancer, although it is still unclear how herpes might be related to the development of cancer.

Clinical effects　The incubation period for genital herpes is 2–6 days after being infected. The signs of the infection are similar in men and women. It is first experienced as itching and irritation at the site of the infection, accompanied by a rash at the site. Blisters then appear in clusters on the genitals (see Fig. 18.5). These blisters soon break and form painful, unpleasant lesions.

FIGURE 18.5
The herpes lesions as they appear on the male penis (top) and the female labia (bottom).

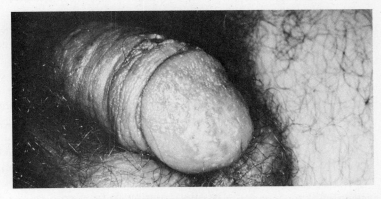

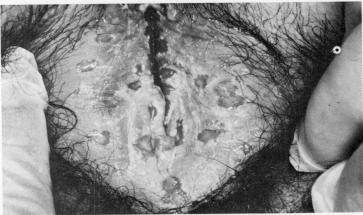

Along with the local discomfort in the genital region, there is usually a more general reaction similar to that for most other viral infections. Fever, weakness, a "sick" feeling, and fatigue are some of the associated symptoms.

The symptoms continue for 3–6 weeks, then disappear, only to reappear at odd intervals for shorter periods of time. With each recurrence the person is again highly infectious. In women, the infection and its recurrences may be totally internal, with no manifestation on the external genitals. Thus, a woman can have the disease and spread it to others without being aware of the fact.

Because of the infection's ability to appear and disappear, couples can keep reinfecting each other over a long period of time. This phenomenon has been called the **herpes ping-pong**, an apt name for an infection that can bounce back and forth between partners, sometimes for years.

Diagnosis   The diagnosis of genital herpes is possible only by observing the physical signs. There is no blood test that can reveal the existence of the infection, so in those cases where there is no discomfort or external signs, the virus will go virtually unnoticed. The fact that it also has an invisible latent phase makes it nearly impossible to know whether someone is carrying the virus. This is particularly a problem for pregnant women.

Treatment   There is no single, effective treatment for herpes simplex type 2. For some sufferers, repeated smallpox inoculations have proved successful. This method is thought to work by arousing the natural autoimmune responses of the body, which then attack the herpes virus. When the infection is at the lesion stage, exposure of the lesions to light after a dye has been applied helps to clear up the local infection, but this approach has created the worry that the virus cells may gather increased potential to produce cancer as a result of the exposure.

Genital herpes has probably been underreported in our society. The lack of knowledge that it is a venereal disease has meant that most people do not know what the uncomfortable infection is. Since it clears up spontaneously, it is often ignored as just a passing irritation. Furthermore, until recently the medical profession expressed little concern about genital herpes because it did not appear to cause further complications. And because there is no adequate treatment, people have even less motivation to report the disease. However, recent awareness of the long-term potential dangers and the resiliency of the virus have created greater concern. The next several years should see increased attention to genital herpes and perhaps the discovery of an effective and safe treatment.

OTHER SEXUALLY TRANSMITTED DISEASES
Trichomoniasis

In this section we shall briefly describe some of the less well-known STDs and some diseases that can be transmitted by both sexual interaction and other means.

As many as 25 percent of all American women may contract **trichomoniasis** at some point in their lives. Men also get the infection but not as frequently. Despite its high incidence, trichomoniasis has not received the same attention as the other STDs. Some experts argue that it is not really an STD, since it can be transmitted in many ways besides sexual encounter.

Trichomoniasis is caused by a protozoan, **Trichomonas vaginalis**, first identified in 1836. This one-celled organism seems to thrive and grow rapidly in moist, warm tissues such as the vagina. Because women frequently do not show symptoms, controlling the spread of this disease has been difficult. When the disease does produce symptoms in women, they consist primarily of a vaginal discharge that can vary from light to heavy and perhaps itching and irritation. Sexual intercourse may be painful. In some cases the pain can be extreme and last for quite some time.

Men also vary in their responses to infection. Some are asymptomatic carriers, while others experience itching and discomfort of the urethra and a slight discharge similar to that caused by gonorrhea.

Much of what is called **nonspecific urethritis**—unidentified irritation of the urethra—is probably trichomoniasis infection. Although the infection can invade organs other than the genitals and urethra, it usually does not.

Diagnosis is established through microscopic examination of cultures grown from vaginal smears or the penile discharge. The parasite can easily be seen when properly stained. The usual treatment is with the drug metronidazole, which is taken orally for 7 days. It is 80 percent effective in both sexes. It is important to do follow-up tests after 3 months, since the organisms are hardy and the few that might survive the metronidazole may reestablish the infection. Not enough of the people who have the infection are treated, probably because of the lack of symptoms in many of the cases. So far trichomoniasis has not been associated with any serious complications.

Moniliasis

Like trichomoniasis, **moniliasis** is a disease that can be contracted through other than sexual transmission. It is an infection caused by the fungus **Candida albicans** and is sometimes referred to as **yeast infection**. This organism usually lives in the bodies of both men and women without producing symptoms. However, when it invades the vaginal area of women, it sometimes produces a white, lumpy discharge that looks something like cottage cheese. The woman experiences irritation, itching, and inflammation of the vaginal area. Intercourse becomes extremely painful. Moniliasis does not appear to have any serious complications, but it is highly uncomfortable and severely limits sexual activity.

Treatment with vaginal creams or suppositories containing the drug **nyastatin** is helpful, but the infection can recur repeatedly, especially during or immediately after menstruation, since menstrual blood is an excellent culture medium.

*Granuloma
inguinale*

Granuloma inguinale is an infection that begins as a red pimple in the genital area and grows to a large, granulated lump that bleeds easily if irritated. The lump appears 1–12 weeks after contact with an infected person. Without treatment it grows larger and spreads. The spread can be quite dramatic and destructive, producing ulceration and scarring of the whole genital area. The causal agent is the bacterium **Donovania granulomatis**, which is usually found in tropical climates. This bacterium can be stained and will show up on slides of material taken from the infected tissue. Treatment with streptomycin or tetracycline is usually effective.

Chancroid

Chancroid is another tropical infection. The causal agent is the bacterium **Hemophilus ducreyi** The major sign of the infection is an ulcerated sore that appears 3–7 days after exposure. Multiple ulcers that are quite painful and unpleasant then develop. The lymph glands in the groin area may become swollen. If the infection is left untreated, gangrene can occur. Sulfa drugs and streptomycin are effective treatments. The incidence of this disease has been declining with improvements in general hygiene.

Lymphogranuloma venereum

The infection called **lymphogranuloma venereum** is caused by the organism **Chlamydia trachomatis**. The disease begins slowly and often goes unnoticed. A small blister appears 5–21 days after contact but heals by itself. Two weeks to a month later, the lymph glands nearest the infection site (usually those in the groin area) swell up. The person may feel quite ill, with flulike symptoms such as fever, chills, headache, joint pain, and upset stomach. If treatment is not initiated, the infection can produce serious effects, including massive swelling of the genitals *(elephantiasis)* and closure of the rectum. This disease is not as easily cured as most of the other STDs. Tetracycline and sulfa drugs appear to be the most effective treatments. Lymphogranuloma venereum was almost unknown in the United States prior to the 1970s, when it was brought home by soldiers returning from Southeast Asia.

Scabies

Popularly known as *"the itch," scabies* is a rash that forms in several areas of the body but particularly in the genital region. It is caused by a highly contagious parasitic mite that burrows under the skin. The rash first appears 4–6 weeks after contact with an infected person. While the mites are most often transmitted during sexual intercourse, any close body contact with an infected person may be enough to pass them along. Treatment consists of careful hygiene and locally applied liquid solution of benzyl benzoate.

Crabs

The **crab louse** or **pubic louse** has a rather fancy name—**Pediculus pubis**— but a louse by any other name is still unpleasant. It causes itching in the pubic hair that can be quite maddening. The parasite can be transferred not only by direct body contact but by bedding, clothing, towels, and other such means. The lice live in the hair roots of the genital region. Treatment is through use of a powder of gamma benzene hexachloride, and complete eradication is likely. This problem is usually more embarrassing than it is dangerous.

The sexually transmitted diseases that we have discussed vary greatly in their symptoms, progressions, treatments, and eventual outcomes. For most of them, the available treatments work well, especially if the problem is diagnosed early enough and the specific causative agent is identified. One potential difficulty is that the person may have more than one STD simultaneously; if the most visible problem is treated, others may remain. Thus, treatment methods must be carefully chosen, and follow-up examinations are important.

A number of diseases and disorders that affect human sexual organs are not transmitted sexually. The sexual system is, after all, as vulnerable to medical problems as any other system of the body. Nevertheless, there appears to be a prevailing view that *all* physical problems involving the sexual system must somehow be sexually transmitted. The resulting accusations, guilt, and confusion about the source of a condition cause a good deal of stress for many individuals. Some people may even hide the medical problem and avoid appropriate treatment because of the negative connotations. It is important, then, that people become aware of the existence of nonvenereal sexual disorders, that they know how to recognize them, and that they seek treatment if they should experience such problems. The diseases included in this category are urethritis, cystitis, vaginitis, and cancer of the sexual organs.

Urethritis

Urethritis is an inflammation of the urethra—the tube that connects the bladder to the outside of the body for the purpose of urination. The infection produces an irritation of the lining of the tube, which results in a burning sensation upon urinating and a desire to urinate when no fluid is in the bladder. The urethra can become so irritated that a **catheter** (thin tube) must be inserted to drain the bladder of urine. The infection can also spread to other organs of the genitourinary system.

Because males have a longer urethra than females, men are more likely to develop urethritis. However, women are vulnerable to the disease because of the location of the urethral opening. Microorganisms from both the vagina and the anus can easily enter the urethral opening and work their way up the tube. As simple a precaution as wiping from front to back after defecating can help prevent infection of the urethra.

During the early stages, the symptoms of urethritis are similar to those of gonorrhea. Thus, people may feel fear or guilt about the infection and not seek treatment. Actually, a wide variety of microorganisms can cause this condition; some are sexually transmitted but many are not.

Treatment of urethritis is best tailored to the specific organism found to be at fault. The culprit can be determined by culturing a smear from the urethral discharge. Increased water intake also helps by diluting the urine so that it does not further irritate the urethra.

Cystitis

The inflammation of the bladder called **cystitis** is, like urethritis, the result of several different causative factors. In fact, urethritis can contribute to bladder infection if it moves up the urethra into the bladder, but other infectious agents can also cause the problem. The symptoms are a burning sensation during urination, a strongly felt urge to urinate even when no fluid is present in the bladder, and severe pains in the abdomen. Women are more vulnerable to bladder infections than men.

Cystitis has often been associated with sexual behavior, since it often occurs in conjunction with increased sexual activity. One type of cystitis common in newlywed women has been given the romantic name *honeymoon cystitis*. This infection is thought to occur as a result of the physical pressure of sexual intercourse, which irritates the bladder by displacing it and which may force bacteria in the urethra up into the bladder.

Cystitis is often erroneously seen as a sexually transmitted infection because women develop it soon after initial sexual experiences or after involvement with a new partner that is accompanied by increased sexual activity. The woman and her partner may both feel that he has infected her with a sexually transmitted disease. The unwarranted shame and guilt that may follow may also interfere with prompt identification and treatment of the cystitis.

Treatment includes increased fluid intake, careful personal hygiene, antibiotics, avoidance of alcoholic beverages, caffeine, and spicy foods, and caution in sexual frequency and position so as to not further irritate the bladder. Women are also encouraged to urinate immediately after intercourse to help prevent infection. While the condition may clear up by itself, the bladder will be weakened and will be more vulnerable to future infections. Treatment is generally successful, although reinfection is not unusual.

Vaginitis

Vaginitis—irritation of the vagina—can develop in a variety of ways. Any of a wide range of organisms already living in the body or new ones entering from outside can grow and cause such irritation. (Many of the STD organisms already discussed can produce vaginitis.)

It seems logical that the best way to prevent such infections would be scrupulous personal hygiene of the genital area. However, several types of vaginitis are the direct result of *excessive* hygiene practices. Douches, soaps, vaginal deodorants, and other substances put into the vagina can all produce chemical changes in the vaginal tissues that lead to conditions favorable for bacterial growth. In addition, sexual intercourse can irritate tissues through too vigorous movement of the penis in the vagina. However, if such irritation does occur from intercourse, it is because the natural ability of the tissue to self-lubricate has been impaired in some way. For example, attempting intromission too early in the woman's sexual excitement response or continuing sex during her resolution phase can interfere with natural lubrication. Other possible causes include increased sexual frequency and hormonal deficiency. Certain contraceptive practices can also cause or complicate vaginitis. The sensitive tissue may react to some of the chemicals in spermicidal foams and jellies, to the materials used to make condoms and diaphragms, to the lubricants used on condoms, or to the irritation caused by leaving a diaphragm in place too long.

The vaginal canal is a very sensitive organ requiring proper care and attention. Yet people commonly use chemical substances and perform physical actions that have the potential for damaging these tissues while taking few precautions. It is important for both partners of a sexually active couple to recognize that delicate tissue is involved and that they should be careful to protect it.

Cancer

Cancer is capable of attacking any part of the human body. The sexual system, however, does appear to be particularly vulnerable to cancer attack. In the United States, breast cancer is the most common form of cancer in women, and prostate cancer is the second most common form of cancer in men (after cancer of the colon). These figures have led to speculation that the sex hormones may somehow be involved in cancer, particularly since women on estrogen replacement therapy seem to run a higher risk of certain kinds of cancer (see Chap. 14). At present the relationship of hormones to cancer is unclear, but the high vulnerability of the sexual system to cancer remains a significant fact.

Prostate cancer   Cancer of the prostate is most common in older men. It is a silent menace, giving few signs of its existence and growth. The early signs are pain or difficulty in urinating and an inability to empty the bladder, resulting in a high frequency of urination. Other signs that might help identify a cancerous process are not likely to appear until the cancer is relatively advanced and the cells have **metastasized** (moved through the bloodstream to other parts of the body). Because of the absence of symptoms and the high incidence of this type of cancer, it is recommended that men over age 50 have a prostate examination once a year. The physician inserts a gloved finger into the rectum and feels the prostate directly, noting its size, shape, and location. Like the **Pap smear** for women, this examination is an important part of preventive health care.

Cancer of the prostate is treated in several ways. Because it is often responsive to sex hormones, it can be treated by administering estrogen and/or reducing androgens. Unfortunately, this treatment has side effects such as reduced sexual interest and possible feminization. The prostate itself may be partially or completely removed, which also has effects on sexual functioning. The degree of postsurgical difficulty is related to how the surgery is done. Potency should not be reduced by removal of the prostate.

Cancer of the prostate, once detected, is likely to be effectively treated, and with proper care neither life nor sexual functioning should be threatened. However, timing is highly important. The earlier the treatment, the better the prognosis.

Testicular cancer   As Box 18.1 points out, cancer of the testis has become an increasing problem in the United States. It is a hidden tumor and can only be discovered in its early stages by self-examination. Procedures for testicular self-examination are described in the box. Any irregularity, change in size, or unusual soreness or pain should be brought to the attention of a physician. Testicular self-examination is as important for men as breast self-examination is for women and should be part of every man's self-care habits.

Cancer of the penis   Cancer of the penis is a relatively rare condition. It appears to be almost totally absent in those peoples of the world who practice circumcision. Whether this a result of hygiene or some other aspect of circumcision has not been established. When penile cancer does occur, it is usually noted early in its growth because it is visible. It can be treated successfully with drugs, radiation, or surgery, with few complications.

BOX 18.1

"If people are mature enough to talk freely about breast cancer, then we are ready for men to do something as important for themselves." This is the view of Dr. Marc B. Garnick, of the Sidney Farber Cancer Institute of Harvard Medical School, who is concerned about our society's lack of knowledge about a growing problem, cancer of the testicles. Although this type of cancer is still fairly rare, its incidence has increased 70 percent since 1972. In fact, it is now the most common cancer in men age 20–35, accounting for 13 percent of all cancer deaths in this age group (Lane and Nagelschmidt, 1981).

Testicular cancer is particularly prevalent in men who were born with an undescended testicle—they have a 40 times greater chance of developing it. This disease is also more likely to strike white, middle-class and upper-class professionals. Incidence in blacks and Orientals of any socioeconomic level is very low. One study found that young college-educated professionals are four times more likely than laborers to have testicular cancer.

The causes of testicular cancer remain unknown. It has been linked to venereal disease and to sports injuries, but researchers deny any such connections. Some Danish scientists have suggested that tight underwear may somehow be involved and are conducting a study to test this idea, but so far it is pure conjecture.

Even though we don't know what causes testicular cancer, it can be cured if caught and treated early enough. Thus, as with breast cancer, early detection is paramount.

Because testicular cancer rarely causes pain, detection must depend on regular self-examination. Unfortunately, too few men are aware of this disease or of the self-examination procedure. The American Cancer Society (ACS) suggests that men conduct such examinations as a normal part of their health-care regimen. Here are the ACS's recommendations:

The best time to examine your testes is right after a hot bath or shower. The heat causes the testicles to descend and the scrotal skin to relax, making it easier to find anything unusual.

Each testicle should be examined with the fingers of both hands. Place your index and middle fingers on the underside of the testicle and your thumb on top. Gently roll your testicle between your thumb and fingers, feeling for a small lump. If you do find anything abnormal, chances are it will be at the front or side of your testicle.

Testicular cancer usually begins with a small, pea-sized tumor or bump on one of the testicles. Other potential symptoms include pain, swelling, discomfort of the testes, problems in urination, and tenderness in the breasts. If you discover any of these symptoms, seek prompt medical attention. They may not mean cancer, but if they do, early treatment can greatly increase the chances of cure. As Garnick points out, "Just ten years ago the chances of surviving testicular cancer would have been as low as ten to forty percent. Death often came within two years of discovery. But today there's a ninety-five to one hundred percent chance of survival if we catch it early enough, while the cancer is still confined to the testicle."

Treatment usually consists of removing the cancerous testicle (the disease rarely affects both testes). This

surgery in most cases does not impair
sexual functioning, since the remaining
testicle is intact. However, fertility
may be reduced.

"Obviously, there's a long way to
go before the men and boys of America
come out of the Dark Ages and realistically confront the threat of testicular
cancer," Garnick concludes. "But I believe that before this decade is out we
shall all be changed by this knowledge.
. . . I see the day not too far from now
when young men will be completely
comfortable in their knowledge of sexual health, just as they are today with
tooth decay prevention."

Breast cancer As we have noted, breast cancer is the most common form
of cancer in women. In fact, it is the major cause of death among women age
40–45. Nevertheless, a woman's chances of getting breast cancer are only about
15 to 1 (Lanson, 1975), although the risk increases as one gets older—72
percent of breast cancers occur in women over 50. The danger of breast cancer,
as with most types of cancer, is greatly reduced when it is detected and treated
early. Of women whose malignancy did not spread beyond the breast, 85
percent are still alive and well 5 years after surgery. Those in whom the cancer
did spread beyond the breast to the lymph nodes have only a 2 to 1 chance of
surviving. Thus, early detection cannot be overemphasized. Box 18.2 describes
a basic method for women to use in making a monthly breast self-
examination.

The usual treatment for breast cancer is **mastectomy**, in which breast
material and surrounding tissues are removed. The extent of the surgery depends on the extent of the tissue involved, the surgeon's opinion as to the
value of one procedure over another, and the desires of the patient. There are
three basic procedures. In **radical mastectomy**, all the involved breast, the
lymph glands, and the supporting muscles are removed. In **partial mastectomy**,
only the breast is removed if the surrounding tissues and structures seem
uninvolved. In **lumpectomy**, only the lump itself is taken. There is a great deal
of debate over which procedure is best. Whatever the case, breast removal is a
highly disruptive experience for the woman, and as much attention should be
paid to her psychological needs and postsurgical adjustment as to the medical
aspects of the condition. In addition to the surgery, hormonal, radiation, and
drug treatment may also be used.

Cervical cancer Cancer of the cervix is the second most frequent type of
cancer in women. It occurs most often in the mid-forties and thus has often
been associated with the beginning of menopause. Like breast and prostate
cancer, it shows little sign of its existence in the first few years of growth.
Because this is the period when treatment would be most valuable, it is
important that women have regular **Pap smears**, in which cervical tissue is
removed and examined for cancerous cells. It is recommended that women
have this test performed yearly, or even more often if a suspicious Pap test has
previously occurred.

"The most dreadful of all diseases to woman is breast cancer. The specter of this disease hovers like a black cloud over all her thoughts and hopes," physician Philip Strax noted in 1974. He suggested that the emphasis on the sexual attributes of the female breast in American society has created a great deal of apprehension and anxiety about breast conditions. He went on to point

Begin your breast check in front of a mirror:

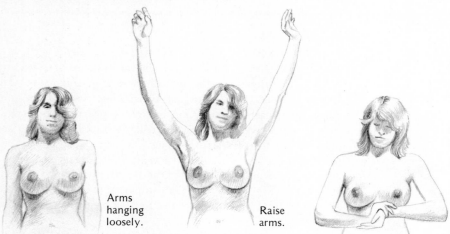

Arms hanging loosely.

Raise arms.

1. Look for any change in the shape or puckering of the skin. Squeeze nipple to check for any discharge.

2. Turn from side to side and look for any changes since last month.

3. Press palms of hands firmly together or place hands on waist and look for changes.

Next, lie down with a small pillow, or large folded towel:

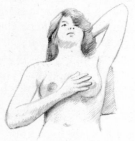
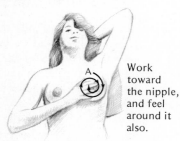

Work toward the nipple, and feel around it also.

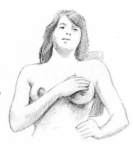

1. Place the folded towel or small pillow under your left shoulder. Put your left hand under your head.

2. Think of your breast as a spiral. Begin at "A" and follow the arrows around the nipple. Feel gently but firmly for a lump or thickening. Also feel under the armpit where the lymph nodes are located.

3. Repeat with the left arm down. Check again.

4. Repeat with other breast.

FIGURE 18.6
Technique for breast self-examination.

Sit up and repeat the procedure for both breasts.

out that the "totally erroneous idea" that the loss of a breast is equivalent to loss of sexual attraction or prowess has been spreading among women who have heard horror stories about gruesome breast disease and disfiguring surgery. He concluded that "a pathological national anxiety bordering on hysteria has come into existence in regard to the breast. Is it any wonder, then, that concern about breast diseases has reached alarming proportions and that a small, nontender lump or a pain or a discharge can produce a state of abject terror" (p. 5)?

Experts such as Strax are worried that this passive fear of breast cancer may actually contribute to the harmfulness of this disease because many women are afraid to examine their breasts ("What if I find a lump?") or to see their doctor if they do find an abnormality ("Maybe it will go away").

The fact is that over 90 percent of all cases of breast cancer are first detected by the woman herself. She notices a lump or abnormality and consults her physician. It is therefore extremely important that all women learn to give themselves a monthly breast self-examination to find any warning signs.

The best time to conduct breast self-examination is a few days after the menstrual period, since many women normally experience breast thickening and tenderness before or during their periods. It is a good idea to perform this technique after a bath or shower, when the skin is wet and smooth. Here is the basic procedure recommended by the University of Massachusetts Health Center/Amherst as shown in Fig. 18.6.

Regular breast self-examination allows you to become familiar with the unique structure and texture of your breasts. As Strax points out, you need to become aware that your breasts actually contain a number of different structures that can be felt as nodules or thickenings. By becoming acquainted with your own breast irregularities, you can be more attuned to any changes. If you do find anything unusual that concerns you, you should not be alarmed. Very few lumps or abnormal discharges are signs of serious growth. Nevertheless, you should see your physician immediately, as only a medical professional can decide whether the condition is abnormal or needs attention.

Regular monthly breast self-examination should be part of every woman's self-care routine. Her life may depend on it.

As with all cancers, the causes of cervical cancer are unknown. However, sexual intercourse may somehow contribute to its occurrence. Women who do not have sexual intercourse (nuns, lesbians) have a much lower cervical cancer rate than those who do engage in coitus, yet they have similar rates of breast, uterine, and ovarian cancer (*Science Notes*, 1969). There is also a higher rate of cervical cancer among women who are more sexually active, who started having sex at a young age, and who have had more partners. As we mentioned earlier, genital herpes has also been associated with cervical cancer and may be the factor that relates sexual intercourse to this type of cancer.

Treatment usually involves partial or total **hysterectomy**, in which the uterus, ovaries, and any other involved tisssues are removed. Drug and radiation therapy may also be used. If the ovaries are removed, the woman may be put on hormone replacement therapy. Identified and treated early enough, cervical cancer can be kept from threatening a woman's life and from interfering with her sexual activity. However, because this type of cancer can create feelings of damaged femininity in the affected woman, appropriate psychological counseling should be part of the recovery process.

For all of the cancers involving the sex organs, serious problems of sexual adjustment often follow treatment, regardless of how successful it has been. Issues of disfigurement, of not feeling like a complete man or woman, and of imagined dangers of sexual intercourse come into play. Surgeons and physicians need to be aware that curing the cancer is only one step back to a normal life for the patient and his or her sexual partner.

GENERAL MEDICAL CONDITIONS AFFECTING SEXUAL BEHAVIOR

Many medical diseases and disorders can affect sexual functioning by producing physical limitations and by creating psychological stresses that make sexual behavior difficult. Among medical problems that can create such physical limitations are heart disease, liver and kidney disease, high blood pressure, diabetes, multiple sclerosis, various types of brain damage (from tumors or strokes), and endocrine disorders.

While each of these medical problems can affect sexual behavior, the person usually adapts to the ongoing medical condition, and his or her sexual interest and functioning return, although the level of sexual interest may be lower than previously. Even many spinal cord injury victims often recover enough to have sexual intercourse, as was depicted in the film *Coming Home*. The sexual needs and capabilities of such handicapped individuals are further explored in Box 18.3.

Serious medical conditions have a tendency to turn people's attention totally toward themselves and their physical problems, which often diminishes their interest in sex and in their sexual partners. Their absorption in their medical problems can be so complete that they may not notice the change in their sexual behavior, although the partner may be experiencing difficulty in trying to adjust to the change. For these reasons, psychological counseling should be part of the treatment for major medical conditions.

Some medical problems create a fear in the patient and the partner that sexual activity will precipitate a recurrence of the illness. This is particularly true of people recovering from such life-threatening conditions as heart attack or stroke. Because they have been told to avoid stress and excitement, they may come to fear that an orgasm will kill them. It is equally frightening for the partner, who may imagine trying to live with the tremendous guilt after having "killed" his or her mate because of sexual "lust." Such people become prisoners of their medical conditions. Help must come from professionals working with such clients who need to actively inquire about the sexual adjustment of the patient if he or she is too embarrassed to bring it up.

BOX 18.3

Sex and the handicapped

The common image of the handicapped person is that of someone who is incompetent, dependent, immature, and asexual. Although in recent years efforts to "mainstream" the handicapped have shown that they can function well in jobs and in society, disabled individuals still tend to be treated as asexual beings, both by others and by the handicapped themselves.

When we speak of the handicapped, we are referring to individuals who have physical disabilities such as deformities, amputations, paralysis, developmental disabilities, and serious chronic diseases. Such handicaps may be present from birth or may have resulted from accidents or progressive disorders occurring in childhood or after puberty. The type of disability and the age at which it occurs both have a bearing on the individual's sexuality.

Children born with handicaps are usually raised as if sexuality does not exist. They tend to be socially isolated and educationally segregated and to be overprotected by parents and teachers. As a result, they are not exposed to the usual socializing experiences by which most children acquire the aspects of their sexual behavior and identity. Even when they reach adolescence their sexuality is usually downplayed. As Glass and Padrone (1978) put it, "Parents tend to keep these young people from sex as long as possible, and to treat them as 'beloved pets' (p. 46). Those who become disabled in adulthood experience problems of body image, self-worth, attractiveness, and performance anxiety in addition to the physical problems created by the disability. Many assume that their sex lives are over simply because they have become handicapped.

Counselors who work with the physically disabled have found, however, that just like all other human beings, the handicapped have sexual needs and that they are quite capable of satisfying those needs. In fact, despite the negative attitudes toward sexuality for the handicapped, 50 percent of the disabled population is sexually active (Anderson and Cole, 1975).

What kinds of sexual behavior are the handicapped capable of? What kinds of problems do they encounter? Most of the research in this area has been done with people who have suffered a spinal cord injury and are either paraplegics (paralyzed from the mid-chest down) or quadraplegics (paralyzed from the neck down). Studies of men with spinal cord injuries have found that 50–90 percent are still capable of erection, although a smaller percentage (5–30 percent) appear able to ejaculate (Higgins, 1979). Because the man has no sensation in the genital area, erection occurs primarily from mechanical stimulation. Although theoretically it seems impossible for orgasm to be experienced, many spinal-injured men and women report orgasms, often achieved through the use of fantasy. As Theodore Cole (1975) explains, "Some paralyzed people report they have the ability to focus on sensations being received from portions of their body still innervated, and, by concentration, to enhance that stimulation and transport it to a part of the body that is anesthetic, such as the genitals. Using this technique, some spinal injured men and women report orgasms not only

once but many times during a single
sexual encounter (p. 393).

When the sexual response cycles of
spinal-cord-injured men and women are
compared to those of able-bodied individuals, they are remarkably similar.
Disabled individuals still experience
many aspects of arousal, including
muscular tension, sex flush, increased
heart rate and blood pressure, vasocongestion of genital tissues, and nipple
erection. Furthermore, spinal-injured
women have intact hormonal systems
and reproductive organs and are fully
capable of having children.

The techniques most often employed in lovemaking with a handicapped person focus on developing new
erogenous zones in areas that are still
responsive to stimulation and on using
oral-genital contact to satisfy the partner. If the man can be manipulated to
erection, intercourse can take place. If
he cannot, the couple can still use a
technique called stuffing, in which the
flaccid penis is placed inside the vagina, often resulting in a semierection
that can help the woman achieve satisfaction.

An important concern of counselors helping to rehabilitate handicapped
people is that of helping such people
realize that they still have sex lives and
sexual options. In the past, professionals working with the disabled avoided
dealing with their patients' sexuality,
but that situation is changing. They are
beginning to realize that sexuality is
such an important part of a person that
encouraging the individual to establish
a healthy sex life is part of the overall
process of adjustment a disabled person
must go through. Counselors are learning to treat sexuality as just one aspect
of the rehabilitation process and are
preparing themselves to answer common questions about sexual capabilities, appropriate techniques, possible
fertility, effects of sexual activities on
medical appliances, physical positions,
and so on. They are also prepared to
speak to the handicapped person's partner to provide information and reassurance.

Cole (1975) summed up the basic
approach needed to be taken by disabled people: "Their ability to communicate wants and feelings with their
partners, their mutual willingness to
experiment with sexual activities
which are pleasing and not exploitive,
emphasis on fantasy, a reasonable program of physical hygiene, and the
knowledge that more sexuality lies
within the head than between the
thighs all help to set the stage for res-
toration of an active and satisfactory
sex life" (p. 395).

Finally, we should mention the problem of pain. Any condition that causes
chronic pain or pain with movement (such as backache) will reduce sexual
behavior. Because pain and sexual arousal are incompatible responses, people
who have intercourse while in pain may actually be aversively conditioning
themselves away from sexual interest. Pain is a complex problem; fortunately,
the recent introduction of pain management clinics in most cities should help
more people to deal with it.

With any serious or chronic medical condition, it is not unusual for the sexual life of the patient to be moved to the background or to be forgotten entirely by the various medical specialists involved in managing the physical problem. The patient is also worried about the medical condition and is often embarrassed to bring up the topic of sex at such a time. Yet a lack of adequate sexual outlets and the subsequent strain on the person's relationships may in fact slow down the medical recovery as well. Thus, helping the patient with his or her sexual adjustment is every bit as important in the course of recovery as the other aspects of his or her care.

SUMMARY

1 Diseases that can be communicated from one person to another during sexual activity are called *sexually transmitted diseases* (STDs), or *venereal diseases* (VD). Rates of STDs in the United States have risen sharply in the past few decades. These increases can be attributed to increased sexual activity, especially among young people, to the greater use of oral contraceptives, and to the appearance of more resistant strains of the disease organisms. Lack of systematic programs of public education has also played a role, as has the inability of public health efforts to keep up with the problem.

2 Control of STDs involves available *clinical treatment* of those who are infected, *epidemiological methods* such as *contact tracing* and *mass screening* to check the spread of the diseases, and *public education* about prevention.

3 *Gonorrhea*, the most common STD, is caused by the bacterium *Neisseria gonorrhoeae*. Transmission is totally through sexual intercourse, since this organism cannot survive outside the body. The symptoms in men are usually a milky discharge from the penis and discomfort in the urethra, but women often show no external clinical signs. This disease can be highly dangerous in both men and women, possibly causing sterility and even death. A pregnant woman can pass the bacterium on to her child during birth, producing multiple damaging effects in the baby. Because gonorrhea is easily cured with penicillin, many people are lax in their precautions against contracting the disease.

4 *Syphilis* is caused by a bacterial *spirochete* called *Treponema pallidum*. Spirochetes usually enter the body through small abrasions or sores during intercourse. Babies may be born with *congenital syphilis* if their mothers have the disease. Syphilis occurs in four basic stages: the *primary stage*, in which a *chancre* is the usual symptom; the *secondary stage*, in which the person has an ugly rash and flulike symptoms; the long *latent stage*, in which the person is symptom-free but the bacteria are doing damage to the internal organs; and the *tertiary stage*, in which degenerative processes emerge *(parenchymatous neurosyphilis)*. Diagnosis of syphilis is accomplished through blood tests. The most effective treatment is penicillin.

5 *Genital herpes*, or *herpes simplex type 2*, is a viral disease of the genitals related to the virus that causes cold sores of the mouth. This virus can be transmitted to babies during birth, and it has been associated with cervical cancer. The disease is characterized by groups of blisters on the genitals in addition to a general viral sickness. The disease can come and go, and couples may reinfect each other in a ping-pong fashion. No effective treatment has yet been found for this problem.

6 Other STDs include *trichomoniasis*, a protozoan disease that affects primarily women and may be transmitted by other than sexual means; *monili-

asis, a fungal infection that can produce a white, lumpy vaginal discharge; *granuloma inguinale,* a tropical bacterial disease; *chancroid,* a tropical infection characterized by ulcerated sores; *lymphogranuloma venereum,* an infection of the lymph glands in the groin; *scabies,* a rash caused by parasitic mites; and *crabs,* an itching in the public region caused by lice.

7 There are several diseases of the sexual organs that are not transmitted sexually. These diseases include *urethritis,* or inflammation of the urethra; *cystitis,* or inflammation of the bladder; and *vaginitis,* or irritation of the vaginal lining. A number of cancers can also affect the sex organs. The main male cancers include prostate cancer, testicular cancer, and cancer of the penis. Regular examination of the prostate by a physician and regular self-examination of the testes can help reduce the seriousness of these problems. The main female cancers include breast cancer and cervical cancer. Breast cancer is usually treated with some sort of *mastectomy;* its severity can be decreased if it is caught early through breast self-examination. Cervical cancer should be checked for regularly through use of *Pap smears.* The usual treatment for cervical cancer is *hysterectomy.*

8 A number of serious medical conditions can interfere with normal sexual functioning. Such conditions not only limit the person's physical behaviors but create stress and distractions. Chronic pain can also interfere with sexual activity.

**ADDITIONAL
READING**

* **Boston Women's Health Book Collective.** *Our Bodies, Ourselves* (2nd ed.). New York: Simon & Schuster, 1976.

   Contains a good discussion of STD in women, especially breast and cervical cancer.

Corsaro, Maria, and Korzeniowsky, Carole. *STD: A Common Sense Guide.* New York: St. Martin's Press, 1980.

   A straightforward, easily understood review of the STDs. Describes symptoms, diagnosis, and treatments in clear, nontechnical language.

Montreal Health Press. *VD Handbook.* Montreal: Montreal Health Press, 1972.

   An excellent discussion of venereal disease written especially for the lay reader.

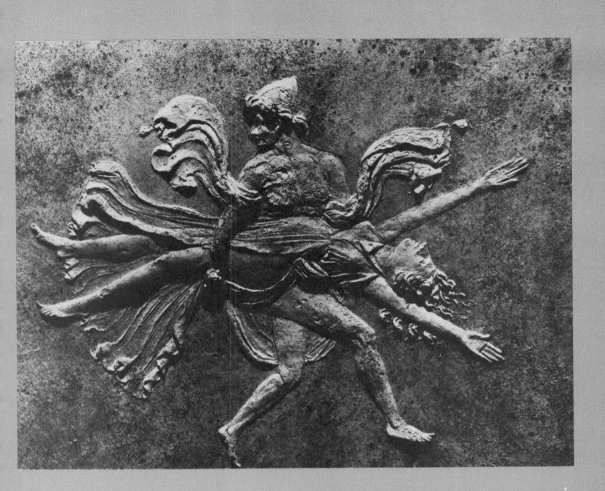

Rape

19

chapter
19

Rape is an act that has existed in all societies throughout recorded history. No sex, race, age group, or socioeconomic class has been exempt. Only in recent years, however, has rape come to be recognized as a crime of major proportion having a tremendous impact on the victims and their families. It has been estimated that a rape occurs on the average of every 12–14 minutes in the United States. Only one-fifth of these rapes are actually reported. In addition, an estimated 20 percent of all rape victims are under 12 years of age.

Despite the traumatic and violent nature of rape, it has been common for society to blame the rape victim and even to sympathize with the rapist. Why? Since the rapist is typically a man and the victim typically a woman, part of this societal reaction may have been shaped by historical views of men and women. Catherine Morrison (1980) has identified several ideas from the past that may have helped form current attitudes and myths about rape. For example, a common early view was that women had no destiny of their own but rather were expected to help a man achieve his destiny. Another early notion was that women belonged to men—that they were men's property. As a result, for thousands of years rape was not considered a crime against a woman but rather a crime against the man to whom she belonged (Brownmiller, 1975). It was also believed that only a virgin could be raped and that a rapist could be absolved by paying the "bride price" to the virgin's father.

Among other views of men and women that contribute to rape myths are the idea that men have strong sex drives that are difficult to control ("Boys will be boys"; "Young men must sow their wild oats") and the notion that women bear the responsibility for maintaining a decorum that will not stimulate men. A number of myths about rape have evolved from these historical views of men and women. Myths concerning the victim include:

"Nice girls don't get raped." Presumably, a "nice" girl is one who is demure rather than flirtatious and who does not wear provocative clothing. However, there is actually little correlation between clothing, flirtatiousness, and rape. All sorts of women—young and old, married and single, prostitutes and nuns—are subject to sexual assault.

"If women would stay home where they belong, they wouldn't get raped." In fact, many rapes take place at home after the rapist has forced or conned his way into the house or apartment.

"Rape is impossible unless the woman wants it." This idea is based on the mistaken assumption that if a woman crosses her legs, penile penetration is impossible. This notion ignores the fact that rapists usually threaten to wound or kill the woman (or her children), can beat the woman into submission, can knock the woman out, or can use accomplices to hold her. Furthermore, rape can be anal or oral in addition to vaginal.

"Most rapes are false accusations reported by women who were spurned by old boyfriends." The evidence suggests that rapists are not usually good friends of the victim, although they may have observed the woman from afar and planned the attack. Furthermore, only 3 percent of reported rapes turn out to be false complaints (Hursch, 1977).

Among myths associated with rapists are:

"Rape is a black man's crime." Although there have been more convictions (not accusations) of black men for the crime of rape, both the rapist and the victim may come from any nationality or race.

"The rapist is a red-blooded male with a healthy sexual appetite who becomes so attracted to a particular woman that he cannot resist his impulse to possess her." This notion, as we shall see, is not supported by interviews with convicted rapists.

"The rapist is a shy, retiring, lonely individual who cannot make normal approaches to women." Again, this view is not supported by the data.

"The rapist is sexually deprived." Actually, a substantial percentage of rapists are married and describe their sex lives as adequate. As one sex offender explained, "The only good thing about our marriage was sex. . . . Sometimes right after I had sex with my wife I would go out and rape someone" (Groth, 1979, p. 23).

Perhaps the greatest rape myth of all concerns the motive behind the rape act. Rape is usually thought of as a sexual crime. Because it involves sexual intercourse, sex is assumed to be the motive. As we shall discover in this chapter, however, it is aggression and power, not sexuality, that are the primary motives of the rapist. Rape is the forceful and sometimes violent negation of one person's will by another. The victim is not treated as a sexual being but rather as an inferior being or object. Rape serves to degrade, hurt, and dehumanize the victim and to otherwise display power over her.

TYPES OF SEXUAL ASSAULT

The occurrence of sexual acts without the consent of the victim constitutes rape. Legally, the term *rape* may also be applied in instances where the victim is unable to consent because of age or because of mental condition. **Statutory rape** is sexual intercourse with a child or teenager below the age at which the law says he or she is capable of consenting. However, the consenting law varies widely from state to state (from age 10 to age 18). In those states with a high consenting age, it is likely that some minors are fully aware of what they are agreeing to do and understand the significance of sexual acts. In such cases, the accused actually may be the victim. Several states are now in the process of lowering the cutoff age for statutory rape.

Burgess and Holmstrom (1979a) have divided sexual assault into three categories, according to the nature of consent: (1) **rape**—sex without consent, (2) **accessory to sex**—inability of the victim to consent, and (3) **sex-stress situations**—sex with initial consent.

Rape—sex without the victim's consent

In rape without consent, an important element is the rapist's ability to gain control over the victim. This control may be gained physically, as in the blitz rape, or through a variety of verbal ploys, as in the confidence rape. The **blitz rape** involves a sudden physical assault on the victim. The rapist usually selects a victim unknown to him—perhaps someone just walking down the street—and attempts to remain anonymous himself. Blitz rapes often occur on dark, isolated streets, where women can be dragged into alleys, or take place in the home after forced entry. In the latter case, the break-in usually occurs at night, and the woman is attacked while asleep in bed. An example of this type of rape was provided by Burgess and Holmstrom (1979a):

> *A 62-year-old woman was brought to the hospital at 8:30 A.M. by the police. She had multiple bruises on her face, neck, chest, and back, as well as a 2-inch stab wound in her abdomen. Her first words to the counselor were, "I thought I was going to be killed. I didn't want to die—I didn't think it was my time, but I remember thinking this is the way I was going to die . . ." The victim said that she had been in her bed sleeping—it was around 3 A.M.—and she woke up to feel someone jumping on her. She said, "I started screaming and he put a blanket over my head. I didn't have it off till he left. He said when he started, "Let's see how you like this." He started doing such crazy things. . . . He kept turning me this way and that. He raped me the regular way. At least he wasn't violent doing that; thank heaven that wasn't crazy. . . . I remember thinking that I never thought such a thing could happen to me. I thought I would die, and his hand kept clamping my neck tighter and tighter. When he finished raping me, he told me to keep the blanket over my head for 20 minutes and said if I took the blanket off, he would finish me. I didn't hear him leave, but every now and then I would call out to see if he was still there. I hoped to get a view of him and kept peeking out of the blanket but couldn't see anything. Finally, I dared to take the blanket off and I called the police. They came right away and I called my daughter. The officer talked to my daughter and said I was lucky to be alive. I could hardly talk and was having a lot of trouble breathing." The victim was unable to identify the assailant, although she did work with the police in hopes of finding a suspect. She definitely would have pressed charges against the assailant. (pp. 4–5)*

In the **confidence rape**, the rapist lures the victim into an unprotected situation under false pretenses and then attacks her. In some cases, the assailant is a friend, an acquaintance, or even a business associate of the victim. In other cases, the rapist is a stranger who may start a conversation with the victim. He may promise to take her somewhere, such as a party, may discuss job opportunities or possible business transactions, or may mention the name of someone the victim knows. All of these ploys are used to establish a degree of confidence and trust with the victim. Then, the rapist lures the victim to an unprotected place and rapes her. The following case demonstrates one kind of confidence rape (adapted from Burgess and Holmstrom, 1979a, p. 7):

> *A woman looked around as she was walking down a New York City street and saw a man on foot and a man on a motorcycle behind her. The man on the motorcycle approached her and hurriedly convinced her that the man on foot was following her. He suggested that she get on his motorcycle and he would drive her to an area where she could hail a cab. After she got on the motorcycle, he raced to a dark alley, threw her on the ground, and raped her.*

In some instances, the confidence rape involves the use of a decoy, often a woman. The task of the decoy is to lure or otherwise attract the victim to the rapist. Decoys are often used in two typical ploys: the hitchhiking situation and the come-to-the-party situation.

In the hitchhiking situation, the rapist may ride around town looking for a hitchhiker as a victim. Because females tend not to accept rides from men, the rapist may use a female accomplice who sits close to him in the front seat. Some hitchhikers may be lulled into thinking they are "safe" in accepting a ride from the couple when, in fact, they are setting themselves up for attack.

In the come-to-the-party situation, a woman decoy initially strikes up a conversation with another woman, perhaps in a singles' bar. As the evening progresses, the decoy mentions a party that she plans to attend and invites the victim to come along. When the victim arrives at the so-called party, she quickly realizes that only men are present and that the decoy has mysteriously disappeared.

Accessory to sex—inability to consent

In this second category, the rapist has sex with a victim who is too young to understand what is going on or who is mentally retarded or mentally ill. Because of the assailant's status (being older, being an authority figure, for example), he is able to gain compliance from the victim. The assailant also makes sure that the victim is rewarded in some way for the compliance. Thus, the experience is not totally unpleasant or intolerable for the victim, and it serves to establish a pattern between victim and attacker that may be repeated over and over again. Burgess and Holmstrom (1979a) have differentiated this type of sexual assault into three categories on the basis of the kinds of rewards that the attacker promises the victim:

1 *Use of material goods, such as candy or money. Some children consent to sexual activities for monetary or material rewards. In effect, they are asked to do something about which they have little knowledge in exchange for something whose value is well established with them. Following the assault, which may involve touching and masturbatory activities more than intercourse, the child may show little or no upset and may not even mention the event to his or her parents.*

2 *Use of psychological needs. Some children may accept sexual overtures because of the implied attention or contact they might receive. Even disoriented, depressed, or lonely adults respond to this need, despite the fact that the contact may be given in a sexually abusive manner.*

3 *Promise of pleasure and falsification of moral standards. Children may be enticed into sexual relationships through the promises of pleasure coupled with moral rightness. The assailant tells the victim that "It's enjoyable" and "There is nothing wrong with doing it." The inital sexual encounter may be brief and may involve only touching and stroking. But as the relationship develops, the adult introduces intercourse. This kind of sexual assault frequently involves the development of a long-term relationship. The child is sworn to secrecy. The experience is usually not physically harmful and may even be enjoyable. However, guilt is strong. This is a common pattern in incestuous relationships between father and daughter.*

*As we mentioned in Chap. 16, incest is much more common in our
society than was previously thought (Sgroi, 1975). Sex offenders of this
type may be tried for rape but are more commonly prosecuted for child
abuse.*

*Sex-stress
situations—sex
with initial
consent*

In sex-stress situations, there is initial consent from the victim, who is
clearly aware that she is agreeing to sexual intercourse. Because of some
dramatic change in the situation, however, the act of intercourse comes to be
treated as a sexual offense. Such changes include development of perverted or
violent behavior in the man, postcoital anxiety in the woman, and disruption
of the act by parents or police.

A situation in which the man began to act perverse and violent is described in the following case history of a woman who met her assailant in a
lounge and agreed to go with him to his apartment for sex (Burgess and
Holmstrom, 1979a):

> *He had given me a good talk. . . . I was horny and feeling neglected, and I
> love my sex. He took me outside and down an alley and threw me on the
> ground. I asked him what he was doing—told him he didn't have to do it
> there if all he wanted was a screw. . . . He pulled everything off me—took
> off all my clothes . . . I told him I wasn't a whore that did it in an alley.
> It didn't stop him. First, he tried natural sex and then he insisted on oral
> sex. . . . He rammed his fists up me twice and bit my breasts. Then he
> stood and urinated all over me and said, "I feel better." He told me not to
> leave; he hit me and said, "You will do what I say." (p. 15)*

In some cases, a woman will become excessively anxious after a sexual
encounter and report the incident as a sexual assault. This is especially common if it has been her first sexual encounter, if she is a teenager, and if she is
afraid of becoming pregnant. The woman may report the incident in order to
receive medical treatment but typically does not identify her "assailant" and is
unlikely to take the case to court (Burgess and Holmstrom, 1980). Clearly this
does not really constitute a sexual offense, but the female may feel forced to
report it as such in order to prevent pregnancy.

In the third possible situation, a female may consent to sex and then
become agitated if the act is interrupted by parents or police. If the female is
legally under age and the male is an adult, the parents may press charges for
statutory rape. It is uncommon for the girl herself to want to press charges. In
such cases the male may actually become the victim if the female "knowing-
ly" consented.

Sexual assault can take many different forms depending on whether the
female is capable of giving her consent and has indeed given her consent to
sexual intercourse. In the remainder of this chapter, we will focus exclusively
on rape (sex without consent) in order to comprehend the nature and consequences of this violent act.

No general picture of the "typical" rapist is readily available today. Mental health programs for the treatment of rapists are new and relatively uncommon, and only a small percentage of rapists are ever tried and convicted; fewer still come under the jurisdiction of mental health professionals. Thus, the following discussion of the rapist's characteristics is based on study of only a small percentage of rapists.

Characteristics of the rapist

As we have seen, the rapist is typically viewed as an oversexed individual belonging to a minority group. In addition, he may be portrayed either as a red-blooded male enticed by the sensuality of the victim or as a bizarre psychotic maniac who stalks his victim. What is the rapist really like? One can begin to glean some information about rapists by examining police records and by reading reports filed by the victims. One of the most extensive demographic studies of rapists and victims comes from a rape prevention project conducted in the 1970s in Denver by Carolyn Hursch (1977). According to her data, the rapist often but not always (1) was young, about 15–30 years old; (2) was from the lower socioeconomic classes; (3) came from no particular ethnic background; and (4) may have had a previous record of minor sexual offenses. (Keep in mind that older or more wealthy rapists might be better able to escape detection and prosecution, thus biasing the results in the direction of young and less well-off offenders.) Hursch also noted that adult victims were more likely to be raped by individuals from their own ethnic group, whereas more cross-ethnic rapes occurred with child victims.

Rape motives

What goes on in the mind of the rapist? What compels him to rape? Is he oversexed or sexually deprived? Interviews and case histories of imprisoned rapists indicate that sexual deprivation and strong sex drives have little to do with rape (Gebhard et al., 1965; Groth, 1979; Groth and Birnbaum, 1980). For example, over one-third of the subjects in Groth and Birnbaum's study were married and sexually active with their wives at the time of the attack. Of those who were not married, many were involved in a sexual relationship at the time of the rape. That is not to say that these relationships were necessarily good ones. But the notion that most rapists are sexually deprived would seem to be patently false.

If sex or the need for sex is not the primary element of rape, what is? Groth and Birnbaum suggest that anger and power are the primary elements of rape and that sex is merely a tool for expressing them. Rape is frequently performed by an individual who is intensely insecure and unable to deal with the stresses and demands of his life. Of course, not all such insecure people become rapists, but insecurity and inability to cope are common attributes of those rapists who have been studied. Another key characteristic of the rapist is his lack of any close individual relationships involving warmth, reciprocity, or sharing. Thus, despite the fact that rapists have access to sex with wives or lovers, the relationship may actually be shallow and superficial.

Rape is now seen primarily as an act of aggression. The rapist, overwhelmed by stress and frustration, uses sexual assault in an attempt to alleviate his frustrations, even if only temporarily. This idea is further supported by findings that rapists have aggressive attitudes toward their victims. These attitudes include the need to dehumanize the victim, to keep her anonymous, and to treat her as an object rather than as a human being.

Groth and Birnbaum have differentiated three patterns or styles of rape: the anger rape, the power rape, and the sadistic rape. The **anger rape** is used to release pent-up feelings of rage. Typically, the rapist reaches a point where he is so angry about presumed injustices at the hands of a woman (mother or wife, for example) that he seeks to hurt, punish, and degrade a female victim. The anger rape is usually unplanned and occurs when the rapist reaches a level of extreme upset, anger, or depression. The rapist looks for the most convenient victim and attacks her. In this case, the man may not be particularly aroused, may not have thought about rape, and may have difficulty maintaining an erection. He is often verbally abusive, shouting obscenities and epithets. The anger rape is usually of short duration.

The key element in the **power rape** is overpowering the victim. It enables the rapist to take control of someone else and thereby reduce his feelings of inferiority and worthlessness. Temporarily, the attacker appears strong, powerful, assertive, and sexually desirable in his own eyes. The power rape is often planned. During the attack, the rapist issues commands to the victim and may ask personal questions. The attack itself may be drawn out. The rapist typically does not find the attack sexually gratifying—it never seems to reach his expectations.

In the **sadistic rape**, the rapist becomes sexually excited by abusing and hurting the victim. The more the victim resists, the more excited he becomes. Torture and bondage are commonly used. In extreme cases, the rapist may murder and mutilate his victim.

*Arousal patterns
in rapists*

Recent reports indicate that the sexual responsiveness of rapists differs from that of nonrapists. Abel and his associates (1977) presented both rapists and nonrapists with vivid, 2-minute audiotaped descriptions of sexual encounters. Some of the tapes were descriptions of mutually enjoyable intercourse, in which the subject interacted with a willing and enthusiastic partner. The other tapes were descriptions of forced intercourse, in which the subject thrust himself violently on a female who attempted to repel his advances. The subjects in the study were asked to imagine themselves as the man described in the tapes. Sexual arousal to the taped descriptions was then measured by recording changes in penis size.

While nonrapists experienced sexual arousal only in response to the tapes of mutually enjoyable sex, rapists were aroused by both types of descriptions (see Fig. 19.1). In addition, the rapists became sexually aroused by purely aggressive acts described on a tape. This finding, while not all that surprising, may have several important consequences for rape prevention and rapist rehabilitation. The abnormal sexual arousal can be used as a marker to identify potential rapists and to assess the effects of various types of therapy.

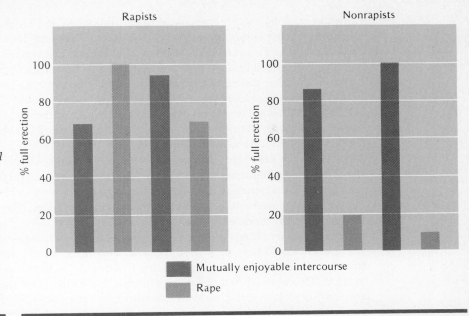

Rapists   Nonrapists

% full erection

FIGURE 19.1
*Rapists are
sexually aroused
by audiotape
descriptions of
rape scenes as well
as by those of
mutually
enjoyable
intercourse.
Nonrapists,
however, are
sexually aroused
primarily by
descriptions of
mutually
enjoyable sex.
(Abel, 1977)*

Mutually enjoyable intercourse

Rape

**REACTIONS TO
RAPE—THE RAPE
TRAUMA
SYNDROME**

In essence, the victim's reaction to rape can be summed up as pervasive, overwhelming *fear*. This fear, in turn, produces a cluster of symptoms that has been called the **rape trauma syndrome** (Burgess and Holmstrom, 1974). The syndrome is divided into an **acute phase** (disorganization) and a **long-term phase** (reorganization). As we shall see, this syndrome may persist for a long time, causing alterations in the victim's relationships, job, residence, social activities, and other aspects of her life in addition to her psychological functioning.

**Acute phase—
disorganization**

People commonly assume that the victim's initial reaction to rape is hysteria. It is not. Women who appear at hospitals for treatment following rape attacks usually have one of two responses: the **expressed reaction** or the **controlled reaction** (Burgess and Holmstrom, 1979b). The woman who shows the expressed response tends to be restless during the interview, becomes tense when asked certain questions, cries as she describes the actions of the rapist, and smiles nervously at other times. The woman who is controlled in her response is calm and subdued. Her feelings are guarded and hidden. Although there is a tendency to assume that the controlled woman is less affected by the rape, this is not generally the case.

During the acute phase, the victim may have difficulty adjusting to her assault and at the time coping with the demands of her life. This phase may last for several days to several weeks. Among the symptoms of disorganization and stress she may exhibit are physical reactions, sleep disturbances, alterations in eating habits, emotional reactions, and obsessive thoughts. It is not surprising for the woman to have a variety of physical complaints after the assault, including trauma to the vaginal area, breasts, and possibly anus as well as more generalized bruises and soreness. She may have trouble falling asleep or may awaken in the middle of the night and be unable to go back to sleep. A period of insomnia seems to occur just when the victim would like to be able to sleep and forget. The victim often stops eating altogether or severely curtails her intake of food. Many women report stomach pains and nausea. In addition, some report that food tastes bad to them.

During the days after the rape, the victim is irritable with others and is hypersensitive to comments or touches. She may develop an intense emotional reaction to characteristics that remind her of the rape or the rapist. She may be unable to get close to other men or to tolerate close contact. The victim is also bombarded with thoughts she cannot shut out. Many of these thoughts are replays of the actual rape. But the woman may also be obsessed with determining how she could have prevented the rape. This is a question many of her friends will also ask her, perhaps hinting that she did not try hard enough to avoid it. This reaction is a peculiarity of rape. If a woman gets into a car accident, is pickpocketed, or loses something, she may be scolded for her carelessness, but it is never assumed that she wanted such a thing to happen. This is not so with rape. Even very sympathetic friends may still hold the victim somewhat responsible for the rape (Hursch, 1977). This notion of victim responsibility is so pervasive that even health care professionals who have been trained to aid the rape victim may attribute greater or lesser responsibility to the victim depending on her attractiveness, the clothes she is wearing, her marital status, her age, and the seriousness of the attack (Alexander, 1980).

*The long-term
phase—
reorganization*

When Burgess and Holmstrom (1979b) interviewed rape victims *4 years* after the rape experience, they found that 26 percent of the victims had not totally recovered, 37 percent had recovered over the span of several years, and the remaining 37 percent had recovered within a few months of the attack. Thus, the long-term phase varies considerably in length from one person to the next. Among the more enduring effects of rape are alterations in physiology, dream disturbances, the development of phobias, loss of sexual desire, and changes in social activity.

Some women appear to experience changes in their reproductive physiology. In particular, their menstrual cycle may become irregular or lengthened. Some women also develop a vaginal discharge. Dream disturbances, often involving unsuccessful attempts to escape an attacker, are common.

Following the global reaction that is typical of the acute phase, the victim may develop a set of irrational but specific fears that may limit her activities. She may be excessively fearful of crowds or of people pressing against her. Conversely, she may develop an intense fear of being left alone. Some fears may be tied to the rape situation. For example, if the rapist had a moustache, the victim may be afraid of all men with moustaches. Some women develop feelings of suspicion and paranoia. They may think that all men are following them or that everyone somehow knows that they are a rape victim. At the beginning of the long-term phase, women are also usually fearful of sex and show a marked lack of sexual desire. As they begin to adjust, their sexuality returns.

During the early part of the long-term phase, the woman may seek to reestablish ties with her family. She may return home, yet not tell her parents about the attack for fear of upsetting them. A common response to rape is to change residences, especially if the rape took place in the home. It is less common but not rare for the woman to change jobs. She may also change her phone number for an unlisted one, not only to prevent the rapist from locating her but to reduce the incidence of obscene calls, to which the victim may now be hypersensitive. The woman may experience difficulty with her social relationships, and in many cases long-term relationships may be terminated as a consequence of the rape trauma.

Factors influencing recovery   As we have seen, there is considerable variation in the length of time it takes for rape victims to recover from the trauma of attack. For some, it may be several months; for others, it may take several years. After interviewing numerous rape victims, Burgess and Holmstrom (1979b) identified a set of factors that can facilitate recovery and another set of factors that may delay it.

Factors aiding recovery   Rape is such a powerful life stress that many women are simply unprepared to cope with it. This is especially the case if the rape victim has never had to deal with any other severe life stress, such as the loss of a loved one. One factor that aids recovery from rape is high self-esteem. Individuals who value themselves as persons tend to overcome rape trauma more quickly than those who do not value themselves so highly. Individuals with high self-esteem view themselves as having a high tolerance for stress and as being strong and calm.

Individuals who make use of coping strategies such as defense mechanisms may also recover more rapidly from the rape experience. Rape victims commonly use four different types of defense mechanisms to reduce their anxiety about the attack: rationalization, minimization, suppression, and dramatization. With **rationalization**, the woman tries to find a reason for the rapist's behavior. She may use his pathology ("He's sick"), her behavior ("I was alone"), his motive ("He wanted to get back at me"), and so on. Just having an explanation may help her keep a reasonable perspective on what has happened to her. Alternatively, the victim may use **minimization** to make the event seem less important. She may minimize the rape in comparison to other rapes ("At least I wasn't killed") or in comparison to her own situation ("My divorce was much more traumatic"). Some women use **suppression**—they put all thoughts or references to the rape out of their minds. They may refuse to discuss it or talk about it. Finally, a woman may **dramatize** her rape experience by talking compulsively about it to different people, essentially reliving the attack. This continuous exposure may make the event seem less horrifying than it was.

Another factor associated with fast recovery is taking action of some kind,

BOX 19.1

The benefits of self-blame

"Although fear (of injury, death, and the rapist) is the primary reaction to rape, self-blame may be second only to fear in frequency of occurrence; perhaps surprisingly, it is far more common than anger" (p. 1801). Social psychologist Ronnie Janoff-Bulman (1979) made this statement after reviewing the literature on rape and noting the pervasiveness of self-blame in the studies of rape victims.

Rape counselors are well aware of this tendency toward self-blame and do their best to reassure the victim that there was nothing she could have done to avoid the rape. However, Janoff-Bulman has come to the conclusion that in many cases self-blame may actually be constructive. She hypothesized that there are two types of self-blame, one that is helpful and one that is maladaptive. The first type she calls "behavioral" self-blame, in which the woman blames herself for having engaged in particular behaviors ("I shouldn't have walked alone at night"). The second type she calls "characterological" self-blame, in which the woman blames herself for being a particular type of person ("I'm so stupid, I deserved to be raped").

To determine what roles these two types of self-blame play in the psychological recovery of rape victims, Janoff-Bulman sent questionnaires to rape crisis centers throughout the United States. She asked what percentage of rape victims seem to blame themselves, at least in part, for the rape, and of these, what percentage seem to be behavioral self-blame and what percentage seem to be characterological. The 38 centers that responded indicated that self-blame occurs among 74 percent of rape victims. On the average, 69 percent were reported as blaming themselves behaviorally ("I shouldn't have let someone I didn't know into the house," "I should not have hitchhiked," "I should have locked my car"), whereas only 19 percent were reported as blaming themselves characterologically ("I'm too trusting," "I'm the kind of person who attracts trouble," "I can't say no"). Furthermore, the centers reported that characterological self-blamers blamed themselves significantly more than did behavioral self-blamers.

According to Janoff-Bulman, behavioral self-blame may actually be an adaptive response, "an attempt to reestablish control following the trauma of rape." When a woman has been raped, she feels unsure of herself and of control over her own life. If she engages in behavioral self-blame, attributing the incident to something she could have done something about, "she is likely to maintain a belief in the future avoidability of a similar misfortune, while simultaneously maintaining a belief in personal control over life outcomes," says Janoff-Bulman. If, however, the victim blames her character, an unchangeable factor, she is less likely to think she has control over future events and may see herself as a chronic victim.

As a result of her research, Janoff-Bulman has recommended that rape counselors recognize the value of behavioral self-blame and that they concentrate on helping the victim to reestablish a belief in her control over outcomes by discussing ways to prevent rape in the future. As Janoff-Bulman puts it, "Too often, behavioral self-blame is regarded as detrimental to mental health. Rather, it may serve as an indicator of the victim's psychological needs at the time" (p. 1808).

such as changing residences or enrolling in a self-defense class. One psychologist has suggested that self-blame may also be a positive factor in rape recovery, as explained in Box 19.1.

Factors delaying recovery   One factor that can definitely delay rape recovery is the occurrence of another rape or assault. Fortunately, such recurrences are rare.

Various chronic life stressors can increase the amount of time for recovery. Poverty is an obvious stressor that impairs recovery, as is a lack of social network—family ties, friends, intimate companions—for emotional support. Low self-esteem is also associated with poor recovery. Individuals with low opinions of themselves may feel that they deserved the rape and may acquire further feelings of helplessness and despair.

The rape victim may use some maladaptive responses to try to adjust to the stress of rape, such as drowning her sorrows in alcohol or numbing her senses with drugs, neither of which reduces her anxiety in the long run nor solves her problem. In general, excessive use of alochol or drugs can markedly delay the victim's recovery. Those individuals who have suicidal tendencies following a rape also tend to be among the slowest to recover.

Finally, certain elements of the attack itself may retard recovery from the trauma. Burgess and Holmstrom (1979a) found that the speed of recovery from a blitz rape depended on where it occurred. Women who were suddenly attacked in their homes, a presumably safe area, recovered more slowly than those who were assaulted in acknowledged unsafe places, such as dark streets, alleyways, empty buildings, and so on. Burgess and Holmstrom found that in the confidence rape speed of recovery was influenced by whether or not the woman had protective company with her at the moment of attack. Women who had believed they were in protective company and were still raped took longer to recover than those who were alone.

Help for victims   Within recent years, community involvement in providing services to help victims recover from rape has increased dramatically. This involvement has generally taken the form of crisis centers operated by women's groups, colleges and universities, or social and welfare agencies. One of the earliest rape crisis centers that gained national attention was formed by a group of women in Washington, D.C., who had either been rape victims or known a rape victim.

The purpose of crisis centers is not only therapeutic but preventive. The centers provide emotional support for victims and their families; information about health care, police, and legal procedures; a 24-hour emergency hotline; and peer counseling by trained personnel. The victim receives help during the medical exam, throughout the legal process if prosecution is instituted, and more generally for as long as the victim needs help to readjust to her life. Thus, such centers help to reduce the severity of the long-term consequences of the rape trauma syndrome.

Rape crisis centers often develop educational programs to make the public more aware of what rape is and why it occurs. Information about safety precautions (such as locks on doors and windows), situations to avoid, and

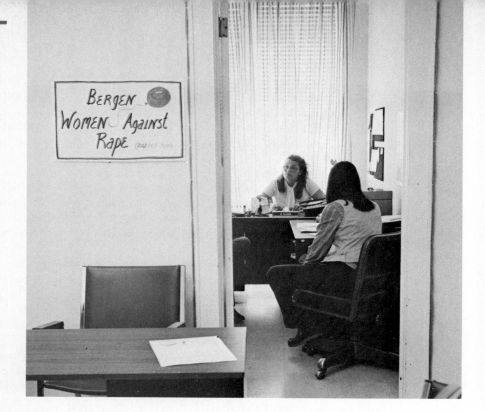

Rape counseling centers, such as the one shown, provide information, legal assistance, and psychological support for rape victims.

other preventive measures may be included in such programs. However, some feel that emphasizing such precautions just reinforces women's feelings of helplessness (Sparks, 1978). Some centers advocate the learning of self-defense techniques and may even offer classes. Whether providing therapeutic or preventive help, rape crisis centers provide a much needed link between the medical-legal system and the victim.

RAPE AND THE LEGAL-SOCIAL SYSTEM

Rape is a violent, traumatic crime, yet it is the most underreported of all serious criminal offenses (FBI, 1973). Why do rape victims fail to report the attack? A number of reactions to the rape experience, such as fear, altruism, embarrassment, and stress, may contribute to the woman's silence.

The fear that the rapist will return to injure them or their family is sufficient to silence many women. This is especially true when the attacker has threatened physical harm if the woman goes to the police and the attack has occurred in the home. However, silence does not necessarily guarantee protection. Some rapists have been known to return to previous victims. According to Hursch (1977), not wanting to hurt an innocent party is another major reason for failure to report rape. Such altruistic behavior is not generally for the benefit of the rapist but for his family or friends, whom the victim may know.

Some women fail to report a rape because they feel that their loved ones may treat them differently. Many victims feel unclean after being raped and worry that their husbands or lovers may have the same reaction. Furthermore, women may keep the rape attack to themselves if they feel it would unduly stress their family. Embarrassment or shame may prevent some women from telling anyone or informing the authorities. This is often characteristic of elderly rape victims, who cannot believe that such a thing has happened to them. Some women, having heard about the stress involved in the judicial process, do not report the rape or else withdraw their rape complaint because they want to avoid any further ordeal. Whatever the reason for failure to report the crime, the rapist is then free to commit future sexual assaults—and the statistics suggest that he will.

If the crime is reported, the woman enters the judicial system. Thus, following the rape, the victim must deal with three situations: (1) the hospital experience, where physical evidence is collected, (2) the filing of a police report, and (3) the prosecution of the attacker. In some cases, the victim may call the police first and then go to the hospital. In other cases, she will go to the hospital emergency room first in order to receive treatment for injury, possible venereal disease, and potential pregnancy. She may then decide to report the crime to police or to remain silent.

The hospital experience

The medical treatment of the rape victim focuses on handling the woman's physical and emotional needs through prompt health care and on collecting the medical evidence necessary for prosecution of the rapist. The first step to adequate health care is a thorough physical exam to determine the nature and extent of any injuries. Those injuries that require immediate attention are quickly treated. The second step is prophylactic treatment for venereal disease or pregnancy if the patient so desires. Because 1 out of every 20 rape victims can expect to contract some form of sexually transmitted disease, doctors often recommend the use of antibiotics as a precautionary measure (Hayman, Lanza, and Fuentes, 1969). Pregnancy is also a possible outcome, especially if the attack occurred in the middle of the woman's menstrual cycle. The most common treatment is the morning-after pill, diethylstilbestrol (DES), which we described in Chap. 8. Because DES can have negative consequences for the developing embryo if pregnancy is not stopped, some doctors do not endorse the use of DES for rape victims, and others recommend it only if the woman is willing to undergo an abortion if pregnancy is not prevented. Other preventive measures include the immediate insertion of an IUD to prevent implantation of a zygote in the uterine lining or the abortion technique called menstrual extraction.

Obtaining the physical evidence of rape is a process that can be hampered by two factors. First, the victim may unknowingly destroy the evidence. In the desire to cleanse her body—to remove the feeling of violation and contamination—the woman may shower, bathe, or douche away the feeling of pain and the evidence simultaneously. To preserve evidence, the victim must go immediately to the hospital and not wash up or change clothes. If a change of clothing is absolutely necessary, the woman should take the other clothes with her. Even the insertion of a tampon can destroy evidence. Second, the procedures necessary for collecting the evidence, while not unusual or painful, may be abhorrent to the victim because of the attack. This problem is emphasized in the comments of one rape victim: "The pelvic exam was quite depressing at the time. To have to get undressed again and get up on the table and go through almost the same thing again of something being stuck into you was awful" (Klapholz, 1980, p. 59). The woman can be better prepared for going through this ordeal if she is told ahead of time about the procedures for collecting semen, pubic hair, fingernail scrapings, and the like.

*The police
investigation*

The police have been stereotyped as unsympathetic to and even suspicious of rape victims. Unless the victim was injured, police officers tended to assume that she had been "asking for it." With the development of special rape investigation units and revised popular attitudes toward rape, however, this image has undergone dramatic changes (Murphy, 1980).

One of the more progressive approaches to rape crimes can be found in Massachusetts. In 1974 the rape law was changed in two important ways. First, instead of requiring that a claim of rape must involve force, the mere threat of bodily injury became sufficient in defining rape. Second, the law was extended to include male as well as female victims. Another piece of legislation in Massachusetts led to major police reforms. Special rape reporting and investigation units were established in every police department, and the units were staffed with officers who had gone through a special training program. These new laws are designed to protect the victim.

*The court
procedure*

The most frustrating aspect of rape prosecution is the long, drawn out court process. Although the process varies somewhat from state to state, it often includes the following steps. The prosecution begins with the *arraignment*, in which the alleged rapist appears before the judge and is informed of the charges made against him. The defendant then either pleads guilty or not guilty, and bail is set. The victim is not required to be present during the arraignment. Next a *probable cause hearing* is held, in which a judge listens to the testimony of the victim and other relevant witnesses in order to determine whether it is likely that a crime has occurred.

The next step is for the *grand jury*, a group of 18–20 people, to examine the prosecutor's evidence and decide whether or not to charge the defendant with the crime. This decision is based on the nature of the prosecutor's evidence and on the statements made by the victim during a meeting of the grand jury. This is a closed meeting attended only by the prosecutor and the victim.

If the defendant is *indicted* (charged) with the crime of rape, the case finally goes to a *jury trial*. In accord with the American legal system, the burden is on the prosecutor to prove beyond a reasonable doubt that the defendant is guilty as charged. The victim is called upon by the prosecutor to testify, but the defendant is not required to say anything or to have any witnesses speak on his behalf. The defense attorney has the right to cross-examine the victim, but the prosecutor cannot question the defendant if he does not testify.

Depending on the nature of the evidence and the circumstances surrounding the attack, the defense attorney may resort to one of two common defenses. In the **identification defense**, the attorney agrees that rape has occurred but argues that his client is not the attacker. With the **consent defense**, the attorney argues that the victim gave her consent and was therefore not forced or threatened into having sex. In the latter case, the attorney may choose to explore the sexual history of the victim. This exploration is governed carefully by state and federal statutes. Questions about the sexual background of the victim can be raised only if the victim knew the defendant or if such testimony would have a bearing on the physical evidence. For example, if sperm were found in the vagina of the victim after the rape, it would be relevant to determine whether the woman had had sexual relations with another man within a short period of time prior to the alleged attack.

The court procedures are lengthy and arduous for everyone concerned. The prosecuting attorney must work closely with rape victims to prepare them for the cross-examination of the defense attorney and to help them understand the nature of evidence and testimony. In addition, victims need to be aware of the delays and postponements that may prevent the case from going to trial for months or even a year. Although these delays are not peculiar to rape trials, they may be particularly distressing for victims who simply want to get the whole thing over with.

RAPE ISSUES

Until recently, rape was a crime that received little attention or publicity. The victim often remained silent, neither reporting the crime nor telling family members. The attacker was free to rape again. Today more attention is being focused on sexual assaults. Rape laws have been changed to aid the victim; rape crisis centers have been established to help the victim return to a normal existence; and rape has become the subject of several television dramas, films, and books, as well as newspaper and magazine articles.

As people have become more informed about rape, several issues have emerged. First, should women resist rape attacks? And if so, what strategies should they use? A second issue is treatment of the rapist. Past emphasis has been on incarceration, not rehabilitation. Is there a therapeutic treatment for rapists? Finally, the public is beginning to recognize that men as well as women can be rape victims. What is male rape and how pervasive is it?

Strategies for protection against attack

Rapes occur so frequently in this country that most women realize they are potential targets for rapists in certain situations. To ignore the issue of rape or to assume that it will only happen to others is foolhardy. Thus, women should actively avoid situations where rape is possible and should have a general plan of action should a rape attempt occur.

Avoidance Hursch (1977) has outlined a set of general rules that may serve to prevent rape attack. These are summarized below.

1 *Don't walk alone at night, especially in unfamiliar neighborhoods.*
2 *If you must walk alone, take the following precautions:*

a   Face traffic. This will make it difficult for a man to jump out of a car to grab you unaware from behind.

b   Don't give directions.

c   Watch doorways and alleyways.

d   If you hear someone following you, turn and face that individual. If it is a rapist, he may back off because he has lost the elements of surprise and anonymity.

e   Carry a weapon designed to impede, not injure, the attacker. In states where it is legal, a can of mace may be suitable. Your goal is to surprise the attacker so that you have sufficient time to escape. It is not advisable to carry a lethal weapon, since the attacker may wrest it away and use it against you. Or you may harm the possible attacker and then have to prove in court that he was going to commit a serious crime against your person.

3   Don't pick up hitchhikers.

4   Don't hitchhike.

5   Do drive with the car doors locked.

6   Do have keys in your hand as you approach your car or your home.

7   Do live in secure residential quarters.

8   Don't work alone in a deserted building.

9   Don't use deserted enclosed stairways.

10   Take a simple self-defense course. It will help you decide on a plan of action and give you the means to implement that plan.

*Classes in
self-defense
training emphasize
a number of
techniques that
can be used to
injure or distract
an attacker long
enough for the
victim to escape.*

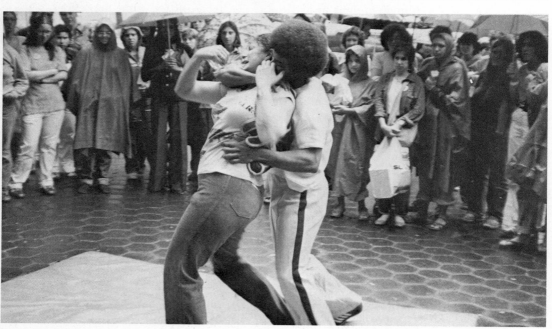

All of these rules are based on the experiences of numerous rape victims and represent the most typical circumstances in which rape occurs.

Resistance If a woman is accosted, she may have only a split second to decide whether to resist or submit to the attacker. Many women are frozen into inaction and are unable to make any decision at all. If a woman decides to resist the attacker, she should do so with the intent of diverting him from his primary goal so that she can escape, since she is unlikely to be able to overpower him physically.

We most commonly think of resistance in terms of physical fighting, but actually women usually resist rapists with verbal ploys. If the attack occurs in the home, they may yell for a nonexistent person; They may tell the rapist that someone is due home in a few minutes; they may say they have VD or some other infectious disease; or they may intimidate the rapist in some manner. For the rapist who expects the victim to say something like, "Please don't hurt me," any other response may catch him off guard. Consider the following example in which the victim was able to intimidate the would-be rapist:

> *A public health nurse left her office late, and was walking toward her car, when a man suddenly appeared beside her, blocked her way, and said, "Move, bitch, into the alley! I'm going to screw you." She stopped short, turned, and looked directly into his face. In a calm voice she said, "If this is the only way you can get a woman, something must be wrong with you. Why don't you come on down to our Mental Health Center in the morning and we'll help you?" The would-be rapist stood perfectly still for a few seconds. Then he averted his eyes from her steady gaze. "Where is it?" he mumbled, his head down and his feet shuffling. (Hursch, 1977, pp. 61–62)*

In some instances, women may use physical resistance to escape from the attack. This is quite a risky tactic, because it may actually increase the attacker's excitement. This is especially true if the rapist is a sadist.

Regardless of whether the resistance is physical or verbal, its timing is crucial to its effectiveness. Resistance has a greater chance of succeeding if it occurs immediately, because it surprises the rapist and takes the control of the situation out of his hands. In situations where the victim initially goes along with the attacker and then resists, the assailant generally becomes violent (Hursch, 1977).

It is difficult to determine whether a victim should decide to resist or submit to sexual attacks. The decision should probably be made on the basis of the circumstances of the attack (indoors or outdoors), the characteristics of the rapist (whether or not he has a weapon, his size, his verbal behavior), and the state of the victim (is she prepared to resist?). Resistance is no guarantee that a woman will escape rape. Indeed, submitting to the attack may actually save her life. Thus, the unpleasant issue of whether to resist or submit is difficult to resolve. Clearly neither choice is desirable, but in a given set of circumstances one may be more appropriate than the other.

*Rehabilitation
of the rapist*

The traditional approach of the legal system has been to punish the rapist with incarceration. And yet 3–4 years in prison is unlikely to help the rapist control his behavior when he is free again. In recent years a few states have established rehabilitation centers for sex offenders. Because such programs are relatively new, a number of therapies are being tried, but their effectiveness is yet to be evaluated.

A treatment used in many other countries, particularly in Europe, is **castration**—removal of the testes. With castration sperm and testosterone production cease, and sexual functioning declines. In Denmark, where a castration law has been in effect since 1929, the treatment is used only at the request of the sex offender and even then only after a special board decides that the offender is likely to benefit from it. The data from Denmark suggest that castration is only beneficial for those people who suffer from abnormally strong sex drives. In these cases, ejaculation rates may decline from 12–24 per day to 3 or 4 times a week following the surgery. Such men are then able to resume normal lives and are unlikely to commit further sex crimes. Nevertheless, the majority of known rapists are not "oversexed," so castration would not be a suitable treatment.

A more promising avenue for rapist rehabilitation may lie with the behavioral therapies. For example, **aversive therapy** has been used to pair visual rape images with unpleasant or noxious stimuli. Other behavioral approaches focus on teaching the rape offender to react differently to stimuli that produce the rape response. Because these therapies have had very little use thus far, their effectiveness cannot yet be evaluated.

What is needed is more information on the rapist—his background, his experiences, and his behavioral tendencies. While we can try to aid the victim as much as possible, perhaps the best help would be to identify the factors that contribute to a person becoming a rapist, to develop procedures for recognizing potential rapists, and to discover and use effective rehabilitation measures.

Male rape

Rape is usually thought of as a crime perpetrated by a man against a woman. But the victim can be either a man or a woman. In homosexual assaults, for example, one man may force another to engage in fellatio or to submit to anal intercourse. **Homosexual rape** in prisons came into national prominence in 1973, when Quaker pacifist Robert Martin held a press conference to describe his experiences in jail (Aiken, 1973, p. 5). Martin had been arrested two weeks before for participating in a peace demonstration in Washington, D.C. Instead of paying a $10 bond, Martin elected to go to jail. In the second week of his incarceration, he was transferred to a different section of the jail: "After entering the cell of some inmates, my exit was blocked and my pants were forcibly taken from me and I was raped. Then, I was dragged from cell to cell all evening" (p. 5). The next night entailed a second round of extensive oral and anal sex. Finally, Martin was able to reach a guard and was then hospitalized for trauma and injury. At the press conference, Martin warned others about the existence of homosexual rape in the jails and the system of dominance that is a part of many prison complexes.

Male rape is not restricted to prison environments. It can occur in the same sorts of situations as rape of women—in secluded areas, deserted buildings, dark alleys, public bathrooms. Male hitchhikers may attack male drivers and vice versa.

The male victim responds to rape in much the same way as the female victim. The male's common reaction is fear, and his tendency is to remain silent about the crime. Male victims also exhibit symptoms characteristic of the rape trauma syndrome, including disturbances in eating, sleeping, and thinking (Burgess and Holmstrom, 1979a). It is only gradually that they return to a normal existence.

The issue of females raping males is one that is seldom considered. For obvious reasons, women cannot force men to engage in sexual intercourse. Fear or threat of force is not conducive to penile erection in most men. However, they may be forced to perform oral sex. The reported incidence of women raping men is extremely low. Whether this is because the phenomenon is indeed rare or because the male is unlikely to report it (and face possible embarrassment and ridicule from peers) is unknown. The information that is currently available is not sufficient to provide any definitive conclusions about the incidence and nature of rapes in which women attack men.

SUMMARY

1   *Rape* is the occurrence of sexual acts without the consent of the victim. The *blitz rape* is a sudden assault on the victim, and the *confidence rape* involves verbal ploys or a decoy to entice the victim into an unprotected situation.

2   A second type of sexual assault is *accessory to sex*, in which the victim is unable to consent because she either is too young or is mentally retarded or disturbed. The attacker may promise the victim material rewards, may appeal to the victim's psychological need for attention, or may promise pleasure and insist there is "nothing wrong with" the behavior.

3   A third type of sexual assault occurs in *sex-stress situations* in which the victim initially consents to sex but the situation suddenly changes, because either the man becomes perverse or violent, the woman experiences postcoital anxiety over possible pregnancy, or the couple are interrupted in the act by parents or police.

4   Little is actually known about the characteristics of the rapist, although many stereotypes appear to be untrue. Rapists are not primarily minority group members, nor are they sex starved, oversexed, or shy, retiring types. The primary motive for rape is not sexual desire but the need to express anger and power. The *anger rape* is an unplanned, quick event used to release pent-up feelings of rage. The *power rape* is more likely to be planned, to be prolonged, and to express the rapist's desire to display control over someone else's life. The *sadistic rape* involves abuse and torture of the victim. Rapists apparently have arousal patterns to sexual stimuli that are different from those of nonrapists.

5   The victim's response to rape consists of a cluster of symptoms referred to as the *rape trauma syndrome*. In the *acute phase* of the syndrome, the victim may exhibit an *expressed reaction* or a *controlled reaction*, suffer from

overwhelming fear, and experience such symptoms as physical problems, sleep disturbances, alterations in eating habits, emotional reactions, and obsessive thoughts. In the *long-term phase*, the victim may experience alterations in physiology, dream disturbances, phobias, loss of sexual desire, and changes in social activity.

6   Factors aiding recovery from rape include previous experience with major life stresses, high self-esteem, use of defense mechanisms, taking action, and, in some instances, self-blame. Factors delaying recovery include repeated rape experiences, chronic life stressors, low self-esteem, maladaptive responses such as drinking and taking drugs, and certain aspects of the attack itself.

7   Rape crisis centers provide services that can help victims recover from their trauma and that help women learn how to prevent rape from occurring or how to deal with rape should it occur.

8   Many women do not report rape out of either fear of retaliation from the rapist, altruism toward the rapist's family, embarrassment, reluctance to go through the long legal process of prosecuting the rapist, or fear that people will treat them differently.

9   If the rape is reported, the woman must go through three major situations: (1) the hospital experience, in which she is treated for any injuries and for potential venereal disease and pregnancy and in which physical evidence for the rape is collected; (2) the police investigation, which is now geared much more toward protecting the victim; and (3) the court procedure, which by its nature is long and drawn out. The victim must be prepared to understand the court procedures and to deal with cross-examination by the defense attorney.

10   How should a woman deal with a rape attack? Many guidelines have been offered for avoiding rape in the first place by taking safety precautions. If a rapist does attack, resistance or compliance depends on many factors, including the circumstances, the characteristics of the rapist, and the state of the victim.

11   Our legal system is currently geared toward punishing rapists, not rehabilitating them. Many treatment methods are currently being tried, but their effectiveness cannot yet be evaluated.

12   Males are also subject to rape, particularly *homosexual rape*. Men react to rape in much the same way as women do—they exhibit many of the same symptoms of the rape trauma syndrome.

**ADDITIONAL
READING**

* ***Brownmiller, Susan.*** *Against Our Will: Men, Women and Rape.* New York: Simon & Schuster, 1975.

    A comprehensive discussion of rape. The arguments are carefully made and well supported.

Groth, Nicholas. *Men Who Rape: The Psychology of the Offender.* New York: Plenum, 1979.

    An in-depth study of men who commit rape, why they do it, and how they might be treated.

Katz, Sedelle, and Mazur, Mary Ann. *Understanding the Rape Victim: A Syntheis of Research Findings.* New York: Wiley, 1979.

    A comprehensive synthesis of research findings in this area. The book is somewhat technical but contains a lot of information.

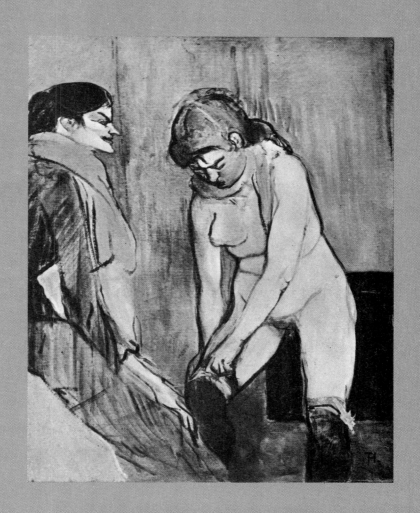

Sex and the law

20

chapter

20

Except for sexual intercourse by a married couple in the man-on-top position, every other sexual act is illegal in at least some jurisdiction of the United States. In effect, then, almost everyone is a law breaker under literal interpretations of the laws governing sexual behavior and is subject to both fines and imprisonment. For the most part, however, sexual offenses between consenting adults are rarely prosecuted. Nevertheless, the existence of the statutes, enforced or not, makes it clear that our society feels justified, even compelled, to control people's sexual behavior through laws.

How did American sex laws come to be so restrictive? We noted in Chap. 2 how religious systems advocating the Judeo-Christian moral codes came to be increasingly concerned about sexual behavior and how many of the religious tenets expressed in the Bible and other church writings became the basis of the laws of Western societies. However, despite the mostly sex-negative attitudes found in the Judeo-Christian tradition, the early laws were not overly restrictive of sexual practices; rather, they were more concerned with the control of antireligious behavior. It took the Puritans to translate moral codes against sexual activities into legal codes. The Puritans were very strict about their lives in general and their sexual lives in particular. Because the church elders were also the only civil authority in the early American colonies, they included their religious rules about sexual behavior in their civil codes and legal constraints.

The Puritan laws still exert a strong influence on the American legal system. Some changes have occurred, and legal reforms are continually being called for, but it is difficult for elected lawmakers to take a liberal stand in an area where morality and legality get so inextricably intertwined. In this chapter we will examine the types of laws against various types of sexual behavior currently on the books. Then we will describe two controversial areas of regulation: prostitution and pornography.

THE VARIETY OF LAWS GOVERNING SEXUAL BEHAVIOR

The current legal system reflects the restrictions imposed on sexual behavior by the many and varied moral views found in our society. The accumulation of these laws, along with the fact that few have ever been repealed, has left us with a confusing array of "offenses" that vary from state to state and even city to city. In order to discuss these various laws, it will be helpful to group them according to the aspect of sexuality they attempt to regulate. There are laws regulating the nature of the sexual activity, the age of the participants, the familial and legal relationships of the sexual partners, procreation, and sexual criminal acts.

Regulation of the nature of sexual interaction

Laws included in this category are those involving "crimes against nature" and those governing rape.

"Crimes against nature" This curious label is invoked when individuals are given jail sentences and fines for sexual behavior that often goes unmentioned or undescribed in the legal proceedings. Laws in this category are sometimes called **sodomy laws**, although other acts besides genital-anal contact are prosecuted under them. The usual sexual behaviors covered by such

laws are oral sex, anal intercourse, sex with animals (zoophilia), and sex with dead bodies (necrophilia).

The vagueness of these laws derives from the fact that when they were enacted such sexual acts were considered too provocative to even be mentioned in police records or legal court transcripts. One judge is quoted as referring to "the abominable crime not fit to be named among Christians . . . the records of the court need not be defiled with the details of the different acts which may go to constitute it" (Ploscowe, 1951, p. 197). Prosecution still occurs with little additional definition of the "crime." Currently, the penalties, which vary from one jurisdiction to another, range from 1 to 20 years in prison and fines of up to $5000.

In actual practice, sodomy laws have been used most often for the prosecution of male homosexuals. Sex with animals and corpses is so rarely reported or prosecuted as to be of little significance. However, the presumably "unnatural acts" of homosexuals are investigated and prosecuted with what many feel is excessive zeal on the part of police and the courts. Homosexuality in and of itself is not a crime and thus is not illegal anywhere in the United States. However, homosexuals are often arrested by police decoys posing as homosexuals and are then prosecuted under the "crimes against nature" laws.

The lack of specification of the "criminal" behavior and the use of police entrapment have caused many reform groups to question the utility of sodomy laws. Some states have tried to indicate more exactly what acts will be prosecuted. Others have simply repealed all such vague laws. It is possible that these laws may be ruled unconstitutional by the Supreme Court because they violate constitutional guarantees about the specificity of charges. In fact, it is surprising that such laws have survived for as long as they have.

It is easy to be unconcerned about "crimes against nature" if we feel that they could never affect us as individuals. But that may be an inappropriate assumption. Take the case of a couple in Indiana, for example. The woman was suing for divorce, and in order to "punish" her husband, she accused him of unspecified sexual practices under the sodomy laws of that state. She indicated that no force was involved and that she was a willing participant, but the acts were nevertheless against the law. When her temper had cooled and she was made to realize the possible penalties if her husband were to be found guilty, she tried to have the charges dropped. But because state laws had been broken, the complaint could not be withdrawn. The husband was subsequently convicted and sentenced to 2–14 years in prison. He served 3 years in the state penitentiary before he was released by an appeals court—and that was only on a technical error in his first trial. Thus, we must also consider ourselves at risk of prosecution if any law, particularly such a vague law, is part of the legal regulations of our community.

Rape   As we indicated in Chap. 19, rape is more often an act of violence and assault than a sexual act, and as such its legal control seems both warranted and necessary. There is one controversial legal problem with rape laws that does require further attention from lawmakers, however. This is the fact that in most states the law does not consider forced sex between husband and wife to be rape. Legal scholars note that this reflects the fact that the original sanctions against rape were really property rights laws, written to protect a man's property (wife or daughter) from forcible use by other men. Thus, a husband "taking" his own property was not considered rape. Once again we find that times have changed but laws have not. The woman's right to be protected against forced sex, regardless of her relationship to the man, needs to be recognized in the rape laws. One recent precedent-setting case in Oregon did involve prosecution of a man for raping his wife, although the man was not convicted. A similar case in Massachusetts did result in conviction. More such cases are likely to be prosecuted in the near future, particularly if the feminist movement continues to draw attention to the issue.

*Regulation of the
age of the
participants*
Laws that fall into this category include those against child molestation and statutory rape laws.

Child molestation   Sexual activities involving children are prohibited by law in all jurisdictions in the United States. The definition of *child*, however, varies greatly from place to place, with the point at which a child becomes a legal adult ranging anywhere from age 14 to 21. **Child molestation** can include any type of sexual approach to a child. Once again, local statutes differ as to what constitutes child molesting. Activities such as touching and fondling may form the basis for a complaint in some localities, while genital contact is part of the definition in others. Arrests and prosecutions are complicated by the fact that the child may have difficulty understanding what has happened, may have problems identifying the offender, and may not make an acceptable court witness. Furthermore, parents and authorities may feel uncomfortable adding the stresses of testifying and cross-examination to the trauma the child may have already suffered.

Child molesting and pedophilia (discussed in Chap. 16) are related but may not be identical. The pedophile is presumed to be motivated by disturbed psychological processes, while the child molester is presumed to be aware of right and wrong and to have criminal intent. There is a fine line here between compulsion and willful action, and it is often difficult for legal authorities and psychological experts to decide which is involved in a particular case.

Of all the various regulations governing sexual behavior, those involving the protection of children and the punishment of those who violate their innocence receive the most widespread public support. Even other criminals rank the child molester as the lowest type of all, and many convicted of this crime must be protected from fellow prisoners once incarcerated. On the other hand, the child molestation laws are often misused. Any approach to a child, even a quite innocent one, may be overreacted to by parents and police. The age, dress, cleanliness, and state of sobriety of a stranger approaching a child may have more to do with the way the approach is interpreted than with the act itself. And, as we noted in Chap. 16, if a man is unable to understand what is happening or is unable to defend himself in court, he may end up in jail even if he had no criminal intentions.

Statutory rape Although we discussed statutory rape in Chap. 19, some of the legal aspects deserve special attention here. Statutory rape laws are intended to prevent an adult from taking unfair sexual advantage of a minor. Force is not the issue here, although that could be part of the act. The important point is that the consent of the minor is irrelevant. A rape is said to have occurred based solely on the existence of the act and the age of the child. Not only is this type of rape complicated by the fact that the age of legal maturity varies from state to state, but the relative ages of the participants can be a factor. There is a great deal of difference between a sexual relationship involving a 17-year-old-boy and a 15-year-old girl and one between a 40-year-old man and a 12-year-old girl. The relative maturity and sophistication of the "child" should also be an important factor in determining whether he or she has been taken advantage of.

Because there have been so many cases that have fallen into the gray areas of statutory rape laws, they are often considered unenforceable. Many groups seeking legal reform have made a number of suggestions for revising these laws. One suggestion, which has been adopted by several states, is to require that there be at least a 4-year difference in age between the participants for a statutory rape charge to be considered. Still another proposal, written into the Model Penal Code of the American Law Institute, is to reduce the age of consent to 10 years of age. If the girl is above age 10, the case would be handled on an individual basis; it might be considered a statutory rape, contributing to the delinquency of a minor, or no legal problem at all.

Regulation of the relationship of the participants

Many laws are concerned with who may or may not engage in sexual activity with whom. Marriage is the basic, permissible relationship for sexual contact in our society, and one's marital status has come to define the legality of certain sexual interactions. Among laws that regulate who may interact with whom are laws against adultery, fornication, cohabitation, bigamy, and incest.

Adultery is consensual sexual intercourse between a married person and someone other than his or her spouse. All states have or have had laws making such behavior illegal. In a 1974 review of the laws, Cohen found that 41 states still had adultery laws on the books. Penalties included a maximum of 5 years in jail and fines of up to $1000. The most common use of adultery laws has been in divorce cases, where such illegal behavior is used as grounds for divorce in states that require one partner to be at fault.

The crime of *fornication* involves sexual intercourse between consenting unmarried adults. In Cohen's survey, 23 states still had laws against fornication. The penalties varied greatly, most being quite light but others surprisingly harsh. Michigan, for example, had penalties of up to 5 years in jail and $2500 in fines.

A third legal regulation involving marital status forbids unmarried individuals of the opposite sex to live together. Most of these laws are unclear as to whether the individuals must be engaging in sexual intercourse in order for a crime to have occurred. In most localities, just the appearance of a "sinful" relationship seems to be enough to violate this law. Cohen found that 26 states had laws against **cohabitation**, with penalties ranging up to 3 years in jail and $500 in fines.

Adultery, fornication, and cohabitation laws are rarely prosecuted. However, they do make ordinary people legally vulnerable. If social values have shifted so that these laws no longer serve a purpose, it seems logical that they be dropped from the books or changed.

Another law involving marriage is the law against **bigamy**—being married to more than one person at the same time. The bigamist is actually committing adultery, since all but the first marriage are null and void. The law in this case, however, is less concerned with the sexual aspects of the multiple marriage than with the issues of legal responsibility, child and spouse support, inheritance, and legitimacy of children by other than the first marriage.

The laws against **incest** are designed to regulate sexual intercourse between blood relatives. All states forbid sexual relations between parents and their children (regardless of age), between brothers and sisters, between grandparents and grandchildren, and between aunts and uncles and their blood-related nieces and nephews. Sexual relations between cousins may or may not be considered incestuous depending on the degree of closeness; definitions vary from state to state. Where did such laws come from? It is difficult to determine. We now know that inbreeding is associated with an increase in the incidence of genetic defects; perhaps this was the basis of some incest laws, even among fairly primitive peoples. Issues of family strife may also have been a source. To have family members competing with each other for sexual favors, often under the same roof, would put enormous stress on the family unit.

Father-daughter incest has been receiving a great deal of attention lately as a result of efforts by feminist groups, as we noted in Chap. 16. From the legal perspective, we must note that laws against incest have not been successful in controlling the problem of father-daughter relations. It is unlikely that a daughter would complain to the police about her father or that she would follow through with prosecution except in extraordinary circumstances. Furthermore, legal authorities seem to make special efforts to avoid the issue. Perhaps the best approach is to consider such incestuous behavior as a type of child abuse and to make available to the family the support services provided under the child abuse legislation enacted in most states.

Regulation of procreation

The Judeo-Christian view that sexual behavior is reserved for procreative functions is reflected in our laws as well as in our religious teachings. There are numerous laws concerned with regulating the individual's freedom to decide whether or not to have children. Included in this category are restrictions on the use of birth control methods, laws against abortion, laws governing sterilization, and laws controlling artificial insemination.

Birth control laws The U.S. Obscenity Act of 1873, known as the **Comstock laws**, classified birth control information as obscene and severely limited the distribution of such information. Under that law it became illegal to send information about contraceptives through the mail. As late as 1965, Massachusetts still had a law making it illegal for married couples to use any birth control device. All such laws were overturned in 1965 by a Supreme Court decision in the case of *Griswald* v. *Connecticut*. In this ruling the Court declared that it is unconstitutional to have laws that restrict the use of, or information about, methods of contraception. The pendulum has swung even further in the liberal direction since 1965, with many states guaranteeing, through law, the availability of contraceptive information and devices to all who wish them—even to minors without their parents' knowledge. These more liberal approaches to contraception were greatly advanced by the Family Planning and Research Act passed by Congress in 1970.

Abortion In legal terms, **abortion** is deliberate termination of a pregnancy. Until relatively recently, abortion was illegal unless specific, agreed-upon medical conditions warranted therapeutic abortion. Despite these laws, abortions were performed. Women who could afford it went to other countries or paid high rates to physicians who performed illegal abortions. Women with little money often ended up having less expensive but dangerous abortions performed by unqualified individuals under nonsterile conditions. Women also tried to abort fetuses on their own, often seriously harming or even killing themselves in the process.

The first wave of changes in abortion laws allowed the mental health of the mother to become an acceptable reason for abortion. Now women who could afford the two or more psychiatric opinions necessary qualified for this type of intervention. The effect of all these laws was to discriminate among women on the basis of socioeconomic group: There were safe abortions for those who could afford them; unsafe, illegal abortions for the less affluent; and the birth of unwanted children for the very poor.

In 1970 New York was the first state to introduce abortion on demand by the mother with no restrictions other than that the fetus be in the first or second trimester of the pregnancy and that the abortion be performed by a licensed, qualified physician. Some states followed suit immediately; most did not. In January 1973 the Supreme Court ruled, with a vote of 7 to 2, that the decision to have an abortion (in the first trimester) is a right of the woman that cannot be interfered with by any state law. This ruling in effect cancelled all state laws prohibiting abortion.

The issue is far from resolved, however. Many antiabortion groups have been working to reverse or at least restrict the laws legalizing abortion. They have been instrumental in introducing laws releasing physicians and nurses from engaging in abortions if it is against their personal principles. They have also been successful in their efforts to restrict public funds for abortions.

Sterilization **Sterilization** is the use of any of a variety of surgical procedures to make a person physically incapable of reproduction. Legal aspects of sterilization have gone in two different directions. On the one hand, laws concerning **compulsory sterilization**, in which people are sterilized without—or even against—their permission, have been part of the legal codes of most states. Such procedures have typically been **eugenic** that is, designed to protect society and the gene pool from production of "defective" members. Those individuals considered for sterilization for this reason included the retarded, epileptics, the "insane," syphilitics, and various criminal offenders. Since World War II, when Germany made sterilization a part of its national policy, there has been a general rescinding of such laws. Nevertheless, there are still some states with eugenic sterilization statutes on their books.

On the other hand, **voluntary sterilization**, in which the person requests the procedure for purposes of birth control, was severely restricted by law. It was not until 1972 that the last state, Utah, finally rescinded its law prohibiting such sterilization. The use of public funds for such operations varies greatly from state to state.

Artificial insemination As we noted in Chap. 7, artificial insemination is the introduction of live sperm into the vagina of a woman. The donor may be the woman's husband, or it may be an anonymous man who has donated to a sperm bank. In the latter case, several legal questions arise. Who is the father of the child? Has adultery taken place? Who is responsible for the child? While these issues are often hypothetical, complications can occur if the couple divorce or if the husband later objects to the procedure. He may argue that he has no responsibility for the child. Inheritance may also be a problem if other family members challenge the legitimacy of the child. To respond to these and other problems, several states have passed laws legitimizing children produced by artificial insemination where both husband and wife have given written consent to the procedure.

Sexual criminal acts

The label **sex offender** has formal legal status in many jurisdictions. It refers to an individual who has been convicted of any "crimes involving the expression of sexual urges" (Sadock, 1976). The term **sexual psychopath** has also been applied to such individuals. These terms imply that the person has uncontrollable sexual desires that will be expressed regardless of legal or social restrictions and with no concern for the wishes of the victim. The results of being labeled thusly can be quite devastating to the person involved.

Although the terms *sex offender* and *sexual psychopath* were originally coined as a means of categorizing individuals as psychologically disturbed rather than purely criminal, they have taken on a meaning much different from that originally intended. The offenses that fall into this category vary from state to state, but would include most of the behaviors discussed in Chaps. 16 and 19. A representative list would have voyeurism, exhibitionism, bestiality, necrophilia, rape, sodomy, child molestation, indecent assault, and incest. The grouping of such a wide variety of individuals with sexual behavior problems, regardless of the nature and degree of the behavior, has resulted in a tendency to treat all members of this group as being capable of the behaviors of the most extreme members; for example, the passive exhibitionist has been equated with the homicidal rapist. Thus, individuals labeled as sex offenders, even if their behavior is as benign as peeking in a window, may be incarcerated for indeterminant lengths of time, may be thought of as both criminal and mentally ill, and may be subjected to such extreme treatments as electroshock therapy, psychosurgery, experimental drugs, and even sterilization. Even when finally released as "cured," these people may have to register with the police in their community as sex offenders and are often treated as prime suspects when any crime with the vaguest sexual overtones is committed in that community.

The problem is that the actual behaviors subsumed under the label of *sex offender* are so different in degree and kind that they defy any single categorization. The generalities that do emerge about individuals with this label are more sociopolitical than pathological; that is, it has been found that they are more likely to be from the lower socioeconomic levels of society and to have low levels of education.

As these facts have become clearer to those in the mental health and legal areas, there has been some movement away from using these damaging labels and toward treating each case more individually. Greater attention has also been paid to humanizing the handling of people who show maladaptive sexual behaviors.

PROSTITUTION

In our society, **prostitution**—the selling of sexual favors for money—is illegal almost everywhere. In recent years there has been much discussion of decriminalizing prostitution. It may be difficult to imagine prostitution as not being illegal because we have been raised in a society where it has always been viewed that way. We have been conditioned to see prostitution as a criminal activity. Yet it is truly a victimless crime. Put in its coldest light, prostitution is a contractual arrangement in which two adults agree on a fee in exchange for sexual services. It is an activity of consenting adults engaging in a behavior by choice and in which no one's rights are violated. In fact, prostitution is a classic example of the free enterprise system at work. Many people feel it should not be considered a crime, and it is not one in many other countries. But the road to decriminalizing prostitution in the United States is a difficult one, even for the most liberal segments of society.

What would be the advantages of decriminalizing prostitution? Even if we believe that the customer is not a victim, we might argue that the prostitute is being victimized. As a society, we might want to prevent individuals from entering the profession, and keeping it illegal would be a deterrent. The fact is, however, that the illegal status of prostitution has never proven to be much of a deterrent. More important, many of the problems of both the prostitute and society are the result of the illegal status of the profession. The prostitute becomes a victim of the police, of the criminal elements of society, and even of her own customers.

The illegal status of prostitution has created a feminist issue of some importance. Because the vast majority of prostitutes are women, while the customers, police, pimps, bar owners, organized crime figures, and others who live off the prostitutes are men, there is a rather obvious sex discrimination issue. Furthermore, since customers are rarely arrested (except to force them to testify against the prostitute), a double standard seems to be operating within the legal system to the obvious disadvantage of women.

Another factor involved in the illegal status of prostitution is sexually transmitted disease. As long as prostitution is kept underground, VD remains difficult if not impossible to control. In countries that have legalized prostitution, women who work as prostitutes are carefully screened for VD.

For these and other reasons, the illegality of prostitution is in fact what creates many of the serious problems associated with it. Reconsideration of the legal status of this, the world's oldest profession, thus seems in order.

The ***streetwalker*** is the most common type of prostitute. She is also, for obvious reasons, the most visible. The streetwalker plies her trade on the streets of most cities. She usually has an area of territory in which she works. She stays near certain corners, cruises various restaurants or bars where she is known, and generally remains visible to clients and "steerers"—individuals who will send customers her way in exchange for tips or kickbacks. While she may have a few regular customers, she depends more on transient visitors to the area. Her clothing is an important form of advertising of both the service

*Types of
prostitutes*

*The streetwalker
is the most visible
and often the most
victimized of the
prostitutes.*

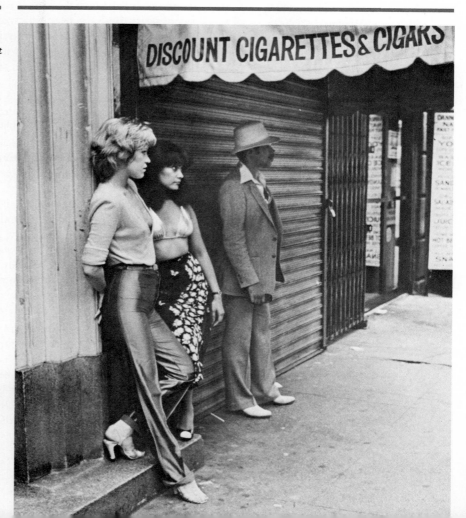

offered and the quality of the goods. The streetwalker must also approach men directly, indicate her willingness to have sex with them, and even briefly describe the nature of the activities in which she is willing to engage. Although prices tend to be standardized in a given locality, there may be some bargaining. It is at this point that the prostitute may be arrested by a vice squad officer on the charge of *soliciting.* Although less likely, the customer may be arrested if the soliciter turns out to be a female police officer. To avoid entrapment, prostitute and client often engage in a complicated dialogue, with each party trying to let the other know what is being offered and requested and each saying as little as possible.

Once a bargain is struck, the woman may take the customer to a room she rents just for the purpose or to her own apartment, or they may go to the man's hotel room or apartment. To earn the necessary income, the streetwalker needs several such customers during her working hours, which include a good part of the daytime as well as the more usual nighttime hours.

The visibility of the streetwalker and her need to approach potential customers makes her the most vulnerable of all prostitutes to arrest. The legal charges vary but can include vagrancy, procuring, disturbing the peace, no visible means of support, and, of course, prostitution. Although these are not serious crimes, they usually involve fines or short jail sentences, which take the woman off the street, require bail, and generally add to the expense and risks of the profession.

The streetwalker is also a target for crimes against her person and property. Because she is likely to have money and because she cannot complain to the police, she becomes an attractive robbery victim. She may also encounter customers who refuse to pay, against whom she again has no legal recourse. Most prostitutes learn quickly to get their money in advance. Most dangerous for the streetwalker is the violent or sadistic customer who wants more than just sex.

All these dangers have led to the existence of an important figure in the world of prostitution: the *pimp.* He is simultaneously the boss and the protector of the prostitute. The pimp takes a percentage of the prostitute's earnings, presumably in exchange for protection, bail bond services, provision of lawyers when necessary, and even paying off the right people to protect "his girls." Some of these relationships are pure business, while others have romantic overtones, more often from the woman's perspective than the pimp's. More often than not, what is supposed to be a symbiotic relationship of mutual gain turns into a parasitic one, in which the pimp lives off the woman's earnings and provides little in return. Today the pimp is a far less common figure than in the past.

Streetwalkers tend to come from poor backgrounds and to be less well educated than the general population. Their customers also tend to come from the lower socioeconomic levels of society.

Many of the laws against prostitution are meant to stop *public solicitation* on the street, or at least to contain it. Even in countries that have decriminalized prostitution, such as Great Britain, such solicitation is usually against the law. The containment approach has been used in many American cities, where streetwalkers are restricted to certain *"combat zones"* in which various illicit activities are tolerated.

At the next higher level of prostitution are the *bar girls* or *B-girls*, who work in bars, cocktail lounges, night clubs, or strip joints and generally do not solicit outside of that setting. The arrangements with the establishments vary but generally involve both a salary and a commission on drinks, as well as tips from the customers. Many B-girls do not actually sell sex but only the *promise* of sex. They get the customer to buy as many drinks as possible before he finds out that nothing more will follow. The drinks the woman orders, which may actually be only weak tea, are charged to the customer as expensive alcoholic beverages. This activity is not actually prostitution but rather a type of confidence game promising something that will not be delivered. Other B-girls, however, *are* prostitutes and use the establishment as a place of contact with customers. The actual sexual interaction may take place in rooms attached to the establishment, or the woman and her client may go elsewhere.

The *brothel prostitute* works out of a house of prostitution. Such whorehouses were familiar fixtures of most communities in earlier times. The typical house had a manager or "madam" who was often the owner and who made the arrangements with the customers. This included collecting the fees, which were then split between the prostitute and the madam. From the perspective of the prostitute, working in such a house offered some strong advantages. The house provided protection from violent or dangerous clients, the companionship of fellow prostitutes, a steady flow of customers, and some insulation from police harassment, as well as many other amenities. On the negative side, the house took a substantial cut of the money earned, usually 40–60 percent of the fee.

Today a modern version of the house of prostitution exists in the form of the *prostitute apartment*. This is a cooperative type arrangement of a group of independent prostitutes who band together and either pay a manager to run the place or are managed by a madam. Some operations serve a walk-in clientele, while others cater to clients who call for appointments with specific women.

The *call girl* is considered to be at the top of the prostitution trade. She is a younger, better looking, better educated, and from a higher socioeconomic background than other types of prostitutes. She usually has a group of steady clients who call her on a regular basis and who may also refer friends or business acquaintances. She spends more time with her clients, may go out with them on "dates," and may even function as a hostess for business or social functions.

The call girl gets her name from the fact that she works primarily by appointment. While her fees are substantially higher than those of other prostitutes, she also has higher expenses (clothes, living accommodations, and so on). The call girl has the least problem with the law, partly because she is the least visible to the police and to the community in general. Her neighbors in her apartment building probably think of her only as that attractive, quiet, *very* popular young woman down the hall.

A relatively new development on the scene is the ***massage parlor prostitute.*** The massage parlor as a front for prostitution is a rather clever and creative approach to the problems we have discussed as being part of the profession. It places the client and the prostitute together in a room with a bed or cot and with the customer undressed, presumably for a legal, socially acceptable activity. There are tremendous advantages to this arrangement not only for the owners, the prostitute, and the customer but for society as well, in that streetwalking is reduced, fewer police are needed, VD is better controlled, and so on.

Massage parlor prostitutes often provide sexual release through masturbating their customers rather than through sexual intercourse. However, the services available frequently extend beyond masturbation to what are euphemistically referred to as "extras." The extras can be anything from mutual massage to oral sex to intercourse. The only limits are those imposed by the establishment and by the prostitute. Extras of course add substantially to the cost of the basic massage.

Two studies of massage parlor prostitutes found them to be slightly higher in socioeconomic background than streetwalkers and a higher percentage of

Massage parlor prostitution has shown a dramatic increase in recent years.

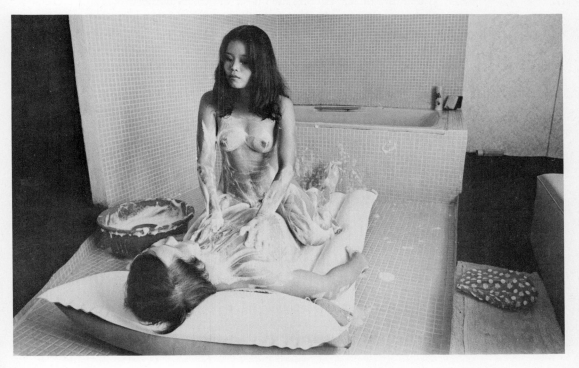

them to be college students and graduates (Bryant and Palmer, 1975; Rasmussen and Kuhn, 1976). Many women were moonlighting housewives with husbands and children at home. Rasmussen and Kuhn found that many denied they were prostitutes at all because they gave only "hand jobs." However, the longer a woman worked at a massage parlor, the more pressured she felt to engage in more extras if she was to keep up with her competition and not get fired.

Massage parlors have a mix of regular and transient clients. In one study employing a masseuse as an observer, it was found that the clients consisted primarily of local businessmen and out-of-town visitors (Armstrong, 1978). She noted that two-thirds of the customers indicated a desire for extras, but only 42 percent actually received any. Those who did not ask for extras may have been naive about the nature of the massage parlor, or they may have been vice squad officers waiting to be solicited.

While far less frequent than female prostitutes, **male prostitutes** do exist in significant numbers in most cities. The largest group serve as sexual partners to other males seeking homosexual relations. Called **hustlers**, they work in a variety of settings, including gay bars, homosexual baths, and on the streets. Some of these male prostitutes have a "call gay" type operation with a group of repeat clients to whom they may be companions as well as sexual partners.

In Chap. 13 we discussed the cruising scene among homosexuals and the easy availability of sex. Among the out-of-the-closet homosexuals in a community, sex for pay is not necessary, and the hustler is not in great demand. However, for homosexuals trying to maintain a heterosexual image or for those heterosexual or bisexual males seeking an occasional homosexual experience, hustlers may be sought out.

Male prostitutes who provide services for women are called **gigolos**. They frequently serve as companions or escorts as well as sexual partners to women. They may be employed by male modeling agencies or escort services that openly advertise the escort part of the service. Women do not usually pick up male prostitutes in clubs or off the street, although this does occur occasionally.

Less is known about male prostitution than female prostitution. This may be because it is a much smaller trade or because female prostitutes are more available for study. Because males are rarely arrested, there is no readily accessible research population. Thus, it may be that male prostitution is more widespread than is currently thought but that it operates beneath the visible surface.

The life of the prostitute

How does a person become a prostitute? Sociologists have been particularly interested in this question, since in most cases it represents voluntary entrance into a socially deviant group. This interest has spurred research in which prostitutes have been interviewed about their life-styles and about the factors that entered into their joining this profession.

Most prostitutes come from the lower socioeconomic levels of society. During adolescence their physical appearance was a definite asset, and they came to view their good looks as a significant part of how they related to the world. Few of the prostitutes interviewed indicated any deliberate, conscious decision to become "hookers." Most reported that they drifted into prostitution gradually, moving from dating, which may have included sex, to sex with strangers for money. In many cases, the novice was encouraged to make the initial step by a friend or acquaintance who was already a prostitute (Bryan, 1967).

Despite the general view that young women are forced into prostitution by pimps or organized crime, being pressed into service was rare among actual reports. Some young women had run away from homes in smaller communities to large urban centers. Without money, skills to earn a living, or a place to live, they were easy prey for pimps who encouraged them to work for them. In some cases, the girls found such men waiting as they got off the bus or train. But these cases were the exception rather than the rule.

Another stereotype is that prostitutes are psychologically disturbed and that they have entered this profession as the result of some defect in their personality development. It has been suggested that prostitutes are incapable of love, are aggressive toward men, or are self-punishing and guilt-ridden. In a similar vein, it has been suggested that prostitutes are latent lesbians who are unaware of their true sexual orientation and are using prostitution to solve their sexual confusion. None of these generalities has been upheld by studies. In general, women who enter prostitution have done so as their own solution to a variety of social and economic problems rather than as a solution to psychological problems.

Interviews with the more experienced and older prostitutes indicated that the life they led was not highly positive. The initial excitement, promises of great amounts of money, and hope for the easy life all soon faded in the day-to-day problems, worries, and fears that are part and parcel of the profession. Most hoped to earn enough money to retire gracefully, while others were hoping for a mythical "sugar daddy" who whould show up to save them. Many found no acceptable way out of "the life" and felt locked into the profession and what they perceived as a dismal future (Jackman, et al., 1963).

Many prostitutes feel that the difficulties of their lives are due to society's reaction to them. An organization made up of prostitutes, COYOTE (Cast Off Your Old Tired Ethics), seeks to improve the current life of the working prostitute and to protect her future. The women in the group seek political power in hopes of decriminalizing their activities and protecting their civil rights. They are also pursuing the economic and retirement issues addressed by other unions. Despite the extensive media coverage that COYOTE attracts to its demonstrations, the organization has not enlisted many of the women on the street, and the goal of a large, powerful prostitutes' union still seems far off.

The clients of the prostitute

The existence of the prostitute is only possible where there is a demand for her services. Yet, as we have seen, her customers are rarely treated as harsly by society. Customers are referred to as "Johns" or "tricks" by the prostitute. They come from all levels of society and have a variety of reasons for seeking

BOX 20.1

Pornography is big business

As of 1978, the pornography business was estimated to gross $4 billion a year in the United States, and many consider that to be a highly conservative estimate. But even at that figure, the pornography industry would have been making about as much as the conventional film and record industries combined (Cook, 1978).

Who is making all this money? A large chunk goes to the men's magazines. The top 10 "skin" magazines (including Playboy, Penthouse, and Hustler) have a combined circulation of over 16 million and make almost $500 million a year. According to Forbes, expensive-looking magazines like Playboy command the highest prices ever charged by large-circulation magazines in publishing history. Because of the high cover price, news dealers have a great incentive to promote these magazines, and today 30 percent of all newsstand sales come from magazines that only 25 years ago would not have been allowed on the stands (Cook, 1978).

Another major part of the porn industry is the "adult" film business, which grosses around $400 million a year. This business went through a radical transformation in the early 1970s when a 35mm hard-core film, Deep Throat, reached a mass audience. This film not only brought the demise of the cheap 16mm film but created a new, more respectable audience for X-rated features. It also began a porn star system by introducing Linda Lovelace, and it put X-rated films into the big money —it has grossed more than $50 million worldwide since its release in 1972. Most porno films make a lot of money —an average of 200 percent return on investment to the makers and a reasonable profit to the exhibitors. These films are also gaining extra life from the home videocassette market, which has become a major consumer of X-rated products.

The biggest part of the X-rated economy in the United States is the network of adult bookstores and peep shows. Although the stores sell lots of paperbacks and magazines, the big money is apparently in the peep shows. A customer drops a quarter in the peep machine and sees the first 2 minutes of a 16-minute film. In order to see the rest of the film, he must continue to drop in quarters at 2-minute intervals. According to one retired Los Angeles vice officer, a single machine takes in $75–$120 a week, which is split 50-50 between the supplier and the store owner.

Other aspects of the pornography industry include sexual toys and marital aids (vibrators, lubricants, S-M equipment) and the mail-order porn business, which spends $50 million a year on advertising alone. As Forbes points out, "The bulk of the sex industry operates underground, where hundreds and thousands of small producers —print shops, film processors, publishers, filmmakers, photographers—feed a vast distribution system" (reported in Cook, 1978, p. 82).

The pornography business has made a lot of people rich, including magazine publishers, filmmakers, distributors, amusement operators, and adult bookstore chain owners. It has also made several lawyers wealthy, since purveyors of pornography continue to be prosecuted at the federal, state, and local levels. As Al Goldstein, flamboyant publisher of Screw magazine has said, "It's a high profit business, pornography, but it's also high risk. My lawyers have made as much as I have."

out sex for money. Men who have a current, active sexual relationship may patronize a prostitute as a source of sexual variety or to engage in behavior that the usual sexual partner refuses or may not like. Some men with wives or girlfriends may seek out a prostitute if they feel their frequency of intercourse at home is not great enough, as when their wife is pregnant or ill. And men who are away from home may seek the services of prostitutes.

For some men, the prostitute may be the only source of sex. They may lack social skills and thus feel too shy to approach women; they may be handicapped and require special help in having sex; or they may be deformed to the point where they feel unable to approach women who are not prostitutes. Some men may be oriented toward sexual behaviors that are difficult to maintain in a continuing relationship, such as sado-masochism. Finally, there are many men who prefer to remain unencumbered by deep relationships and seek out prostitutes to avoid the commitment often implied in sexual relationships with nonprostitutes.

How many men patronize prostitutes? It is difficult to estimate. Kinsey (1948) came up with a figure of 69 percent of all white males having had some experience with prostitutes. Many feel this was an overestimate, even for a time when sexual attitudes were more repressive. The Hunt (1974) report found that approximately 20 percent of men under age 35 had had at least 1 interaction with a prostitute.

The client is still the most important uninvestigated factor in understanding the maintenance of prostitution. Although we usually think of controlling prostitution by arresting and prosecuting the women, control should be directed at the *demand* rather than the *supply*.

OBSCENITY AND PORNOGRAPHY

Pornography is big business, not only in this country but all over the world. As Box 20.1 points out, pornographic films, books, and paraphernalia are enjoying great popularity in this country. What laws govern our exposure to such sexual materials?

Obscenity laws

In the seventeenth century, as a result of puritanical rule in England, the first banning of obscenity occurred when profanity was outlawed. Similar laws to maintain religious rule and ban material that was antireligious appeared in America in the 1700s. Sexually explicit materials became included in such bans, since they were considered antireligious.

The first obscenity trial in the United States was conducted in 1815, when a man was charged with displaying a painting of a nude woman. Another trial in 1821 led to a conviction for selling sexually explicit literature—the now-famous *Fanny Hill* case. In 1842 the federal government passed a law forbidding importation of obscene material from other countries. Next came the famous **Comstock laws**, which made it illegal to send obscene materials through the mail. These laws, and their underlying theme that sexually explicit materials "corrupt and deprave" those exposed to them, have dominated legal thinking since that time. The argument is that obscene materials must be controlled and that those who produce and distribute them must be punished because the material harms the individual and leads him to antisocial actions. In legal terms, this constitutes a "clear and present danger" and permits legal interventions to protect society from "dangerous" obscene materials.

A major problem with these laws was that none of them clearly and precisely defined what was obscene. Thus, anyone could be prosecuted at any time, depending on the whim of the prosecuting authorities. In 1957 the landmark case of *Roth* v. *the United States* was ruled on by the Supreme Court. The argument raised in this case was that obscenity laws violated the constitutional guarantees of free speech and press. The suit was lost. The Court declared that obscentiy was *not* protected by these constitutional guarantees. However, the Court felt obliged to provide a way of defining obscenity, so it stipulated that three criteria must be met for material to be considered obscene: (1) it must appeal to the "prurient" interest in sex; (2) it must be "offensive" in that it affronts "contemporary community standards" of what is acceptable sexual material; and (3) it must be "utterly lacking in redeeming social value."

Despite this attempt to define obscenity, there are in fact few explicit criteria for either prosecutors or defenders to use as guidelines. Too much is still left to the interpretation of prosecutors, judges, and juries. The result has been continuing confusion in obscenity cases, with trials and appeals constantly reversing one another.

The period since *Roth* v. *the United States* has been understandably confusing. Congress became concerned enough over the problem to establish a Commission on Obscenity and Pornography in 1967. The commission, which was appointed by President Lyndon Johnson, concerned itself with many aspects of the issue but particularly focused on the actual effects of pornography on people exposed to it. The findings and recommendations of the committee, which we will discuss shortly, were presented to President Richard Nixon,

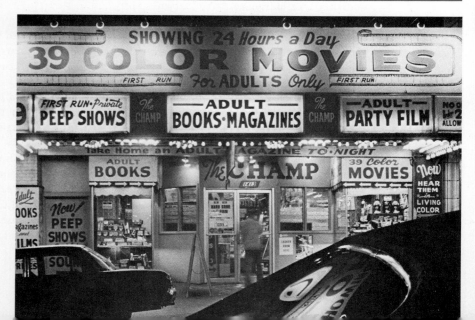

A typical "combat zone" scene of stores that sell pornography.

who categorically rejected them. He refused to accept the commission's conclusion that the legal responses to pornography were excessive in light of the
minimal danger of the material.

The Supreme Court added still another level of confusion to the legal
morass in their 1973 decision in the case of *Miller* v. *California*. This decision
revised the federal guidelines of the Roth decision and in effect moved the
judgment of what is obscene back to local communities. The Court's rewor-
ing of the Roth definition of obscenity makes prosecution more likely and puts
the burden of proof of the serious intent of any work on the shoulders of the
defendant. This move was seen as a swing back toward more conservative and
restrictive controls. And, in fact, there has been an increase in prosecutions for
obscenity in the last decade. It is obvious that the United States is still
struggling with the problems of defining and managing sexual materials and
that the most recent laws are inadequate in responding to the needs of society.
Communities vary so greatly in their approach to the problem that nationally
distributed magazines, for example, are likely to be prosecuted in a few local
areas that have particularly restrictive definitions of obscenity. Some attempt
must be made to find a general standard that would reduce such discrepancies.
For the present, however, confusion reigns.

**The effects of
pornography**

Basic to all the legal arguments about obscenity is the idea that people are
somehow damaged as the result of exposure to obscene materials. If there is no
negative effect from pornographic material, the laws protecting us from exposure are unnecessary and, since they interfere with the freedoms of speech and
press, cannot be defended. If there is indeed danger from such material, it is
necessary to define what materials are dangerous and to separate them from
those that present no such danger.

One of the central charges of the U.S. Commission on Obscenity and
Pornography was to provide an answer to this question of the potential danger
of obscene materials. The investigators for the commission reviewed the available scientific literature, the current experimental studies, and the opinions of
professionals who were experts on the subject. They conducted surveys of
social scientists and of the general public and sought direct information by
sponsoring experimental studies. They also looked rather closely at the experiences of Denmark, a country that had suspended all controls on pornography
in 1965.

The massive amount of data and opinion was summarized in the commission's report (1970). The report concluded that there was no support for the
belief that exposure to erotic material is a significant factor in producing
criminal sexual behavior in adults. The report pointed out that no lasting
changes could be found in those adults exposed to such material and that the
short-term effect of overexposure is satiation and boredom—not arousal to
commit sex crimes. As to the effect of erotic material on children, the commission felt that there were not enough data to make a judgment. They did find
that the general public was strongly opposed to allowing children free access to
pornographic materials.

The commission made the following recommendations, based on the investigations:

1 *All restrictions on adult access to pornographic materials should be elminated.*
2 *There should be control of children's access to such materials.*
3 *Unwanted public exposure to such materials should be controlled by rules governing public display and advertising.*
4 *Massive sex education programs should be instituted to counter the need for pornography and to change fundamental attitudes about sexuality.*
5 *Further and more extensive studies should be done on the effects of pornography.*

Although President Nixon rejected these recommendations, the commission's report is still an influential document in understanding some of the issues concerning pornography and is continuing to have an impact on local and federal responses to the problem.

Several investigators have followed up on the commission's call for additional research and have tended to support the commission's conclusions. One area of research has focused on the varying responses of men and women to pornography. Contrary to the stereotype that men are more sexually aroused by erotic materials than woman, studies have shown that most men and women are aroused by sexually explicit material of all types, although women may be more responsive to literary presentations, whereas men may be more responsive to visual presentations (Schmidt, Sigusch, and Schafer, 1973).

One of the studies conducted for the commission concerned the response of married couples to extensive exposure to pornographic materials. Mann and his associates (1973) showed movies to married couples every night for 4 weeks. Some of the films were erotic; some were not. The couples kept records of the frequency and nature of their sexual activities during the experimental period. Analysis of the records showed that the erotic films did stimulate sexual activity at first. However, satiation and boredom soon set in. The couples did not mimic the sexual behaviors they saw in the films but generally stayed with the sexual behaviors that were typical for them.

Another approach to assessing the possible dangerous effects of pornography has been to study individuals convicted of sexual crimes to see what function exposure to pornographic materials may have played in their pasts. Such studies have revealed that there had been *less* exposure to pornography among the sex offenders than there had been in matched samples of other types of criminals. In fact, the sex offenders showed rather prudish attitudes toward such materials and found them unpleasant. Pornography had not played an important role in their upbringing, in their lives at the time they committed the sex-related crimes, or in their current lives in jail (Goldstein and Kant, 1973).

The largest "experiment" of all on the effects of pornography involved Denmark's rescinding of all laws against obscenity in 1965. In effect, the country totally decriminalized the production and distribution of pornographic materials. When Kutchinsky (1973) examined the statistics for sex-related crimes prior to and following this action, he found that there was not only no increase in the incidence of sex-related crimes but that after 1965 several categories of sex crimes actually decreased significantly. Interestingly, sales of pornographic materials slowed considerably after the initial rise following the law change. Much of the pornography produced in Denmark is now sold to visitors rather than to the Danes.

The contemporary American scene is a confusing mixture of increased censorship *and* increased explicitness of the sexual material available for sale. Because of the legal confusion created by the 1973 Supreme Court decision, responsible individuals are tending to avoid the problem by not presenting sexual materials at all, while those who are less responsible, who are more concerned with capitalizing on the confusion, are rushing into the vacuum with highly explicit and tasteless materials. The irony of the current wave of conservatism in this area is that it is suppressing the beauty of artistic presentations of an important aspect of human life while creating a market for a much more unpleasant type of sexual material.

SUMMARY

1   Laws governing sexual behavior include those regulating the nature of sexual activity, the age of participants, familial and legal relationships of sexual partners, procreation, and sexual criminal acts.

2   Regulations of the nature of sexual interaction include those governing "crimes against nature" (*sodomy laws*) and rape. The sodomy laws are extremely vague and are rarely enforced, except in the case of homosexuals.

3   Regulations governing the age of the participants include those against child molestation and statutory rape. *Child molestation* is defined differently in different jurisdictions depending on what age is considered the cutoff point for childhood and what activities are considered molestation. Statutory rape laws also vary depending on the definition of age of consent and on the relative ages of the participants.

4   Laws governing the relationship of the participants include those against *adultery, fornication, cohabitation, bigamy,* and *incest.* Regulation of procreation includes law governing use and dissemination of contraceptives, laws regulating abortion, and laws regarding *sterilization* (both *compulsory* and *voluntary*) and artificial insemination.

5   Miscellaneous sexual criminal acts, from voyeurism to pedophilia, are often lumped into the category of sexual offenses, and the convicted criminal is referred to as a *sex offender* or *sexual psychopath.* Grouping a wide diversity of individuals into such a stigmatizing category has resulted in mistreatment of those who have committed minor offenses. Handling such crimes on an individual basis would be preferable.

6   Although *prostitution*—the selling of sexual favors—is illegal in most of the United States, there is a movement to decriminalize it. Such decriminalization would reduce victimization of the prostitute, free the legal system to deal with crimes that have victims, and help to reduce the incidence of venereal diseases.

7   The main types of prostitutes are the *streetwalker* (who may have a *pimp* as boss and protector), the *bar girl (B-girl)*, the *brothel prostitute*, the *call girl*, and the *massage parlor prostitute*. There is also a small number of *male prostitutes* who may be *hustlers*, with homosexual men as clients, or *gigolos*, with women as clients. Unlike the stereotype of women being forced into prostitution by pimps or organized crime, most women drift into the profession gradually, attracted by the promise of high income and an easy life.

8   Clients of prostitutes may be men with regular sex partners who are seeking sexual variety or additional sex, men away from home, men who lack the social skills to develop relationships, handicapped individuals, men with unusual sexual orientations, and men who have no interest in ongoing sexual relationships.

9   Laws against obscenity and pornography in America essentially began with the *Comstock laws*, which prohibited the sending of obscene materials through the mail. The idea behind such laws was that sexually explicit materials "corrupt and deprave" people exposed to them, creating a "clear and present danger" to society. In 1957, the Supreme Court defined obscenity in its ruling in the case of *Roth* v. *United States*. However, this definition was still vague, and the legal issues of pornography and obscenity continued to be confusing. In 1973 the Supreme Court moved the judgment of what is obscene back to the communities, creating even greater confusion.

10   In its 1970 report, the U.S. Commission on Obscenity and Pornography concluded that there is no evidence to show that exposure to eplicit sexual materials is a significant factor in producing criminal sexual behavior in adults. The commission recommended that all restrictions on adult access to pornographic materials be lifted but that children's access be controlled. President Nixon rejected the recommmendations.

11   Additional research on the effects of pornography have shown that men and women show similar arousal to erotic materials and that both tend to become satiated and bored with excessive exposure to such materials. Studies of individuals convicted of sex crimes have found that they have actually had less exposure to pornographic materials than have other criminals. Legalization of pornography in Denmark appears to have resulted in reduced incidence of sex crimes.

**ADDITIONAL
READING**

Evans, Hilary. Harlots, Whores, and Hookers: A History of Prostitution. New York: Taplinger, 1979.
>   *A history of prostitution from classical times to the present. Interesting and well written.*

* **Geis, Gilbert.** *Not the Law's Business? An Examination of Homosexuality, Abortion, Prostitution, Narcotics, and Gambling in the United States.* New York: Schocken, 1979.
>   *An excellent discussion of laws concerning "victimless" crimes. The book makes a number of thought-provoking points.*

* **The Report of the Commission on Obscenity and Pornography.** New York: Bantam Books, 1970.
>   *The report of a presidential commission appointed to study the issue of obscenity and pornography in our society. Quite readable and includes a review of the history of pornography as well as the legislative recommendations made by the committee.*

Sexual Law Reporter. (1800 North Highland Ave., Suite 106, Los Angeles, CA 90028)
>   *A bimonthly publication that summarizes both judicial and legislative actions affecting sex laws.*

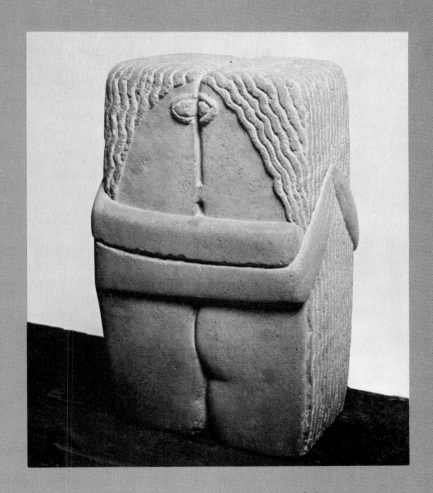

The future of human sexuality

chapter
21

In the film *Sleeper*, Woody Allen depicts a future in which, among other things, people can enter a cabinet similar to a telephone booth, the "orgasmatron," to receive electronically induced orgasms. Although Allen's imaginative invention is presented for comic effect, some feel it is no more fanciful an idea of things to come than those proposed by serious scientists. It is, however, somewhat more unusual than most predictions coming from scientific sources.

Forecasting future developments is not just an exercise in speculation. Human behavior, sexual and otherwise, is likely to follow from current trends. And while there may be problems in envisioning the future, it is important to try, for if we do not anticipate our future, we are more likely to become the victims of change rather than the directors of that change. Changes in our society are now occurring so rapidly and have such great impact on our lives that science must offer whatever help it can in smoothing transitions to the future.

In this chapter we will be gazing into our crystal ball to see what the future has in store for human sexuality. In order to hold reign on our imaginations and to stay somewhat more reality-based than Woody Allen's orgasmatron, we will focus our discussion on four areas that are likely to be important in shaping these future developments: (1) technological advances in conception and in contraceptive knowledge, (2) changes in social factors of importance to sexual behavior, (3) advances in research on sexual behavior, and (4) the dissemination of knowledge about sexuality.

TECHNOLOGICAL ADVANCES IN CONCEPTION AND BIRTH CONTROL

Human sexual behavior has always had to be controlled and modified by the procreative needs of the family and of society. Technological developments in the control of birth have already changed that relationship dramatically. Emerging advances in conception and birth control show every indication of even more dramatic changes in the future.

Advances in conception

As technological developments continue in the area of conception, the bearing of children is becoming more and more separated from sexual interaction. Where once sexual intercourse and procreation were nearly synonymous, they are now almost separate topics. One set of developments contributing to this separation is the increasing ability to scientifically predict conception, thus making it easier to control. Another set of developments is the increasing ability to modify both the roles of the partners in conception and the biological act itself.

One of the most striking advances has been the development of techniques for conceiving humans in test tubes rather than in the mother. In this process, discussed in Chap. 7, the fertilized egg is transplanted into the uterus of a woman for the remainder of its prenatal development. Although the usual host is the egg donor—the biological mother—and the usual sperm donor is the mother's husband, any combination of biological and foster parents is possible with this procedure. The biological contributors may not necessarily be the same man and woman who eventually raise the child. The egg and sperm could come from one set of contributors; the child could be nurtured in the uterus of a third person; and the newborn could be raised by still others. One vision of the future might include "baby farming," involving various combinations of test-tube and transplant techniques. In such cases, problems of parenting responsibilities, lineage, inheritance, and so on could become highly complicated. How far off is the reality of this image? It's difficult to say, but there are already several healthy test-tube babies growing up in the world today.

Another technological change separating conception from sexuality is the use of **surrogate mothers**. Many women have already served as surrogates for infertile women by being artificially inseminated with sperm from the husband and carrying the child to term. The child is then adopted by the couple. In a more futuristic version of surrogation, transplant procedures could be used to move an already fertilized egg from a fertile biological mother to the uterus of a surrogate, who would nurture the child to full term. This procedure would be used in the cases of women whose own uterus is hostile to fetal development or who have a history of miscarriage. Although such embryo transplants are most likely to be performed for medical reasons, our scenario for the future might well include women who wish to raise their own biological children but

*America's first
test-tube baby.
There is obviously
no less parental
pride in these
parents for their
child.*

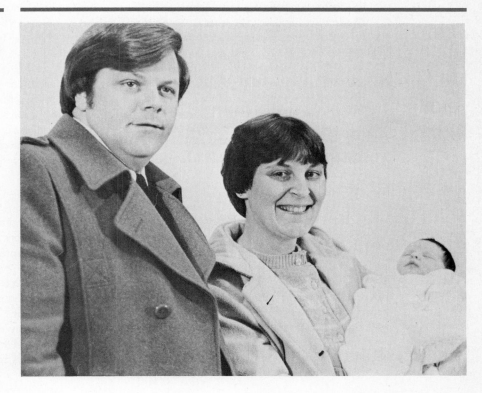

whose careers or personal desires make pregnancy undesirable. Once again, issues of parental responsibility and questions of custody if the surrogate mother wants to keep the child raise numerous legal and moral issues. And these issues and questions are already upon us, with the first birth (in November 1980) of a baby from what the press referred to as "rent-a-womb."

Other advances have been made in the area of artificial insemination. This method is currently used if the husband is infertile or if the husband's sperm requires a condensing procedure to increase the chances of conception. One interesting possibility for contraception-conception is for a husband to "bank" sperm while he is young, have the sperm frozen, obtain a vasectomy so there is no concern about unwanted pregnancies, and still father his own biological child several years later through artificial insemination. One of the major implications of artificial insemination is that it makes sexual intercourse unnecessary for procreation—an idea that challenges a number of traditional views in our society.

Finally, at the very fringe of science is the technique of **cloning**—reproduction of a new organism from one "parent." In effect, a genetic carbon copy of the parent is produced from a single cell. Since the genetic material of parent and offspring is exactly the same, there is no variation in inherited characteristics. Although no advanced animal life forms have yet been cloned, the technology for doing so seems to be moving into the realm of possibility. If cloning ever reaches the human level, it will raise several important questions: Who would be chosen for such reproduction? Who would do the choosing? What effect would cloning have on society?

One highly publicized approach to efforts to control the genetic makeup of offspring was one sperm bank's efforts to recruit "superior" men, such as Nobel Prize winners, as donors. Most of the potential donors refused the honor. The public reaction against this bizarre elitism was understandable. The entrepreneurs who initiated this program, aside from being poorly attuned to the values of a democratic society, were demonstrating great naiveté as to the relative contribution of genes to a person's visible accomplishments in the world.

Another development with implications for the future of human conception is the recent work on **recombinant DNA** In such research, genetic materials from one organism are inserted into the genes of another organism. So far, this work has been done with only the simplest of organisms, but it is fascinating to speculate as to what it might mean if the techniques were to be applied to human organisms.

*The future of
contraception*

Although the technological developments in conception have important implications for sexual behavior, preventing conception has even greater potential impact. Contemporary couples may desire pregnancy one or two times in their lives; for every other sexual interaction, they will be trying to *avoid* conceiving a child. Currently available methods are reasonably effective, but most have undesirable side effects. What types of contraceptives that overcome these problems might we see in the future?

Male contraceptives   Although vasectomy is the most direct and effective
method of male contraception, it is not commonly used. One problem that has
kept many couples from choosing vasectomy is its lack of reversibility in most
cases. Thus, current work has focused on the development of reversible vasectomy techniques. One avenue being explored is mechanically blocking the
male tubes rather than cutting them. Experiments using various surgical clips,
valves, and dissolvable substances have been conducted. One device even uses
a magnetically activated valve that can be opened or closed from outside the
body. However, the varous mechanical devices have generally proved wanting.
Greater success has been achieved with newer microsurgery processes. It is
reasonable to expect that there will be a truly reversible vasectomy in the
future.

Research on chemical interference with sperm production or sperm maturation has been going on for several years. The problem is to find a chemical
agent that kills sperm without side effects to the man and without genetic
alteration of the sperm that might lead to defective offspring should a pregnancy occur. Thus far, all chemicals tried have failed to meet one or the other of
these criteria. One drug that looked very promising when tried with prison
inmates turned out to be incompatible with alcohol use. In trials with nonin-
mates, it was discovered that if the drug was taken while the man had alcohol
in his body, he experienced nausea, vomiting, and other violent side effects.
Another chemical, called Inhibin, a natural substance produced by the testes to
shut down sperm production, shows greater promise for development as a safe
male contraceptive in the future.

Female contraceptives   The amount of research on female contraception
continues to be far greater than that on male contraception. Many feel this
reflects a bias among investigators who expect women to carry the burden of
contraception. However, scientists in this area defend themselves by pointing
out that the male system is less modifiable than the woman's and that the
large doses of drugs required to inhibit sperm production also tend to inhibit
the male sex drive. They also argue that with women the problem is how to
suppress one egg per month, while with men it is how to suppress the production of millions of sperm each day. Some researchers have gone as far as
arguing that more emphasis is placed on female contraception methods because more is known about the action of female hormones as a result of
research with the Pill. This argument actually puts women in double jeopardy:
Because they were singled out for unequal responsibility in the past, this
inequality must continue in the future.

Some researchers suggest that the female system, being more complex and
consisting of several structures that are involved in the conception and development of an embryo, gives them more flexibility in the ways they can
interfere with the process. Perhaps. But vasectomy of the male is much easier
than tubal ligation of the female, yet many times more women have had tubal
ligations compared to the number of men who have had vasectomies. It is
obvious that the decision of who is to bear responsibility for birth control is

affected by sex-role factors. Before any changes can occur in equalizing the responsibility, there will have to be changes in the general sociopolitical climate as well as in technological areas.

There have indeed been some promising technological advances in female birth control methods. Among nonhormonal approaches, there has been renewed interest in the rhythm method. If the prediction of ovulation could be made highly reliable, rhythm would become the method of choice for women who prefer a natural approach. Although at this point no reliable method has emerged, several tests based on body chemicals or processes have been reported as showing promise.

Along other lines, safer and easier abortion methods have been developed and are already in use. One approach being studied is self-administered abortion, in which the woman would introduce a chemical into her uterus by douching that would cause expulsion of the embryo. Despite the current ease and safety of abortion methods, most women would still prefer to prevent pregnancy rather than deal with the moral and health issues of terminating a pregnancy.

Research on various types of IUDs is also continuing in an attempt to refine them and make them safer. One possibility is a chemically laden capsule that makes the uterine wall inhospitable but does not carry with it the physical difficulties of the stiff, plastic IUDs. Such a capsule would be inserted once a month and would prevent pregnancy during that period. Although the capsule does involve chemical intervention, it would work locally rather than centrally in the female system, which would give it important advantages over the Pill. The capsule is still being investigated, so it is not yet known whether it will prove successful and safe.

As we noted in Box 8.2, a number of avenues are being explored in the development and refinement of barrier methods of contraception, such as cervical caps, sponges, and so on. A different type of barrier method being explored is closing off the fallopian tubes by methods other than tubal ligation. Zatuchni (1980) describes current work on an adhesive tissue that is injected into the tube to close it off permanently. A nonpermanent method, in which surgical plugs are placed in the fallopian tube, is also being tested.

One new approach that is both a male *and* female method consists of a condom that is worn during intercourse and that disintegrates in the vagina, depositing a spermicidal chemical. The male can thus control the deposit of the chemical, but it is still the woman who must experience any problems created by it.

Hormonal methods of contraception will probably continue to be favored throughout most of the world in the foreseeable future. Refinements of current technology seem to be the thrust of today's research. The primary focus is to find the minimal dosage and correct balance of hormones for effective contraception with the fewest possible side effects. And the search is continuing for a pill that need be taken only once a week or once a month.

Research has also focused on ways of administering hormones besides the oral route. This approach is being pursued particularly in those countries where oral contraceptives have not been effective in reducing birth rates because women have problems taking the pills on a regular basis. Alternatives include injections that are given once a month or even less often, steroid implants, chemically impregnated vaginal rings, and even inhalable contraceptives.

SOCIOCULTURAL
CHANGES

The term *sociocultural* is actually a shorthand label for the numerous nonbiological factors that are likely to contribute to future changes in sexual behavior. To be totally accurate, we should probably label these factors as being "socio-politico-economic-psycho-cross-cultural." Well, you get the picture: Many forces within the society affect human sexual behavior, and changes in them will affect the future directions of that behavior. Although this has always been the case, there has never been a time in human history when these forces have been so strong and changing so rapidly. The result is that we live in a society that is advancing at such a dizzying rate that severe strains are being put on our ability to cope with the change.

Alvin Toffler, in his books *Future Shock* (1970) and *The Third Wave* (1980), has described the kinds of strains that this rapid change is producing. Among the most important changes that are likely to have a major impact on sexual behavior are (1) rapid and far-reaching changes in sex roles of men and women, (2) influence of the feminist movement, (3) changes in our views of marriage and parenthood, and (4) changes in attitudes toward sexuality. Although we have examined all these forces to some extent elsewhere in this book, here we will look at how they may affect future sexual behavior.

*Changes in
sex-role-related
behavior*

Changes in sex (gender) roles have been most clearly expressed in changes in the woman's role. Women have already entered the work force in large numbers, and the 1980s began with one out of every two households containing a working wife. Women have achieved equality with men in college attendance, and educational levels of men and women have narrowed so that there is less educational difference between them than ever before. Many other changes of a similar nature indicate that women are moving closer to traditional male roles and activities.

It is reasonable to expect the movement of women into some of the traditional masculine areas to be met with a corresponding movement of men into some of the traditional female activities. For example, it might be expected that men would begin to become more involved in child care and household responsibilities. Yet this is not the case. There has, in fact, been little movement of men into traditionally female areas (Weitz, 1977; Kaplan and Bean, 1976; Tavris and Offir, 1977). The result has been that women have had to *add* their new roles and activities to already existing feminine responsibilities. A woman may be going out to work or to school with all the same pressures and problems as her husband but still is expected to come home to prepare meals,

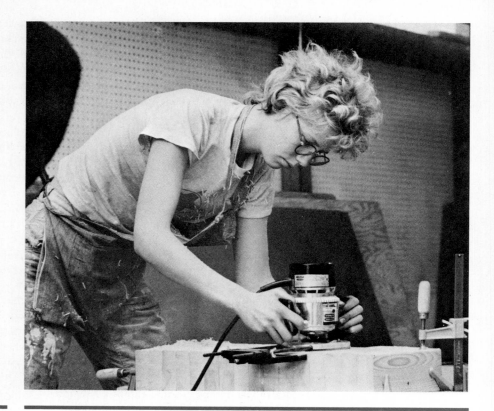

clean house, manage children, and generally be in charge of other aspects of family life. Weitz found that this scenario was true in several societies she studied, including the USSR, China, and Israel.

Changing sex-role behavior has thus meant that women are adding new dimensions to their roles but that men are not experiencing reciprocal change. This is even more clear in the area of sexual interaction. Whereas surveys are finding that women are moving closer to men in sexual behavior (frequency of intercourse, and so on), the male profiles have shown much less change. This lack of corresponding change may indicate that a serious clash of the sexes in sex-role-related areas is due in the near future.

One type of sexual problem that may arise from evolving sex roles has been labeled the *new impotence* by Ginsberg, Frosch, and Shapiro (1972). These therapists noted that many of their recent cases involved men who were experiencing erectile problems during sexual encounters with assertive women. They considered these cases to be casualties of the effort of traditionally oriented males to adapt to more sexually active, secure, and assertive contemporary women. However, other clinicians feel this problem has been seriously overestimated.

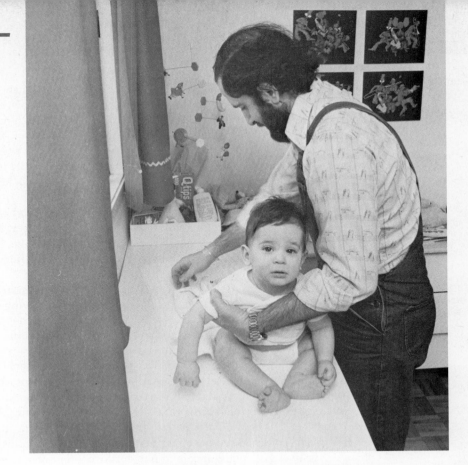

*Gender role
behaviors are
changing in our
society.*

One of the tasks of the social sciences is to recognize the potentially problematic situations that may be developing as a result of change and to help create an atmosphere in which such change can be absorbed and more easily accepted by people. They have their task cut out for them in helping people realize the fact that women are changing and that men must adapt to these changes if a long period of confusion, conflict, and stress is to be avoided.

*The influence of
feminism*

Feminism, the philosophy of the women's rights movement, has already had an enormous impact on society. Many of the sex-role changes we have already noted developed out of this new (or renewed) feminist perspective. The 1980s and 1990s will certainly see even greater activity from feminist groups in demanding equality for women in a wide variety of areas. While there are many different factions within the feminist movement, all agree that things must continue to change if women are to realize their individual potential. The groups differ, however, on how radical the change should be and how quickly it should be achieved. Many feminists note that despite their efforts and much rhetoric by influential leaders in this country, there has been little real change. Kaplan (1976) summarized the feelings of many women with her comment that "we are pessimistic but not without hope" (p. 391).

The changes in sexual behavior promoted by the feminists are generally in the direction of sexual equality. In the feminist version of utopia, sexual encounters would be between two totally equal people, as much involved with each other as with their own needs and desires. The woman would not have to feel responsible for the man's satisfaction nor feel that she is a passive recipient of his "gift" of love. The man would be free of the responsibility of bringing the woman to orgasm and would not see her orgasm as his "badge of success" as a man.

There would appear to be advantages for both sexes in the changes toward equality in sexual relationships advocated by feminists. However, the traditional roles are so deeply ingrained that change does not come easily. Existing roles, attitudes, and behaviors would have to be dramatically altered to even begin to approach the feminist ideal.

*Changes in
marriage and
parenthood*

As the 1980s began, there was one divorce for every two marriages, and the increased spiral in the divorce rate showed no signs of slowing. This is not necessarily a reflection of dissatisfaction with the state of marriage, however, since most of those who divorce also remarry. The problem seems to lie in the traditional view of marriage as a lifelong commitment to one partner. The divorce and remarriage pattern may reflect the rapid changes people must absorb in other aspects of their lives; that is, they may find it most appropriate to have different spouses at different stages in their lives. Margaret Mead felt that this type of **serial monogamy** would become even more typical in the future and that it is not inappropriate to the way of life that must be lived in our fast-paced society. One type of partner may be very good for us during one phase of our lives but totally inappropriate during another phase. For example, two people may form an excellent, mutually beneficial relationship during the young, career-growth years when both of them are working toward advancement in their professions. However, this may not be a good alliance for raising children at a later time. Both may want a partner who is more willing to be involved in child rearing while they continue their career development. Thus, both might gain from a change in partner at this stage in their lives. In later years, when retirement becomes a major focus, still another partner might be more ideal than either of the earlier mates.

But what if one partner is satisfied with the relationship while the other is dissatisfied? There is no easy resolution to this problem. However, the previous solution of our society—locking the dissatisfied partner into the marriage relationship—certainly did not work, as divorce, desertion, wife abuse, and other such statistics tell us.

If serial monogamy or some similar change involving several different partners becomes the marriage pattern of the future, sexual behavior will certainly be affected dramatically. Many of the problems of sexual relationships today arise from the boredom that sets in when a couple's lovemaking becomes ritualized and nearly automatic. In a system allowing regular changing of marriage partners, boredom would seem to be less of an issue. In fact, the potential for partner changes may actually keep the current partners more involved with each other. Individuals would have to actively keep their partners interested in the relationship rather than depend on the rules of society to keep them together, as is the case with traditional marriage. Marital sex might also take on some of the characteristics of nonmarital sex, which derives much of its intensity and diversity from partners actively trying to hold on to each other. The irony of this situation is that the potential ease of changing partners may actually reduce the need or the desire to do so. Monogamy may thus be strengthened by loosening the traditional bonds tying the partners together and guaranteeing their marriage.

There are many other possible shapes that marriage may take in the future. What does seem clear is that the traditional marriage must adapt to the forces currently challenging every assumption upon which marriage as we have known it is based. To some extent, traditional marriage has been incompatible with an active and satisfying sexual life by making sex part of a nonnegotiable, "no-cut" contract. Sexual satisfaction has always been something of an invisible force in the survival of marriages. In the next few years it promises to be a much more visible force, either helping to maintain marriage in some form that we recognize or leading to the development of something new.

Parenthood has also been an important source of definition of sexual behavior. Comfort (1972) noted that the developed countries of the world are moving toward zero population growth, meaning that "few people will have more than two children and many will have none" (p. 282). This trend affects many of our traditional views of the family. People will rarely engage in sexual intercourse for the purpose of procreation, and they will be less bound to each other "for the sake of the children." With only one or two children, if any, the parents will have a relatively short child-care period in their adult lives. Thus, the central focus of life for most people in the future will no longer be parenting activities.

What are the roles of marital partners to be if not mother and father? Without those roles to define the family relationship, what is a family? It is likely that the reason for couples to stay together will have to be motivated by the value of the relationship itself rather than by "keeping the family together." If this is the case, the sexual satisfaction of any couple will be an important component in maintaining their relationship. Compared to the sexual functioning of today's couples, future sexual functioning in marriage must be much more interactive, mutually satisfying, and capable of maintaining the couple's interest in each other if they hope to stay together as a "family."

While we can only speculate on how this changing nature of the family unit will be expressed, it is clear that many of the patterns are changing without awareness on the part of most people in our society. Many people find themselves with one foot planted firmly in the traditional marriage roles defined by parenthood while the other foot is tentatively reaching into a future where totally new views and values will be required. The problem is that these two orientations are moving apart rapidly, and individuals must soon decide which foot to move if they are to avoid being pulled apart.

Large-scale attitude surveys can give us a few insights into the important directions sexual behavior is likely to take in the future. In other chapters we reviewed many of the major surveys made before 1980. During 1980 two popular women's magazines, *Cosmopolitan* and *Redbook*, conducted major surveys of the sexual behavior of their readers. Although the problems inherent in the survey method are compounded when the survey sample is narrowed to the readership of a specific magazine and even further to those who voluntarily return their responses, it is still worthwhile to look at some of the results reported.

Both *Redbook* (Sarrel and Sarrel, 1980) and *Cosmopolitan* (Wolfe, 1980) had large returns. *Redbook* received replies from 20,000 women and 6,000 men; *Cosmopolitan* received responses from a whopping 106,000 women. Although all the results have not yet been reported, initial analyses contain some interesting findings.

Both surveys showed a trend of continuing liberalization of attitudes among women in general. However, the differences between the results of the two surveys are so striking as to make one wonder just what the contemporary woman is really like. The "Cosmo" woman is described as younger, better educated, and more liberated than women in the general population. Even so, the responses seem even more liberal than might be expected by that profile. As an example, here are some of the preliminary *Cosmopolitan* findings:

At least half of the sample said they had had an extramarital affair.
60 percent wanted more sex in their lives.
74 percent felt it is possible to have a good sexual relationship without love.
47 percent had had sexual intercourse with more than one man on the same day.
70 percent had had sexual intercourse on a first date.
85 percent had participated often in fellatio and cunnilingus.
15 percent had regularly had anal sex.
23 percent had had sexual relations with more than one partner at the same time. (pp. 254–265)

Although these behaviors and attitudes are far more liberal than might be expected, the results are even more surprising when we consider the size of the sample.

Because the 1980 *Redbook* survey did not ask the same questions in the same way as the *Cosmopolitan* questionnaire, no direct comparisons are possible. However, examining the general areas of sexual behavior in both surveys reveals the *Redbook* readers to be a far more conservative group of people. Nevertheless, the changes from the 1975 *Redbook* survey to the 1980 one were consistently in a more liberal direction. There was greater interest in sexual relationships, more sexual activity, greater sexual satisfaction, and an increased desire for a more active role in one's own sexual fulfillment. Sexual experimentation was higher, and guilt was lower. Thus, the trend among *Redbook* readers was in the same direction as that of the Cosmo girls, although the degree of change reported was much more moderate.

What implications do these surveys have for our predictions about the future of sexual behavior? We will probably see a continued liberalization of sexual attitudes and behaviors for all people, but with a sharper rise in the change curve for women. This will lead to a further narrowing of the differences between men and women in their sexual attitudes, desires, activities, and satisfaction, both in and outside marriage. There will be fewer feelings that constraints are being imposed by society and a greater sense of freedom to experiment in the sexual sphere. On the negative side, there is a growing trend toward impersonal sexual encounters, and both men and women report feeling forced to include intercourse in the early part of relationships. This represents a trend toward sex for its own sake without deep relationships—a trend viewed with mixed feelings. Overall, however, it looks as though in the future more people will have satisfying sex lives than in the past and present.

RESEARCH
DIRECTIONS

Much of this text has been concerned with reviewing, analyzing, and discussing the contributions that various sciences have made to our knowledge of human sexuality. The questions that scientists are currently exploring are likely to be the areas of importance in the not too distant future. At a conference on New Directions in Sex Research sponsored by the National Institutes of Health in 1974, many of the major figures in contemporary sex research summarized the work to date in their respective areas and then discussed the directions research would probably take (Rubinstein, Green, and Brecher, 1976). Among the general areas discussed were the ethics and the likely subject matter of future research.

With regard to ethics, the participants noted that studying sexual behavior continues to be a sensitive research area as far as the general public is concerned. Many researchers have worked hard to keep their research on the highest plane. Awareness of subjects' rights and of the potential harm to subjects, both physically and psychologically, has been of prime importance. Violations of subjects' rights could beckon the repressive forces that are always in the wings where investigations of sexual behavior are concerned.

The subject matter of future sexual research is what interests us the most, given our desire to see where scientific research is likely to add to our current knowledge. The report of the conference listed five areas that are deserving of greater research efforts: (1) gender role and gender identity studies, (2) research on the effects of changes in contemporary morés, (3) studies of sexual minorities (homosexuals, bisexuals, and so on), (4) studies of therapy for sexual dysfunction, and (5) research on sexual functioning among the physically handicapped. In addition to these areas of applied research, the conference also emphasized two areas of basic research worthy of extra effort and support: study of the neurophysiology of sexual response and of the biochemistry of sexual response. Finally, the conference report stated that an open mind must be maintained for the unforseeable research areas that might emerge and become "worthy gambles" in terms of furthering our understanding of sexual behavior.

The conference report represents an interesting attempt to look into the future of research explorations. A review of the 1980 volumes of the *Journal of Sex Research* and the *Archives of Sexual Behavior* indicates that the vast majority of studies now indeed fall into the general categories identified by the conference as deserving of future emphasis. Some areas not included in the conference lists that are represented by emerging research and that are likely to have future importance include the effects of various drugs on sexual arousal, further work on conception and birth control, and basic research on mechanisms of arousal.

DISSEMINATION OF
INFORMATION
ABOUT HUMAN
SEXUALITY

All the activity of accumulating knowledge about human sexuality would be of little value if the next and most crucial step were not taken: disseminating that information to the public in a meaningful and effective manner. If this information were only passed back and forth among interested scientists, therapists, and others, or if we were to accumulate facts only for the purpose of storing them away in learned treatises, little would be accomplished in increasing society's knowledge and understanding of sexual functioning.

We have noted throughout this book that many sexual adjustment problems result from a lack of factual information, which forces people to operate on pure conjecture or downright misinformation. It is our belief that the most effective "sex therapy" and the best approach to prevention of problems is to provide people with the best and most reliable information available. Of all the future scenarios we could generate, the most optimistic is one in which people are well equipped with sound knowledge about sexual functioning, have an open and accepting attitude toward their own and others' sexuality, and are encouraged to feel that there is always more to learn and to pursue that knowledge at every opportunity.

The dissemination of information about sexual behavior is referred to as *sex education*. This term, unfortunately, carries with it the image of public school programs for adolescents. It is actually more appropriate to consider sex education as applying to all people, regardless of the target age group or the institutional structure under which a program is conducted. In 1964 a group of concerned professionals established the Sex Information and Education Council of the U.S. (SIECUS) to make information available to the whole society, from preschool through adulthood. Kirkendall (1965) included the following major points in his summary of the goals and objectives put forth by the group:

1   *To provide the individual with an adequate knowledge of his own physical, mental, and emotional maturation processes as related to sex.*
2   *To eliminate fears and anxieties relative to individual sexual development and adjustments.*
3   *To develop objective and understanding attitudes toward sex in all of its various manifestations—in the individual and in others.*
4   *To give the individual insight into his relationships to members of*

both sexes and to help him understand his obligations and responsibilities to others.

5   To provide an appreciation of the positive satisfaction that wholesome
human relations can bring to both individual and family living.

6   To build an understanding of the need for the moral values that are
essential to rational decision making.

7   To provide enough knowledge about the misuses and aberrations of
sex to enable the individual to protect himself against exploitation
and against injury to his physical and mental health.

8   To provide an incentive to work for a society in which such evils as
prostitution and illegitimacy, archaic sex laws, irrational fears of sex,
and sexual exploitation are nonexistent.

9   To provide the understanding and conditioning that will enable each
individual to use his sexuality effectively and creatively in his several
roles as spouse, parent, community member, and citizen. (p. 42)

These goals stress the importance of knowing one's own physical, mental,
and emotional processes as related to sexuality, not only because knowledge
provides a basis for adequate sexual adjustment but also because it helps
banish fears and anxieties. The goals also emphasize understanding diverse
sexual orientations. People fear and hate things that they do not understand.
With knowledge comes demystification, dispelling of hate, reduction of discrimination, and acceptance.

Several of the goals on the SIECUS list acknowledge the great value of an
informed citizenry in changing the sexual values of society in a more sex-
positive direction. However, listing the goals of an ideal sex education approach is just a beginning. When and how should different materials be
learned? Who should teach them? These are major issues yet to be resolved.

Sex education programs, particularly those based in public schools, rarely
find ready acceptance in communities. Surveys show that a majority of parents

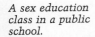

*A sex education
class in a public
school.*

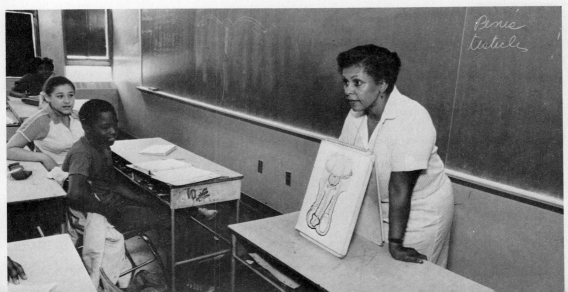

favor sex education. Nevertheless, a vocal and organized minority often emerges to oppose such programs. The same fears and anxieties that educators hope to wipe out by disseminating information prevent that educational effort from gaining easy access to the members of the community. The parents seem to be saying, "I'm not going to teach this stuff to my kids, and I'll be damned if I'll let you do it either." The professional hoping to begin a sex education program for children or adolescents must keep in mind that such seeming irrationality stems from fear and must be dealt with as such.

Sex education for adults is a more complex issue. The goals usually involve reducing fears and anxieties, providing information not previously available to the target group, and providing a base for the enhancement of the emotional and sexual attachments the person now has or will form in the future. There is an important secondary bonus to having a society of informed individuals: They become the *source* of education and enhancement of the sexual lives of others, especially their own children. Formal programs of sex education would probably not be needed in a society in which the great majority of people have reached some adequate level of sexual knowledge and adjustment. The fact that our society is so desperately in need of remedial sex education programs is only another indication of just how far we fall short of this ideal, informed society.

We envision a society in which the full potential for this physical, emotional, and interactional dimension of people can be realized. How do we attain this goal? We have argued from the beginning of this text that knowledge is the foundation for that ideal society and that the dissemination of sexual knowledge to all is of central importance. It is only through inquiry into sexual matters, generation of *real* knowledge through the most reliable and valid methods of investigation, and dissemination of that information in an effective and sensitive manner that we can achieve the goal of a society in which sexuality can reach its full potential.

SUMMARY

1   Among technological advances in the area of conception are test-tube babies, *surrogate motherhood*, artificial insemination, and *cloning*. Many of these techniques carry with them complex legal and moral implications.

2   Among techniques being explored in the area of contraception are reversible vasectomies, a male Pill, improved abortion methods, capsule IUDs, surgical plugs for the fallopian tubes, and a condom that dissolves into spermicidal chemicals. Researchers are also looking for improved hormonal methods and different ways of administering them.

3   *Sociocultural* changes that will affect sexual behavior include changes in male-female sex-role behavior, increased influence of *feminist* philosophy, increased incidence of *serial monogamy*, fewer children, and liberalization of sexual attitudes.

4   Research directions that indicate future areas of importance in sexual behavior include study of: (1) gender roles and gender identity, (2) effects of

changes in morés, (3) sexual minorities, (4) therapy for sexual dysfunction, (5)sexual functioning of the physically handicapped, (6) the neurophysiology of the sexual response, and (7) the biochemistry of sexual response.

5   The accumulation of knowledge about sexual functioning is useless unless the information is disseminated. One organization concerned with such *sex education* is SIECUS, which emphasizes learning about one's own sexuality, eliminating fears and anxieties, understanding and accepting those with other orientations, and changing the attitudes of society as a whole so that it is more sex-positive. If adults were to have a greater understanding of sexual functioning based on accurate information, formal sex education programs would be unnecessary.

Glossary

KEY TO PRONUNCIATION

a   *a* as in *back*
ah   *a* as in *ha*
aw   *aw* as in *shawl* or *a* as in *tall*
ay   *ay* as in *play*
e   *e* as in *set*
ee   *ee* as in *see*

iy   *i* as in *kite*
i   *i* as in *sit*
oh   *o* as in *boat*
oo   *oo* as in *soon*
ow   *ow* as in *how*
yu   *ew* as in *few* or *you* as in *you*
uh   vowels in unstressed syllables pronounced "uh" as the *a* in *about*

Exceptions are sometimes made when syllables are clearly pronounceable.
Example: her

abortion [ah-BOR-shun] Termination of a pregnancy may be spontaneous or induced by physicians.

accessory to sex Sexual assault on a victim, such as a minor, who is by definition unable to consent.

actual use effectiveness rate Practical effectiveness of a birth control method, having taken human error into account.

acute phase In rape trauma syndrome, the initial phase of disorganization after the attack.

adultery [uh-DUL-tuh-ree] Consensual sexual intercourse between a married person and someone other than his or her spouse.

agape [ah-GAH-pay] Altruistic, unselfish love.

amenorrhea [ay-men-uh-REE-uh] Failure of menstruation to occur.

amniocentesis [am-nee-o-sen-TEE-sis] Procedure by which fetal cells are extracted from the amniotic sac and tested for genetic disorders.

amnion [AM-nee-ahn] Inner membrane of the implanted blastocyst.

ampulla [am-PUL-uh] Enlarged area of the vas deferens used to store sperm. Also refers to the portion of the fallopian tube after the infundibulum.

anaclitic [an-uh-KLIT-ik] *depression* Depression resulting from maternal deprivation.

anal [AY-nul] *-genital sex* Insertion of the penis into the rectum of the partner.

anal [AY-nul] *stage* Second psychosexual stage in which libido is focused on the organs and activities of elimination.

androgyny [an-DRAH-juh-nee] The idea that a flexible blend of masculine and feminine traits is the optimal sex-role orientation.

androstenedione [an-dro-STEEN-diy-ohn] Androgen produced by the adrenal gland.

anger rape Rape motivated by the need to express pent-up feelings of rage at women.

anonymity [an-uh-NIM-ih-tee] Procedure by which a subject's identity is disguised in research.

anovulatory [an-OV-yu-luh-tor-ee] *cycles* Menstrual cycles in which no egg is released.

anterior pituitary [pi-TOO-uh-tehr-ee] Forward lobe of the pituitary gland, which affects sexual behavior.

areola [uh-REE-oh-luh)] Area of dark skin around the nipple of the breast.

asceticism [a-SEHT-uh-sism] Nonsexuality.

asexual [ay-SEKS-yu-ul] *homosexual* Homosexual who seldom engages in any one type of sexual activity and who generally regrets his or her sexual orientation.

atresia [ah-TREE-zee-ah] Deterioration of partially mature ova in the follicles of the ovaries.

attraction The study of why people like each other.

aversive therapy Therapy that pairs an arousing but unwanted stimulus with an unpleasant (aversive) stimulus.

bar girl See *B-girl.*

Bartholin's [BAR-to-linz] *glands* Pair of glands located just inside the labia minora on either side of the introitus that produces a small amount of fluid during sexual arousal.

basal [BAY-sul] *body temperature* Rhythm method of birth control based on monitoring the body temperature to detect ovulation.

behavioral Psychological approach based on learning or conditioning theory.

behavioral deficit Lack of adaptive learning in a particular area.

behavioral-learning theories See *behavioral*.

behavior therapy techniques Therapy techniques based on learning and conditioning theories that seek to change maladaptive behavior via the process of relearning.

bestiality [bes-chee-AL-uh-tee] See *zoophilia*.

beta subunit HCG radioimmunoassay [ray-dee-o-im-yu-no-AS-ay] Recently developed pregnancy test that can detect pregnancy as early as 8 days after conception.

B-girl Prostitute who works out of a bar or club. Also called *bar girl*.

bigamy [BIG-uh-mee] Being married to more than one person at the same time.

Billings method See *cervical mucus secretion method*.

bisexual [biy-SEKS-yu-ul] Person who finds both sexes equally attractive as sexual partners.

blaming the victim Blaming the victim of a crime for having caused the crime.

blastocyst [BLAS-to-sist] Hollow ball of cells formed out of the morula on the fourth day after conception.

blitz rape Rape via a sudden physical assault.

body Main part of the uterus. Also refers to the shaft of the penis.

Braxton Hicks contractions Occasional painless uterine contractions, which may occur during the third trimester of pregnancy.

breasts Areas of fatty tissue over the chest that contain the mammary glands.

breech presentation Buttocks-first position of the fetus at the start of labor.

brothel [BRAH-thul] *prostitute* Prostitute who works in a house of prostitution.

bulbocavernosus [bul-bo-kav-er-NO-sus] Exterior muscle surrounding the introitus that opens and closes the introitus.

butch See *dyke*.

calendar method Rhythm method of birth control that uses a calendar to monitor the menstrual cycle.

call girl Prostitute who works primarily by appointment with a select group of regular clients.

Candida albicans [KAN-di-dah al-bi-kans] Fungus that produces moniliasis.

case study In-depth study of an individual.

castration [kas-TRAY-shun] Surgical removal of the testes.

casual dating Courtship that involves little commitment and is primarily recreational in nature.

catheter [KATH-uh-ter] Thin tube used to drain urine from the bladder.

caudal [KAW-dul] *block* See *spinal block*.

cephalic [suh-FAL-ik] *presentation* Head-first position of fetus at the start of labor.

cervical [SER-vi-kul] *mucus secretion method* Rhythm method of birth control based on examination of changes in the cervical mucus to detect ovulation.

cervical os [SER-vi-kul ohs] Small opening at the center of the cervix.

cervix [SER-viks] Neck of the uterus, which projects into the vagina.

cesarean [suh-ZEHR-ee-un] *section* Delivery of a baby via a surgical incision in the abdominal and uterine walls.

chancre [SHANG-ker] Small sore caused by a viral infection.

chancroid [SHANG-kroid] Sexually transmitted disease.

child molestation Any type of sexual approach aimed at a child.

Chlamydia trachomatis [khlah-MID-ee-ah trah-KO-mah-tis] Organism that causes lymphogranuloma venereum.

chorion [KOR-ee-ahn] Outer membrane of the implanted blastocyst.

chromosomes [KRO-mo-sohmz] Thin, strandlike structures in the nucleus of a cell that carry the genes.

circumcision [ser-kum-SIZ-yuhn] Surgical removal of the foreskin of the penis.

circumferential penile transducer [pee-niyl-trans-DOOS-er] Device that measures the degree of penile erection.

classical conditioning Learning, through repeated pairings, to associate a response with a stimulus that does not usually produce that response.

climacteric [kliy-MAK-tuh-rik] Aging process of the reproductive system in females that occurs approximately between the ages of 45 and 60; also used to refer to the aging process of the reproductive system in males.

clinical treatment Medical treatment.

clitoris [KLIT-uh-rus] Small shaftlike structure that juts out from the vulva just below the mons pubis. Stimulation of the clitoris produces orgasm.

cloasma [klo-AYS-ma] Darkened spots on the face produced by estrogen.

clomiphene citrate [KLO-mi-feen SIT-rayt] Common fertility drug.

cloning [KLO-ning] Reproduction of an organism from a single parent cell.

close-coupled homosexuals Homosexual couples with long-term, marriagelike relationships.

closet queens Homosexuals who have never divulged their orientation to anyone except their immediate partners.

cognitive [KAHG-ni-tiv] *aversion* Aversion therapy using mental images as the aversive stimulus.

cohabitation Liaison in which the partners live together.

coital [KO-ut-ul] *abstinence* Ban on coitus often prescribed as part of sex therapy.

coitus interruptus [KO-ut-us in-ter-up-tus] Withdrawal of the penis from the vagina just prior to ejaculation to prevent pregnancy.

combat zones Specific areas in cities or towns in which illicit activities are tolerated.

combination pill Birth control pill containing both estrogen and progesterone.

coming-out process Self-labeling and entrance by an individual into the homosexual community.

companionate love Love experiences marked by feelings of affection and attachment, without the extremes of passionate love.

compulsory sterilization Sterilization against a person's will.

Comstock laws Early set of antipornography laws.

conception Point at which an ovum is penetrated by a sperm, and an embryo begins to develop.

condom [KAHN-dum] Birth control device consisting of a thin sheath of material that fits tightly over the erect penis.

confidence rape Rape in which the rapist lures the victim to an unprotected setting under false pretenses.

congenital adrenal hyperplasia [kun-JEN-uh-tul a-DREE-nul hiy-per-PLAY-zee-uh] *(CAH)* Condition in which a genetic female develops ovaries and masculine genitals because of abnormal functioning of the adrenal gland.

congenital syphilis [kun-JEN-uh-tul SI-fuh-lis] Syphilis contracted by the fetus of an infected mother.

consent defense Common rape defense which argues that the victim in fact gave consent and that therefore no rape occurred.

contact tracing Finding all the sexual contacts of a STD-infected individual from the time of the infection onward.

contraceptive [kahn-truh-SEP-tiv] Something that prevents conception.

control group Subjects in an experiment who are not given the experimental treatment.

controlled reaction Rape victim's suppression of feelings under a calm and subdued exterior following the rape.

coronal [kor-OH-nul] *ridge* Ridge that separates the glans from the body of the penis.

corpora cavernosa [KOR-por-uh kav-er-NO-suh] Twin cylinders of spongy tissue in the penis, which become engorged with blood during an erection. Also present in the clitoris.

corpora spongiosum [KOR-por-uh spun-jee-O-sum] Cylinder of spongy tissue in the penis, which becomes engorged with blood during an erection.

corpus albicans [KOR-pus AL-bi-kans] Structure that replaces the corpus luteum after 12 days if pregnancy has not occurred.

corpus luteum [KOR-pus loo-TEE-um] Yellowish structure formed out of an empty follicle after ovulation has occurred, which secretes hormones.

correlation research Research that measures the relationship between two variables but cannot determine causality.

correlation coefficient Statistic that measures the strength of the relationship between two variables.

cortex Outer layer of the ovary that contains the follicles. Also refers to a part of the primitive gonadal tissue.

couvade [koo-VAHD] Sympathetic pregnancy in which husband develops symptoms similar to those of pregnant wife.

covert [KOV-ert] *sensitization* Form of cognitive aversion.

Cowper's [KOW-perz] *glands* Small glands on either side of the base of the penis which secrete an alkaline fluid during sexual arousal that lubricates and reduces the acidity of the urethra.

crab louse See *Pediculus pubis.*

cremaster [kree-MAS-ter] *muscle* Muscle that raises and lowers the testes in response to changes in temperature.

cremaster [kree-MAS-ter] *reflex* Reflexive raising and lowering of the testes in response to temperature changes.

crown-to-rump measurement Length of the embryo as measured from the top of the head to the rump.

CR measurement See *crown-to-rump measurement.*

cruising Searching for casual sexual partners by homosexuals.

cryptorchidism [krip-TOR-ki-dizm] Condition in which the testes fail to descend via the inguinal canal into the scrotum.

culpotomy [kawl-PO-to-mee] Tubal ligation performed via vaginal incision.

cunnilingus [kun-i-LING-gus] Stimulation of the female's genitals by the partner's mouth.

cystitis [sis-TIY-tis] Inflammation of the bladder.

dartos [DAHR-tohs] *muscle* Muscle that expands and contracts the scrotum in response to changes in temperature and sexual stimulation.

dependent variable Variable that is measured in an experiment to assess the effects of the independent variable.

detumescence [dee-too-MES-ens] Loss of erection.

diaphragm [DIY-a-fram] Used as a method of birth control, it is a dome-shaped latex cup that is covered with spermicidal jelly or cream and inserted into the vagina prior to intercourse.

diethylstilbestrol [diy-eth-il-stil-BES-trol] *(DES)* See *morning-after pill.*

dilatation Expansion of cervical opening.

dilation and curettage [kyu-RET-uj] *(D and C)* Method of abortion in which a sharp metal curette is used to scrape out the contents of the uterus.

dilation and evacuation (D and E) Method of abortion used in early part of second trimester that is a combination of vacuum curettage and dilation and curettage methods.

dildo [DIL-doh] Artificial penis substitute.

dissatisfied heterosexual See *sexual preference disturbance.*

dissatisfied homosexual See *ego-dystonic homosexuality.*

Donovania granulomatis [dahn-o-VA-nee-ah gran-yu-LO-ma-tis] Bacterium that causes granuloma inguinale.

douching [DOO-shing] Rinsing or cleansing of the vaginal canal.

Down's syndrome Genetic disorder involving physical abnormality and mental retardation.

dramatize Psychological defense mechanism used to reduce anxiety via a compulsive retelling of the source of the stress in an attempt to desensitize the individual to it.

dropping See *engagement.*

dyke [diyk] Lesbian who assumes a traditionally masculinized gender role.

dysfunctional homosexual Homosexual who is sexually active with a number of partners but who feels much regret about his or her homosexual activities.

dysmenorrhea [dis-men-uh-REE-uh] Painful menstruation.

dyspareunia [dis-per-OO-nee-ah] Painful intercourse.

eclampsia [eh-KLAMP-see-uh] State of convulsions and coma. Possible outcome of untreated toxemia.

ectoderm [EK-to-derm] Embryonic tissue that forms the nervous system, sensory organs, and the skin.

ectopic [ek-TAHP-ik] *pregnancy* Condition in which a fertilized egg becomes implanted in an area other than the uterus.

edema [e-DEE-muh] Swelling of the limbs as a result of water retention.

effacement Extent to which the cervix is incorporated into the lower part of the uterus and thins out in preparation for birth.

eggs See *ova.*

ego-dystonic [dis-TAH-nik] *homosexuality* Homosexuals who are not comfortable with their sexual preference and wish to change it.

ejaculation [ee-JAK-yu-lay-shun] Expulsion of semen from the penis.

ejaculatory [ee-JAK-yu-luh-tor-ee] *duct* Short duct at the end of the vas deferens, which empties into the urethra.

ejaculatory [ee-JAK-yu-luh-tor-ee] *incompetence* See *inhibited male orgasm.*

Electra [e-LEK-truh] *complex* Conflict occurring during phallic stage, in which girls experience penis envy (according to Freud).

elephantiasis [eh-luh-fan-TIY-uh-sis] Massive swelling of the genitals due to untreated lymphogranuloma venereum.

emission [ee-MI-shun] First stage of ejaculation when semen is forced to the base of the urethra.

endocrine [EN-do-krin] Glands that manufacture and secrete hormones.

endoderm [EN-do-derm] Embryonic tissue that gives rise to the digestive and respiratory systems.

endometriosis [en-do-mee-tree-OH-sis] Growth of endometrial tissue in places other than the uterus.

endometrium [en-do-MEE-tree-uhm] Inner layer of the uterine wall, which is rich in blood vessels that carry nutrients from mother to fetus.

engagement Turning of the fetus in the uterus 3 weeks prior to birth to position the fetus for a head-first delivery.

environmentalists Scientists who emphasize the importance of early experience and environmental influences in the determination of behavior.

epidemiological [ep-i-dem-ee-o-LAJ-i-kul] *method* Method that deals with incidence, distribution, and control of disease in a population.

epididymes [epi-DID-i-meez] Tubes running from the testes to the vas deferens, which receive sperm from the testes and store them for ripening.

epidural [ep-i-DOO-rul] *block* See *spinal block*.

episiotomy [ee-piz-ee-AHT-o-mee] Incision made to widen the vaginal opening to let the baby pass during birth without tearing the skin.

erogenous [i-RAHJ-uh-nus] *zones* Areas of the body that produce sexual excitement when stimulated.

eros [I-rohs] Love based on physical attraction.

estrogen [ES-troh-jen] *deficiency hypothesis* Hypothesis that menopausal symptoms are due to the lowered estrogen levels in menopausal women.

estrogen [ES-troh-jen] *replacement therapy (ERT)* Use of estrogen preparations by postmenopausal women to alleviate menopausal symptoms.

estrogens [ES-troh-jenz] Group of related hormones that produce female sex characteristics.

estrous [ES-trus] *cycle* Sexual cycle found in females of lower mammalian species.

eugenic [yu-JEN-ik] Aimed at improving the gene pool of a population.

eunuch [YU-nuk] Castrated male.

excitement First stage of human sexual response marked by increasing vasocongestion in the genital regions.

exclusive dating Courtship in which there is exclusive involvement with the other.

exhibitionism Exposure of one's sexual organs to an unconsenting other.

experimental group Subjects in an experiment who are given the experimental treatment.

experimental method Method of science aimed at studying causes in which there are at least two groups, one who receives a treatment and the other who does not.

experimenter bias Expectations of the experimenter, which distort the objective recording of data.

expressed reaction Rape victim's overt restlessness, anxiety, and depression after the rape.

expulsion Contraction of urethral bulb and penis, which forces semen out of the meatus.

extinction Repeated presentation of a conditioned stimulus without the unconditioned stimulus in order to break the link between the two; or the nonreinforcement of a previously reinforced response.

extramarital sex See *adultery*.

extrinsic [ek-STRIN-sik] *theories* Theories of sexual development that focus on environmental forces that shape gender role and sexual patterns.

fading Behavioral technique in which a response is allowed to occur but is gradually transferred to a new stimulus.

fallopian [fuh-LO-pee-un] *tubes* Pair of tubes that transfer mature eggs from the ovaries to the uterus.

fellatio [fuh-LAY-shee-o] Stimulation of the penis by the partner's mouth.

female-superior position Coitus with the female on top.

feminism Philosophy of the women's rights movement.

femme [fem] Lesbian who assumes traditionally feminized gender role.

fertility Capacity to produce offspring.

fertility workup Medical assessment aimed at identifying and rectifying causes of a couple's infertility.

fertilization See *conception*.

fetal [FEE-tul] *alcohol syndrome* Condition present in a certain percentage of babies born to alcoholic mothers. Characterized by physical deformities and mental retardation.

fetishism [FET-ish-izm] Sexual variance in which sexual arousal occurs in response to inanimate objects.

fibrinogenase [fiy-BRIN-o-jen-as] Secretion from the prostate which produces a temporary coagulation of the semen within the vagina so that the sperm do not leak out.

fimbriae [FIM-bree-ee] Hairlike projections at the edges of the infundibulum of the uterus.

fixation Failure to resolve the conflicts involved in a particular psychosexual stage.

follicles [FAH-li-kulz] Vesicles on the cortex of the ovary, which contain immature egg cells.

follicle-stimulating [FAH-li-kul STIM-yu-layt-ing] *hormone (FSH)* Hormone that regulates the development of eggs and sperm.

follicular [fah-LIK-yu-ler] *phase* Stage of the menstrual cycle in which an egg matures within an ovary.

foreplay Lovemaking activities that occur as a prelude to coitus.

foreskin See *prepuce.*

fornication [for-ni-KAY-shun] Crime of sexual intercourse between consenting, unmarried adults.

free association Psychodynamic technique in which the client is to say freely whatever comes into his or her mind without reservation.

French kissing Kissing in which the lips are separated and the tongue enters the mouth of the partner.

frenulum [FREN-yu-lum] Fold of skin that connects the prepuce with the underside of the glans in males and the clitoris in females.

frigidity Obsolete term for inadequate female sexual functioning.

functional analysis Behavioral assessment procedure that seeks to identify the specific antecedents and consequences of a particular behavior.

fundus [FUN-dus] Upper, widest part of the uterus.

gain-loss theory Theory of attraction suggesting that relative increases and/or decreases in rewards from another are more important regulators of attraction than absolute levels of rewards.

gametes [GAM-eets] Mature reproductive cells: sperm in men and eggs in women.

gay bar Bar that serves a primarily homosexual clientele.

gay Turkish bath Clubs catering to male homosexuals seeking immediate sexual encounters.

gender [JEN-der] *identity* Person's own view of his or her gender as being male or female.

gender identity disorder Diagnostic category that includes transsexuals and gender identity disturbances in children.

gender identity disturbance See *transsexual.*

gender role Constellation of behaviors that are characteristic of each sex.

general paresis [puh-REE-sis] Obsolete term for parenchymatous neurosyphilis.

genes [jeenz] The basic hereditary units.

genital [JEN-uh-tul] *folds* Part of the rudimentary external genitals.

genital herpes [HER-peez] See *herpes simplex type 2.*

genitals [JEN-uh-tulz] External sex organs of either sex.

genital stage Final psychosexual stage in which libido is directed toward sexual pleasure with others.

genital swelling Part of the rudimentary external genitals.

genital tubercle [TOO-ber-kul] Part of the rudimentary external genitals.

gestation [jes-TAY-shun] Period of pregnancy from conception to birth.

gigolos [JIG-uh-loz] Male prostitutes who cater to women.

"give-to-get" principle Attending to the sexual needs of the partner so that he or she will attend to you.

glans [glanz] Head or tip of the penis or clitoris.

gonadal [go-NAD-ul] *tissue* Generalized genital tissue in the embryo that eventually becomes either the testes or ovaries.

gonadotrophin- [go-nad-o-TRO-fin] *releasing hormone (GnRH)* Hormone that controls the production of follicle-stimulating hormone (FSH) and luteinizing hormone (LH).

gonads [GO-nadz] Internal sex glands of either sex (testes or ovaries).

gonorrhea [gahn-uh-REE-uh] Most common sexually transmitted disease.

granuloma inguinale [gran-yuh-LO-muh ing-gwi-NAY-ee] Sexually transmitted disease.

group marriages Formal marriages in which there are three or more partners.

habitual abortion Three or more miscarriages in a row.

Hegar's [HAY-garz] *sign* Change in the consistency of the lower part of the uterus that indicates pregnancy.

Hemophilis ducreyi [hee-MO-fil-us du-KRAY-ee] Bacterium that causes chancroid.

hermaphroditism [her-MA-fro-diyt-izm] Condition in which an individual develops both male and female sexual structures.

herpes [HER-peez] *ping-pong* Reciprocal reinfection of herpes simplex type 2 in a sexually active couple.

herpes simplex [HER-peez SIM-pleks] *type 2* Sexually transmitted viral infection.

heterosexual [het-er-o-SEKS-yu-ul] Adult of either sex whose preferred sexual partner is a member of the opposite sex.

heterosocial skills Social skills that aid successful functioning in a heterosexual environment.

homoerotic [ho-mo-ee-RAH-tik] *expression* Expression of men's sensual desire for men.

homophobia [ho-mo-FO-bee-uh] Anxiety and fear of homosexuality.

homosexual [ho-mo-SEKS-yu-ul] Adult of either sex whose preferred sexual partner is a member of the same sex.

homosexual community Homosexual subculture existing parallel to, but separate from, the heterosexual world.

homosexual rape Forcing a member of the same sex to engage in sexual acts.

hormone [HOR-mohn] *replacement therapy* Use of externally administered sex hormones to replace those lost through castration, ovariectomy, or menopause.

hormones [HOR-mohnz] Chemicals produced by various glands in the body that enter the bloodstream and regulate physiological functioning.

hormone therapy Injection of hormones of the opposite sex as part of sex-reassignment therapy.

hot flash Common symptom of menopause.

Huehner test Test that examines the cervical mucus for the presence of sperm after intercourse.

human chorionic gonadotropin [ko-ree-ON-ik gohn-ad-o-TROP-in] *(HCG)* Hormone suspected of causing morning sickness.

human sexual response The cycle of sexual arousal and resolution in humans.

hustlers Male prostitutes who cater to a homosexual clientele.

H-Y antigen [AN-ti-jun] Substance produced by the chromosomes that causes the development of testes.

hymen [HIY-mun] Thin, nonfunctional membrane that partially covers the introitus in most virgin females.

hypersexuality Insatiable sexual desire.

hypertension High blood pressure.

hypothalamus [hiy-po-THAL-uh-mus] Small area of the brain that controls the regulation of the sex hormones.

hysterectomy [his-tuh-REK-tuh-mee] Surgical removal of the uterus.

hysterosalpingogram [his-ter-o-sal-PING-go-gram] Test to see if the fallopian tubes are open.

hysterotomy [his-tuh-RAH-tuh-mee] Method of abortion that involves major abdominal surgery in which the fetus is excised from the uterus and removed through an incision in the abdominal wall.

identification Resolution of Oedipus complex, in which boy eliminates anxiety and guilt toward the father by seeking to become just like him.

identification defense Common rape defense which argues that the accused has been misidentified as the rapist.

implantation Attachment of the blastocyst to the endometrium—the onset of pregnancy.

impotence [IM-put-ens] Obsolete term for male inhibited sexual excitement.

incest [IN-sest] Sexual relations with a blood relative.

incubation [in-kyu-BAY-shun] *period* Amount of time it takes for symptoms to appear after infection has occurred.

independent variable Treatment variable that is manipulated in an experiment.

indifferent period Period of embryonic development during which the genital system is generalized, that is, before sexual differentiation begins.

informed consent Procedure by which a client or research subject is fully informed of and consents to the nature and procedure of a treatment or research before it is delivered.

infundibulum [in-fun-DIB-yuh-lum] Cone-shaped end of the fallopian tubes located near the ovaries.

inguinal [ING-gwi-nul] *canal* Passageway by which the testes descend from the abdomen of the fetus into the scrotum.

inhibited ejaculation See *inhibited male orgasm*.

inhibited female orgasm Sexual dysfunction in which the female does not experience orgasm.

inhibited male orgasm Sexual dysfunction in which the male is unable to ejaculate while in the vagina.

inhibited sexual desire General lack of interest in all of the sexual aspects of life.

inhibited sexual excitement (ISE) In males, inability to achieve or maintain sufficient erection to engage in coitus; in females, lack of responsiveness to sexual stimulation during sexual encounter.

insertee [in-ser-TEE] Passive partner in homosexual couple.

inserter Active partner in homosexual couple.

interpretation Psychodynamic technique in which the therapist indicates the unconscious meaning of the client's actions.

interstitial [in-ter-STISH-yul] Cells in the testes that produce testosterone.

interstitial cell stimulating hormone (ICSH) See *luteinizing hormone.*

interview Method of research that involves verbally questioning people.

interviewer biases Expectations and opinions of the interviewer that interfere with the collection of objective data.

intramural [in-tra-MYU-rul] *portion* Last section of the fallopian tubes, which is contained in the walls of the uterus.

intrauterine [in-tra-YU-tuh-rin] *device (IUD)* Mechanical form of birth control consisting of small device placed in the uterus.

intrinsic [in-TRIN-sik] *theories* Theories of gender role development that emphasize the importance of internal (physiological or developmental) factors.

introitus [in-TRO-i-tus] Entrance to the vagina.

intromission [in-tro-MI-shun] Insertion of the penis into the vagina.

isosexual [iy-so-SEKS-yu-ul] Of the same sex.

isthmus [IS-mus] Term used to describe the narrow parts of the fallopian tubes and the uterus, through which the eggs and sperm must travel.

"the itch" See *scabies.*

Kegel exercise Repeated contractions of the pubococcygeal muscle. Used to improve vaginal elasticity and strength.

Klinefelter's syndrome [KLIYN-fel-terz SIN-drohm] Sex chromosome pattern of XXY or XXXY.

labia majora [LAY-bee-uh muh-JOR-uh] Outer fatty folds of skin, or "lips," of the vulva.

labia minora [LAY-bee-ah muh-NOR-uh] Inner, smaller lips of the vulva.

labor The birth process.

Lamaze [luh-MAAZ] *method* Method of natural childbirth.

lanugo [luh-NOO-go] Downy hair that grows on the body of the fetus.

laparoscopic [lap-ah-RAHS-ko-pik] *tubal sterilization* Tubal ligation performed via abdominal incision and using a laparoscope.

latent homosexual Individual with homosexual preferences who does not act on them.

latent stage Fourth psychosexual stage, in which libido is latent and not localized in any area of the body. Also refers to stage of syphilis during which there are no visible symptoms.

learned maladaptive behavior Behavior that has been learned but is problematic.

leather shop See *sex shop.*

lesbian [LEZ-bee-un] Female homosexual.

Leydig's [LIY-digz] *cells* See *interstitial cells.*

liaison [LEE-ay-zahn] Sexual relationship formed outside of a mateship.

libido [luh-BEED-o] Freud's term for sexual, or life, energy.

lightening See *engagement.*

long-term phase In rape trauma syndrome, the phase of reorganization following the acute reaction to the rape.

ludis [LOO-dis] Love that is perceived as a game or conquest.

lumpectomy [lump-EK-to-mee] Surgical removal of a breast lump.

luteal [LOOT-ee-ul] *phase* Stage of the menstrual cycle in which the corpus luteum is formed and the uterus is prepared to nourish a fertilized egg.

luteinizing [LOOT-ee-un-iyz-ing] *hormone (LH)* Hormone that regulates the production of estrogen and testosterone.

lymphogranuloma venereum [lim-fo-gran-ye-LOH-muh veh-NEE-ree-um] Sexually transmitted disease.

male prostitutes Men who sell sexual favors.

male-superior position Coitus with the male on top.

mammary [MA-muh-ree] *glands* Mammalian organs that produce milk that is used to nourish offspring.

mania [MAY-nee-uh] Obsessive love marked by extremes of jealousy and despair.

masochism [MA-so-kizm] Derivation of sexual pleasure from the infliction of pain on oneself.

massage parlor prostitute Prostitute who works in a phoney massage parlor that is really a cover for prostitution.

mass screening Checking members of the general population for a disease.

mastectomy [mas-TEK-to-mee] Surgical removal of the breast and surrounding tissue.

masturbation [mas-ter-BAY-shun] Self-stimulation of the genitals.

maternal deprivation Lack of emotional care from a constistent mother figure when young.

mateship Formalized, socially sanctioned sexual unions, such as marriages.

meatus [mee-AY-tus] Opening in the glans of the penis through which urine and semen pass.

medulla [muh-DUL-uh] Inner layer of the ovary. Also refers to a part of the primitive gonadal tissue.

membranous urethra [MEM-bruh-nuss yu-REE-thruh] Short part of the urethra between the prostatic urethra and the penile urethra.

menarche [men-AR-ke] First menstrual period.

menopause [MEN-o-pawz] Cessation of menstruation during the climacteric.

menstrual [MEN-stroo-ul] *cycle* The reproductive cycle of human and some other primate females, which is marked by the presence of menstruation.

menstrual extraction Method of abortion in which menstrual fluid is sucked out without the use of dilation or anesthesia.

menstrual phase Stage of the menstrual cycle in which the vascular lining of the uterus is shed through the cervix and vagina if conception has not occurred.

menstruation [men-stroo-AY-shun] The sloughing off and discharge through the vagina of the inner vascular layer of the endometrium.

mesoderm [MEZ-uh-derm] Embryonic tissue that gives rise to the muscles, skeleton, circulatory, excretory, and reproductive systems.

metastasized [muh-TAS-tuh-siyzd] Spread of cancer via the bloodstream to other parts of the body.

minilaparotomy [mi-ni-lap-ah-RAHT-o-mee] Tubal ligation performed via abdominal incision.

minimization Psychological defense mechanism used to reduce anxiety via a belittling of the cause of the stress.

minipill Birth control pill containing low doses of progesterone and no estrogen.

miscarriage Spontaneous death and expulsion of the fetus.

mittelschmerz [MIT-tul-shmehrtz] Cramping felt by some women at ovulation.

modeling technique Demonstration, in person or on film, of an adaptive behavior.

moniliasis [mo-ni-LIY-ah-sis] Sexually transmitted disease.

mons pubis [mahnz-PYOO-bus] Fatty pad of tissue located on frontal part of the vulva.

mons veneris [mahnz VEHN-uh-rus] See *mons pubis*.

morning-after-pill Birth control pill taken after unprotected intercourse that contains high levels of estrogen to prevent egg implantation.

morning sickness Nausea that occurs between the sixth and twelfth week in about half of all pregnant women.

morula [MOR-yuh-luh] Ball of 16 cells formed out of the developing fertilized egg on the third day after conception.

morula stage Stage of pregnancy at which morula is formed.

mucosa [myu-KO-sah] Soft mucus membrane that makes up the innermost layer of the fallopian tubes and the vagina.

Mullerian [myul-EER-ee-en] *ducts* Fetal precursors to the fallopian tubes and uterus.

Mullerian-inhibiting substance Substance produced by the testes that causes the Mullerian ducts to degenerate in the male.

multilateral family Group marriage formed out of several pair-bonded couples in which resources, work, and child rearing are all handled communally.

multipara [mul-TIP-ah-ra] Woman giving birth to second or later baby.

muscularis [muhs-kyu-LAH-ris] Second layer of the fallopian tubes, which moves the egg through the tube via wavelike contractions.

myometrium [miy-o-MEE-tree-um] Second layer of the uterine wall, which is made up of smooth muscle tissue used to expel the fetus.

myotonia [miy-uh-TO-nee-uh] Muscle contractions.

nativists Scientists who emphasize the importance of biological variables in the determination of behavior.

natural childbirth Childbirth accomplished without the aid of drugs and using special techniques of breathing and relaxation to aid the delivery.

naturalism The doctrine that scientific laws can adequately account for all phenomena.

necrophilia [nek-ro-FIL-ee-uh] Desire for sexual intercourse with a corpse.

negative feedback loop Hypothalamic-pituitary-gonadal circuit that controls the levels of gonadal hormones.

Neisseria gonorrhoeae [niy-SEER-ah gahn-o-REE-ee] Bacterium that causes gonorrhea.

neural [NYU-rul] *groove* First major organ system formed in the embryo. Precursor to the spinal cord and brain.

new sex therapy Approach to the treatment of sexual dysfunctions that blends psychodynamic and behavioral approaches.

nondemand pleasuring Sensate focus with no demand for intercourse.

nonspecific urethritis [yu-ri-THRIY-tus] Irritation of the urethra whose cause is unidentified.

nulliparous [nuhl-LIP-pah-rus] Female who has never given birth.

nyastatin Drug used to treat moniliasis.

nymphomaniac [nim-fo-MAY-ni-ak] Hypersexual female.

Oedipus [ED-i-pus] *complex* Conflict occurring during phallic stage in which a boy sees his father as a rival for the attention of his mother, and both fears him and has fantasies of killing him.

observation Direct scrutiny of a situation.

open-coupled homosexuals Homosexual couples with sexually open, nonexclusive, relationships.

open marriage Marriage in which each partner is free to seek sexual partners other than the spouse.

operant [AH-puh-runt] *conditioning* Learning via the systematic application of reinforcement.

oral stage First psychosexual stage, in which libido is focused on the mouth.

orchidectomy [or-ki-DEK-to-mee] See *castration.*

orgasm [OR-gaz-um] Brief, intensely pleasurable period when the sexual tension produced by vasocongestion and myotonia is released.

orgasmic [or-GAZ-mik] Third stage of the human sexual response, in which orgasm occurs.

orgasmic dysfunction See *inhibited female orgasm.*

orgasmic platform Swelling of the tissues surrounding the outer third of the vagina during the plateau stage.

orgasmic reconditioning Sex therapy technique used in cases of inhibited female orgasm.

orgastic dysfunction See *inhibited female orgasm.*

osteoporosis [ahs-tee-o-po-RO-sis] Disease in postmenopausal women in which the bones become brittle because of lowered estrogen levels.

ova [o-vuh] Female reproductive cells; eggs.

ovarian [o-VAR-ee-un] *ligaments* Bands of tissue connected to the uterus and abdominal wall that hold the ovaries in place.

ovariectomy [o-var-ee-EK-tuh-mee] Surgical removal of the ovaries.

ovotestes [o-vo-TES-teez] Pair of combined gonads in true hermaphrodites.

ovulation [o-vyu-LAY-shun] Release of a mature ovum from a follicle in an ovary.

ovulatory [o-vyu-luh-tor-ee] *phase* Stage of the menstrual cycle in which an egg is released from the ovary and begins to travel down the fallopian tube.

oxytocin [ahk-si-TOS-un] Drug that promotes uterine contractions and restricts blood loss, often used during dilatation and evacuation method of abortion.

pansexual Arousable by both sexes.

Pap smear Test for cancer of the cervix.

parenchymatous neurosyphilis [par-an-KIM-uh-tus nyu-ro-SIF-uh-lis] Degenerative disease of the brain caused by advanced syphilis.

parous [PA-rus] Female who has given birth.

partial mastectomy [mas-TEK-to-mee] Surgical removal of the breast without disturbing the underlying tissue.

partialism Fetish for a particular part of the body.

participant observation Collection of data about a group by someone who joins and participates in the activities of that group.

parturition [pahrt-uh-RISH-un] Childbirth.

passionate love Love experiences that are marked by extremes of feeling, such as elation, possessiveness, and jealousy.

Pediculus pubis [peh-DIK-yuh-lus PYOO-bus] Louse that causes the crabs.

pedophilia [peh-do-FIL-ee-ah] Desire for children as the preferred sexual object.

peer review Review of an experimental design by other researchers to ensure its compliance with ethical standards.

Pelvic inflammatory disease (PID) Infection of the uterus and fallopian tubes.

penile urethra [PEE-niyl yu-REE-thruh] Portion of the urethra extending from the root of the penis to the meatus.

penis [PEE-nis] Pendulous, rodlike male organ used for copulation and the elimination of urinary waste.

penis envy Theory that phallic-stage girls blame their lack of a penis on their mothers and become attracted to their fathers.

performance anxiety Fear of sexual failure that interferes with normal sexual response.

pergonal [PER-go-nal] Common fertility drug.

phallic [FAL-ik] *stage* Third psychosexual stage, in which libido is focused on the genitals.

phobic [FO-bik] *reactions* Irrational fears.

physical aversion Aversive therapy that uses physical sensations as the aversive stimulus.

pimp Boss and protector of a prostitute.

pituitary [pi-TOO-i-tehr-ee] An endocrine gland that produces several hormones which stimulate the production of other hormones in the body.

placebo [pla-SEE-bo] Inert substance, often administered to the control group in an experiment.

placebo effects Experimental effects produced by an inert substance or treatment.

placenta [pla-SEN-tuh] Organ connecting the fetus and uterine wall, through which the fetus receives oxygen and nutrients and eliminates waste products.

plateau Second stage of the human sexual response, in which vasocongestion and myotonia peak in preparation for orgasm.

postpartum [post PAHR-tum] *depression* Depression experienced by a mother after the birth of her baby.

potent [POH-tunt] Obsolete term used to indicate a male with adequate sexual functioning.

power rape Rape motivated by a need to degrade and control the victim.

pragma [PRAG-muh] Practical love.

preadolescence Ages 8–11.

precipitating event Event that seems to have brought about the development of a psychological disorder.

preeclampsia [pree-ee-KLAMP-see-ah] Woman showing symptoms of toxemia.

premarital sex Sexual activity among people who are below the expected age of marriage.

premature Baby born during the seventh or eighth month of pregnancy who also weighs less than 2500 grams (approximately 5.4 pounds).

premature ejaculation Sexual dysfunction in which the male reaches orgasm too quickly.

premenstrual [pree-MEN-stroo-ul] *tension* Syndrome of depression, anxiety, and low self-esteem that some women report as occurring just prior to menstruation.

prenatal period Period of time that begins with conception and ends with birth.

prepuce [PREE-pyoos] Layer of skin that covers the glans of the penis in males and the clitoris in females.

primary amenorrhea Cases in which menstruation has not occurred by age 18.

primary inhibited orgasm Case in which male has never experienced ejaculation during coitus.

primary inhibited sexual excitement Cases of inhibited sexual excitement in which there has never been adequate sexual functioning.

primary spermatocyte [sper-MAT-uh-siyt] Immature sperm cell.

primary stage First stage of syphilis, characterized by a chancre.

primipara [pree-MIP-ah-ra] Woman giving birth to her first baby.

primitive spermatogonia [sper-mat-uh-GO-nee-uh] See *spermatogenic cells*.

progesterone [pro-JES-tuh-rohn] Female sex hormone produced by the ovaries and corpus luteum.

progestin-induced hermaphroditism [proh-JES-tun in-DOOSED her-MA-fro-diyt-izm] Condition in which a genetic female develops ovaries and masculine genitals because of ingestion of progestin by the mother during pregnancy.

prolactin [pro-LAK-tin] Hormone that stimulates breast development during pregnancy to prepare for breast-feeding.

promiscuity [prah-mis-KYU-uh-tee] Indiscriminant involvement with a large number of sexual partners.

prostaglandins [pros-tah-GLAN-dinz] Complex fatty acids that are found in many body tissues and are involved in the onset of labor and the degeneration of the corpus luteum.

prostate [PRAHS-tayt] Gland located below the bladder that provides a nutrient fluid that makes up the bulk of the semen and nourishes the sperm.

prostatectomy [prahs-tuh-TEK-tuh-mee] Surgical removal of the prostate gland.

prostatic urethra [prah-STAT-ik yu-REE-thruh] The portion of the urethra that passes through the prostate.

prostitute [PRAH-sti-toot] *apartment* Cooperative arrangement of a group of independent prostitutes who band together.

prostitution [prah-sti-TOO-shun] Selling of sexual favors for money.

proteinuria [pro-teen-YU-ree-ah] Excretion of protein in the urine.

pseudocyesis [soo-do-siy-EE-sis] Condition in which a woman may experience all the signs of pregnancy without actually being pregnant.

pseudohermaphroditism [soo-do-her-MA-froh-diyt-izm] Condition in which the sexual characteristics of an individual are mismatched, most commonly involving a discrepancy between the gonads and external genitals.

psychic [SIY-kik] *energy* Psychological energy.

psychoanalytic [siy-ko-an-uh-LI-tik] See *psychodynamic*.

psychodynamic [siy-ko-diy-NAM-ik] Psychological approach based on the work of Freud.

psychosexual [siy-ko-SEKS-yu-ul] *stages* Series of developmental stages postulated by Freud as the basis of psychological and sexual development.

puberty [PYU-ber-tee] Physical changes that occur during the process of sexual maturation.

pubic [PYU-bik] *louse* See *Pediculus pubis*.

pubic symphysis [SIM-fuh-sis] Point at which the pubic bones fuse together beneath the mons pubis.

public solicitation See *soliciting*.

pubococcygeus [pu-bo-kahk-SIJ-ee-us] Muscles surrounding the outer third of the vaginal barrel.

pudendal [pyu-DEN-dul] *block* Regional anesthetic that numbs the external genitals.

pudendal cleft Space between the labia majora and labia minora.

questionnaire Set of questions designed as a research method to elicit answers to specific questions.

quickening Fetal movement in the uterus.

radical mastectomy Surgical removal of the breast, lymph nodes, and supporting muscles.

random sample Sample of subjects in which each member of the population from which the sample is drawn has an equal chance of being selected for the sample.

rape trauma syndrome [TRAH-muh SIN-drohm] Cluster of psychological symptoms, including anxiety, anger, and depression, often present in rape victims.

rationalization Psychological defense mechanism used to reduce anxiety via a search for a rational reason for the source of the anxiety.

rear-entry position Coitus with the male facing the female's back.

reciprocity [reh-si-PRAH-si-tee] Tendency to like those who like you.

recombinant [ree-KAHM-buh-nunt] *DNA* Insertion of genes from one organism into the genes of another organism.

refractory [re-RAK-tuh-ree] *period* Period following orgasm during which males are not sexually responsive.

regression Return under stress to the coping mechanisms of an earlier psychosexual stage as the result of fixation in that stage.

regular dating Courtship in which a couple see each other frequently but not exclusively.

reinforcer Consequences (objects or events) that modify the probability of the occurrence of the behavior they follow.

relearning Replacement of dysfunctional behavior with functional behavior—the goal of behavioral therapy.

repressed Unconscious.

resolution Final stage of the human sexual response marked by the decline of vasocongestion and myotonia.

retarded ejaculation See *inhibited male orgasm*.

retrograde ejaculation [RE-tro-grayd ee-jak-yu-LAY-shun] Rare condition in which sperm are carried backward in the ejaculatory ducts rather than out through the meatus during ejaculation.

retrograde menstruation [RE-tro-grayd men-stroo-AY-shun] Forcing of menstrual fluid up through the fallopian tubes and out into the abdomen.

rewards See *reinforcers*.

Rh factor Blood factor found in humans.

rhythm method Birth control method based on monitoring the stages of the menstrual cycle.

root Point at which the penis is attached to the abdomen.

Rubin test Test that determines if the fallopian tubes are open.

rudimentary external genitals External embryonic structures that later become the penis and scrotum or clitoris and vagina.

sadism [SAY-dism] Derivation of sexual pleasure from inflicting pain on another.

sadistic [suh-DIS-tik] *rape* Rape in which the rapist becomes sexually excited by the pain and suffering inflicted on the victim.

sadomasochist [sayd-o-MAS-uh-kist] Person who alternates sadistic and masochistic roles with his or her sexual partner.

satyriasis [sayt-uh-RIY-uh-sis] Hypersexuality in males.

scabies [SKAY-beez] Sexually transmitted disease caused by infestation by a parasitic mite.

scrotum [SKROHT-um] Sack that contains the testes.

secondary amenorrhea Cases in which menstruation has ceased for at least 1 year.

secondary inhibited orgasm Case in which the male was formerly able to ejaculate during coitus but can no longer do so.

secondary inhibited sexual excitement Cases of inhibited sexual excitement in which there has been a history of adequate sexual functioning that is then replaced by a pattern of inhibited sexual excitement.

secondary sexual characteristics Physical changes that occur during puberty, such as pubic hair and the growth of breasts.

secondary spermatocyte [sper-MAT-uh-siyt] Immature sperm cell.

secondary stage Stage of syphilis following the primary stage. The secondary stage is characterized by a rash over the entire body and in the mouth.

semen [SEE-mun] Mixture of sperm and fluids expelled from the penis during ejaculation.

seminal plasmin [SEM-un-ul-PLAZ-mun] Naturally occurring antibiotic in the semen.

seminal vesicles [SEM-un-ul VES-i-kulz] Twin glands in the male on either side of the prostate that secrete fluid into the vas deferens to aid sperm motility.

seminiferous tubules [sem-uh-NIF-uh-rus TOO-byulz] Structures in the testes that produce the sperm.

senile vagina [SEE-niyl va-JIY-nuh] See *vaginal atrophy*.

sensate [SEN-sayt] *focus* Mutual pleasuring in which each partner takes turns actively producing erotic sensations in the other, who remains passive.

serial monogamy [mo-NAH-gah-mee] Sequential marriages with different partners.

Sertoli [ser-TO-lee] *cells* Cells in the seminiferous tubules that nurture the sperm.

sex assignment End point of the process of sexual differentiation, when a physician or other expert declares the sex of the infant.

sex chromosomes In humans, the twenty-third pair of chromosomes, which carry the genetic information required for sexual differentiation.

sex flush Rashlike reddening of the skin during the plateau phase of the human sexual response.

sex offender Individual convicted of an illegal sexual expression or action.

sex reassignment Hormonal and surgical procedures that change a person's anatomical sex.

sex-role typing Process by which children acquire the values, motives, and behaviors that their culture ascribes to their sex.

sex shop Shop that sells sexual paraphernalia, especially of the sadomasochistic variety.

sex-stress situation Sexual assault following initial consent that is later withdrawn before or during the sex act.

sexual differentiation The process by which an organism develops the anatomical and physiological characteristics of its sex.

sexual dysfunction Inability to engage in or enjoy sexual encounters.

sexually transmitted diseases (STD) Diseases that are transmitted via sexual contact.

sexual minorities Individuals who engage in sexually variant activities.

sexual orientation Sexual responsiveness to the same or opposite sex, for example, heterosexuality, homosexuality, or bisexuality.

sexual orientation continuum Scale of sexual orientation developed by Kinsey, which ranges from purely homosexual on one end to purely heterosexual on the other.

sexual preference disturbance Person who is unhappy with his or her sexual preference.

sexual releasers Stimuli that elicit instinctual chains of sexual behavior.

sexual surrogates [SER-o-gaytz] Individuals with no prior relationship to the client who are willing to go through sexual experiences with the client as part of sex therapy.

sexual variances Patterns of sexual behavior that differ markedly enough from the usual cultural patterns to be considered abnormal.

shaft Lower part of the clitoris which is surrounded by the prepuce.

shoulder presentation See *transverse presentation.*

side effects Undesirable effects of a contraceptive device.

side-to-side position Coitus with the male and female facing each other while lying on their sides.

situational orgasmic dysfunction Case in which a woman experiences orgasm under certain specific conditions but not others.

sixty-nine Simultaneous cunnilingus and fellatio.

Skene's [skeenz] *glands* Glands located within the labia minora on either side of the urinary opening that secrete fluid to keep the urethral opening moist.

smegma [SMEG-mah] Cheeselike material secreted by glands beneath the foreskin of uncircumcised males.

social reinforcers Interpersonal cues that signal attitudes toward another person, such as smiles and frowns.

social script Cognitive plan that guides a person's actions, expectations, and understanding in a certain social situation.

sociocultural Shorthand label for the numerous nonbiological factors that are likely to contribute to future changes.

sodomy [SAH-do-mee] *laws* Laws prohibiting oral and anal sex, zoophilia, and necrophilia.

soliciting Crime of offering to sell sexual favors.

spasm [spazm] Involuntary muscle contraction.

spectator role Self-awareness during sexual activity that interferes with sexual response.

sperm Male gamete that is capable of fetilizing the ovum.

spermatids [SPER-mah-tidz] Immature sperm cells.

spermatogenesis [sper-maht-uh-JEN-uh-sus] Process of sperm production.

spermatogenic [sper-maht-uh-JEN-ik] *cells* Cells in the seminiferous tubules that give rise to the sperm cells.

spermatozoa [sper-maht-uh-ZO-uh] Mature sperm cells.

spermicidal [sper-mi-SIY-dal] *foam* Birth control device consisting of foam that is sprayed into the vagina before intercourse, killing sperm on contact.

spinal block Regional anesthetic that numbs from the belly to the thighs.

spirochete [SPIY-ruh-keet] Family of bacteria that includes Treponema pallidum (syphylis).

spontaneous abortion See *miscarriage.*

squeeze technique Squeezing the penis just below the coronal ridge to delay ejaculation. Used to treat premature ejaculation.

start-stop technique Stimulation of the male to a point just short of orgasm, then stopping until arousal subsides, then stimulating again, and so on. Used to treat premature ejaculation.

statutory rape Sexual intercourse with a minor.

steady dating Courtship in which there is a stronger relationship than in regular dating but not exclusivity.

sterilization Use of a surgical procedure to make a person physically incapable of reproduction.

storge [STOR-gay] Quiet and affectionate love.

streetwalker Prostitute who acquires customers by solicitation on the street.

subject bias Expectations and opinions that can distort the answers a subject gives.

subject sampling Selecting a small number of individuals from a larger population to represent that population in a study.

suppression Psychological defense mechanism used to reduce anxiety via a disregarding of all thoughts and feelings associated with the source of the anxiety.

surrogate [SER-o-gayt] See *surrogate mother*.

surrogate mother Woman who becomes pregnant and carries a baby to term for another woman who is unable to conceive.

swinging Mate swapping for the purpose of recreational sexual intercourse.

symptom Indicator of underlying problem.

syphilis [SI-fuh-lis] Sexually transmitted disease.

syphilitic psychosis [si-fuh-LIT-ik siy-KO-sis] See *parenchymatous neurosyphilis*.

systematic desensitization Behavioral treatment designed to remove phobic fear via a graduated exposure to the feared stimulus.

teratogens [ter-ah-TOJ-ens] Substances that can alter the structural development of the embryo or fetus and produce congenital defects.

tertiary syphilis [TER-shee-ehr-ee SI-fuh-lis] Advanced syphilis.

testes [TES-teez] The male sex glands located in the scrotum, which produce male hormones and gametes.

testicular [teh-STIK-yu-ler]-*feminizing syndrome* Condition in which a genetic male develops testes and feminine external genitals because of insensitivity of the gonadal tissue to the effects of testosterone.

testosterone [teh-STAHS-tuh-rohn] Hormone that produces male sex characteristics.

theoretical effectiveness rate Effectiveness rate of a birth control method under optimal conditions.

third-stage (or tertiary) Most advanced stage of syphilis. The symptoms include loss of muscle function, loss of speech, convulsions, paralysis, intellectual deficits, memory loss, and, eventually, madness.

toxemia [tahk-SEE-mee-uh] Potentially fatal condition of unknown cause associated with excessive weight gain by the mother in the third trimester of pregnancy.

transient [TRANCH-unt] *homosexuality* Occasional homosexual activity by a person who is predominantly heterosexual.

transsexual [trans-SEKS-yu-ul] Individuals who feel that they are of the gender opposite their biological sex.

transverse [trans-VERS] *presentation* Side-first position of the fetus at the start of labor.

transvestism [trans-VES-tizm] Sexual arousal from dressing in the clothing of the opposite sex.

transvestite [trans-VES-tiyt] Person who derives pleasure from dressing in the clothes of the opposite sex.

Treponema pallidum [trep-o-NEE-mah PAL-i-dum] Bacterium responsible for syphilis.

tribadism [TRIB-ad-iz-um] Lesbian sexual technique in which one woman lies on top of the other and there is mutual stimulation of each other's clitoris via pelvic rubbing.

Trichomonas vaginalis [tri-KOH-mo-nas vaj-in-AL-is] Protozoan that causes trichomoniasis.

trichomoniasis [trik-o-mo-NIY-ah-sis] Sexually transmitted disease.

true hermaphrodite [her-MA-fro-diyt] Individual who has both testes and ovaries, or a pair of combined gonads, called ovotestes.

tubal abortion Condition in which an embryo from tubal pregnancy is forced out of the end of the tube into the abdomen.

tubal ligation [li-GAY-shun] Method of sterilization in which a section of each of the fallopian tubes is removed and the remaining ends are closed off.

tubal pregnancy Ectopic pregnancy implanted in the fallopian tubes.

tubal rupture Condition in which tubal pregnancy results in a bursting of the fallopian tube.

tunica albuginea [TOO-ni-kah al-byu-JIN-ee-ah] Thin, white sheath that encapsulates each of the testes and divides them into several lobes.

Turner's syndrome Condition in which an individual has only one sex chromosome.

undescended testes See *cryptorchidism*.

urethra [yu-REE-thruh] Passageway for sperm and urine, which runs from the prostate down the length of the penis.

urethral [yu-REE-thrul] *opening* Urinary opening in females located below the clitoris and between the labia minora.

urethritis [yu-ri-THIYT-us] Inflammation of the urethra.

uterus [yu-tuh-rus] Pear-shaped organ in the abdomen of the female that contains and nourishes a developing fetus.

vacuum curettage [kyu-RET-uj] *method* Method of abortion in which a hollow plastic tube is inserted into the uterus and the contents are sucked out.

vagina [vuh-IY-nuh] Flexible canal in the female extending from the cervix to the vulva. Accepts the penis during intercourse and forms a passageway for the fetus at birth.

vaginal atrophy [VAJ-i-nul AT-ro-fee] Thinning of the vaginal walls during the climacteric.

vaginal photoplethysmograph [VAJ-i-nul fo-to-pleh-THIYZ-mo-graf] Device that measures changes in the vagina associated with sexual arousal.

vaginismus [vaj-i-NIZ-mus] Sexual dysfunction in which the muscles of the vagina contract involuntarily, making penile entry difficult or impossible.

vaginitis [vaj-uh-NIYT-us] Irritation of the vagina.

vas deferens [vas DEF-uh-renz] Sperm ducts in the male that run from the epididymes to the seminal vesicles and urethra.

vasectomy [vas-EK-to-mee] Surgical severing of the vas deferens that prevents sperm from entering the penis, thus rendering the male sterile.

vasocongestion [vay-o-kahn-JES-chun] Buildup of blood and fluid in a particular area of the body.

venereal [veh-NIR-ee-ul] *disease* Obsolete term for sexually transmitted disease (STD).

verifiable data Data that can be independently replicated by other experimenters.

vernix caseosa [VER-niks cas-ee-O-suh] Protective coating that covers the skin of the fetus.

voluntary sterilization Sterilization with consent.

voyeurism [vwah-YUHR-iz-um] Sexual variance in which the primary or exclusive source of sexual arousal is watching other people in various stages of undress or engaging in sexual activities.

vulva [VUHL-vuh] Entire external genital region of the female.

Wasserman [WAH-ser-mun] *test* Blood test used to diagnose syphilis.

withdrawal See *coitus interruptus.*

Wolffian [WUHL-fee-un] *ducts* Fetal precursors of the epididymes, vas deferens, ejaculatory ducts, and urethra.

work through Process in psychodynamic therapy of identifying intrapsychic conflicts and resolving them.

yeast infection See *moniliasis.*

XXX chromosomal [kro-mo-SO-mul] *pattern* Chromosomal pattern in which a female has an extra X chromosome.

XYY chromosomal [kro-mo-SO-mul] *pattern* Chromosomal pattern in which a male has an extra Y chromosome.

zoophilia [zo-o-FIL-i-uh] Desire for animals as the preferred sexual object.

References

Abel, G. G., Barlow, D. H., Blanchard, E. B., and Guild, D. The components of rapists' sexual arousal. *Archives of General Psychiatry*, 1977, **34**, 895–903.

Abrams, M. Birth control: The new breakthroughs. *Harper's Bazaar*, April 1980.

Adams, C. R. An informal preliminary report on some factors relating to sexual responsiveness of certain college wives. In M. F. DeMartino (Ed.), *Sexual behavior and personality characteristics*. New York: Grove Press, 1966.

Adams, D. B., Gold, A. R., and Burt, A. D. Rise in female-initiated activity at ovulation and its suppression by oral contraceptives. *The New England Journal of Medicine*, 1978, **299**, 1145–1150.

Adams, V. Getting at the heart of jealous love. *Psychology Today*, May 1980, 38–47+. (a)

Adams, V. Sex therapies in perspective. *Psychology Today*, August 1980, 35–36. (b)

Addiego, F., Belzer, E. G., Comolli, J., Moger, W., Perry, J. D., and Whipple, B. Female ejaculation: A case study. *The Journal of Sex Research*, 1981, **17**, 13–21.

Aiken, D. L. Ex-sailor charges jail rape, stirs up storm. *The Advocate*, September 26, 1973, 5.

Alexander, C. S. Responsible victim—nurses' perceptions of victims of rape. *Journal of Health and Social Behavior*, 1980, **21**, 22–33.

Alexander, N. J., Wilson, B. J., and Patterson, G. D. Vasectomy: Immunologic effects in rhesus monkeys and men. *Fertility and Sterility*, 1974, **25**, 149–156.

Altrocchi, J. Abnormal behavior. New York: Harcourt Brace Jovanovich, 1980.

Anderson, T. P., and Cole, T. M. Sexual counseling of the physically disabled. *Postgraduate Medicine*, July 1975, **58**, 117–123.

Armstrong, E. A. Massage parlors and their customers. *Archives of Sexual Behavior*, 1978, 7(2), 117–125.

Aronson, E. The social animal. San Francisco: Freeman, 1972.

Aronson, E., and Linder, D. Gain and loss of esteem as determinants of interpersonal attractiveness. *Journal of Experimental Social Psychology*, 1965, **1**, 156–172.

Asmussen, I. Arterial changes in infants of smoking mothers. *Postgraduate Medical Journal*, 1978, **54**, 200–204.

Baker, S. W., and Ehrhardt, A. A. Prenatal androgen, intelligence and cognitive sex differences. In R. C. Friedman, R. M. Richart, and R. L. Vandeweile (Eds.), *Sex differences in behavior*. New York: Wiley, 1974.

Baker, T. G. A quantitative and cytological study of germ cells in human ovaries. *Proceedings of the Royal Society* (Biology), 1963, **158**, 147.

Bakke, J. L. A double-blind study of a progestin-estrogen combination in the management of menopause. *Pacific Medicine and Surgery*, 1965, **73**, 200–205.

Bakwin, H. Erotic feelings in infants and young children. *American Journal of Diseases of Children*, 1973, **126**, 52–54.

Bandura, A. Social learning through imitation. In M. R. Jones (Ed.), *Nebraska Symposium on Motivation*. (Vol. 10.) Lincoln, Nebraska: University of Nebraska Press, 1962.

Bandura, A. The principles of behavior modification. New York: Wiley, 1969.

Bandura, A., Ross, D., and Ross, S. A. Imitation of film-mediated aggressive models. *Journal of Abnormal and Social Psychology*, 1963, **66**, 3–11.

Barclay, A. M. Sexual fantasies in men and women. *Medical Aspects of Human Sexuality*, 1973, **7**, 209–212.

Bardwick, J. M. Psychology of women: A study of biocultural conflicts. New York: Harper & Row, 1971.

Barlow, D. H. Increasing heterosexual responsiveness in the treatment of sexual deviation: A review of the clinical and experimental evidence. *Behavior Therapy*, 1973, **4**, 655–671.

Barlow, D. H., and Agras, W. S. Fading to increase heterosexual responsiveness in homosexuals. *Journal of Applied Behavior Analysis*, 1973, **6**, 355–366.

Barlow, D. H., Agras, W. S., and Reynolds, E. J. Direct and indirect modification of gender specific motor behavior in a transsexual. Paper presented at the annual meeting of the American Psychological Association, Honolulu, 1972.

Barlow, D. H., Reynolds, E. J., and Agras, S. Gender identity change in a transsexual. *Archives of General Psychiatry*, 1973, **28**, 569–576.

Bart, P. B. Depression in middle-aged women. In V. G. Gornick and B. K. Moran (Eds.), *Women in sexist society*. New York: Basic Books, 1971.

Beach, F. *Human sexuality in four perspectives,* Baltimore: Johns Hopkins University Press, 1976.

Beck, S. B., Ward-Hull, C. I., and McLear, P. M. Variables related to women's somatic preferences for the male and female body. *Journal of Personality and Social Psychology,* 1976, **34,** 1200–1210.

Behrman, S. J., and Kistner, R. W. (Eds.). *Progress in infertility.* Boston: Little, Brown, 1968.

Bell, A., and Weinberg, M. *Homosexualities: A study of diversity among men and women.* New York: Simon & Schuster, 1978.

Bell, R. R., and Bell, P. L. Sexual satisfaction among married women. *Medical Aspects of Human Sexuality,* 1972, 136–144.

Belson, A. Erotic fantasies: The new therapy. *Harper's Bazaar,* April 1980, 153+.

Belzer, E. G. Orgasmic expulsions of women: A review and heuristic inquiry. *The Journal of Sex Research,* 1981, **17,** 1–12.

Bem, S. L. The measurement of psychological androgyny. *Journal of Clinical and Consulting Psychology,* 1974, **42,** 155–162.

Bem, S. L. Androgyny vs. fluffy women and chesty men. *Psychology Today,* September 1975, 59–62.

Benedek, T. *Psychosexual functions in women.* New York: Ronald Press, 1952.

Bengis, I. *Combat in the erogenous zone.* New York: Knopf, 1972.

Bennett, R. Forum penile study. *Forum: The International Journal of Human Relations,* 1972, **1,** 36–41.

Bernstein, B. E. Effect of menstruation on academic performance among college women. *Archives of Sexual Behavior,* 1977, **6,** 289–295.

Berry, J. W. Temne and Eskimo perceptual skills. *International Journal of Psychology,* 1966, **1,** 207–229.

Bieber, I., Dain, H., Dince P., Drellich, M., Grand, H., Gundlach, R., Kremer, M., Rifkin, A., Wilbur, C., and Bieber, T. *Homosexuality: A psychoanalytic study of male homosexuals.* New York: Basic Books, 1962.

Block, E. Quantitative morphological investigations of the follicular system in women: Variations at different ages. *Acta Anatomy,* 1952, **14,** 108–123.

Block, J. H. Another look at the sex differentiations in the socialization behaviors of mothers and fathers. In F. Wenmark and J. Sherman (Eds.), *Psychology of women: Future directions of research.* New York: Psychological Dimensions, 1978.

Block, J. H., Block, J., and Harrington, D. M. The relationship of parental teaching strategies to ego resiliency in preschool children. Paper presented at the Meeting of the Western Psychological Association, San Francisco, 1974.

Boston Women's Health Book Collective. *Our bodies, ourselves.* (2nd rev. ed.) New York: Simon & Schuster, 1976.

Bowlby, J. Separation anxiety. *International Journal of Psychoanalysis,* 1960, **41,** 89–93.

Brackbill, Y. Obstetrical medication and infant behavior. In J. D. Osofsky (Ed.), *Handbook of infant development.* New York: Wiley, 1978.

Branden, N. *The psychology of romantic love.* Los Angeles: Tarcher, 1980.

Brasch, R. *How did sex begin?* New York: McKay, 1973.

Brecher, R., and Brecher, E. (Eds.). *An analysis of human sexual response.* New York: Signet, 1966.

Bremer, J. *Asexualization: A follow-up study of 244 cases.* New York: Macmillan, 1959.

Broderick, C. B. Sexual development among preadolescents. *The Journal of Social Issues,* 1966, **22,** 6–21.

Bronfenbrenner, U. Freudian theories of identification and their derivatives. *Child Development,* 1960, **31,** 15–40.

Brooks, J., Ruble, D., and Clarke, A. College women's attitudes and expectations concerning menstrual-related changes. *Psychosomatic Medicine,* 1977, **39,** 288–298.

Brown, W. A., Monti, P. M., and Corriveau, D. P. Serum testosterone levels and sexual activity and interest in men. *Archives of Sexual Behavior,* 1978, **7,** 97–103.

Brownmiller, S. *Against our will.* New York: Simon & Schuster, 1975.

Bryan, J. Apprenticeships in prostitution. In Gagnon, J. H., and Simon, W. (Eds.), *Sexual deviance.* New York: Harper & Row, 1967.

Bryant, C. D., and Palmer, C. E. Massage parlors and "hand whores": Some sociological observations. *Journal of Sexual Research,* 1975, **11,** 227–241.

Bryson, J. B. Situational determinants of the expression of jealousy. In H. Sigall, *Sexual jealousy.* American Psychological Association, Symposium, San Francisco, August 1977.

Bullough, V. L. *Sexual variance in society and history.* New York: Wiley, 1976.

Bullough, V. L. Age at menarche: A misunderstanding. *Science,* 1981, **213,** 365–366.

Burgess, A. W., and Holmstrom, L. L. Rape trauma syndrome. *American Journal of Psychiatry,* 1974, **131,** 981–986.

Burgess, A. W., and Holmstrom, L. L. *Rape: Crisis and recovery.* Maryland: Robert J. Brady Co., 1979. (a)

Burgess, A. W., and Holmstrom, L. L. Adaptive strategies and recovery from rape. *American Journal of Psychiatry,* 1979, **136,** 1278–1282. (b)

Burgess, A. W., and Holmstrom, L. L. Rape typology and the coping behavior of rape victims. In S. L. McCombie (Ed.), *The rape crisis intervention handbook.* New York: Plenum, 1980.

Burnside, I. M. Sexuality and the older adult: Implications for nursing. In I. M. Burnside (Ed.), *Sexuality and aging.* Los Angeles: University of Southern California Press, 1975.

Butler, E. W. *Traditional marriage and emerging alternatives.* New York: Harper & Row, 1979.

Butler, R. N., and Lewis, M. I. *Sex after sixty: A guide for men and women in their later years.* New York: Harper & Row, 1976.

Byrne, D. Attitudes and attraction. *Advances in Experimental Social Psychology,* 1969, **4,** 36–89.

Byrne, D. *The attraction paradigm.* New York: Academic, 1971.

Catterall, R. D. *A short textbook of venereology.* Philadelphia: Lippincott, 1974.

Catterall, R. D. *Sexually transmitted diseases.* New York: Academic Press, 1976.

Chertok, L. Vomiting and the wish to have a child. *Psychosomatic Medicine,* 1963, **25,** 13–18.

Chevalier-Skolnikoff, S. Male-female, female-female, and male-male sexual behavior in the stumptail monkey with special attention to female orgasm. *Archives of Sexual Behavior,* 1974, **3,** 95–115.

Chodoff, P. A critique of Freud's theory of infantile sexuality. *American Journal of Psychology,* 1966, **123,** 507–518.

Christenson, C. V. *Kinsey: A biography.* Indiana University Press, 1971.

Cimbalo, R., Faling, V., and Mousaw, P. The course of love: A cross-sectional design. *Psychological Reports,* 1976, **38,** 1292–1294.

Clanton, G., and Smith, L. G. *Jealousy.* Englewood Cliffs, N.J.: Prentice-Hall, 1977.

Clarke, A. E., and Ruble, D. N. Young adolescents' beliefs concerning menstruation. *Child Development,* 1978, **49,** 231–234.

Clayton, R., and Voss, H. Shacking-up: Cohabitation in the 1970's. *Journal of Marriage and the Family,* 1977, **39**(2), 273–283.

Cole, T. M. Sexuality and physical disabilities. *Archives of Sexual Behavior,* 1975, **4,** 289–403.

Comfort, A. *Sex in society.* London: Duckworth, 1963.

Comfort, A. *The joy of sex.* New York: Crown, 1972.

Comfort, A. *A good age.* New York: Simon & Schuster, 1976.

Constantine, L., and Constantine, J. *Group marriage.* New York: Collier Books, 1973.

Consumers Union. Estrogen replacement therapy. In *The medicine show* (rev. ed.). New York: Pantheon Books, 1980.

Cook, J. The X-rated economy. *Forbes,* September 18, 1978, 81–92.

Cutler, W. B., and Garcia, C. R. The psychoneuroendocrinology of the ovulatory cycle of women: A review. *Psychoneuroendocrinology,* 1980, **5,** 89–111.

Dalton, K. *The premenstrual syndrome.* Springfield, Ill.: Thomas, 1964.

Dalton, K. *The menstrual cycle.* New York: Pantheon Books, 1969.

Daly, M., and Wilson, M. *Sex, evolution, and behavior.* N. Scituate, Mass.: Duxbury Press, 1978.

Dank, B. Six homosexual siblings. *Archives of Sexual Behavior,* 1971, **1,** 193–204.

Davenport, W. Sex in cross-cultural perspective. In F. A. Beach (Ed.), *Human sexuality in four perspectives.* Baltimore: Johns Hopkins University Press, 1977.

Davidson, G. C. Homosexuality: The ethical challenge. *Journal of Consulting and Clinical Psychology,* 1976, **44,** 157–162.

Davidson, J. M., Comargo, C. A., and Smith, E. R. Effects of androgen on sexual behavior in hypogonadal men. *Journal of Clinical Endocrinology and Metabolism,* 1979, **48,** 955–958.

Davidson, P. O. (Ed.). *The behavioral management of anxiety, depression, and pain.* New York: Brunner Mazel, 1976.

Davis, K. B. *Factors in the sex life of 2200 women.* New York: Harper & Row, 1929.

DeMartino, M. How women want men to make love. *Sexology,* October 1970, 4–7.

Deutscher, I. The quality of postparental life. *Journal of Marriage and the Family,* 1964, **26,** 263–268.

Deveraux, W. P. Endometriosis: Long-term observation with particular reference to incidence of pregnancy. *Obstetrics and Gynecology,* 1963, **22,** 444.

Diagnostic and statistical manual of mental disorders (3rd ed.). Washington: American Psychiatric Association, 1980.

Dick-Reade, G. *Natural childbirth.* London: Heinemann, 1933.

Dick-Reade, G. *Childbirth without fear* (2nd rev. ed.). New York: Harper & Row, 1944.

Dickinson, R. L., and Beam, L. *A thousand marriages.* Baltimore: Williams & Wilkins, 1931.

Dion, K. K., and Berscheid, E. Physical attraction and peer perception among children. *Sociometry,* 1972, **37,** 1–12.

Dion, K. K., Berscheid, E., and Walster, E. What is beautiful is good. *Journal of Personality and Social Psychology,* 1972, **24,** 285–290.

"Dr. Kinsey," editorial in the *New York Times,* August 27, 1956.

Douglas, J. W. B., and Blomfield, J. H. *Children under fire.* London: George Allen & Unwin Ltd., 1958.

Douglas, J. W. B. *The home and the school: A study of ability and attachment in the primary school.* London: MacGibbon & Kee, 1964.

Driscoll, J. P. Transsexuals. *Transaction,* March–April 1971, 28–31.

Duberman, L. *Marriage and other alternatives.* New York: Praeger, 1977.

Dweck, C. S., and Goetz, F. E. Attributions and learned helplessness. In J. H. Harvey, W. Ickes, and R. F. Kidd (Eds.), *New directions in attribution research.* Hillsdale, N.J.: Lawrence Erlbaum, 1977.

Edwards, C. P., and Whiting, B. Sex differences in children's social interactions. Unpublished report to the Ford Foundation, 1977.

Ehrhardt, A. A., and Baker, S. W. Fetal androgens, human central nervous system differentiation and behavior, sex differences. In R. C. Friedman, R. M. Richart, and R. L. Vandervile (Eds.), *Sex differences in behavior.* New York: Wiley, 1974.

Ehrhardt, A. A., Epstein, R., and Money, J. Fetal androgens and female gender identity in the early treated adrenogenital syndrome. *Johns Hopkins Medical Journal,* 1968, **122,** 160–167.

Ehrhardt, A. A., and Meyer-Bahlburg, H. F. L. Effects of prenatal sex hormones on gender related behavior. *Science,* 1981, **211,** 1312–1318.

Ehrhardt, A. A., and Money, J. Progestin induced hermaphroditism: IQ and psychosexual identity in a study of 10 girls. *Journal of Sex Research,* 1967, **3,** 83–100.

Eichenlaub, J. E. *The marriage art.* New York: Dell, 1961.

Elias, J., and Gebhard, P. Sexuality and sexual learning in childhood. *Phi Delta Kappan,* 1969, **L,** 401–405.

Ellis, A. Masturbation. In M. F. De Martino (Ed.), *Sexual behavior and personality characteristics.* New York: Grove, 1966.

Ellis, H. *Studies of the psychology of sex.* New York: Mentor Books, 1954.

Emmerich, W. Parental identification in young children. *Genetic Psychology Monographs,* 1959, **60,** 257–308.

Emmerich, W., Goldman, K. S., Kirsh, B., and Sharabany, R. Development of gender constancy in economically disadvantaged children. Report of the Princeton, N.J., Educational Testing Service, 1976.

"Estrogen therapy: Still deliberating." *Science News,* October 13, 1979, 246–247.

"Estrogen therapy and breast cancer," *Science News,* May 3, 1980, 278–279.

Faiman, C., and Winter, J. S. D. Diurnal cycles in plasma FSH, testosterone, and cortisol in men. *Journal of Clinical Endocrinology and Metabolism,* 1971, **33,** 186–192.

Federal Bureau of Investigation. *Uniform crime reports,* 1973.

Feldman, M. P., MacCulloch, M. J., Mellor, V., and Pinchof, J. The application of anticipatory avoidance learning to the treatment of homosexuality, III: The sexual orientation method. *Behavior Research and Therapy,* 1966, **4,** 111–117.

Fennema, E. Mathematics, spatial ability and the sexes. Paper presented at the meeting of the American Educational Research Association Annual, Chicago, 1974.

Filler, W., and Drezner, N. The results of surgical castration in women under forty. *American Journal of Obstetrics and Gynecology,* 1944, **47,** 122–124.

Flanagan, J. C. Trends in male/female performance on cognitive ability measures. American Institutes for Research, 1978.

Fleming, A. T. New frontiers in conception. *New York Times Magazine,* July 20, 1980, 14–20.

Ford, C. S., and Beach, F. A. *Patterns of sexual behavior.* New York: Harper & Row, 1951.

Forest, M., Saez, J., and Bertrand, J. Assessment of gonadal function in children. *Pediatrician,* 1973, **2,** 102–128.

Forest, M., Sizonenko, P., Cathiard, A., and Bertrand, J. Hypophyso-gonadal function in humans during the first year of life 1: Evidence for testicular activity in early infancy. *Journal of Clinical Investigation,* 1974, **53,** 819–828.

Fortino, D. New pill for men. *Harper's Bazaar,* June 1979, 129, 144.

Fox, C. A. Studies on the relationship of plasma testosterone levels and human sexual activity. *Journal of Endocrinology,* 1972, **52,** 51–58.

Francher, J. S., and Henkin, J. The menopausal queen: Adjustment to aging and the male homosexual. *American Journal of Orthopsychiatry,* 1973, **43,** 621–674.

Frank, E., Anderson, C., and Rubinstein, D. Frequency of sexual dysfunction in "normal" couples. *New England Journal of Medicine,* July 20, 1978, **299,** 111–115.

Frank, R. T. The hormonal causes of premenstrual tension. *Archives of Neurology and Psychiatry,* 1931, **26,** 1053–1057.

Freedman, M. Homosexuals may be healthier than straights. *Psychology Today,* 1975, **8**(10), 28–32.

Freud, A. As cited in L. A. Kirkendall and I. Rubin, *Sexuality and the life cycle.* In *Human Sexuality 77/78.* Guilford, Conn.: Dushkin Publishing Group, 1977.

Friedman, R. C., Wolleson, F., and Tendler, R. Psychological development and blood levels of sex steroids in male identical twins of divergent sexual orientation. *Journal of Nervous and Mental Diseases,* 1976, **163,** 282–288.

Friesen, H. G. Human placental lactogen and human pituitary prolactin. *Clinical Obstetrics and Gynecology,* 1971, **14,** 669–684.

Gagnon, J. H. *Human sexualities.* Glenview, Ill.: Scott, Foresman, 1977.

Gagnon, J. H., and Simon, W. (Eds.). *Sexual deviance.* New York: Harper & Row, 1967.

Gagnon, J. H., and Simon, W. *Sexual conduct: The social sources of human sexuality.* Chicago: Aldine, 1973.

Galenson, H. Discussion (Early sexual differences and development, P. B. Neubauer). In E. Adelson (Ed.), *Sexuality and psychoanalysis.* New York: Brunner-Mazel, 1975.

Ganong, W. F. *Review of medical physiology.* Los Altos, Calif.: Lange Medical Publication, 1967.

Gartrell, N. K., Loreaux, L., and Chase, T. N. Plasma testosterone in homosexual and heterosexual women. *American Journal of Psychiatry,* 1977, **134,** 1117–1119.

Gebhard, P. H. Factors in marital orgasm. *Journal of Social Issues,* 1966, **22,** 88–95.

Gebhard, P. H. The acquisition of basic sex information. *Journal of Sex Research,* 1977, **13,** 148–169.

Gebhard, P. H., Gagnon, J. H., Pomeroy, W. B., and Christenson, C. V. *Sex offenders: An analysis of types.* New York: Harper & Row, 1965.

German, J., Simpson, J. L., Chaganti, R. S. K., Summitt, R. L., Reid, L. B., and Merkatz, I. R. Genetically determined sex reversal in 46 XY humans. *Science,* 1978, **202,** 53–56.

Gilmartin, B. G. That swinging couple down the block. *Psychology Today,* February 1975, 54–58.

Ginsberg, G. L., Frosch, W. A., and Shapiro, T. The new impotence. *Archives of General Psychiatry,* 1972, **26**(3), 218–220.

Glass, D. D., and Padrone, F. J. Sexual adjustment in the handicapped. *Journal of Rehabilitation,* January–March 1978, 43–47.

Golde, P., and Kogan, N. A sentence completion procedure for assessing attitudes toward old people. *Journal of Gerontology,* 1959, **14,** 355–360.

Goldstein, M. J., and Kant, H. *Pornography and sexual deviance.* Berkeley, Calif.: University of California Press, 1973.

Golub, S. The effect of premenstrual anxiety and depression on cognitive function. *Journal of Personality and Social Psychology,* 1976, **34,** 99–104. (a)

Golub, S. The magnitude of premenstrual anxiety and tension. *Psychosomatic Medicine,* 1976, **38,** 4–12. (b)

Gordon, M. B., and Fields, E. M. Observations on the effect of chronic gonadotropin and male sex hormone on eunuchoidism. *Journal of Clinical Endocrinology,* 1943, **3,** 589–595.

Gordon, R. E., Kapostins, E. E., and Gordon, K. K. Factors in postpartum emotional adjustment. *Obstetrics and Gynecology,* 1965, **25,** 158–166.

Gordon, T. P., and Bernstein, I. S. Seasonal variation in the sexual behavior of all-male rhesus troops. *American Journal of Physical Anthropology,* 1973, **38,** 221–226.

Gorski, R. A. Sexual differentiation of the brain. In D. T. Krieger and J. C. Hughs (Eds.), *Neuroendocrinology.* Sunderland, Mass.: Sinauer Associates, 1980.

Goy, R. W., Wolf, J. E., and Eisele, S. G. Experimental female hermaphroditism in rhesus monkeys: Anatomical and psychological characteristics. In J. Money and H. Musaph (Eds.), *Handbook of sexology.* New York: Excerpta Medica, 1977.

Green, R. *Sexual identity conflict in children and adults.* New York: Basic Books, 1974.

Griswold v. Connecticut, 1965, 381 U.S., 479; 484.

Grobstein, C. External human fertilization. *Scientific American,* June 1979, **240,** 57–67.

Groth, A. N. The rapist's view. In A. W. Burgess and L. L. Holmstrom (Eds.), *Rape: Crisis and recovery.* Bowie, Md.: Robert J. Brady, 1979.

Groth, A. N., and Birnbaum, H. J. The rapist: Motivations for sexual violence. In S. L. McCombie (Ed.), *The rape crisis intervention handbook.* New York: Plenum, 1980.

Halverson, H. Genital and sphincter behavior of the male infant. *Journal of Genetic Psychology,* 1940, **56,** 95–136.

Hamilton, E. Emotions and sexuality in the woman. In H. A. Otto (Ed.), *The new sexuality.* Palto Alto, Calif.: Science and Behavior, 1971.

Hampson, J. L., and Hampson, J. G. The ontogenesis of sexual behavior in man. In W. C. Young (Ed.), *Sex and internal secretions.* Baltimore: Williams & Wilkins, 1961.

Hand, J. R. Surgery of the penis and urethra. In M. F. Campbell and J. H. Harrison (Eds.), *Urology.* Vol. 3. Philadelphia: Saunders, 1970.

Hanson, R. W., and Adesso, U. S. A multiple behavioral approach to male homosexual behavior: A case study. *Journal of Behavior Therapy and Experimental Psychiatry,* 1972, **3**, 323–325.

Hariton, E. B. The sexual fantasies of women. *Psychology Today,* 1973, **6**, 39–44.

Harlow, H. F., and Harlow, M. K. The affectional systems. In A. M. Schrier, H. Harlow, and F. Stollnitz (Eds.), *Behavior of nonhuman primates.* New York: Academic Press, 1965.

Harmatz, M. *Abnormal psychology.* Englewood Cliffs, N.J.: Prentice-Hall, 1978.

Harris, L. *The myth and reality of aging in the U.S.* Washington, D.C.: Louis Harris and Associates for the National Council on Aging, 1976.

Harry, J., and DeVall, B. *The social organization of gay males.* New York: Praeger, 1978.

Haseltine, F. P., and Ohno, S. Mechanisms of gonadal differentiation. *Science,* 1981, **211**, 1272–1278.

Hassett, J. A new look at living together. *Psychology Today,* December 1977, 82–83.

Hatcher, R. A., Stewart, G. K., Stewart, F., Guest, F., Stratton, P., and Wright, A. H. *Contraceptive technology.* (9th rev. ed.) New York: Irvington, 1978.

Hatcher, R. A., Stewart, G. K., Stewart, F., Guest, F., Stratton, P., and Wright, A. H. *Contraceptive technology.* (10th rev. ed.) New York: Irvington, 1980.

Hayman, C. R., Lanza, C., and Fuentes, R. Sexual assault on women and girls in the District of Columbia. *Southern Medical Journal,* 1969, **62**, 1227–1231.

Hecks, P. *The joys of open marriage.* Chatsworth, Calif.: Books for Better Living, 1974.

Heiman, J. A psychophysiological exploration of sexual arousal patterns in females and males. *Psychophysiology,* 1977, **14**, 266–274.

Heller, C. G., and Neison, W. O. Hyalinization of seminiferous tubules and clumping of Leydig cells: Notes on treatment of clinical syndrome with testosterone propionate, methyl testosterone, and testosterone pellets. *Journal of Clinical Endocrinology,* 1945, **5**, 27–33.

Hellerstein, H. K., and Friedman, E. H. Sexual activity and the postcoronary patient. *Medical Aspects of Human Sexuality,* 1969, **3**, 70–74.

Henig, R. M. The case for mother's milk. *New York Times Magazine,* July 8, 1979, 39–41.

Henry, J. B., Choi, Y. J., Sandler, M., and Hubbel, C. Immunological consequences of vasectomy. Presented at the 13th International Congress of the International Society of Blood Transfusion, Washington, D.C., August 1972.

Herbert, J. Sexual preference in the rhesus monkey. *Macaca mulatta,* in the laboratory. *Animal Behavior,* 1968, **16**, 120–128.

Herbert, J. Hormones and reproductive behavior in rhesus and talapoin monkeys. *Journal of Reproduction and Fertility,* 1970, **11**, 119–140.

Herbst, A. L., Kurman, R. J., and Scully, R. E. Vaginal and cervical abnormalities after exposure to stilbestrol in utero. *Obstetrics and Gynecology.* 1972, **40**, 287–298.

Herbst, A. L., Kurman, R. J., Scully, R. E., and Poskanzer, D. C. Clear-cell adenocarcinoma of the vagina in young females. *New England Journal of Medicine,* 1973, **287**, 1259–1264.

Herbst, A. L., Robboy, S. S., Scully, R. E., and Poskanzer, D. C. Clear-cell adenocarcinoma of the vagina and cervix in young girls: Analysis of 170 registry cases. *Journal of Obstetrics and Gynecology,* 1974, **119**, 713–724.

Hersey, R. B. Emotional cycles in man. *Journal of Mental Science,* 1931, **77**, 151–169.

Hetherington, E. M., Cox, M., and Cox, R. Divorced fathers. *The Family Coordinator,* 1976, **25**, 417–428.

Hetherington, E. M., and Parke, R. D. *Child psychology: A contemporary approach.* New York: McGraw-Hill, 1979.

Higgins, G. E., Jr. Sexual response in spinal cord injured adults: A review of the literature. *Archives of Sexual Behavior,* 1979, **8**, 173–193.

Higham, E. Sexuality in the infant and neonate: Birth to two years. In B. B. Wolman and J. Money (Eds.), *Handbook of human sexuality.* Englewood Cliffs, N.J.: Prentice-Hall, 1980.

Hill, C. T., Rubin, Z., and Peplau, L. A. Breakups before marriage: The end of 103 affairs. *Journal of Social Issues,* 1976, **32**, 147–168.

Hite, S. *The Hite report.* New York: Macmillan, 1976.

Hite, S. *The Hite report on male sexuality.* New York: Knopf, 1981.

Homans, G. C. *Social behavior: Its elementary forms.* New York: Harcourt Brace Jovanovich, 1961.

Hooker, E. The adjustment of the male overt homosexual. *Journal of Projective Techniques,* 1957, **21**, 18–31.

Horner, M. S. Toward an understanding of achievement-related conflicts in women. *Journal of Social Issues,* 1972, **78**, 157–176.

Howard, I. L., Piptzin, M. B., and Reifler, C. B. Is pornography a problem? *Journal of Social Issues,* 1973, **29**, 133–145.

Huff, R. W. Changes in menstruation. In R. W. Huff and C. J. Pauerstein (Eds.), *Human reproduction.* New York: Wiley, 1979.

Hulka, J. F. Current status of elective sterilization in the United States. *Fertility and Sterility,* 1977, **28,** 515–520.

Hunt, M. *The affair.* New York: Harcourt Brace Jovanovich, 1969.

Hunt, M. *Sexual behavior in the 1970's.* Chicago: Playboy Press, 1974.

Hurlock, E. B. *Child development,* New York: McGraw-Hill, 1950.

Hursch, C. J. *The trouble with rape.* Chicago: Nelson-Hall, 1977.

Hyde, J. S., and Rosenberg, B. G. *Half the human experience: The psychology of women.* Lexington, Mass.: Heath, 1976.

Imperato-McGinley, J., Guerrero, L., Gautier, T., and Peterson, R. E. Steroid 5 alpha reductase deficiency: An inherited form of male pseudohermaphroditism. *Science,* 1974, **186,** 1213–1215.

Israel, S. L. *Diagnosis and treatment of menstrual disorders and sterility.* (5th ed.) New York: Harper & Row, 1967.

Ivey, M., and Bardwick, J. M. Patterns of affective fluctuation in the menstrual cycle. *Psychosomatic Medicine,* 1968, **30,** 336–345.

J. (Pseud.). *The sensuous woman.* New York: Dell, 1969.

Jacklin, C. N., and Maccoby, E. E. Social behavior at 33 months in same-sex and mixed-sex dyads. *Child Development,* 1978, **49,** 557–569.

Jacklin, C. N., Snow, M. E., and Maccoby, E. E. Tactile sensitivity and strength in newborn boys and girls. *Infant Behavior and Development,* 1980, **3,** 387–394.

Jackman, N. R., O'Toole, R., and Geis, G. The self-image of the prostitute. *Sociological Quarterly,* 1963, **4**(2), 150–161.

Jaffe, R. B., HoYuen, B., Keye, W. R., Jr., and Midgley, A. R., Jr. Physiologic and pathological profiles of circulating human prolactin. *American Journal of Obstetrics and Gynecology,* 1973, **117,** 757–759.

Janoff-Bulman, R. Characterological versus behavioral self-blame: Inquiries into depression and rape. *Journal of Personality and Social Psychology,* 1979, **37,** 1798–1809.

Jay, K., and Young, A. *The gay report.* New York: Summit Books, 1979.

Jarvik, L. F., Klodin, V., and Matsuyama, S. S. Human aggression and the extra Y chromosome: Fact or fantasy. *American Psychologist,* 1973, **28,** 674–682.

Johnson, D. F., and Phoenix, C. H. Hormonal control of female sexual attractiveness, proceptivity and receptivity in rhesus monkeys. *Journal of Comparative and Physiological Psychology,* 1976, **90,** 473–483.

Johnson, V. E., and Masters, W. H. Intravaginal contraception studies, phase 1 anatomy. *Western Journal of Surgical Obstetrics and Gynecology,* 1963, **70,** 202–207.

Jones, E. E. *Ingratiation.* Englewood Cliffs, N.J.: Prentice-Hall, 1964.

Jong, E. *Fear of flying.* New York: Holt, Rinehart and Winston, 1973.

Jost, A. Hormonal factors in the sex differentiation of the mammalian foetus. *Philosophical Transactions of the Society of London,* Ser. B., 1970, **259,** 119–131.

Jost, A. A new look at the mechanisms controlling sex differentiation in mammals. *Johns Hopkins Medical Journal,* 1972, **130,** 38–53.

Kahn, S. S. *The Kahn report on sexual preferences.* New York: St. Martin's Press, 1981.

Kallman, F. J. Comparative twin study on the genetic aspects of male homosexuality. *Journal of Nervous and Mental Disease,* 1952, **115,** 283–298. (a)

Kallman, F. J. Twin and sibship study of overt male homosexuality. *American Journal of Human Genetics,* 1952, **4,** 136–146.

Kaplan, A. Androgyny as a model of mental health for women: From theory to therapy. In A. Kaplan and J. P. Bean (Eds.), *Beyond sex role stereotypes.* Boston: Little, Brown, 1976.

Kaplan, A., and Bean, J. (Eds.). *Beyond sex role stereotypes.* Boston: Little, Brown, 1976.

Kaplan, H. S. *The new sex therapy.* New York: Brunner-Mazel, 1974.

Kardiner, A. *The individual and his society.* New York: Columbia University Press, 1939.

Karnaky, K. J. Diagnosis and treatment of endometriosis. *American Journal of Obstetrics and Gynecology,* 1971, **111,** 598–599.

Kegel, A. M. Sexual functions of the pubococcygeus muscle. *Western Journal of Surgery,* 1952, **60,** 521–524.

Kelly, J. The aging male homosexual: Myth and reality. *Gerontologist,* 1977, **17,** 328–332.

Kenkel, W. F. *Society in action.* (2nd ed.) New York: Harper & Row, 1980.

Kimmel, D. C. Life-history interviews of aging gay men. *International Journal of Aging and Human Development,* 1980, **10,** 239–248.

Kinsey, A. C., Pomeroy, W. B., and Martin, C. E. *Sexual behavior in the human male.* Philadelphia: Saunders, 1948.

Kinsey, A. C., Pomeroy, W. B., Martin, C. E., and Gebhard, P. H. *Sexual behavior in the human female.* Philadelphia: Saunders, 1953.

Kirkendall, L. A. *Sex education.* SIECUS Study Guide No. 1. New York: Sex Information and Education Council of the United States, 1965.

Klapholz, H. The medical examination: Treatment and evidence collection. In S. L. McCombie (Ed.), *The rape crisis intervention handbook.* New York: Plenum, 1980.

Kleeman, J. A boy discovers his penis. *Psychoanalytic Study of the Child,* 1965, **20,** 239–266.

Klinck, L. Menopause: The estrogen controversy. *Harper's Bazaar,* November 1979, 183–243.

Knobil, E., Plant, T. M., Wildt, L., Belchetz, P. E., and Marshall, G. Control of the rhesus monkey menstrual cycle: Permissive role of hypothalamic gonadotropin-releasing hormone. *Science,* 1980, **207,** 1371–1373.

Knox, D. *Exploring marriage and the family.* Glenview, Ill.: Scott, Foresman, 1979.

Kohlberg, L. Cognitive development and analysis of children's sex role concept and attitudes. In E. E. Maccoby (Ed.), *The development of sex differences.* Stanford, Calif.: Stanford University Press, 1966.

Kolata, G. Homones and brain development. *Science,* September 7, 1979, 985–987.

Kolb, L. C. *Modern clinical psychiatry.* Philadelphia: Saunders, 1963.

Kosner, A. What sex therapists are learning. *McCalls,* August 1979, 85+.

Krafft-Ebing, R. V. *Psychopathia sexualis.* New York: Pioneer Publications, 1950 (original published 1886).

Kreitler, H., and Kreitler, S. Children's concepts of sexuality and birth. In R. S. Rogers (Ed.), *Sex education.* London: Cambridge University Press, 1974.

Kugelmass, S., and Lieblich, A. Impact of learning to read on directionality in perception: A further cross-cultural analysis. *Human Development,* 1979, **22,** 406–415.

Kutchinsky, B. The effect of easy availability of pornography on the incidence of sex crimes: The Danish experience. *Journal of Social Issues,* 1973, **29,** 163–181.

Lamb, M. E. (Ed.). *The role of the father in infant development.* New York: Wiley, 1976.

Lane, R. M., and Nagelschmidt, S. M. Testicular threat. *Omni,* July 1981, 16, 123.

Lanson, L. *From woman to woman.* New York: Knopf, 1975.

LaTorre, R. A., and Kear, K. Attitudes toward sex in the aged. *Archives of Sexual Behavior,* 1977, **6,** 203–213.

Leboyer, F. *Birth without violence.* New York: Knopf, 1975.

Lee, J. A. Styles of loving. *Psychology Today,* 1974, **8**(5), 43–51.

Leifer, M. Psychological changes in pregnancy. *Genetic Psychology Monographs,* 1977, **95,** 55–96.

Lester, D. Incest. *Journal of Sex Research,* 1972, **8,** 268–285.

Lester, D. *Unusual sexual behavior.* Springfield, Ill.: Thomas, 1975.

Levin, R. J. The Redbook report on premarital and extramarital sex: The end of the double standard? *Redbook,* October 1975, 38–44, 190–192.

Levin, R. J., and Levin, A. Sexual pleasure: The surprising preferences of 100,000 women. *Redbook,* September 1975, 51–58.

Levinger, G. Toward the analysis of close relationships. *Journal of Experimental Social Psychology,* 1980, **16,** 510–544.

Levinger, G., and Snoek, J. D. *Attraction in relationship: A new look at interpersonal attraction.* Morristown, N.J.: General Learning, 1972.

Levitt, E. E., and Klassen, A. Public attitudes toward homosexuality. *Journal of Homosexuality,* 1974, **1**(1), 29–45.

Lewis, M., and Kagan, J. Studies in attention. *Merrill-Palmer Quarterly,* 1965, **2,** 95–127.

Licklider, S. Jewish penile carcinoma. *Journal of Urology,* 1961, **86,** 98.

Lips, A. M., and Colwill, N. L. *The psychology of sex differences.* Englewood Cliffs, N.J.: Prentice-Hall, 1978.

Lloyd, T. S. The mid-thirties syndrome. *Virginia Medical Monthly,* 1963, **90,** 51.

LoPiccolo, J., and Lobitz, W. C. The role of masturbation in the treatment of sexual dysfunction. *Archives of Sexual Behavior,* 1972, **2,** 163–171.

LoPiccolo, J., and Lobitz, W. C. The role of masturbation in the treatment of orgasmic dysfunction. In J. LoPiccolo and L. LoPiccolo (Eds.), *Handbook of sex therapy.* New York: Plenum, 1978.

Lubin, B. Mood and somatic symptoms during pregnancy. *Psychosomatic Medicine,* 1975, **37,** 136–146.

Luce, G. *Biological rhythms in psychiatry and medicine.* New York: Dover, 1970.

Luttge, W. G. The role of gonadal hormones in the sexual behavior of the rhesus monkey and the human: A literature survey. *Archives of Sexual Behavior,* 1971, **1,** 61–88.

McAdoo, B. C., Doering, C. H., Kraemer, H. C., Dessert, N., Brodie, H. K. H., and Hamburg, D. A. A study of the effects of GnRH on human mood and behavior. *Psychosomatic Medicine,* 1978, **40,** 199–209.

MacArthur, R. Sex differences in field dependence for the Eskimo. *International Journal of Psychology,* 1967, **2,** 139–140.

McCance, R. A., Luff, M. C., and Widdowson, E. E. Physical and emotional periodicity in women. *Journal of Hygiene,* 1937, **37**, 571–605.

McCauley, C., and Swann, C. P. Male-female differences in sexual fantasy. *Journal of Research in Personality,* 1978, **12**, 76–86.

McClure, H. M., Ridley, J. H., and Graham, C. E. Disseminated endometriosis in a rhesus monkey. *Journal of the Medical Association of Georgia,* 1971, **60**, 11–13.

Maccoby, E. E. *Social development.* New York: Harcourt Brace Jovanovich, 1980.

Maccoby, E. E., and Jacklin, C. N. *The psychology of sex differences.* Stanford, Calif.: Stanford University Press, 1974.

McKinlay, S. M., and Jeffreys, M. The menopausal syndrome. *British Journal of Preventive and Social Medicine,* 1974, **28**, 108.

Macklin, E. Non-marital heterosexual cohabitation. *Marriage and Family Review,* March–April 1978, **1**, 1–12.

MacLeod, J., and Gold, R. Z. The male factor in fertility and infertility, IV: Semen quality and certain other factors in relation to ease of conception. *Fertility and Sterility,* 1953, **4**, 10–33.

MacLusky, N. J., and Naftolin, F. Sexual differentiation of the central nervous system. *Science,* 1981, **211**, 1294–1303.

Macy, C., and Falkner, F. *Pregnancy and birth, pleasures and problems.* New York: Harper & Row, 1979.

Male pill. *Science,* June 1979, 74+.

Mann, J., Sidman, J., and Starr, S. Evaluating social consequences of erotic films: An experimental approach. *Journal of Social Issues,* 1973, **29**, 113–131.

Manning, F., Wyn Pugh, E., and Boddy, K. Effect of cigarette smoking on fetal breathing movements in normal pregnancies. *British Medical Journal,* 1975, **1**(5957), 552–553.

Marano, H. Breast or bottle: New evidence in an old debate. *New York,* October 29, 1979, 56–60.

Marshall, W. A., and Tanner, J. M. Variations in patterns of pubertal changes in girls. *Archives of Disturbed Children,* 1969, **44**, 291–303.

Marshall, W. A., and Tanner, J. M. Variations in the patterns of pubertal changes in boys. *Archives of Disturbed Children,* 1970, **45**, 13–23.

Martin, C. E. Sexual activity in the aging male. In J. Money and H. Musaph (Eds.), *Handbook of sexology.* Amsterdam: ASP Biol. Med. Press, 1977.

Martin, J. A. A longitudinal study of the consequences of early mother-infant interaction. A microanalytic approach. *Monographs of the Society for Research in Child Development,* 1980.

Martinson, F. *Infant and child sexuality.* St. Peter, Minn.: The Book Mark, 1973.

Martinson, F. M. Eroticism in infancy and childhood. *The Journal of Sex Research,* 1976, **2**, 251–262.

Martinson, F. M. Childhood sexuality. In B. B. Wolman and J. Money (Eds.), *Handbook of human sexuality,* Englewood Cliffs, N.J.: Prentice-Hall, 1980.

Marx, J. L. Dysmenorrhea: Basic research leads to a rational therapy. *Science,* 1979, **205**, 175–176.

Masica, D. N., Money, J., and Ehrhardt, A. A. Fetal feminization and female gender identity in the testicular feminizing syndrome of androgen insensitivity. *Archives of Sexual Behavior,* 1971, **1**, 131–142.

Masters, W. H., and Johnson, V. E. *Human sexual response.* Boston: Little, Brown, 1966.

Masters, W. H., and Johnson, V. E. Ten sex myths exploded. *Playboy,* December 1970, 124ff.

Masters, W. H., and Johnson, V. E. *Human sexual inadequacy.* Boston: Little, Brown, 1970.

Masters, W. H., and Johnson, V. E. *The pleasure bond.* Boston: Little, Brown, 1974.

Masters, W. H., and Johnson, V. E. *Homosexuality in perspective.* Boston: Little, Brown, 1979.

Mastroianni, L. Fertility disorders. In S. Romney, M. J. Gray, A. B. Little, J. A. Merrill, E. J. Qulligan, and R. Stander (Eds.), *Gynecology and obstetrics: The health care of women.* New York: McGraw-Hill, 1975.

Mead, M. *Sex and temperament in three primitive societies.* New York: Morrow, 1935.

Mead, M. Cultural determinants of sexual behavior. In W. Young (Ed.), *Sex and internal secretions.* Vol. II. Baltimore: Williams & Wilkins, 1961.

Mead, M., and Newton, N. Fatherhood. In S. A. Richardson and A. F. Guttmacher (Eds.), *Childbearing: Its social and psychological aspects.* Baltimore: Williams & Wilkins, 1967.

Meeker, C. I., and Gray, M. J. Birth control, abortion and sterilization. In S. L. Romney, M. J. Gray, A. B. Little, J. A. Merrill, E. J. Quilligan, and R. Stander (Eds.), *Gynecology and obstetrics: The health care of women.* New York: McGraw-Hill, 1975.

Melville, K. *Marriage and family today.* (2nd ed.) New York: Random House, 1980.

Meyer, J. K., and Reter, D. J. Sex reassignment. *Archives of General Psychiatry,* 1979, **36**, 1010–1015.

Meyer, R. J., Roelofo, H. A., Bluestone, J., and Redmond, S. Accidental injury to the preschool child. *Journal of Pediatrics,* 1963, **63**, 95–105.

Meyer-Bahlburg, H. F. L. Sexuality in early adolescence. In B. B. Wolman and J. Money (Eds.), *Handbook of human sexuality*. Englewood Cliffs, N.J.: Prentice-Hall, 1980.

Michael, R. P., Herbert, J., and Welegalla, J. Ovarian hormones and grooming behavior in the rhesus monkey (*Macaca mulatta*) under laboratory conditions. *Journal of Endocrinology*, 1966, **36**, 263–279.

Michael, R. P., Herbert, J., and Welegalla, J. Ovarian hormones and the sexual behavior of the male rhesus monkey (*Macaca mulatta*) under laboratory conditions. *Journal of Endocrinology*, 1967, **39**, 81–98.

Michael, R. P., and Welegalla, J. Ovarian hormones and sexual behavior of the female rhesus monkey (*Macaca mulatta*) under laboratory conditions. *Journal of Endocrinology*, 1968, **41**, 407–421.

Miller v. California, 1973, 413 U.S., 15.

Miller, J. A. Unisex birth control chemical. *Science News*, May 24, 1980, **117**, 331–334.

Miller, P. Y., and Simon, W. Adolescent sexual behavior: Context and change. *Social Problems*, 1974, **22**, 58–76.

Mishell, D. R., Jr., Wide, L., and Gemzell, C. A. Immunologic determination of human chorionic gonadotropin in serum. *Journal of Clinical Endocrinology and Metabolism*, 1963, **23**, 125–131.

Money, J. Sexology: Behavior, cultural, hormonal, genetic, etc. *The Journal of Sex Research*, 1973, **9**, 1–10.

Money, J. Hormones, gender identity and behavior. In B. F. Eleftheriou and R. C. Spratt (Eds.), *Hormonal correlates of behavior*. New York: Plenum, 1975.

Money, J., and Ehrhardt, A. A. *Man and woman, boy and girl*. Baltimore: Johns Hopkins Press, 1972.

Money, J., and Schwartz, M. Dating, romantic and nonromantic friendships and sexuality in 17 early treated adrenogenital females, ages 16–25. In P. A. Lee, L. P. Plotnick, A. A. Kowarski, and C. J. Migion (Eds.), *Congenital adrenal hyperplasia*. Baltimore: University Park Press, 1976.

Moos, R. H. *Preliminary manual for the mental distress questionnaire*. Stanford, Calif.: Stanford University. School of Medicine, 1969.

Moramarco, S. S. Giving birth at home. *Family Health*, March 1979, 25–30.

Morris, D. *The naked ape*. New York: Dell, 1969.

Morrison, C. H. A cultural perspective on rape. In S. L. McCombie (Ed.), *The rape crisis intervention handbook*. New York: Plenum, 1980.

Morton, R. S. *Sexual freedom and venereal disease*. London: Peter Owen, 1971.

Murdock, G. P. *Ethnographic atlas*. Pittsburgh: University of Pittsburgh Press, 1967.

Murphy III, P. J. The police investigation. In S. L. McCombie (Ed.), *The rape crisis intervention handbook*. New York: Plenum, 1980.

Neugarten, B. L. Women's attitudes towards the menopause. *Vita Humana*, 1963, **6**, 140–151.

Newcomb, T. M. The prediction of interpersonal attraction. *American Psychologist*, 1956, **11**, 575–586.

Newcomb, T. M. *The acquaintance process*. New York: Holt, Rinehart and Winston, 1961.

Newmark, S. R., Rose, L. I., Todd, R., Birk, L., and Naftolin, F. Gonadotropin, estradiol, and testosterone profiles in homosexual men. *American Journal of Psychiatry*, 1979, **136**, 767–771.

Newton, N. A. Childbearing in broad perspective. In Boston Children's Medical Center, *Pregnancy, birth and the newborn baby*. New York: Delacorte Press, 1972.

Norwood, C. A humanizing way to have a baby. *Ms.*, May 1978, 89–92.

Novell, H. A. Psychological factors in premenstrual tension and dysmenorrhea. *Clinical Obstetrics and Gynecology*, 1965, **8**, 222–232.

Nyberg, K. L., and Alston, J. P. An analysis of public attitudes toward homosexual behavior. *Journal of Homosexuality*, 1977, **2**(2), 99–107.

O'Conner, J., and Stein, L. Results of treatment in functional sexual disorders. *New York State Journal of Medicine*, 1972, **72**, 1927–1929.

Ohno, S. *Sex chromosomes and sex-linked genes*. New York: Springer-Verlag, 1967.

Ohno, S. The role of H-Y antigen in primary sex determination. *Journal of the American Medical Association*, 1978, **239**, 217–220.

Olds, S., et al., *Obstetric nursing*. Menlo Park, Calif.: Addison-Wesley, 1980.

O'Neill, G., and O'Neill, N. *Open marriage: A new life style for couples*. New York: M. Evans, 1972.

Opting for androgyny. *Human Behavior*, November 1978, 51.

O'Reilly, J. Isolating the chocolate factor. *Ms.*, August 1980, 44–46.

Osofsky, J. D., and Osofsky, H. J. The psychological reactions of patients to legalized abortions. *American Journal of Orthopsychiatry*, 1972, **42**, 48–60.

Ostow, M. *Sexual deviation: Psychoanalytic insight*. New York: Quadrangle, 1974.

Ovid. *The art of love*. Trans. by Rolfe Humphries. Bloomington, Ind.: University of Indiana Press, 1957.

Paige, K. E. Effects of oral contraceptives on affective fluctuations associated with the menstrual cycle. *Psychosomatic Medicine*, 1971, **33**, 515–537.

Parsons, T. Family structure and the socialization of the child. In T. Parsons and R. Bales (Eds.), *Family socialization and interaction process.* New York: Free Press, 1955.

Pauly, I. Male psychosexual inversion: Transsexualism: A review of 100 cases. *Archives of General Psychiatry,* 1965, **13,** 172–181.

Pavlov, I. P. *Conditioned reflexes.* New York: Oxford University Press, 1927.

Pearlman, C. K. Frequency of intercourse in males at different ages. *Medical Aspects of Human Sexuality,* 1972, 92–113.

Peplau, L. A. What homosexuals want. *Psychology Today,* March 1981, 28–38.

Peplau, L. A., Rubin, Z., and Hill, C. T. Sexual intimacy in dating relationships. *Journal of Social Issues,* 1977, **33,** 86–109.

Perloff, W. H. Role of the hormones in human sexuality. *Psychosomatic Medicine,* 1949, **11,** 133–139.

Perry, J. D., and Whipple, B. Pelvic muscle strength of female ejaculators: Evidence in support of a new theory of orgasm. *The Journal of Sex Research,* 1981, **17,** 22–39.

Persky, H., Lief, H. I., Strauss, D., Miller, W. R., and O'Brien, C. P. Plasma testosterone levels and sexual behavior of couples. *Archives of Sexual Behavior,* 1978, **7,** 157–173.

Pfeiffer, E. Sexual behavior in old age. In E. Busse and E. Pfeiffer (Eds.), *Behavior and adaptation in late life.* Boston: Little, Brown, 1969.

Pfeiffer, E. Sex and aging. In L. Gross (Ed.), *Sexual issues in marriage.* New York: Spectrum, 1975.

Pfeiffer, E., and Davis, G. C. Sexual behavior in middle life. *American Journal of Psychiatry,* 1972, **128,** 82–87.

Pfeiffer, E., Verwoerdt, A., and Wang, H. Sexual behavior in aged men and women; I: Observations on 254 community volunteers. *Archives of General Psychiatry,* 1968, **19,** 753–758.

Phoenix, C. H. Effects of dihydrotestosterone on sexual behavior of castrated male rhesus monkeys. *Physiology and Behavior,* 1974, **12,** 1045–1055.

Phoenix, C. H. Sexual behavior of castrated male rhesus monkeys treated with 19 hydroxytestosterone. *Physiology and Behavior,* 1976, **16,** 305–310.

Phoenix, C. H. Steroids and sexual behavior in castrated male rhesus monkeys. *Hormones and Behavior,* 1978, **10,** 1–9.

Phoenix, C. H., Slob, A. K., and Goy, R. W. Effects of castration and replacement therapy on sexual behavior of adult male rhesuses. *Journal of Comparative and Physiological Psychology,* 1973, **84,** 472–481.

Plato. *Symposium.* Trans. by Benjamin Jowett. Indianapolis: Bobbs-Merrill, 1956.

Playboy Magazine, May 1979, 75–106.

Ploscowe, M. *Sex and the law.* New York: Ace Books, 1951, 1962.

Pomeroy, W. *Dr. Kinsey and the Institute for Sex Research.* New York: Harper & Row, 1972.

Presser, H. B., and Bumpass, L. L. The acceptability of contraceptive sterilization among U.S. couples: 1970. *Family Planning Perspectives,* 1972, **4**(3), 18–26.

Preston, R. C. Reading achievement of German and American children. *School and Society,* 1962, **90,** 350–354.

Prince, V., and Butler, P. Survey of 504 cases of transvestism. *Psychological Reports,* 1972, **31,** 903–917.

Rakoff, A. E. Ovarian failure. *Obstetrics and Gynecology,* 1977, **24,** 10.

Ralph, J. B., Goldberg, M. L., and Passow, A. H. *Bright underachievers.* New York: Teachers College, 1966.

Rapp, F. Herpes viruses, venereal disease and cancer. *American Scientist,* 1978, **66,** 670–672.

Rasmussen, P. K., and Kuhn, L. The new masseuse: Play for pay. *Urban Life,* 1976, **5**(3), 271–292.

Rebirth for midwifery. *Time,* August 29, 1977, 66.

Rees, L. Psychosomatic aspects of the premenstrual tension syndrome and its treatment. *Journal of Mental Science,* 1956, **99,** 62–73.

Reinisch, J. M. Prenatal exposure of human foetuses to synthetic progestin and oestrogen affects personality. *Nature,* 1977, **266,** 561–562.

Reiss, I. L. *The social context of premarital sexual permissiveness.* New York: Holt, Rinehart and Winston, 1967.

Reiss, I. L. *The family system in America.* New York: Holt, Rinehart and Winston, 1971.

Reiss, I. L. Premarital sexuality: Past, present, and future. In I. L. Reiss (Ed.), *Readings on the family system.* New York: Holt, Rinehart and Winston, 1972.

The report of the commission on obscenity and pornography. Washington, D.C.: U.S. Government Printing Office, 1970.

Restak, R. The sex-change conspiracy. *Psychology Today,* December 1979, 20–25.

Rinehart, W., and Winter, J. Injectable progestins—Officials debate but use increases. *Population Reports,* Series K, no. 1 (March 1975), K1–K16.

Robbins, M. B., and Jensen, G. D. Multiple orgasms in males. *Journal of Sex Research,* 1978, **14,** 211–226.

Romney, S. L., Gray, M. J., Little, A. B., Merrill, J. A., Quilligan, E. J., and Stander, R. *Gynecology and obstetrics: The health care of women.* New York: McGraw-Hill, 1975.

Rose, R. M., Gordon, T. P., and Bernstein, I. S. Plasma testosterone levels in the male rhesus: Influences of sexual and social stimuli. *Science,* 1972, **178,** 643–645.

Rosencrane, H. A factor analysis of attitudes toward the elderly. *Gerontologist,* 1969, **9,** 55–59.

Rossi, A. S. Sex equality: The beginnings of ideology. *The Humanist,* September/October 1969, 3–16.

Roth v. U.S., 1957, 354 U.S., 476.

Rubenstein, C. Reining in androgyny. *Psychology Today,* March 1980, 27.

Rubin, J. *Sexual life after sixty.* New York: Basic Books, 1965.

Rubin, R. Attainment of the maternal role, Pt. 1; Processes. *Nursing Research,* 1967, **16,** 237–245.

Rubin, R. T., Reinisch, J. M., and Haskett, R. F. Postnatal gonadal steroid effects on human behavior. *Science,* 1981, **211,** 1318–1324.

Rubin, Z. Measurement of romantic love. *Journal of Personality and Social Psychology,* 1970, **16,** 265–273.

Rubin, Z. Disclosing oneself to a stranger: Reciprocity and its limits. *Journal of Experimental Social Psychology,* 1975, **11,** 233–260.

Rubinstein, E. A., Green, R., and Brecher, E. (Eds.). *New directions in sex research.* New York: Plenum, 1976.

Ruble, D. N. Premenstrual symptoms: A reinterpretation. *Science,* 1977, **197,** 291–292.

Sadock, B. J., and Sadock, V. A. Techniques of coitus. In B. J. Sadock, H. Kaplan, and A. Freedman (Eds.), *The sexual experience.* Baltimore: Williams & Wilkins, 1976.

Sadock, B. J., Kaplan, H., and Freedman, A. *The sexual experience.* Baltimore: Williams & Wilkins, 1976.

Sadoff, R. Sex and the law. In B. Sadock, H. Kaplan, and A. Freedman, *The sexual experience.* Baltimore: Williams & Wilkins, 1976.

Saghir, M. T., and Robinson, E. *Male and female homosexuality: A comprehensive investigation.* Baltimore: Williams & Wilkins, 1973.

Sarrel, P., and Sarrel, L. The *Redbook* report on sexual relationships. *Redbook Magazine,* October 1980, 73–80.

Saxton, D. W. The behavior of infants whose mothers smoke in pregnancy. *Early Human Development,* 1978, **2,** 363–369.

Scarf, M. The promiscuous woman. *Psychology Today,* July 1980, 78–87.

Schildkraut, M. S. An updated look at the estrogen scare. *Good Housekeeping,* March 1979, 227–228.

Schlessinger, A. An informal history of love U.S.A. *Saturday Evening Post,* December 1966.

Schlessinger, B., and Miller, G. A. Sexuality and the aged. *Medical Aspects of Human Sexuality,* 1973, **3,** 46–52.

Schmidt, G., Sigusch, V., and Schafer, S. Responses to reading erotic stories: Male-female differences. *Archives of Sexual Behavior,* 1973, **2,** 181–199.

Schultz, T. Birth control not for women only? *Family Health,* May 1980, 44.

Science notes. *Sexology,* September 1969, 14.

Sears, R. R., Maccoby, E. E., and Levin, H. *Patterns of childrearing.* Evanston, Ill.: Row, Peterson, 1957.

Seigelman, M. Psychological adjustment of homosexual and heterosexual men: A cross national replication. *Archives of Sexual Behavior,* 1978, **7,** 1–11.

Seitchik, J. Labor. In R. W. Huff and C. J. Pauerstein (Eds.), *Human reproduction: Physiology and pathophysiology.* New York: Wiley, 1979.

Sevely, J. L., and Bennett, J. W. Concerning female ejaculation and the female prostate. *Journal of Sex Research,* 1978, **14,** 1–20.

Sgroi, S. Molestation of children: The last frontier in child abuse. *Children Today,* 1975, **44,** 19–24.

Shepard, M. K. Reproductive endocrinology. In R. W. Huff and C. J. Pauerstein (Eds.), *Human reproduction.* New York: Wiley, 1979.

Sherman, J. *On the psychology of women: A survey of empirical studies.* Springfield Ill.: Thomas, 1971.

Shettles, L. B. Predetermining children's sex. *Medical Aspects of Human Sexuality,* 1972, **6,** 72.

Shope, D. F. *Interpersonal sexuality.* Philadelphia: Saunders, 1975.

Silny, A. J. Sexuality and aging. In B. B. Wolman and J. Money (Eds.), *Handbook of human sexuality.* Englewood Cliffs, N.J.: Prentice-Hall, 1980.

Silvers, W. K., and Wachtel, S. S. H-Y antigen: Behavior and function. *Science,* 1977, **195,** 956–960.

Sintchak, G., and Geir, J. H. A vaginal plethysmograph system. *Psychophysiology,* 1975, **12,** 113–115.

Sipova, I., and Starka, L. Plasma testosterone values in transsexual women. *Archives of Sexual Behavior,* 1977, **6,** 477–481.

Skinner, B. F. *The behavior of organisms.* Englewood Cliffs, N.J.: Prentice-Hall, 1938.

Smith, P. K., and Daglish, L. Sex differences in parent and infant behavior in the home. *Child Development,* 1977, **48,** 1250–1254.

Smith, S. L. Mood and the menstrual cycle. In E. J. Sachar (Ed.), *Topics in psychoendocrinology.* New York: Grune & Stratton, 1975.

Snyder, E. E., and Spreitzer, E. Attitudes of the aged toward nontraditional sexual behavior. *Archives of Sexual Behavior*, 1976, **5**, 249–254.

Sommer, B. The effect of menstruation on cognitive and perceptual-motor behavior: A review. *Psychosomatic Medicine*, 1973, **35**, 515–534.

Sopchak, A. L., and Sutherland, A. M. Psychological impact of cancer and its treatment, VII: Exogenous sex hormones and their relation to lifelong adaptations in women with metastatic cancer of the breast. *Cancer*, 1960, **13**, 528–531.

Sorenson, R. *Adolescent sexuality in contemporary America.* New York: Harcourt Brace Jovanovich, 1973.

Spada, J. *The Spada report.* New York: Signet Books, 1979.

Sparks, C. H. *Response to intrafamily violence and sexual assault.* Washington, D.C.: Center for Women Policy Studies, February 1978.

Spengler, A. Manifest sadomasochism of males: Results of an empirical study. *Archives of Sexual Behavior*, 1977, **6**, 441–455.

Spitz, R. Anaclitic depression. In *Psychoanalytic Study of the Child.* Vol. 2. New York: International University Press, 1946.

Spitz, R. A. Autoeroticism: Some empirical findings and hypotheses on three of its manifestations in the first year of life. *The Psychoanalytic Study of the Child*, 1949, **3**, 4.

Stoller, R. *Sex and gender: The transsexual experience.* New York: Jason Aronson, 1976.

Stoller, R. J. *Sex and gender: On the development of masculinity and femininity.* New York: Science House, 1968.

Strax, P. *Early detection: Breast cancer is curable,* New York: Harper & Row, 1974.

Strayer, F. F. Peer attachment and affiliative subgroups. In F. F. Strayer (Ed.), *Ethological perspectives on preschool social organization.* Memo de Recherche No. 5, Université du Quebec, A. Montreal. Department of Psychologe, Avril 1977.

Streissguth, A. P., Landesman-Dwyer, S., Martin, J. C., and Smith, D. W. Teratogenic effects of alcohol in humans and laboratory animals. *Science*, 1980, **209**, 353–361.

Subak-Sharpe, G. The venereal disease of the new morality. *Today's Health Magazine*, March 1975, 40–45, 55.

Talese, G. *Thy neighbor's wife.* New York: Doubleday, 1980.

Tanner, J. M. Growing up. *Scientific American*, September 1973, **229**, 34–43.

Tanner, J. M. Growth and endocrinology of the adolescent. In L. I. Gardner (Ed.), *Endocrine and genetic diseases of childhood and adolescence.* (2nd ed.) Philadelphia: Saunders, 1975.

Tauber, E. S. Effects of castration on the sexuality of the adult male. *Psychosomatic Medicine*, 1940, **2**, 74–87.

Tavris, C., and Offir, C. *The longest war: Sex differences in perspective.* New York: Hartcourt Brace Jovanovich, 1977.

Tavris, C., and Sadd, S. *The Redbook report on female sexuality.* New York: Dell, 1975.

Tavris, C., and Sadd, S. *The Redbook report on female sexuality.* New York: Delacorte Press, 1975, 1979.

Tavris, C., and Sadd, S. *The Redbook report on female sexuality.* New York: Dell, 1978.

Tennov, D. *Love and limerence—the experience of being in love.* New York: Stein & Day, 1979.

Terman, L. M. *Psychological factors in marital happiness.* New York: McGraw-Hill, 1938.

"TSE," American Cancer Society pamphlet. New York: American Cancer Society.

Thompson, S. K. Gender labels and early sex-role development. *Child Development*, 1975, **46**, 339–347.

Tiger, L. Male dominance? Yes, alas. A sexist plot? No. *New York Times Magazine*, October 25, 1970, 35–37; 124–127; 132–138.

Toffler, A. *Future shock.* New York: Random House, 1970.

Toffler, A. *The third wave.* New York: Morrow, 1980.

Tolis, G. Prolactin: Physiology and pathology. In D. T. Krieger and J. C. Hughes (Eds.), *Neuroendocrinology.* Sunderland, Mass.: Sinauer Associates, 1980.

Townes, B. D., Ferguson, W. D., and Gilliam, S. Differences in psychological sex adjustment, and familial influences among homosexual and nonhomosexual populations. *Journal of Homosexuality*, 1976, **1**, 261–272.

Trethowan, W. H., and Conlon, M. F. The couvade syndrome. *British Journal of Psychiatry*, 1965, **111**, 57–66.

Trien, S. F. When it's time for a bottle, *Parents Magazine*, October 1977, **52**, 51.

Tripp, C. *The homosexual matrix.* New York: McGraw-Hill, 1974.

Udry, J. R., and Morris, N. M. Distribution of coitus in the menstrual cycle. *Nature*, 1968, **220**, 593–596.

Udry, J. R., and Morris, N. M. Human sexual behavior at different stages of menstrual cycles. *Journal of Reproduction and Fertility*, 1977, **51**, 419–425.

Vance, E. G., and Wagner, N. N. Written descriptions of orgasm: A study of sex differences. *Archives of Sexual Behavior*, 1976, **5**, 87–98.

Vasectomy: Follow-up of 1000 Cases. Cambridge, England: Simon Population Trust, 1969, **12,** 1–17.

Vasectomy: What are the problems? *Population Reports*, Series D, January 1975.

Vener, A. M., and Stewart, C. S. Adolescent sexual behavior in middle America revisited: 1970–1973. *Journal of Marriage and the Family*, 1974, **36,** 728–735.

Verwoerdt, A., Pfeiffer, E., and Wang, H. Sexual behavior in senescence, II: Patterns of sexual activity and interest. *Geriatrics*, 1969, **24,** 137–154.

Viorst, J. *Yes married.* New York: Saturday Review Press, 1972.

Wagner, N., and Solberg, D. Pregnancy and sexuality. *Medical Aspects of Human Sexuality*, 1974, **8,** 44–79.

Waldrop, M. F., and Halverson, C. F., Jr. Intensive and extensive peer behavior: Longitudinal and cross-sectional analysis. *Child Development*, 1975, **46,** 19–26.

Walen, S., Hauserman, N., and Lavin, P. *Clinical guide to behavior therapy.* Baltimore: Williams & Wilkins, 1977.

Wallechinsky, D., and Wallace, I. A survey of sex surveys. In *The people's almanac.* Garden City, N.Y.: Doubleday, 1975.

Wallen, K., and Goy, R. W. Effects of estradiol benzoate, estrone, and propionates of testosterone or dihydrotestosterone on sexual and related behaviors of ovariectomized rhesus monkeys. *Hormones and Behavior*, 1977, **9,** 228–248.

Waller, W. The rating and dating complex. *American Sociological Review*, 1937, **2,** 727–737.

Walsh, P. C., Madden, J. D., Harrod, M. J., Goldstein, J. L., MacDonald, P. C., and Wilson, J. D. Familial incomplete male pseudohermaphroditism, type 2: Decreased dihydrotestosterone formation in pseudovaginal perineoscrotal hypospadias. *New England Journal of Medicine*, 1974, **291,** 944–949.

Walster, E., Aronson, V., Abrahams, D., and Rottmann, L. Importance of physical attractiveness in dating behavior. *Journal of Personality and Social Psychology*, 1966, **4,** 508–516.

Walster, E., and Walster, G. W. *A new look at love.* Reading, Mass.: Addison-Wesley, 1978.

Walster, E., Walster, G. W., Piliavin, J., and Schmidt, L. Playing hard to get: Understanding an elusive phenomenon. *Journal of Personality and Social Psychology*, 1973, **26,** 113–121.

Ward, W. *Disadvantaged children and their first school experience.* ETS Headstart longitudinal study: Development of self-regulatory behaviors PR-73-18. Princeton, N.J.: ETS, 1973.

Warren, C. *Identity and community in the gay world.* New York: Wiley, 1974.

Wasow, M., and Loeb, M. B. Sexuality in nursing homes. *Journal of American Geriatric Society*, 1979, **27,** 73–79.

Wax, J. Sex and the single grandparent. In S. H. Zarit (Ed.), *Readings in aging and death: Contemporary perspectives.* New York: Harper & Row, 1977.

Waxenberg, S. E. Some biological correlates of sexual behavior. In G. Winokur (Ed.), *Determinants of human sexual behavior.* Springfield, Ill.: Thomas, 1963.

Waxenberg, S. E., Drellich, M. G., and Sutherland, A. M. The role of hormones in human behavior: I. Changes in female sexuality after adrenalectomy. *Journal of Clinical Endocrinology and Metabolism*, 1959, **193** 193–197.

Weideger, P. *Menstruation and menopause.* New York: Knopf, 1976.

Weinberg, M. S., and Williams, C. J. *Male homosexuals: Their problems and adaptations.* New York: Oxford University Press, 1974.

Weitz, S. *Sex roles.* New York: Oxford University Press, 1977.

Wessman, A. E., and Ricks, D. F. *Mood and personality* New York: Holt, Rinehart and Winston, 1966.

Whitehead, R. E. Women pilots. *Journal of Aviation Medicine*, 1934, **5,** 47–49.

Whitehurst, R. N. Living together unmarried on campus. Unpublished paper, University of Windsor, Ontario, Canada, 1974.

Whiting, B. B., and Edwards, C. P. A cross-cultural analysis of sex differences in the behavior of children aged three through eleven. *Journal of Personality and Social Psychology*, 1973, **91,** 171–188.

Whiting, B. B., and Whiting, J. W. M. *Children of six cultures.* Cambridge, Mass.: Harvard University Press, 1975.

Wickham, M. The effects of the menstrual cycle on test performance. *British Journal of Psychology*, 1958, **49,** 39–41.

Wiggins, J. S., Wiggins, N., and Conger, J. C. Correlates of heterosexual somatic preference. *Journal of Personality and Social Psychology*, 1968, **10,** 32–90.

Wilson, G. D. *The secrets of sexual fantasy.* London: Dent, 1978.

Wilson, J. D., George, F. W., and Griffin, J. E. The hormonal control of sexual development. *Science*, 1981, **211,** 1278–1284.

Witkin, H. A., Mednick, S. A., Schulsinger, F., Bakkestrom, E., Christiansen, K. O., Goodenough, D. R.,

Hirschhorn, K., Lundsteen, C., Owen, D. R., Philip, J., Rubin, D. B., and Stocking, M. Criminality in XYY and XXY men. *Science*, 1976, **193**, 547–555.

Witters, W. L., and Jones-Witters, P. *Human sexuality: A biological perspective.* New York: Van Nostrand, 1980.

Wittig, M. A., and Petersen, A. C. (Eds.). *Sex-related differences in cognitive functioning.* New York: Academic Press, 1979.

Wolfe, L. *Playing around: Women and extramarital sex.* New York: New American Woman, 1975.

Wolfe, L. The sexual profile of that Cosmopolitan girl. *Cosmopolitan*, September 1980, 254–257, 263–265.

Wolfe, L. The good news: The latest expert word on what it means to be single. *New York*, December 28, 1981, 33–36.

Wolkind, S., and Zajicek, E. Psycho-social correlates of nausea and vomiting in pregnancy. *Psychosomatic Research*, 1978, **22**, 1–5.

Wolpe, J., and Lang, P. J. A fear survey schedule for use in behavior therapy. *Behavior Research and Therapy*, 1964, **2**, 27–30.

Wolpe, J., and Lazarus, A. *Behavior therapy techniques.* New York: Pergamon Press, 1966.

World Health Organization. Steroid contraception and the risk of neoplasia. *Technical Report Series.* No. 614. Geneva: World Health Organization, 1978.

Yalom, I. D., Green, R., and Fish, N. Prenatal exposure to female hormones: Effect on psychosexual development in boys. *Archives of General Psychiatry*, 1973, **28**, 554–561.

Yen, S. S. C. The biology of menopause. *Journal of Reproductive Medicine*, 1977, **18**, 287–296.

Yen, S. S. C. Neuroendocrine regulation of the menstrual cycle. In D. T. Kreiger and J. C. Hughs (Eds.), *Neuroendocrinology.* Sunderland, Mass.: Sinauer Associates, 1980.

Yen, S. S. C., Rebar, R. W., and Quesenberry, W. Pituitary function in pseudocyesis. *Journal of Clinical Endocrinological Metabolism*, 1976, **43**, 132–136.

Zajicek, E., and Wolkind, S. Emotional difficulties in married women during and after the first pregnancy. *British Journal of Medical Psychology*, 1978, **51**, 379–385.

Zajonc, R. B. Attraction, affiliation, and attachment. In J. F. Eisenberger and W. S. Dillon (Eds.), *Man and beast: Comparative social behavior.* Washington, D.C.: Smithsonian Institution, 1971.

Zatuchni, G. I. *Parade Magazine* interview, November 1980, 30.

Zilbergeld, B., and Evans, M. The inadequacy of Masters and Johnson. *Psychology Today*, August 1980, 29–43.

Zimbardo, P. G. *Shyness.* Reading, Mass.: Addison-Wesley, 1978.

Zimring, J. G. Sexual problems of the geriatric patient. *N.Y. State Journal of Medicine*, 1979, **79**, 752–753.

Index